Lung Disease STATE OF THE ART

1975-1976

Lung Disease STATE OF THE ART

Edited by
JOHN F. MURRAY
Professor of Medicine
University of California
San Francisco

1975-1976

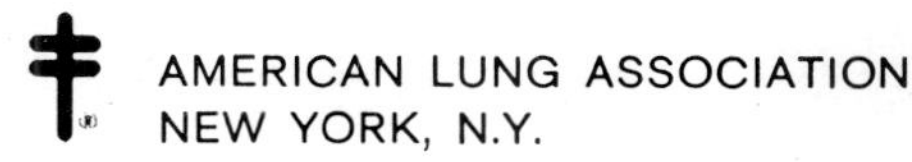AMERICAN LUNG ASSOCIATION
NEW YORK, N.Y.

ISBN 0-915116-01-4

Printed in the United States of America

Selected articles from American Review of Respiratory Disease,
Journal of the American Thoracic Society

American Lung Association
1740 Broadway
New York, New York 10019

#9804

Contributors

MORTON ZISKIND
ROBERT N. JONES
HANS WEILL
    Tulane University School of Medicine, New Orleans, Louisiana

W. K. C. MORGAN
N. L. LAPP
    West Virginia University Medical Center, Morgantown, West Virginia

MARGARET R. BECKLAKE
    McGill University, Montreal, Quebec, Canada
    Royal Victoria Hospital, Montreal, Quebec, Canada

H. BENFER KALTREIDER
    University of California, San Francisco, California
    Veterans Administration Hospital, San Francisco, California

D. M. WILLIAMS
    Stanford University School of Medicine, Stanford, California

J. A. KRICK
    Palo Alto Medical Research Foundation, Palo Alto, California

J. S. REMINGTON
    Alamo Medical Clinic, Alamo, California

HENRY N. WAGNER, JR.
    The Johns Hopkins Medical Institutions, Baltimore, Maryland

ALLAN J. HANCE
RONALD G. CRYSTAL
    National Heart, Lung, and Blood Institute, Bethesda, Maryland

ROBERT E. WOOD
THOMAS F. BOAT
CARL F. DOERSHUK
    Rainbow Babies and Childrens Hospital, Cleveland, Ohio

K. FRANK AUSTEN
    Harvard Medical School, Boston, Massachusetts
    Robert B. Brigham Hospital, Boston, Massachusetts

ROBERT P. ORANGE
    The Hospital for Sick Children, Toronto, Ontario, Canada

J. PEPYS
    Brompton Hospital, London, England

B. J. HUTCHCROFT
    Charing Cross Hospital, London, England

KAI REHDER
ALAN D. SESSLER
H. MICHAEL MARSH
    Mayo Clinic and Mayo Foundation, Rochester, Minnesota

Preface

Last year, the American Thoracic Society and American Lung Association published "Lung Disease: State of the Art, 1974-1975." This book contained the first fourteen articles of the State of the Art series that began as a new feature in the *American Review of Respiratory Disease* in 1974. The first volume was published and distributed on a trial basis and plans for subsequent issues were to depend on the response to the first one. The price was kept as low as possible to encourage purchase by persons interested in respiratory disease, particularly medical students and house officers. The experiment has been a success, at least as determined by sales and reader interest. Thus, the editor and members of the Policy Committee are pleased to offer the second volume of what we hope will be an annual publication.

As I explained in the preface to the first edition, the purpose of the "State of the Art" articles is to provide physicians and scientists with concise, comprehensive, and authoritative reviews of selected topics within the broad field of lung disease. Because it is impossible to cover all possible aspects of lung disease in a single year, subjects are chosen in which important new developments or discoveries have been made that should be brought to the attention of concerned persons. The authors of this year's series of articles, like last year's, were selected on the basis of their knowledge and expertise in different specialized branches of pulmonary medicine and its related basic science disciplines.

In this volume, readers will find discussions about recent discoveries that pertain to the scientific basis and pathophysiology of common and important lung diseases, a description of new diagnostic methods, and an analysis of various therapeutic options. There is much that should be of interest and value to clinicians and scientists who are generalists as well as specialists. Everyone will learn something from "Lung Disease: State of the Art, 1975-1976."

John F. Murray, Editor
American Review of Respiratory Disease

Lung Disease

STATE OF THE ART
1975-1976

State of the Art

Silicosis[1-3]

MORTON ZISKIND, ROBERT N. JONES, and HANS WEILL

Contents

History

The effects of silicosis, the chronic fibrosing disease of the lungs produced by prolonged and extensive exposure to free crystalline silica, have been recognized for centuries. Pulmonary disease produced by dust is mentioned by Agricola in his *Treatise on Mining* (1556) and is described in stonecutters by van Diemerbroeck (1672) and Ramazzini (1713) (1). The physical evidence of previous occupational exposure to sources of free silica abound in old mines, abandoned quarries, and ancient flint tools and weapons (2). The disease can be acquired during direct operations with siliceous materials or in mineral extraction in which the free silica is contained in the residual rock. The exposure in such operations produces contact with high concentrations of dangerous fibrogenic material. Technologic advances that have supplied powerful sources of energy to industry have greatly increased the dust exposure of the worker. The pneumoconioses became more frequent and developed more rapidly after the introduction of steam machinery into factories at the turn of the nineteenth century. Zenker (1866) gave the general name pneumoconiosis to the group. Kussmaul (1866) demonstrated silica within the lungs. The specific name silicosis (Latin, *silex*, flint) was applied by Visconti (1870) (3). Intensive mining using pneumatic drills and modern energy sources made mining even more dangerous at the turn of this century. The gold mines in South Africa were opened in 1886 and clinical disease and pathology were described in this location in 1902 (3). Haldane (1902, 1914) stated that silica created the dust hazards for tin miners, and Collis (1915) proposed the theory that crystalline silica was the cause of most serious lung disease and predisposition to tuberculosis related to dust exposure (1). Increasing interest in industrial hygiene led to more intensive study of traditional trades carrying a dangerous free silica exposure, such as work in potteries, quarries, brick yards, and foundries. The frequency of the disease in metal grinders was known in the early nineteenth century. The high risk of work with granite was recognized almost a century later (4). Rapidly developing disease ("acute silicosis") was reported in scouring powder workers in 1929 after a short, intense exposure to high concentrations of free silica (5). The same course of illness has been described in tunnelers (6) and sandblasters (7).

1 From the Pulmonary Disease Section, Department of Medicine, Tulane University School of Medicine, New Orleans, La.

2 Supported in part by USPHS Grant T 12 HE 05829-6, National Institutes of Health; Grant OH 00387-03, National Institute for Occupational Safety and Health; and NHLI SCOR Grant P 17 HL 15092-02.

3 Requests for reprints should be addressed to Dr. Morton Ziskind, 1700 Perdido Street, New Orleans, La. 70112.

The great increase in frequency of pneumoconiosis in coal miners and associated workers in this century led to special studies that have advanced our understanding of the pathogenesis, pathology, roentgenographic appearances, and progression of silicosis (8). Epidemiologic studies of involved workers have thrown light on the determinants of group disease (9). The relation of dust exposure to tissue reaction as visualized on chest roentgenograms and alterations in pulmonary function is under continuing study. Experiences with the coal workers has established the importance of the concept of mixed dust exposure and has made it possible to some degree to distinguish changes produced by prolonged coal dust exposure from those created by free silica (10). This concept has been of great importance in deciding the part that silica plays in the development of diffuse pulmonary fibrosis and pleural changes. It appears that admixed free silica accounts for the pulmonary disease produced by bentonite and montmorillonite. To a lesser degree, free silica may produce disease in workers exposed to talc and kaolin. In those instances where the workers are exposed to industrial combinations of asbestos and sand, variable degrees of nodular silicosis have developed. Mixing of substances containing free silica with other dusts or chemical substances has maintained the silica hazard in industry. Understanding of chemical changes has demonstrated that certain substances become increasingly dangerous in the course of industrial processes. The heating of diatomaceous earth produces high concentrations of cristobalite and tridymite which are forms of crystalline silica more dangerous than the commonly encountered quartz (11). In the course of industrial development throughout the world, problems of production have led to the revival of dangerous industrial processes. Abrasives for the cleaning of metal surfaces before painting are in constant demand in construction and shipbuilding. In older industrial regions, the use of sandblasting for such purposes has been forbidden by law (United Kingdom, 1949, and European Economic Community, 1966). Sand as an abrasive has been extensively used in the United States in shipbuilding operations and in preparation and maintenance of oil rigs for offshore drilling since the termination of World War II. This has produced a resurgence of accelerated silicosis in sandblasters, leading to a large number of injuries and legal claims. Health and financial costs have therefore increased and have engendered a great need for modern protective devices and preventive work practices. Protective measures adopted in the past have almost eliminated clinical silicosis in quarry workers (12) and metal miners (13). At this time, the use of metal grit and coal ash residue promises to eliminate silicosis in abrasive blasters.

The early literature on silicosis is relatively limited. Important accounts were supplied by writers working for official institutions in South Africa (14), Australia (15), and Great Britain (16). In the United States, the earliest reports came from the U. S. Public Health Service (17). A pioneer monograph on roentgenology in pneumoconiosis was written by Americans (18). The early situation in the roentgenography of silicosis is described with personal reminiscences by Cole in a valuable and entertaining book (19). Descriptions of the pathologic features of silicosis are encountered in the works of Gardner (20), Gloyne (21), and the South Africans, Simson and Strachan (22). The earliest works on general studies of miners' diseases are given in varying detail by Rosen (23) and Meiklejohn (24). The enlarging literature contains valuable accounts of national experiences with silicosis. A French monograph (25) and a large Swedish text (26) described the situation before 1960. In the encyclopedic volumes on occupational health and safety published by the International Labour Organization (27), there are substantial sections devoted to silicosis. Valuable material will be found in the latest edition of Hamilton and Hardy's textbook (11). The experience of the U. S. Public Health Service is brought up to date in the recent criteria document on crystalline silica published by the National Institute of Occupational Safety and Health (28). There is a large section on silicosis that includes historic data in Hunter's *The Diseases of Occupation* (2). Modern clinical accounts of silicosis are found in 2 excellent recent books by Parkes (29) and Morgan and Seaton (30). In Baum's textbook (31), Kleinerman writes a full account of silicosis and the other pneumoconioses. A monograph on experimental pneumoconiosis includes extensive material on silicosis (1). The proceedings of the International Pneumoconiosis Conference (32) and of the International Symposia on Inhaled Particles and Vapors (33) review current epidemiologic, experimental, and environmental work.

Geology and Occupational Sources

Most of the earth's crust consists of compounds

of silicon and oxygen. The place of silicon in the inorganic world is similar to that of carbon in the organic sphere. The compound that is responsible for the development of silicosis is silicon dioxide, which occurs in nature in 3 different crystalline forms: quartz, with hexagonal crystals; cristobalite, with cubic crystals; and tridymite, with hexagonal crystals. Quartz, a hard, colorless substance, is the most common of all minerals and is a constituent of many rocks, such as granite and sandstone. The structure of quartz is described as consisting of SiO_4 tetrahedra, with each oxygen atom serving as the corner of 2 of the tetrahedra. To break a crystal of quartz, it is necessary to divide some silicon-oxygen bonds. The structure of quartz accounts for the hardness of the mineral (34).

The uncombined forms of silicon dioxide are called, collectively, "free silica" to distinguish them from silicates, which contain cations. The silicates are found in chains and in more complex structures.

The ubiquitous presence of silicon dioxide in the earth's crust is the prime factor responsible for the frequent contact of workers of various occupations with the substance. The silica-rich rock or mineral may be directly quarried for purposes of construction or may be the matrix in which a desired material is embedded. Residual rock is sometimes used for industrial purposes, notably in construction; but when the special properties of free silica are needed for abrasives, relatively pure forms of the crystalline material are used. Crypto-crystalline flints have been used since pre-recorded history, and with other materials containing silicon dioxide in high concentrations are used in those industries in which hard, heat-resistant materials are required for production of pottery and porcelain and in casting metals. Crystalline silica may be present in lesser concentrations (up to 10 to 24 per cent) when silicates such as fuller's earth and bentonite are mined. The noncrystalline (or amorphous) forms of silica are regarded as having little or no fibrogenic properties but may acquire these if heated or calcined.

The history of industrial development shows how the silica hazard has increased with the application of new and more powerful sources of mechanical energy to the earth's crust. In mining and quarrying, the introduction of pneumatic drills and blasting increased production and produced larger dust clouds that contained high concentrations of respirable particles ($<$ 10 μm in diameter). The danger of using such methods in enclosed spaces while handling substances containing high concentrations of crystalline free silica is demonstrated in tunneling and in sandblasting (35, 36). Rapid development of complicated silicosis was vividly illustrated at Gauley Bridge, W. Va., in 1931 (6). Unprotected tunnelers encountered a vein of quartz and developed fatal silicosis after short exposures, in some cases less than one year. The same pattern of rapidly developing disease occurred in abrasive powder workers, who also worked in enclosed spaces with no respiratory protection.

Free silica is widely used in industry, but the dust risk may be unsuspected because of its admixture in rock structure or clay. Combination of free silica with other minerals is a common industrial practice: The silica is often added to asbestos in asbestos-cement mixtures for the production of pipe, tile, and roofing, and to cement and concrete for use in heavy construction.

The following list of principal industrial sources of free silica is modified from Parkes (29):

(1) Mining, quarrying, and tunneling. The mining of gold, tin, copper, and mica produces a dust containing high concentrations of free silica. Sandstone is a rich source of quartz that may be encountered in the development of gold mines. Quarrying of quartz leads to exposure to dust containing 10 to 30 per cent of free silica. The quartz content of dust from quarried slate may approach 20 to 30 per cent. Tunneling through stone containing quartz or digging graves in sandstone has been associated with the production of silicosis.

(2) Stonecutting, dressing, polishing, and cleaning monumental masonry. In this work, the stones used, sandstone and granite, contain high concentrations of quartz and are dangerous because of both the silica content and the difficulty in protecting the worker, who is in close contact with the material and frequently removes his protective devices to inspect his work. Pneumatic hand tools are used for cutting and smoothing; abrasive blasting for lettering and decoration increases the risk of the procedure.

(3) Abrasives and abrasive blasting. Sandstone grindstones are now rarely used, but sandpaper and scouring powders still contain flints and quartz. The use of abrasive soaps and scouring powders was recently discontinued in the United Kingdom. The risk from abrasive blasting is greatest when sand propelled by compressed air is used. This has been largely re-

placed by steel grit in the United Kingdom. However, shot blasting of sand molds on metal castings creates dust containing high concentrations of respirable free silica.

(4) Glass manufacture. Limited use of sand in slurries to grind glass has continued in the operations of small companies.

(5) Foundry work. The free silica used in foundry work contaminates the atmosphere because of the development of molds containing sand and clay. The work is carried out at high temperatures and there is some conversion of quartz to cristobalite. There is a trend toward sand substitutes that do not contain quartz; olivine is said to be in general use in Sweden. The widespread use of sand molds and the use of blasting, hammering, and chiseling create a dusty environment containing iron oxide and quartz and lead to a form of pneumoconiosis to which silica probably makes the most important contribution.

(6) Pottery, porcelain, and lining bricks. The combination of materials containing free silica in concentrations varying from 2 per cent to 30 per cent and the high temperatures used creates a serious silicosis risk.

(7) Boiler scaling. High energy sources are used in this work creating mixed dust clouds with variable concentrations of respirable quartz particles.

(8) Vitreous enameling. All such occupations produce contact with significant amounts of free silica. Because of the use of high temperatures and pneumatic air jets or other high pressure techniques, a dusty environment is produced that will expose workers to excessive concentrations of free silica.

Characterization of Exposure

The development of silicosis depends on the inhalation of respirable free silica particles < 10 μm in diameter. The size range for maximal alveolar deposition is 1 to 3 μm. Free silica concentrations vary greatly in materials that enter into industrial processes. Concentrations usually exceed 60 per cent in sand, but this material is not hazardous under ordinary conditions because the particles are coarse and unrespirable. Where powerful desert winds whip up sandstorms, clinical silicosis does not occur; definite hyaline nodules have not been demonstrated in the lungs of inhabitants of the desert.

The silica content of natural substances can be studied in several ways. The traditional method in petrology is to use the polarizing microscope to examine small particles of the material (37). In analysis of finely divided material, roentgenographic diffraction may be used if the sample contains more than 200 μg of free silica, but the error of current methods is about 30 per cent (38). In the absence of other silicon compounds (silicates or amorphous silica), a wet chemical method can be used in which hydrochloric and hydrofluoric acids separate the free silica, which is read by colorimetry (39). Infrared spectrophotometry is also used in analysis of dust containing free silica (40).

Measurement of the degree of exposure to respirable free silica is necessary to determine the risk of disease within the industrial environment. Standards have been published through the years that were originally based on a unit of one million respirable particles in a cubic foot of air (mppcf). Current standards are usually expressed in milligrams of respirable dust per cubic meter. The current threshold limit value for respirable dust containing free silica (American Conference of Government Industrial Hygienists, 1973) is (1) $\dfrac{300}{\% \text{ quartz} + 10}$ in mppcf, or (2) $\dfrac{10}{\% \text{ quartz} + 2}$ in mg per m³. This calculated threshold limit value is divided by 2 if the dust contains cristobalite or tridymite instead of quartz. For respirable nuisance particulates containing less than 1 per cent of quartz, the threshold limit value is 30 mppcf or 10 mg per m³. A new standard for silica exposure has recently been proposed (28).

A number of methods have been used to measure the concentration of dust in the atmosphere. These include (1) settlement by gravity or centrifugation, (2) filtration, (3) impingement, (4) electric precipitation, and (5) thermal precipitation.

The method of impingement was modified successively to serve as a field method for sampling industrial dusts. An early technique was the konimeter method, in which the dust particles were sucked onto a plate covered with a thin film of petroleum. The number of particles collected within a given time was calculated by magnification of a microscopic grid. Readings of this instrument were high because fragmentation of particles by impingement exaggerated the relative dust hazard. A related instrument, the impinger, was originally described in 1932 (41); more recently, it has been modified by Greenburg and Smith to produce a practical field instrument known as the midget impinger, in which particles were entrapped by high velocity impingement and collected in water and alcohol. In the portable midget impinger, particles impinge at a velocity of 70 per sec, and the air flow for sampling is 0.1 cu ft per min. The instrument can be operated by hand or by electric pump, with the particles being collected in a liquid volume of 10 ml. The midget impinger reduced the risk of shattering large particles or the loss of particles after impingement, but aggregated particles that broke up on contact with the fluid within the collection chamber increased the dust count.

The instrument that is in general use in field operations today is the personal gravimetric dust sampler. The sampler is composed of a cyclone assembly and filter holder containing a pre-weighed millipore filter that is attached to a battery-powered pump. In the Mine Safety Appliance sampler, the pump draws air through the assembly at a flow rate of 1.7 liter per min. Non-respirable particles > 10 μm are discarded and the smaller particles adhere to the filter (42). The total weight of dust on the filter is established and the weight of the sample is obtained by subtraction. The dust is analyzed by one of the methods previously described.

Pathogenesis

Events in the pathogenesis of silicosis include (1) inhalation of silica particles, their penetration to the lung periphery, and their retention; (2) ingestion of the particles by macrophages; (3) death of the macrophages; (4) release of the contents of the killed cells, including silica particles; (5) ingestion of silica by other macrophages and their deaths; (6) gradual accumulation of other cells; (7) production of collagen; (8) hyalinization; and (9) (possibly) complication.

Particles deposited in alveoli are readily ingested by macrophages, the process resulting in creation of a phagosome from invaginated cell membranes. Silica particles at first lie within the phagosomes, which receive enzymes from the lysosomes. Within hours, however, the phagosome ruptures and silica particles can be demonstrated lying free in the cytoplasm (43). The lysosomal enzymes, discharged into the cytoplasm in activated forms, are probably responsible for the rapid death of the macrophage and extracellular loss of its contents, including the particulate silica (44). More macrophages accumulate in the area, ingest the silica, and are killed. This cytotoxic effect of silica is a necessary step in the production of silicotic fibrosis. For a variety of mineral dusts, good correlation between macrophage toxicity and fibrogenicity has been demonstrated (45, 46).

The relative ease and speed with which one may expose macrophages to dust and detect phagosomal rupture and cell death have led to a number of studies of the relative cytotoxicity of various dusts. This assay system circumvents problems of particle penetration and retention in studies of relative pathogenicity and allows studies relating particle size and composition to actual cell toxicity (47). A number of substances are ingested by macrophages and lie undigested in phagosomes but fail to alter permeability of the phagosomal membrane. Macrophages may become "choked" with such dusts and yet retain mobility as well as structural integrity. Carborundum and diamond dust fail to show macrophage toxicity, although they are angular and sharp (48). These experiments, in fact, demonstrate on a cellular level the basis of earlier animal studies that disposed of the "angularity theory" of silicogenesis. Stishovite, a rare form of crystalline free silica, also accumulates harmlessly in macrophages and fails to produce fibrosis (49). This material is octahedral; only the tetrahedral forms of silicon dioxide possess cytotoxic and fibrogenic properties. Coesite is another high temperature, high pressure form of silica. Quartz is more soluble than coesite, but the 2 minerals possess equal fibrogenic activity (50). In other experiments, differing quartz specimens with similar particle sizes and solubilities have shown significant differences in fibrogenicity (51). The foregoing have led to the rejection of the solubility theory of silicogenesis and to increased interest in stereochemical hypotheses. The importance of silanol groups on the surfaces of silica particles has recently been emphasized (51). The formation of hydrogen-bonded complexes between silica particles and active groups of the phagosomal membranes (such as quaternary and phosphate ester groups of phospholipids) may be the mechanism producing rupture of the phagosome (52). The hydrogen donor hypothesis has another attractive feature, namely, that most of the compounds that protect against experimental silicosis behave as hydrogen acceptors (53, 54). Experiments relating the particle size of colloidal silica to its activity in rupturing erythrocyte membranes lend support to a stereochemical rather than a simple "energy-transfer" explanation for membrane toxicity. The larger particle sizes of colloidal silica are more hemolytic; 3 μm particles lack hemolytic effect and, in fact, protect against the effects of subsequent exposure to the larger particle sizes even after repeated washing of the treated erythrocytes. The implication is that the smaller particles can become firmly attached to the cell membrane but lack sufficient surface area to effect membrane rupture (54). Further support for a stereochemical hypothesis comes from the fact that stishovite, lacking cytotoxic or fibrogenic properties, does possess surface silanol groups (51). Apparently, the octahedral configuration of stishovite prevents the orientation of silanol groups that produces membrane disruption. The proposed membrane toxicity of particulate silica is thus more geometric than energetic; however, this does not require that the silica be in crystalline form (55, 56).

Other recent work has examined the induction of fibrosis by products of dusted macrophages. In these experiments, macrophages are harvested from dusted animals or are exposed to particulate silica *in vitro*. The cells may then be lysed by ultrasound and separated into fractions that are subsequently injected subcutaneously into animals of the same species to assay for fibrogenicity. Control experiments have shown that residues from lysed nondusted macrophages produce little if any fibrosis. To exclude a direct effect of silica the mineral was added to the residue of lysed but undusted macrophages, and this mixture also produced little fibrosis. Using these methods, Heppleston and Styles (45) found a fibrinogenic factor in the supernate of a centrifuged suspension of dusted lysed macrophages. They considered this factor soluble. Kilroe-Smith and associates (57) used similar experimental methods but much higher speeds of centrifugation. They found the fibrinogenic activity in the residue, not the supernate. This fibrogenic factor was not a lipid, because it was not extracted by methanol-chloroform; the factor was also resistant to treatment with acetic-trichloracetic acid.

Further work on macrophages *in vitro* has demonstrated a toxic basis for the impaired resistance of silicotic patients to certain infections. *Mycobacterium tuberculosis* grows more rapidly in macrophages that are fed sublethal doses of quartz particles, and the bacilli are released more rapidly into the surrounding medium (58).

At this point, it is useful to consider some differences between these experimental models and human silicosis. The models require high silica doses, administered for relatively brief exposure times, to produce rapid biologic responses. These are exactly opposite to the usual conditions leading to human silicosis. Differences in individual exposures, in anatomic and physiologic factors governing particle retention, in exposures to other noxious agents, and in host responses to retained silica must separately and together be important determinants of which exposed persons will actually develop disease. Experimental models may therefore exclude some mechanisms that ultimately prove to be of considerable importance in human silicosis. Although these models have provided useful data on limited aspects of silicosis and have indicated promising areas for new research efforts, they have yet to provide an inclusive theory of silicogenesis. Recent work has challenged the apparent simplicity of explaining fibrogenesis by a factor released from dusted cells (59).

Autoimmunity may be important in several phases of development of silicosis. Interest in immunologic mechanisms is based on several observations: (*1*) silicotics show increased prevalence of autoantibodies (60–63); (*2*) silicotic lesions contain plasma cells and immune globulins (64–66); (*3*) gamma globulins are increased in the plasma of silicotics (64); (*4*) there is an increased prevalence of autoimmune diseases in silicosis (67–69); (*5*) the presence of a collagen disease may influence the course of the pneumoconiosis (70). Immune mechanisms probably do not participate in the killing of macrophages by silica, or in the induction of fibrosis by the residues of the dusted macrophages. Immune reactions may, however, be responsible for providing a large and continuing supply of macrophages to the area and may thus occupy a central role in the pathogenesis. Established silicotic nodules (in rats) may become more active in the presence of remote tuberculous foci (71), and Caplan's observations (70) suggest a similar effect of immune globulins in man. Another area of possible importance is the role of lipids in silicosis. The initial attack of silica on the phagosomal membrane may involve hydrogen bonding to lipids. The finding that lipid residues of dusted macrophages lack fibrogenicity does not vitiate the importance of lipids in the intact animal. Lipids may have an active part in macrophage accumulation and may also have passive effects in rendering silica particles less wettable (72). In any case, striking alterations in lipid content (and metabolism) characterize silicotic tissues (73).

Pathology

Three types of tissue reaction have been distinguished (74): chronic, in which moderate exposure extends for a period of 20 to 40 years; accelerated, with increased particle dose for a period of 5 to 15 years; and diffuse, in which there is a heavy alveolar deposition of particles for a period of less than 5 years.

Chronic reactions are encountered in industries in which the proportion of quartz in respirable dust is less than 30 per cent. In such cases, the nodules are seen after approximately 20 years of exposure. These are usually rounded but may take oval or slightly lobulated forms. The distribution is uneven, with lesions usually more prominent within the upper lobes, probably relating to better clearance of dust from the lung bases. Studies of postmortem material have shown that practically all of the silica particles visualized within the lungs are 1 to 2 μm in diameter. Careful studies of human and experimental material have demonstrated that the particles can reach the supporting tissue of the finer air spaces either through macrophages or less commonly as a result of the movements of the lungs. The particles pass toward the hilar lymph nodes, where free silica is concentrated. The death of macrophages usually leads to the formation of nodules containing free silica in the fixed interstitial tissue near the respiratory bronchiole. Here the nodules lie in relation to bronchioles and small arteries. They are also found near the lymphatics of the small veins. In chronic disease, the nodules surround a central hyaline zone that contains a variable amount of dust. This is in turn surrounded by a concentric zone of cellular connective tissue that contains no particles; it is surrounded by a halo of dust containing crystalline silica in a zone of irregularly dispersed connective tissue, which also contains crystalline silica. It is from the peripheral zone that silica is carried to enlarge the nodules and set up new silicotic nodules. A typical hyaline nodule is shown in figure 1.

Variations in the formation of the nodules have been noted. Alveolar wall involvement can lead to denudation of the overlying layer and the formation of a lumpy cellular lesion protuding into the alveoli (figure 2) that resembles bronchiolitis fibrosa obliterans (75). In the simple stage of silicosis, with few nodules larger than 5 mm, the surrounding air spaces are usually not violated. The hyaline material shows some resemblance to amyloid (74). Serum globulins within the hyaline material have been demonstrated by Vigliani and Pernis (64).

Silicosis is often complicated by the formation of massive fibrotic lesions that usually develop within the upper lobes. They are composed of nodules matted together by fibrosis and contain obliterated blood vessels and bronchi. Ischemic slit-like cavities may be demonstrated, but in the past the most important type of cavitation reported was produced by associated tuberculosis.

In coal miners with rheumatoid arthritis, Caplan (70) noted an increased prevalence of massive fibrosis. The larger masses were associated

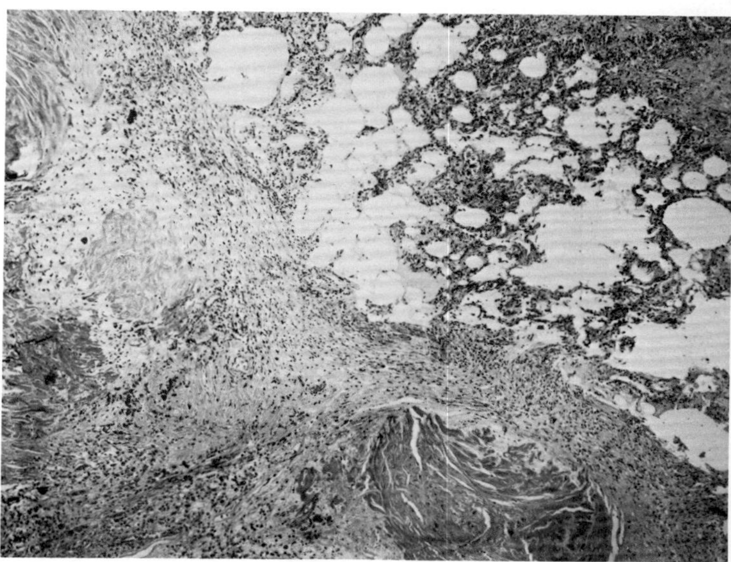

Fig. 1. Classical silicotic hyaline nodules associated with adjoining parenchymal scarring and limited lymphoid exudate (Original magnification: × 40).

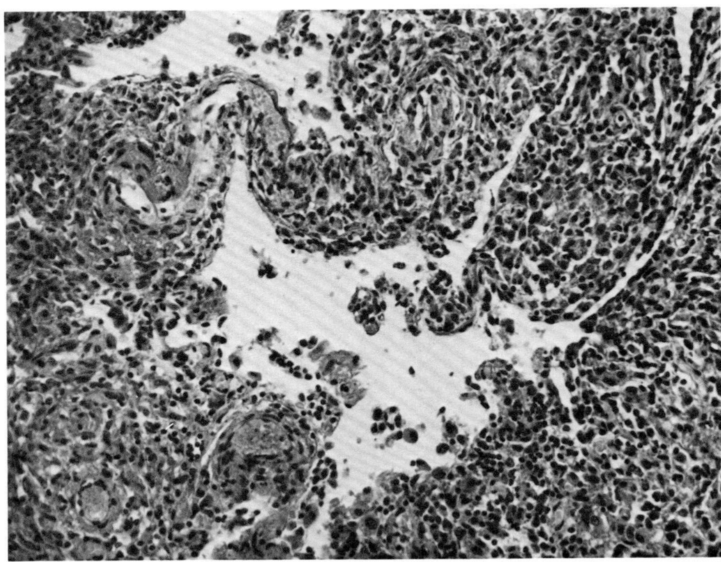

Fig. 2. Diffuse alveolar wall thickening by histiocytes with air space encroachment (Original magnification: × 140).

with a crop of round, rapidly developing opacities larger than simple silicotic nodules. Cavitation and calcification in the larger nodules has been described. Pathologic examination has demonstrated that Caplan's nodules contain necrotic materials surrounded by palisading connective tissue cells as seen in rheumatoid subcutaneous nodules. Complicated silicosis is characterized by distortion of the structure of the lungs with contraction of upper lobes and the development of emphysematous changes in the lower lobes, often with large bullae. Pleural adherence is common in this form of the disease. The enlarged lymph nodes often contain peripheral layers of calcium producing the fairly characteristic eggshell appearance. The masses can occupy one-third or more of the upper lobes. The disease has been noted to cross the interlobar fissure. The amount of dust within the masses is variable. In tuberculosis, occasional caseating granulomas may be found, but the histologic reactions may be nonspecific. There are numerous complications of silicosis. Cor pulmonale has been frequently mentioned but is not often confirmed on pathologic examination. Calcified lymph nodes, often the result of previous tuberculous infection, have produced the following changes in neighboring structures: the superior vena cava syndrome, esophageal compression, perforation of the bronchial tree with infection and hemorrhage, and paralysis of the phrenic nerve and, less often, the recurrent laryngeal nerve (76).

Data concerning the residual ash from silicotic lungs have been published (37, 77). The upper limit of normal content of free silica in human lungs is 0.2 g, whereas in disease, the quantity of free silica may rise to 15 to 20 g. McCrae showed that in the normal person the average percentage of silica in ash was 14.7 per cent. This rose to the range of 29.4 to 48 per cent in patients with silicosis. The silicon percentage of dry matter was 4.7 in the most severe cases (78). Patients with silicosis usually had at least twice as much free silica in their lungs, in percentages of dry matter, than did normal persons. Others have shown that the lungs of normal persons contain less than 0.12 per cent silica but that the fibrosis in silicotuberculous patients is excessive for the amount of silica in their lungs (79). The importance of the silica content in relation to fibrosis has been shown by Rossiter: The amount of visible reaction on the chest roentgenograms was related to the total amount of coal dust, except in those instances in which the percentage of free silica was increased (80).

The changes that have been described in chronic silicosis are also seen in accelerated silicosis, but the rate of progression is more rapid and the lesions usually become visible on chest roentgenograms after 4 to 8 years of exposure. Much of the information on this group has been obtained from studies of sandblasters. In these men, well-formed nodules developed, but there was a tendency for nodules to form in relation to the walls of the alveolar space, instead of near the respiratory bronchiole at the orifice of the acinus (81). The disease leads more frequently to massive fibrosis, and the large opacities are seen more often in the middle and basal portions of the lungs than in chronic silicosis. Cavitation is as frequently the result of atypical mycobacterial infection as of human tuberculosis (82). Ischemic cavitation may also occur.

"Acute" silicosis is a rare condition related to exposure to heavy concentrations of respirable free silica in enclosed spaces with minimal protection. The disease develops rapidly and clinical features appear after an exposure of approximately 1 to 3 years. On autopsy, there is consolidation with maintained lung volume. The lungs have a grayish white airless appearance with thickening related to diffuse interstitial fibrosis. The nodulation and massive changes of the more chronic forms of silicosis are not grossly demonstrable.

Because of terminal pulmonary edema or exudation, fluid flows from the cut surfaces. The disease is usually complicated by mycobacterial or other infections that produce thickened and adherent pleura. A striking microscopic change is the presence of acidophilic fluid, containing fine granules and many macrophages, within the alveolar spaces (figure 3). There is also cuboidal transformation of the alveolar cells. Interstitial fibrosis is prominent, but silicotic nodules are poorly demarcated and small (6). The fluid within these spaces contains lipids and proteins and gives a strongly positive reaction to periodic Schiff reagent (7). Quartz crystals are present within the lungs and the hilar lymph nodes. The cells seen within the alveolar spaces are macrophages, but it is possible that in the course of the disease, type 2 pneumocytes are desquamated into the alveolar spaces as well.

The reaction of silica has been elucidated by experimental exposure of laboratory animals. Silica has been introduced into the respiratory tract by dusting or by direct intratracheal injection. Subcutaneous, intravenous, and intraperitoneal routes of administration have been used. Silica has even been placed in the anterior chamber of the eye. Important studies have been carried out on macrophages exposed to free silica in tissue culture media. Lesions produced in animals have been studied for silica content by the sensitive spectrophotometric colorimetric method in which silicomolybdate is formed.

A number of animal models have been used for these studies. Examinations at various intervals have demonstrated the course of silicotic lesions. Typical compact nodules have been produced in rats after exposure in dust chambers for periods as long as one year (83). Collagenous nodules have also been produced in chronically dusted monkeys (84). In the hamster, nodulation

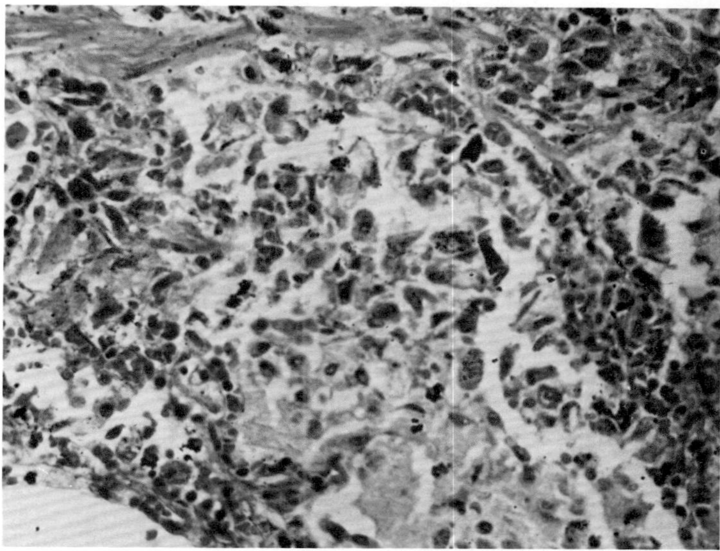

Fig. 3. Silico-proteinosis. The alveolus is filled with macrophages associated with pigment granules and proteinaceous material. The alveolar margins are demarcated by congested capillaries.

occurs early, is widespread, and is associated with diffuse pulmonary fibrosis. This is probably related to numerous foci in lymphoid tissue scattered throughout the lungs (85). Intratracheal injection of a massive dose of free silica usually produces acute cellular reaction, which fills the air spaces and only later leads to the formation of nodules and fibrosis. This reaction is well illustrated in the guinea pig (86). The sequence of focal collection of dust cells followed by the concentration of fibroblasts leading to definite collagen nodules has been demonstrated in monkeys chronically exposed to small particles of quartz, 3 μm or less. Under similar conditions, amorphous fused silica dust produced only limited fibrosis.

The resistance to mycobacteria of dusted animals, often guinea pigs and rats, has been studied by experimental methods. The native resistance of both species was altered by silica. The disease was produced more readily by virulent organisms and by attenuated strains that ordinarily would not produce infection. *Mycobacterium marinum* produced progressive disease in guinea pigs after their exposure to silica by both intratracheal injection and dusting techniques.

Clinical Features

Silicosis is usually a chronic disease, and the principal symptoms develop late; it is rare for the chest film to become positive before 20 years of exposure. In the past, the average duration of life after first exposure has been approximately 40 years for those whose exposure to free silica was moderate, as in foundrymen, quarrymen, miners, and potters (87). An earlier, more rapid onset of the disease would be an indication of heavier exposure due to unusual circumstances of employment (lack of protection and work in enclosed spaces), or an infectious or immunologic complication.

The earliest symptoms in chronic cases are cough and expectoration, which can usually be explained by a history of cigarette smoking extending back to early youth. The principal symptom of established silicosis is shortness of breath on effort. This is usually associated with roentgenograms showing complicated, rather than simple pneumoconiosis. Significant dyspnea on effort is almost invariably related to massive changes within the lungs, contraction of lobes, or cavitation of infectious or ischemic origin. Distortion of the bronchial tree under these circumstances leads to increased cough and expec-

toration, but these symptoms will be more severe if cavities are present. Hemoptysis and chest pain due to infection are not uncommon. Weight loss is a characteristic finding in silicotuberculosis and other types of infective pneumoconioses. Mycotic infections, including nocardiosis, cryptococcosis, and sporotrichosis, have complicated this pneumoconiosis. Infections are particularly common when silicosis is accelerated or acute.

Respiratory failure is the most important consequence of complicated silicosis. Ventilatory failure may be aggravated by the development of pneumothorax, which resists successful treatment because of the difficulty in obtaining reexpansion of the shrunken, fibrotic lung and in sealing the leak in the poorly retractile tissue.

There have been a number of reports dealing with the increased prevalence of scleroderma in pneumoconiosis and silica exposure. In our experience, autoimmune disease has often been associated with the accelerated type of silicosis seen in sandblasters: About 10 per cent developed connective tissue disorders, including scleroderma, rheumatoid arthritis, and systemic lupus erythematosus. The role of the complicating disease is uncertain but is usually associated with more rapid progression of roentgenographic and functional abnormalities. It is in these cases that some response to adrenal corticosteroids may be noted. The evolution of silicosis associated with auto-immune disease can be very rapid, producing marked structural and functional changes within the course of 1 or 2 years.

In accelerated silicosis, the major features of the disease are identical to the chronic disease, but the chest roentgenogram usually becomes positive within 4 to 8 years of first dust exposure. The over-all course of deterioration is rapid and the average exposure to free silica is approximately 10 years in fatal cases of sandblasters' silicosis. Mycobacteriosis affects 25 per cent of the workers; half of these infections are due to atypical organisms. In Wisconsin, the common atypical mycobacterium complicating silicosis is *M. intracellulare* (Battey bacillus) (88). This is the organism usually associated with rural residence. In the coastal zones, and near the larger cities of the southwest, *M. kansasii* has been the atypical mycobacterium usually associated with silicosis.

Most of the disease described above has been related to high doses of free crystalline silica. Smaller doses of quartz produce a rather mild disease of long duration. This may occur in patients exposed to minor amounts of quartz contaminating other minerals.

Silicoproteinosis is the name applied to a variant of rapidly developing silicosis in which there are characteristic histologic changes. It is the result of heavy exposure to respirable silica dust. Dyspnea on effort may develop within 6 months of first exposure. There is associated weakness and weight loss and, in more severe cases, cyanosis and diffuse rales. Complication by mycobacterial infection is the rule, but in one case treated with steroids there was terminal nocardiosis. Progressive deterioration may be temporarily and partially suppressed by corticosteroids. Death is due to intractable hypoxemia.

The prevalence of mycobacterial infections may be declining for chronic silicosis but remains high for the accelerated and acute forms. The roentgenographic appearance varies from characteristic cavitary infiltrates to massive disease, with or without cavitation, in which tuberculous elements may be difficult to distinguish. In those with positive sputum cultures, the rate of sputum conversion is high; but the massive disease and conglomerate lesions will often progress despite appropriate chemotherapy (89).

A number of investigators indicate that tuberculosis tends to complicate silicotic disease of long standing and that it tends to be more severe in the more rapidly progressive types of the disease. Can prior silica exposure, insufficient to produce nodulation on the chest roentgenogram, predispose a person to tuberculosis? In persons who have had years of silica exposure and negative roentgenograms, active tuberculosis may suddenly appear. In some instances, the disease may continue to progress and produce massive lesions without visible associated nodular foci. Macrophages are of undoubted importance in immunity to mycobacterial infections; it is precisely these cells that demonstrate exquisite susceptibility to the toxic effect of particulate silica. Watkins-Pitchford (90) found an association between work as a gold miner for 3 to 5 years and the subsequent development of tuberculosis, even though silicosis was not demonstrated on the chest roentgenograms. This potentially important observation has not been confirmed. The progressive and massive changes produced by mycobacterial infection in silicosis have not been described for mycotic superinfection. A study of the relation of silicosis and silica exposure to histoplasmosis would be of theoretic and practical interest.

There is no indication that silicosis is associated with increased risk for the development of cancer of the respiratory or other systems. When there is combined exposure to silica and other substances such as arsenic, nickel, or chromate, the increased susceptibility to cancer appears to be related to the other material. There is no indication of a synergistic increase of susceptibility to cancer after exposure to such other dusts and silica.

Diagnosis

The diagnosis of silicosis usually depends on historical and roentgenographic evidence. A history of significant exposure to free silica is required. This is usually obvious, but occasionally the source of silica may not be apparent, particularly in mixed exposure. In the case of brickyard workers, the exposure to silica brick that lines the kilns may be overlooked; the clay bricks contain little or no free silica. In another instance, an apparently safe amorphous silica (e.g., diatomaceous earth) may be rendered toxic by heating to near or above the temperature of crystallization (55).

Roentgenographic changes provide the evidence that exposure has in fact produced lung disease. The individual elements that combine to form the pathology of silicosis are seen on chest roentgenograms as characteristic shadows. The roentgenographic features of silicosis have been known for more than 50 years (18, 19, 91). In the simple forms of the disease, rounded nodules are the basic elements (figure 4). In the complicated forms, massive densities predominate (figure 5). Because of the diagnostic and epidemiologic value of distinguishing these changes, there has been a continuous effort to standardize descriptions of the abnormal shadows. Originally, the descriptions were based on patterns composed of small rounded opacities, as seen typically in silicosis and coal worker's pneumoconiosis. It was later recognized that mixed disease was common and that a more useful classification should also include the small irregular opacities produced by asbestos and other noxious inhalants (92). The current Union International Contra Cancre–International Labour Organization classification provides for identification and grading of both rounded and irregular opacities. Four grades of profusion (0-1-2-3) are used. After assigning a grade, the reviewer has an opportunity to reconsider his or her original choice and to designate a second grade of greater, equal, or lesser magnitude, as

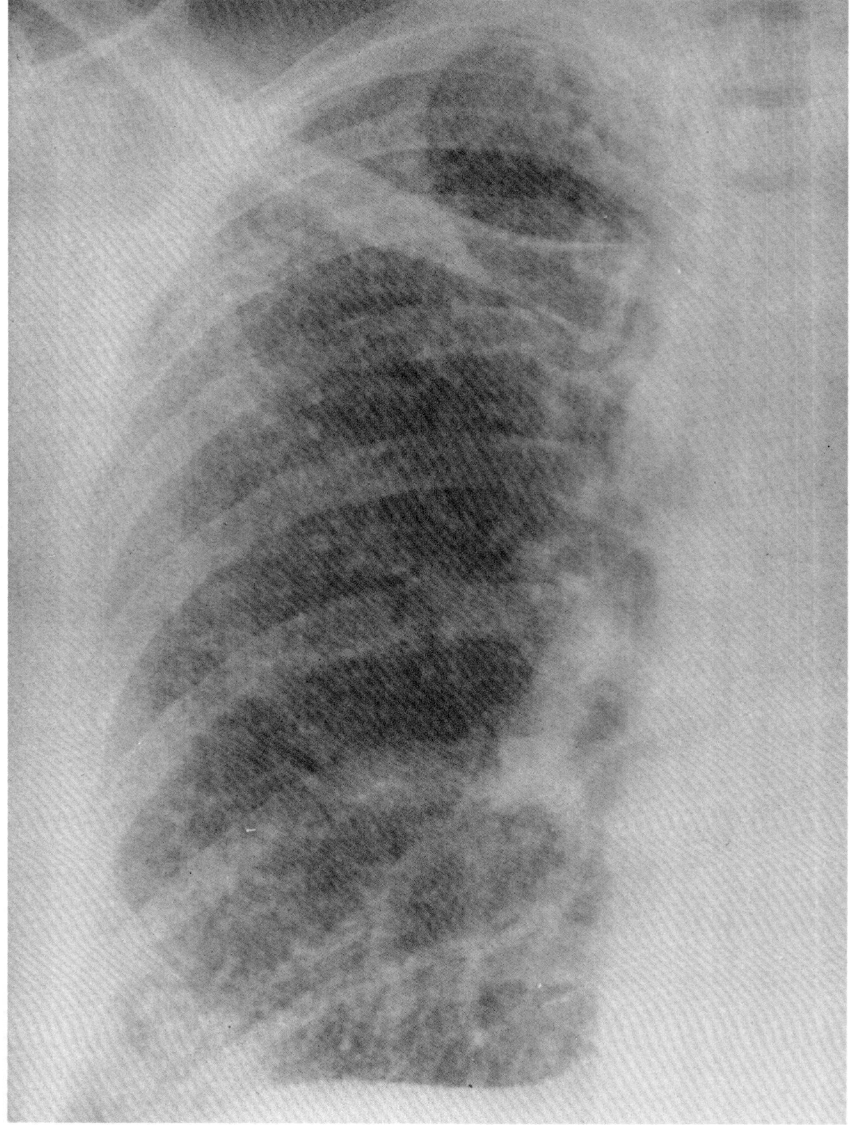

Fig. 4. Simple nodular silicosis.

appropriate. In this manner, 12 possible sub-categories of profusion can be selected, producing a 12-point scale that results in greater precision and sensitivity when a panel of readers is used (93). The resulting data can then be compared with exposure, clinical, functional, and pathologic data (94). In addition to this grading of simple opacities, the current scheme allows description of complicated disease on the basis of the size of opacities > 1 cm. The classification also provides for grading of pleural changes, a modification of special value in dealing with the effects of asbestos exposure.

The lesions of silicosis are usually more prominent within the upper lung fields. They may be difficult to distinguish in the early forms of the simple disease and at this stage may be more readily detected on 15° oblique projections (95). The same effect may be obtained on standard oblique views or on lateral views in which the fine lesions are superimposed. The nodules, which are rounded and fairly uniform in size in simple disease, may later show coalescence as a result of infection or the beginning of massive fibrosis. As mentioned above, the development of massive change may itself be an indication of complication by mycobacterial infection. In miners with rheumatoid arthritis, massive changes are more prevalent and opacities of one to several centimeters may enlarge more rapidly than expected. A third form of rheumatoid pneumoconiosis is rapid enlargement of disseminated small opacities (96).

Roentgenographic progression of simple disease, or from simple to complicated disease, can usually be expected within 5 years (26). Masses usually occur within the upper lobes and are often associated with contraction of the lobes, elevation of the lung roots, and the development of emphysematous changes at the bases.

Although calcification of pulmonary nodules is rare, lymph nodes may calcify, producing an "eggshell" appearance. Enlargement of lymph nodes is common and may occur before pulmonary nodulation. Within the mediastinum enlargement may be extreme, leading to compression of the superior vena cava and the esophagus (76). Massive disease with contraction of the upper lobes is frequently associated with thickening of the pleura, and with pleural adhesions. Pneumothorax is not unusual in silico-tuberculosis or massive fibrosis and is often a pre-terminal complication.

The so-called acute form of the disease is characterized by widespread involvement of both lungs. The air spaces are filled; there are associated interstitial changes, with poorly defined nodulation demonstrable at the periphery. The lung volumes are obviously small and the diaphragm is high. Although infection is often present, cavities can rarely be demonstrated, and the infectious exudates are concealed within the larger exudates produced by reaction to the dust. This applies to fungal as well as mycobacterial infections; nocardia can complicate silicoproteinosis as well as idiopathic pulmonary alveolar proteinosis.

In mixed exposures to respirable silica and asbestos, patients may show roentgenographic changes associated with either or both types of dust. It is not unusual to see both rounded and irregular opacities within the lung fields, as well as fibrous and calcified pleural plaques (97).

Exposed workers without roentgenographic

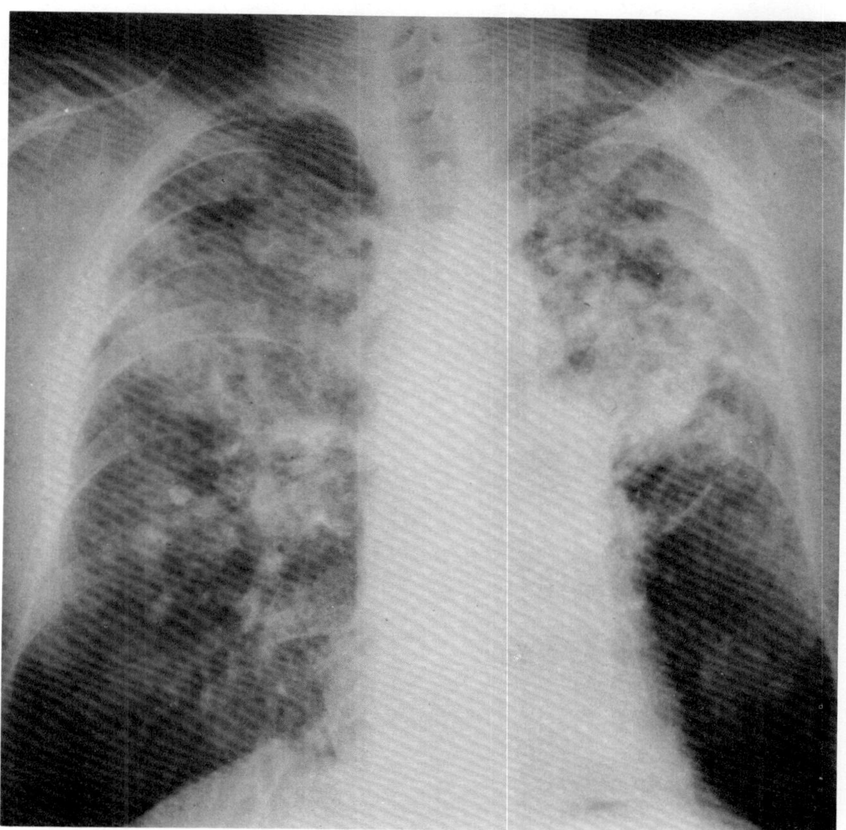

Fig. 5. Complicated silicosis with conglomerate massive shadows.

abnormalities should receive regular follow-up examination, because well-established nodulation may become evident within a year. This may occur even though silica exposure has terminated.

Silicosis must be differentiated from disorders producing similar roentgenographic abnormalities. Sarcoidosis shares with silicosis a tendency to produce widespread nodulation, often more profuse in the upper zones, and hilar lymphadenopathy. Advanced cases of sarcoidosis may also show small lung volumes, conglomerate densities, and emphysematous changes. Sarcoidosis may exhibit characteristic extrapulmonary clinical findings and often shows roentgenographic improvement with corticosteroid treatment. Massive opacities of silicosis have been mistaken for cancer and vice versa. It should be noted that clubbing of the digits is most unusual in silicosis. Diffuse carcinomatosis and simple silicosis may have similar roentgenographic appearances, but the patient suffering from carcinomatosis ordinarily shows severe clinical and lung functional abnormalities. Infectious granulomas may provide problems of differential or simultaneous diagnosis. Large opacities in the upper zones that are clearly separated from the pleura (producing the characteristic "angel's wings" appear-

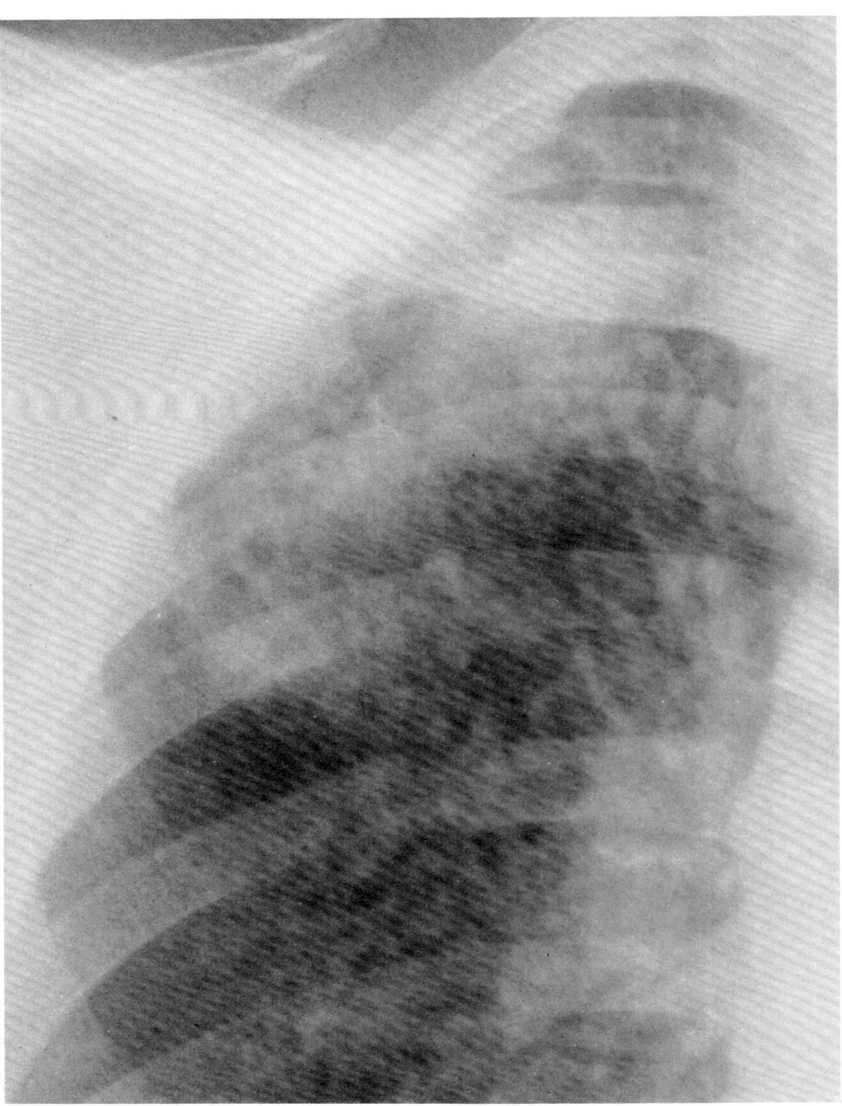

Fig. 6. Conglomerate shadow, often described as "angel's wing" appearance.

ance) favor a diagnosis of silicosis (figure 6). With similar densities in mycobacterial infection, greater contact with the pleural surface is expected; remote pleural reactions favor a diagnosis of mycobacterial infection. The simultaneous diagnosis of silicosis and mycobacteriosis can be extremely difficult. The silicotic nodules may be caught up in the tuberculous process, and emphysematous basilar changes may spread the remaining nodules, making them difficult to detect. In the presence of massive tuberculous changes, silicosis may be suspected only when there is widespread uniform small nodulation, remote from the tuberculous foci. Other pneumoconioses may mimic the roentgenographic appearance of silicosis. In this connection it should be remembered that welders, for example, may work near sandblasters and develop silicosis (figure 7), siderosis, or both.

Ordinarily, a lung biopsy is not required to establish the diagnosis of silicosis; the combination of a history of significant silica exposure and a characteristic roentgenogram will suffice.

Biopsy must sometimes be undertaken in exposed persons because the roentgenographic abnormality is thought to be atypical. This has been the case in some patients who have diffuse alveolar filling or diffuse interstitial reactions as the result of heavy dust exposure (figure 8). Biopsy may be needed when there is complicating auto-immune disease, or in other cases showing progressive and rapid deterioration (figures 9A, 9B). Biopsy may also be needed where there has been exposure to more than one type of dust. Under any of the above circumstances, histologic information may be of crucial importance in legal proceedings.

When lung biopsy is required, an open chest procedure is preferable. Needle biopsy is inadvisable because of coexisting emphysematous changes. Needle and transbronchoscopic biopsies do not yield sufficient tissue for the special studies that are often necessary. Conventional histologic examination is sufficient for diagnosis when it shows the cellular reaction and hyaline nodules in differing stages of formation.

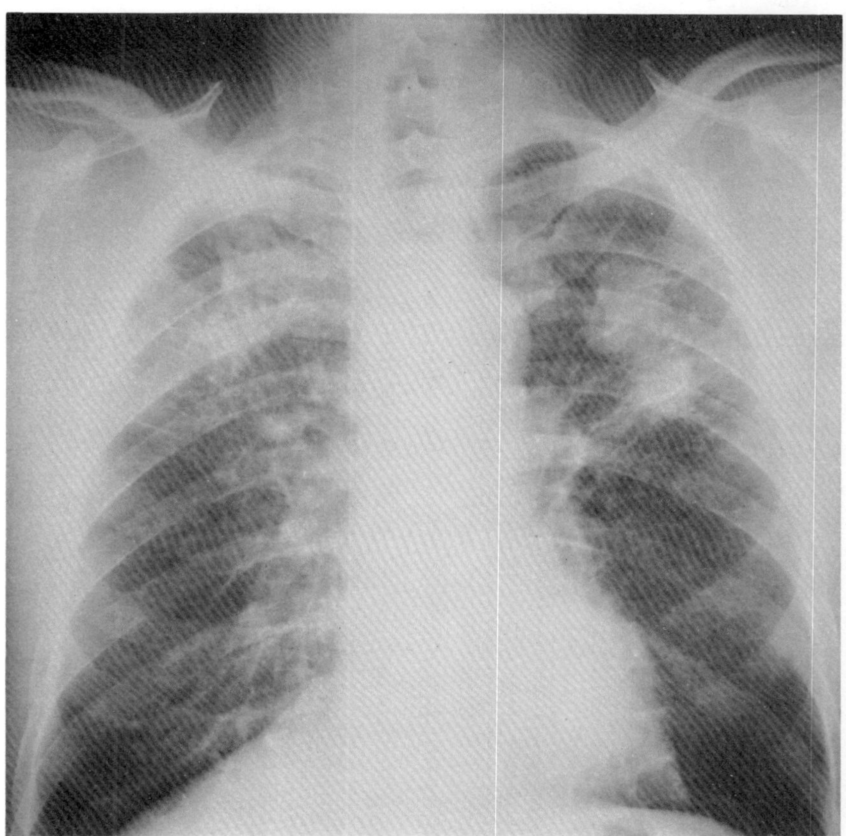

Fig. 7. Welder with complicated silicosis who was employed in sandblasting operations.

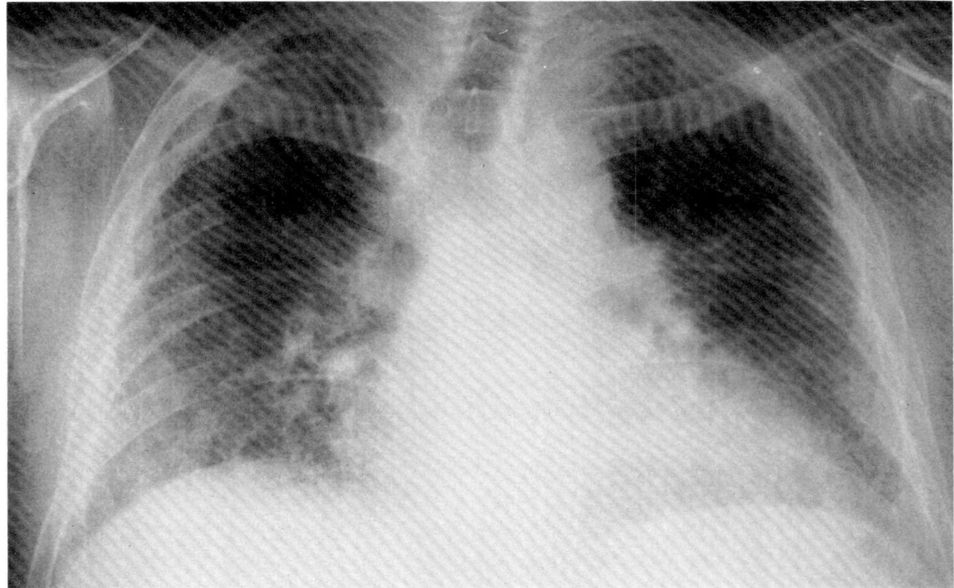

Fig. 8. "Acute" silicosis showing diffuse infiltration obscuring the vascular pattern. Lung volumes are reduced.

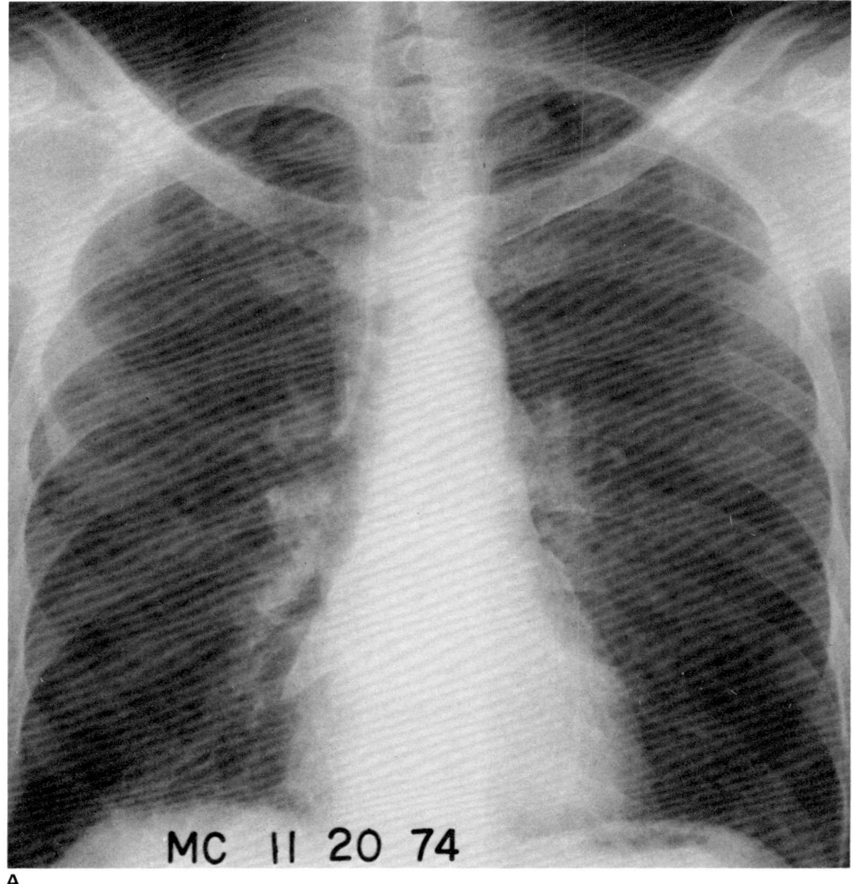

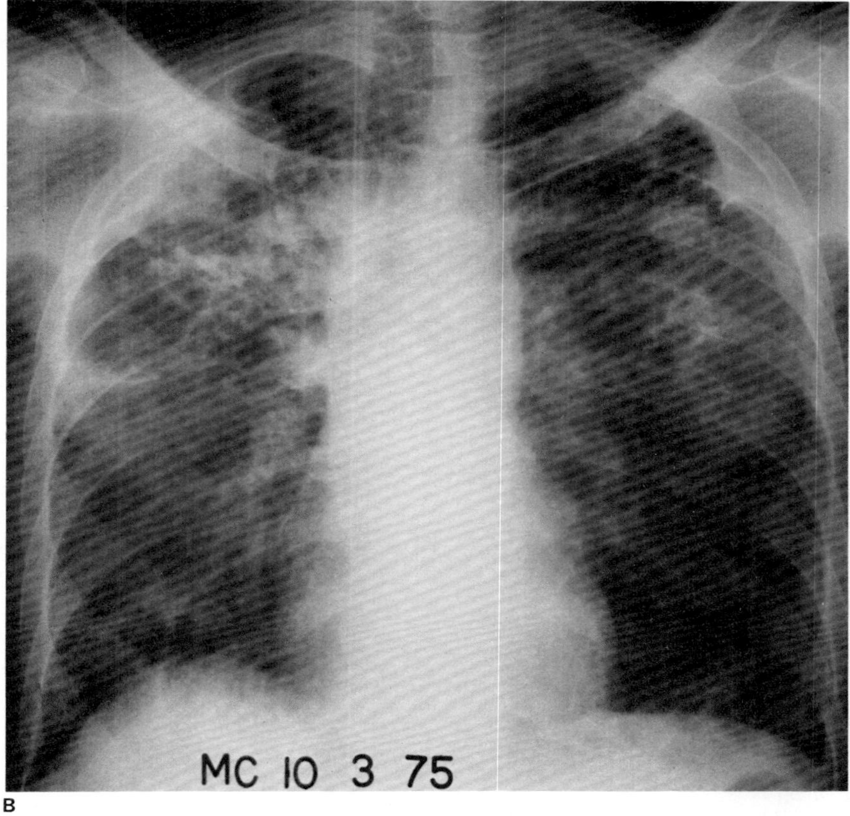

Fig. 9. Sandblaster with scleroderma exhibiting rapid progression of silicosis in less than one year.

When the tissue pattern is not characteristic, examination under polarized light may demonstrate doubly refractile particles of silica. When further characterization is required, fine particles of quartz can be demonstrated by scanning electron microscopy. The presence of excess silicon may be demonstrated by x-ray energy spectrometry. High silicon-sulphur ratios determined by this method are diagnostic for pneumoconiosis and are strongly suggestive of silicosis. When tissues contain silicates rather than free silica, x-ray energy spectrometry may disclose the presence of unusual amounts of associated elements such as calcium, magnesium, or iron (98). These elegant methods should be applied to all biopsy and autopsy specimens from dust-exposed persons that show obscure or atypical changes on routine tissue examination. These methods will not only provide improved diagnosis in individual cases but will widen our awareness of known hazards and disclose unsuspected sources of dust exposure.

Lung Function

It is difficult to propound general statements about lung function in silicosis. This is due to the wide variety of clinical and pathologic forms of the disease. This variation is due partly to the exposure variables of intensity and duration and to the type of silicious dust. Infections and immune reactions may complicate the disease and affect lung function. The effects of age and tobacco are not easily assessed, because most silicotics are older men who have smoked for many years.

To add to the confusion, most of the cross-sectional studies of lung function and silicosis have examined miners, quarrymen, or foundry workers. Mixed dust exposures are the rule in those occupations, and free silica usually comprises less than half of the total and respirable dust exposure. Industrial bronchitis is common in such populations, and symptoms and functional abnormalities may correlate better with smoking than with dust exposure (99–101).

Heavy exposures to relatively pure, respirable free silica, on the other hand, produce the less common accelerated or acute forms of silicosis (87, 102–104). These forms are rapidly progressive, and lung function data differ from that found in the more ordinary form of silicosis (105). Animal studies are even more limited in applicability: Enormous doses of dust are generally given in a short period, or in a single dose. The experimental pathology frequently differs greatly from human tissue changes, thwarting from the outset any attempt to relate directly the animals' functional change to the human disease. The foregoing seem to express an "uncertainty principle" wherein the more confident one is that he is studying pure silicosis, the less confident he may be in applying his results to the ordinary human disease.

It is not surprising, then, to find apparent contradictions in the literature of lung function. Investigators have focused on the fibrotic or emphysematous aspects of silicosis (106–111). Lung diffusing capacity in various studies has shown a rather wide range of correlations with other measures of functional impairment (112–119). Static and dynamic compliance are often reduced in silicosis (120–121). The difficulty of applying invasive tests (such as compliance and arterial gas studies) to working populations has retarded study of the early phases of development of pneumoconioses. Arterial oxygen tensions may be normal both at rest and during exercise (122). Measurement of resistance of the lower airways requires a plethysmograph, substantial time, and good subject cooperation, so has not been widely applied to exposed populations. The procedure yields limited additional information when the forced expiratory spirogram is abnormal. Pulmonary mixing is impaired in a large percentage of silicotics but is more sensitive to bronchitis (123).

These varied functional abnormalities are easier to understand if the lung pathology is reviewed. Focal dust collections are often peribronchiolar, in excellent location for producing a disturbance of ventilatory distribution, and, later, obstruction of the acinus. Focal fibrosis can obliterate peripheral airways. Overall, more generalized fiberosis tends to reduce lung size, whereas obstruction of expiration leads to enlargement of lung volume. When conglomerate masses form, they not only produce restriction per se (as does any space-occupying lesion), but they commonly distort, compress, and even obliterate larger airways. Vessels are similarly affected. The discontinuous, asymmetric lung changes in silicosis contrast with those in asbestosis and explain the wider range of functional abnormalities in silicosis.

Despite the complex pathophysiology, howev-

er, the following statements seem to have wide support. (1) In simple silicosis, clinical tests of ventilatory function are often normal (30, 100, 111, 120, 124). We found this to be true even for a group of sandblasters with heavy exposure to pure quartz: The relative youth of that group (mean age, 37 years) probably minimized the effect of smoking (105). (2) Series of symptomatic silicotics will include patients with restriction, obstruction, and mixed patterns of ventilatory impairment (105, 111, 122). (3) Complicated cases show reduced diffusing capacities and exercise-induced hypoxemia (125). (4) Lung compliance is usually reduced (120). (5) Terminal cases have severe restrictive impairments. (6) Severe hypoxemia dominates the last phase of the disease.

Selection of lung function tests has recently been reviewed (126, 127). Aside from simple spirometry, a test may have differing utility in clinical, survey, or disability evaluation testing. No functional measurement, or combination of measurements, is specific for silicosis. Serial testing of silicotics is highly desirable because the course of progression in the ordinary form of this disease has not received adequate study.

Treatment

Unfortunately, there is no specific treatment for silicosis and current therapy is directed entirely at complications. Anti-tuberculosis drugs are effective in sterilizing the sputum of infected patients, but massive changes have frequently progressed after institution of the appropriate drugs. Drug treatment should begin with suspicion of infection and should not await confirmation by cultures. A positive tuberculin test constitutes strong evidence of mycobacterial infection. The high proportion of atypical mycobacteria warrants the initial use of 3 anti-tuberculous drugs, including rifampin. The physician should not be anxious to discontinue treatment after 2 years, especially if there is cavitation or continued roentgenographic progression. The physician must also be alert to the possibility of other infections and vigorous in their treatment. When auto-immune diseases complicate silicosis, corticosteroids should be tried. When obstruction forms part of the functional impairment, bronchodilators may be used; a surprising percentage of obstructed patients will show significant improvement. Pneumothorax is treated with chest tube drainage, but with poor results in the advanced case. Heart failure is treated in the ordinary way, but this may produce only modest relief of chronic dyspnea. Digitalis should be used carefully to avoid complicating rhythm disturbances. Phlebotomy is rarely required. The need for supplemental oxygen is a prominent feature of the later stages of the disease. Ventilatory failure, unless precipitated by acute infection or sedation, is a terminal event.

A number of compounds have received experimental study in prevention or treatment of silicosis. Of these, polyvinyl pyridine N-oxide has shown the greatest promise; a related drug is receiving clinical trial (29).

Prevention

Where silica exposure is moderate, as in mines, quarries, potteries, and foundries, workers may be protected by improving ventilation and by the use of wet techniques. In some cases, materials may be substituted for those containing free silica. In many instances, however, such substitutes are not available or suitable or are adopted slowly because of their costs. Respirators are required when the concentration of respirable free silica exceeds the threshold limit value by more than 5 times. At such levels, dust masks can be useful if the work is carried out for short periods of time. When the work is prolonged, such respirators produce too great a resistance to air flow and become intolerable. All masks used in work with free silica must completely exclude the ambient, unfiltered air. Defects along the seams and eyeglasses greatly reduce the value of the masks. With very high concentrations of free silica, as produced by blasting with white sand, workers require air-supplied abrasive blasting hoods. These devices must be checked to be sure that the air flowing through the hoods is not contaminated by dust or oil, that the pressure is reduced sufficiently to prevent excessive noise within the hood, and that the flow rate is still high enough to exclude entry of ambient air. Flow rates should be in the range of 3 to 6 cu ft per min. Work practices should prescribe the wearing of hoods during periods of blasting and for sufficient time afterwards to allow dispersal of the dangerous cloud of suspended respirable silica. Associated workers should (but often do not) wear appropriate protective equipment.

One can be optimistic about the eventual control of silicosis despite national statistics from industrial countries that show thousands of new cases as late as 1965 (27). Recent results from the United Kingdom and from certain industries in the United States indicate that the disease can be controlled. With better control of the environment and the observance of modern standards for air quality, workers will be exposed to lower concentrations of free silica. This approach will eliminate most of the cases produced by the traditional sources of silicosis. For dangerous operations such as sandblasting, the only effective solution can be the substitution of less noxious abrasive materials. New potential sources of exposure will appear with additional uses for silica. The risk of silicosis will always be present in mining; recent advances in mine safety should be universally applied. With continued progress in occupational health, it is our hope that silicosis will become a medical curiosity rather than an important cause of disability and premature death.

Acknowledgment

The writers thank Dr. Herbert Ichinose for supplying photomicrographs.

References

1. Zaidi, S. H.: Experimental Pneumoconiosis, Johns Hopkins Press, Baltimore, 1969.
2. Hunter, D.: The Diseases of Occupations, Little, Brown, and Company, Boston, 1955, p. 841.
3. Silicosis and Asbestosis, A. J. Lanza, ed., Oxford University Press, New York, 1938, p. 5.
4. Hosey, A. D., Trasko, V .M., and Ashe, H. B.: Control of Silicosis in Vermont Granite Industry: Progress Report, Publication 557, U. S. Department of Health, Education, and Welfare, Washington, D. C., 1957, p. 10.
5. Middleton, E. L.: The present position of silicosis in industry in Britain, Br Med J, 1929, 2, 485.
6. Gardner, L. U.: Pathology of the so-called "acute" silicosis, Am J Public Health, 1933, 23, 1240.
7. Buechner, H. A., and Ansari, A.: Acute silico-proteinosis, Dis Chest, 1969, 55, 174.
8. McKerrow, C.: Silicosis and coalworkers' pneumoconiosis, in *Clinical Aspects of Inhaled Particles*, D. C. F. Muir, ed., F. A. Davis & Co., Philadelphia, 1972, pp. 156–172.
9. Cochrane, A. L.: Epidemiology of coalworkers' pneumoconiosis, in *Industrial Pulmonary Diseases*, E. J. King and C. M. Fletcher, ed., J and A Churchill, Ltd., London, 1960, pp. 221-231.
10. Gough, J., and Heppleston, A. G.: The pathology of the pneumoconioses, in *Industrial Pulmonary Disease*, E. J. King and C. M. Fletcher, ed., J and A Churchill Ltd., London, 1960, pp. 23–36.
11. Hamilton, A., and Hardy, H. L.: Industrial Toxicology, ed. 3, Publishing Sciences Group, Inc., Acton, Mass., pp. 429-440.
12. Theriault, G. P., Burgess, W. A., DiBerardinis, L. J., and Peters, J. M.: Dust exposure in

the Vermont Granite Sheds, Arch Environ Health, 1974, *28*, 12.

13. Flinn, R. H., Bruton, H. P., Doyle, H. N., Cralley, L. J., and Harris, R. L.: Silicosis in the Metal Mining Industry, Public Health Service Publication No. 1076, U. S. Department of the Interior, Bureau of Mines, U. S. Government Printing Office, Washington, D. C., 1963.

14. Watkins-Pitchford, W.: The silicosis of the South African gold mines and the changes produced in it by legislative and administrative efforts, Ind Hyg, 1927, *9*, 109.

15. Report of Technical Commission of Inquiry: The Prevalence of Miner's Phthisis and Pneumoconiosis in the Metalliferous Mines at Broken Hill, No. 6 Report, Department of Labor and Industry, New South Wales, Australia, Dec. 1, 1921.

16. Collis, E. L.: Industrial Pneumoconiosis with Special Reference to Dust Phthisis, Milroy Lectures, 1915, H.M.S.O., London, 1919.

17. Lanza, A. J., and Childs, S. B.: Miners' Consumption: A Study of 433 Cases of the Disease Among Zinc Miners in Southwestern Missouri, U. S. Public Health Service Bulletin, No. 85, Washington, D. C., 1917.

18. Pancoast, H. K., and Pendergrass, E. P.: Pneumoconiosis (Silicosis): A Roentgenological Study with Notes on Pathology, Paul B. Hoeber, Inc., New York, 1926.

19. Cole, L. G.: "Lung Dust Lesions (Pneumoconiosis) versus Tuberculosis," American Medical Films, Inc., White Plains, N. Y., 1948.

20. Gardner, L. U.: Experimental pathology, in *Silicosis and Asbestosis*, A. J. Lanza, ed., Oxford University Press, New York, 1938, pp. 257–345.

21. Gloyne, S. R.: Pathology, in *Silicosis and Asbestosis*, A. J. Lanza, ed., Oxford University Press, New York, 1938, pp. 198–256.

22. Simson, F. W., and Strachan, A. S.: Silicosis and tuberculosis: Observations on the origin and character of silicotic lesions as shown in cases occurring on the Witwatersrand, Publications of the South African Institute for Medical Research, XXXVI, 1935, *6*, 367.

23. Rosen, G.: The History of Miners' Diseases, Schuman's, New York, 1943.

24. Meiklejohn, A.: History of lung diseases of coalminers in Great Britain: Part II, 1875–1920, Br J Ind Med, 1952, *9*, 93.

25. Sadoul, P., and Dusapin, M.: L'Expertise de la Silicose Pulmonaire, Masson et Cie, Nancy, France, 1959.

26. Ahlmark, A., and Nystrom, A.: Silicosis and Other Pneumoconioses in Sweden, Svenska Bokforlaget, Stockholm, 1960.

27. Encyclopedia of Occupational Health and Safety, International Labour Organization, Geneva, Switzerland, 1971, p. 1309.

28. Occupational Exposure to Crystalline Silica: HEW Publication No. (NIOSH) 75–120, U. S. Dept. H.E.W., P.H.S., C.D.C., Washington, D.C., 1974.

29. Parkes, W. R.: Occupational Lung Disorders, Butterworths, London, 1974, p. 166.

30. Morgan, W. K. C., and Seaton, A.: Occupational Lung Diseases, W. B. Saunders Co., Philadelphia, 1975, p. 80.

31. Kleinerman, J.: Industrial pulmonary diseases: Silicosis, asbestosis, and talc pneumoconiosis, in *Textbook of Pulmonary Diseases*, ed 2, G. L. Baum, ed., Little, Brown, and Co., Boston, 1974, pp. 489–507.

32. Proceedings of the IVth International Pneumoconiosis Conference, Bucharest, 27 Sept.–2 Oct., 1971, Apimondia Publishing House, Bucharest, Hungary.

33. Inhaled Particles III, W. H. Walton, ed., Unwin Brothers, Ltd., Old Woking, Surrey, England, 1971.

34. Pauling, L.: General Chemistry, ed. 2, W. H. Freeman and Co., San Francisco, 1953.

35. Samimi, B., Weill, H., and Ziskind, M.: Respirable silica dust exposure of sandblasters and associated workers in steel fabrication yards, Arch Environ Health, 1974, *29*, 61.

36. Bobear, J. B., Hanemann, S. J, and Beven, T.: Silicosis in Lousiana: New or unrecognized hazard, J Louisiana Med Soc, 1962, *114*, 391.

37. Drinker, P., and Hatch, T.: Industrial Dust: Hygienic Significance, Measurement and Control, ed. 2, McGraw-Hill Book Co., New York, 1954, p. 208.

38. Allen, G. C., Samimi, B., Ziskind, M., and Weill, H.: X-ray diffraction determination of α-quartz in respirable and total dust samples from sandblasting operations, Am Industr Hyg Assoc J, 1974, *35*, 711.

39. Talvitie, N. A.: Determination of free silica-gravimetric and spectrophotometric procedures applicable to airborne and settled dust, Am Ind Hyg Assoc J, 1964, *25*, 169.

40. Cares, J. W., Goldin, W. A., Lynch, J. J., and Burgess, A. S.: The determination of quartz in airborne respirable granite dust by infrared spectrophotometry, Am Ind Hyg Assoc J, 1973, *34*, 298.

41. Greenburg, L., and Bloomfield, J. J.: Impinger dust sampling apparatus as used by the U. S. Public Health Service, U. S. Public Health Rep, 1932, *47*, 654.

42. Ayer, H. E., and Sutton, G. W.: Size-selective gravimetric sampling in dusty industries, Am Ind Hyg Assoc J, 1968, *29*, 336.

43. Allison, A. C., Harrington, J. S., and Birbeck, M.: An examination of the cytotoxic effects of silica on macrophages, J Exp Med, 1966, *124*, 141.

44. Allison, A. C.: Lysosomes and the toxicity of

particulate pollutants, Arch Intern Med, 1971, *128*, 131.

45. Heppleston, A. G., and Styles, J. A.: Activity of a macrophage factor in collagen formation by silica, Nature, 1967, *214*, 521.

46. Marks, J., and Nagelschmidt, G.: Study of toxicity of dust with use of in vitro dehydrogenase technique, Arch Ind Health, 1959, *20*, 283.

47. Kysela, B., Kirakova, D., Holusa, R., and Skoda, V.: The influence of the size of quartz dust particles on the reaction of lung tissue, Ann Occup Hyg, 1973, *16*, 103.

48. Luhr, H. G.: Comparative studies on phagocytosis of coal powders of various carbonification grades, also of quartz and diamond powders in tissue cultures, Arch Gewerbepath, 1958, *16*, 355.

49. Brieger, H., and Gross, P.: On the theory of silicosis. III. Stishovite, Arch Environ Health, 1967, *15*, 751.

50. Brieger, H., and Gross, P.: On the theory of silicosis. I. Coesite. Arch Environ Health, 1966, *13*, 38.

51. Stober, W., and Brieger, H.: On the theory of silicosis. IV. The topochemical interaction, Arch Environ Health, 1968, *16*, 706.

52. Nash, T., Allison, A. C., and Harrington, J. S.: Physico-chemical properties of silica in relation to its toxicity, Nature, 1966, *210*, 259.

53. Schlipköter, H. W.: Possibilities of causal prophylaxis and therapy of pneumoconiosis, Arch Environ Health, 1970, *21*, 181.

54. Hailey, J. D., and Margolis, J.: Hemolytic activity of colloidal silica, Nature, 1966, *189*, 1010.

55. Swensson, A.: Tissue reaction to different types of amorphous silica, in *Inhaled Particles and Vapours II*, C. N. Davies, ed., Pergamon Press, London, 1967, pp. 95–102.

56. King, E. J., Mohanty, G. P., Harrison, C. V., and Nagelschmidt, G.: The action of different forms of pure silica on the lungs of rats, Br J Ind Med, 1953, *10*, 9.

57. Kilroe-Smith, T. A., Webster, I., Van Drimmelen, M., and Marasas, L.: An insoluble fibrogenic factor in macrophages from guinea pigs exposed to silica, Environ Res, 1973, *6*, 298.

58. Allison, A. C., and Hart, P. D.: Potentiation by silica of the growth of *Mycobacterium tuberculosis* in macrophage cultures, Br J Exp Pathol, 1968, *49*, 465.

59. Richards, R. J., and Wusteman, F. S.: The effects of silica dust and alveolar macrophages on lung fibroblasts grown in vitro, Life Sci, 1974, *14*, 355.

60. Lippmann, M., Eckert, H. L., Hahon, N., and Morgan, W. K. C.: Circulating antinuclear and rheumatoid factors in coal miners, Ann Intern Med, 1973, *79*, 807.

61. Jones, R. N., Turner-Warwick, M., Ziskind, M., and Weill, H.: High prevalence of antinuclear antibodies in sandblasters' silicosis, Am Rev Respir Dis, 1976, *113*, 393.

62. Kang, K. Y., Yagura, T., and Yamamura, Y.: Antinuclear factor in pneumoconioses (letter to the editor), N Engl J Med, 1973, *288*, 164.

63. Burrell, R. G., Wallace, J. P., and Andrews, C. E.: Lung antibodies in patients with pulmonary disease, Am Rev Respir Dis, 1964, *89*, 697.

64. Vigliani, E. C., and Pernis, B.: Immunological aspects of silicosis, Adv Tuberc Res, 1963, *12*, 230.

65. Ceppellini, R., and Pernis, B.: Presence of plasma globulins in the hyaline tissue in cases of silicosis, Nature, 1958, *181*, 55.

66. Wagner, J. C., and McCormick, J. N.: Immunological investigations of coalworkers' disease, J R Coll Physicians Lond, 1967, *2*, 49.

67. Bramwell, B.: Diffuse sclerodermia: Its frequency; its occurrence in stonemasons; its treatment by fibrolysin—elevations of temperature due to fibrolysin injections, Edinburgh Med J, 1914, *12*, 387.

68. Erasmus, L. D.: Scleroderma in gold miners on the Witwatersrand, with particular reference to pulmonary manifestations, S Afr J Lab Clin Med, 1957, *3*, 209.

69. Rodnan, G P., Benedek, T. B., Medsger, T. A., Jr., and Cammarata, R. J.: The association of progressive systemic sclerosis (scleroderma) with coal miners pneumoconiosis and other forms of silicosis, Ann Intern Med, 1967, *66*, 323.

70. Caplan, A.: Certain unusual radiological appearances in the chest of coalminers suffering from rheumatoid arthritis, Thorax, 1953, *8*, 29.

71. Levis, F., Olivieri, A., and Pernis, B.: Sul decorso della silicosi polmonare sperimentale in ratti con infezione tubercolare spontanea, Med Lav, 1958, *49*, 725.

72. Ross, P., and de Treville, R. T.: Experimental "acute" silicosis, Arch Environ Health, 1968, *17*, 720.

73. Heppleston, A. G., Fletcher, K., and Wyatt, I.: Changes in the composition of lung lipids and the turnover of dipalmitoyl lecithin in experimental alveolar lipoproteinosis induced by inhaled quartz, Br J Exp Pathol, 1974, *55*, 384.

74. Spencer, H.: The Pathology of the Lung, ed. 2, Pergamon Press, Oxford, 1968, p. 385.

75. Policard, A., and Collet, A.: Etude au microscope electronique de reactions cellulaires experimentales a la silice, in *Die Staublungerkrankungen*, vol. 3, K. W. Jotter and W. Klosterkotter, ed, Verlag von Dr. Dietrich Steinkopf, Darmstadt, West Germany, 1958, pp. 368–373.

76. Arnstein, A.: Non-industrial pneumoconiosis, pneumoconiotuberculosis, and tuberculosis of the mediastinal and bronchial lymph glands in old people, Tubercle, 1941, *22*, 281.

77. Nagelschmidt, G.: The relation between lung

dust and lung pathology in pneumoconiosis, Br J Ind Med, 1960, *17*, 247.

78. McCrae, J.: The Ash of Silicotic Lungs, South African Institute of Medical Research, Publication 3, Johannesburg, South Africa, 1913.

79. Fowweather, F. S.: Silica content of normal and silicotic lungs and its bearing on the problem of silicosis, Chem Ind, 1934, *53*, 713.

80. Rossiter, C. E.: Relations between content and composition of coalworkers' lungs and radiological appearances, Br J Ind Med, 1972, *29*, 31.

81. Spencer, H.: Chronic interstitial pneumonia, in *The Lung*, A. A. Liebow and D. E. Smith, ed., Williams and Wilkins Co., Baltimore, 1968, pp. 134–150.

82. Bailey, W. C., Brown, M., Buechner, H. A., Weill, H., Ichinose, H., and Ziskind, M.: Silico-mycobacterial disease in sandblasters. Am Rev Respir Dis, 1974, *110*, 115.

83. Heppleston, A. G.: The disposal of dust in the lungs of silicotic rats, Am J Pathol, 1962, *40*, 493.

84. Caucer, H., and Negmann, N.: Neue Untersuchungen auf dein Gebiete der Elektro-Aerosol Inhalation, Staub, 1953, *33*, 293.

85. Gross, P., and Brieger, H.: Silicotic bronchiolitis obliterans: A focal clearance failure, in *Inhaled Particles and Vapours*, C. N. Davies, ed., Pergamon Press, London, 1967, pp. 105–108.

86. Gardner, L. U.: Experimental production of silicosis, U. S. Public Health Rep, 1935, *50*, 695.

87. Merewether, E. R. A.: The risk of silicosis in sandblasters, Tubercle, 1936, *17*, 385.

88. Rosenzweig, D. Y.: Silicosis complicated by atypical mycobacterial infections, in *Transactions of the 26th V. A.–Armed Forces Pulmonary Disease Research Conference*, U. S. Government Printing Office, Washington, D. C., 1967, p. 47.

89. Keers, R. Y.: The treatment of silicotuberculosis, in *Health Conditions in the Ceramic Industry*, C. N. Davies, ed., Pergamon Press, Oxford, 1969, pp. 63–69.

90. Watkins-Pitchford, W.: quoted in: Experiences in administration of South African Silicosis Act, Ind Doctor, 1924, *2*, 124.

91. Jarvis, D. C.: A roentgen study of dust inhalation in the granite industry, Am J Roentgenol, 1921, *8*, 244.

92. Jacobson, G., and Gilson, J. C.: Present status of the UICC/Cincinnati classification of radiographic appearances of the pneumoconioses, Report of meeting held at Pneumoconiosis Research Unit, Cardiff, Wales, April 13–15, 1971, Ann NY Acad Sci, 1972, *200*, 552.

93. Liddell, D.: Validation of classifications of pneumoconiosis, Ann NY Acad Sci, 1972, *200*, 527.

94. Gaensler, E. A., Carrington, C. B., Coutu, R. E., Tomasian, A., Hoffman, L., and Smith, A. A.: Pathological, physiological and radiological correlations in the pneumoconioses, Ann NY Acad Sci, 1972, *200*, 574.

95. Pendergrass, E. P.: The Pneumoconiosis Problem, Charles C Thomas, Springfield, Ill., 1958, pp. 49–51.

96. Caplan, A., Payne, R. B., and Withey, J. L.: A broader concept of Caplan's syndrome related to rheumatoid factors, Thorax, 1962, *17*, 205.

97. Weill, H., Waggenspack, C., Bailey, W., Ziskind, M., and Rossiter, C.: Radiographic and physiologic patterns among workers engaged in manufacture of asbestos cement products, J Occup Med, 1973, *15*, 248.

98. Funahashi, A., Pintar, K., and Siegesmund, K. A.: Identification of foreign material in lung by energy dispersive x-ray analysis, Arch Environ Health, 1975, *30*, 285.

99. Golli, V., Berila, I., and Popescu, I.: L'influence du tabagisme sur la fonction ventilatoire chez les fondeurs, Bull Soc Sci Med Grand Duche Luxemb, 1974, *111*, 223.

100. Ulmer, W. T.: Chronic obstructive airways disease in pneumoconiosis in comparison to chronic obstructive airways disease in non-dust exposed workers, Bull Physiopathol Respir (Nancy), 1975, *11*, 415.

101. Muir, D. C. F.: Pulmonary function in miners working in British collieries: Epidemiological investigations by the National Coal Board, Bull Physiopathol Respir (Nancy), 1975, *11*, 403.

102. Fulton, W. B., Butters, F. E., Dooley, A. E., Koppenhaver, F. B., Matthews, J. L., and Kirk, R. M.: A Study of Silicosis in the Silica Brick Industry, Commonwealth of Pennsylvania, Department of Health, Bureau of Industrial Hygiene, Harrisburg, Pa., 1941, p. 60.

103. Vigliani, E. C., and Mottura, G.: Diatomaceous earth silicosis, Br J Ind Med, 1948, *5*, 148.

104. Ziskind, M., Weill, H., Anderson, A. E., Samimi, B., Neilson, A., and Waggenspack, C.: Silicosis in Shipyard Sandblasters, No. 8, Preprints of Conference Papers, International Shipyard Health Conference, University of Southern California School of Medicine, Los Angeles, Dec. 13-15, 1973, pp. XIV-1 to XIV-4.

105. Jones, R. N., Weill, H., and Ziskind, M.: Pulmonary function in sandblasters' silicosis, Bull Physiopathol Respir (Nancy), 1975, *11*, 589.

106. Baldwin, E. deF., Cournand, A., and Richards, D. W., Jr.: Pulmonary insufficiency. II. A study of thirty-nine cases of pulmonary fibrosis, Medicine, 1949, *28*, 1.

107. Wright, G. W., and Filley, G. F.: Pulmonary fibrosis and respiratory function, Am J Med, 1951, *10*, 642.

108. Zohman, L. R., and Williams, M. H., Jr.: Cardiopulmonary function in pulmonary fibrosis, Am Rev Respir Dis, 1959, *80*, 700.

109. Frost, J., and Georg, J.: The clinical evaluation of disability in silicosis, Acta Med Scand, 1953, *147*, 349.

110. Chatgidakis, C. B.: Silicosis in South African white gold miners. A comparative study of the disease in different stages, Med Proc, 1963, *9*, 383.

111. Sartorelli, E.: Assessment of lung function in pneumoconiosis, in *Respiratory Function Tests in Pneumoconioses*, Report and related papers of a meeting of experts, Occupational Safety and Health Series No. 6, International Labor Office, Geneva, Switzerland, 1966, pp. 27–92.

112. Renzetti, A. D., Jr., Kobayashi, T., Bigler, A., and Mitchell, M. N.: Regional ventilation and perfusion in silicosis and in the alveolar-capillary block syndrome, Am J Med, 1970, *49*, 5.

113. Nissardi, G. P., Sanna-Randaccio, F., Torrazza, P. L., and Gariel, G.: Lung diffusing capacity on effort in normal and silicotic subjects, Lav Um, 1965, *17*, 397.

114. Bouhuys, A.: Breathing: Physiology, Environment, and Lung Disease, Grune and Stratton, New York, 1974, p. 107.

115. Cotes, J. E., and Rivers, D.: Relation entre la fonction alveolo-capillaire, le pronostic et les descouvertes d'autopsie dans les pneumopathies chroniques, Poumon Coeur, 1960, *16*, 1121.

116. Kanagami, H., Katsura, T., Shiroishi, K., Baba, K., and Ebina, T.: Studies on the pulmonary diffusing capacity by the carbon monoxide breath holding technique. II. Patients with various pulmonary diseases, Acta Med Scand, 1961, *169*, 595.

117. Cugell, D. W., Marks, A., Ellicott, M. F., Badger, T. L., and Gaensler, E. A.: Carbon monoxide diffusing capacity during steady exercise, Am Rev Tuberc, 1956, *74*, 317.

118. Teculescu, D. B., and Stanescu, D. C.: Carbon monoxide transfer factor for the lung in silicosis, Scand J Respir Dis, 1970, *51*, 150.

119. Refsum, H. E.: Pulmonary gas exchange during and after exercise of short duration in silicosis, Scand J Clin Lab Invest, 1972, *29* (Supplement 121, p. 1).

120. Teculescu, D. B., Stanescu, D. C., and Pilat, L.: Pulmonary mechanics in silicosis, Arch Environ Health, 1967, *14*, 461.

121. Vecchione, C., and Mole, R.: The compliance in the silicotic subject, Poumon Coeur, 1967, *23*, 713.

122. Becklake, M. R., du Preez, L., and Lutz, W.: Lung function in silicosis of the Witwatersrand gold miner, Am Rev Tuberc, 1958, *77*, 400.

123. Teculescu, D., Muica, N., and Preda, N.: Impairment of pulmonary mixing in simple and complicated silicosis, Bull Physiopathol Respir (Nancy), 1975, *11*, 447.

124. Council on Occupational Health: The pneumoconioses: Diagnosis, evaluation and management, Arch Environ Health, 1963, *7*, 130.

125. Bates, D. V., Macklem, P. T., and Christie, R. V.: Respiratory Function in Disease, ed. 2, W. B. Saunders Co., Philadelphia, 1971, p. 584.

126. Weill, H.: Pulmonary function testing in industry, J Occup Med, 1973, *15*, 693.

127. Cotes, J. E.: Respiratory and cardiac function tests in relation to occupational lung diseases, Bull Physiopathol Respir (Nancy), 1975, *11*, 561.

Respiratory Disease in Coal Miners[1]

W. K. C. MORGAN and N. L. LAPP

Although the earliest known reference to coal mining is found in the Saxon chronicle of Peterborough (A.D. 852), it was not until the early 1800s that reports of occupational lung disease in coal miners started to make their appearance (1). Laennec (2) was the first to separate melanotic cancer of the lungs from "la matière noire pulmonaire," or exogenous deposits of pigment. In the nineteenth century, a variety of names were attached to the several diseases that afflict coal miners. These included miner's asthma, miner's phthisis, spurious melanosis, and silicosis; but despite the varied nomenclature, most authorities believed that there was but a single disease produced by the inhalation of coal mine dust. It was not until the first decades of the twentieth century that newer techniques, such as chest radiography, histologic examination of tissues, and the identification of the tubercle bacillus, allowed a separation to be made of the various causes of the several respiratory diseases that occur in coal miners. In the past 50 years, much has been done to unravel the varied conditions that are included in the term miner's asthma, and in this regard the recent introduction of the nonspecific and meaningless catch phrase "Black Lung" is to be deplored. For those interested in the history of coal miner's lung disease, an excellent description is found in a series of papers by Meiklejohn (3–5).

The inhalation of coal mine dust may lead to the development of 3 pulmonary conditions: (*1*) coal worker's pneumoconiosis (CWP), (*2*) silicosis, and (*3*) industrial bronchitis. Although there is some doubt that CWP and silicosis can

be present in the same subject, some degree of industrial bronchitis usually coexists with both of the former conditions. We will first consider the over-all effects of coal mining on respiratory health, and then elaborate separately on the effects of CWP and industrial bronchitis. Although silicosis is still the most common occupational lung disease and, as such, deserves a review in its own right, it is of relatively minor import for coal miners, and for this reason will not be included in this paper.

Composition of Coal and Mining Methods

Coal may be found as surface outcrops, and also in underground seams, the depths of which vary from a few feet to more than a mile below ground level. The deeper the seam, the higher the temperature in the mine. For geologic purposes, coal is customarily "ranked" according to certain properties. Thus, anthracite is ranked highest and is followed in descending order by bituminous coal, sub-bituminous coal, and lignite. The highest-ranked coals are the hardest, contain the least volatile matter, and provide the greatest amount of heat in British thermal units, when burned. Anthracite is found mainly in eastern Pennsylvania, and large bituminous coal deposits are found in Appalachia, the Midwest, including Illinois, Indiana, and Oklahoma, and the Far West, in particular, Utah, Colorado, and Montana. Some lignite is also found in the Dakotas.

The height of the seams varies between 1.5 feet in parts of Appalachia to 100 feet in Colorado and Utah. The anthracite seams in Pennsylvania are not located at an even depth, and owing to faults in the earth's crust, run up and down in a series of "switchbacks." The height

---

[1] From the Division of Pulmonary Diseases, West Virginia University Medical Center, Morgantown, W. V. 26506.

of the seam and possibly the rank of the coal being mined have an important influence on the type of dust to which the miner is exposed, and also probably on his likelihood of developing CWP and silicosis (6). Thus, anthracite and other miners who work in low seams are more likely to extend their mining and drilling operations to adjacent rock strata that, in many instances, are composed of rock containing a high percentage of free silica.

Underground Work Force

Some knowledge of the underground work force in the various jobs involved in coal mining is necessary to understand the several health hazards to which coal miners are exposed. All men who work in a coal mine, whether underground or on the surface, are regarded as miners. The area at which coal is cut is known as the coal face and is the most dusty part of the mine. It is at the face that the cutting machines and continuous miners are in operation. The operators of these machines and their helpers are exposed to the highest concentrations of coal mine dust (7). Only slightly less exposed are roof bolters, loading machine operators, and shot firers. Because the roof bolter inserts a 5-foot-bolt into the roof by means of a high-speed drill, he may be exposed to dust from rock strata outside of the coal seam that often contains appreciable quantities of crystalline silica.

After the coal has been cut and detached, it is loaded onto a transportation system before being moved from the face. This is usually done with a shuttlecar that scurries back and forth from the face to the system. The latter usually consists of a small electrically operated train or a conveyor belt. The haulage system is operated by a motorman and a brakeman, who frequently put sand on the rails to obtain traction. Accordingly, the sand is frequently effectively aerosolized. Miners employed on transportation are exposed to smaller coal dust concentrations, but occasionally they develop classic silicosis owing to this practice. Further back from the coal face, and only intermittently exposed to coal dust, are a group of miners who maintain the utilities, track, and cage. Most are mechanics and electricians, but some men dust the entrance ways with rock dust to prevent explosions. Finally, a small proportion of men work on the surface at the tipple or at the portal. In both the United States and Britain, there is a tendency for men as they become older to move back from the coal face and to work at one of the jobs mentioned

above. Somewhat incongruously, the jobs that require the least physical exertion are those at the face, because this area of the mine is the most mechanized.

Epidemiology of Respiratory Disease in Coal Miners

Reliable data concerning the prevalence of various diseases in the U. S. coal mining population have been scanty and unreliable until recently. For many years, it was believed that coal miners had a higher prevalence of lung disease than did the general population (8). Several respiratory conditions have been reported to occur with greater frequency in coal miners. In some instances, e.g., CWP, there is a direct relationship between the inhalation of coal dust and the disease that results; however, most of the alleged excesses of morbidity and mortality are consequences of nonspecific airway obstruction associated with chronic bronchitis and emphysema. Coal dust plays a very minor role in the etiology of these disorders (9).

The association between respiratory disease death rates and occupation was noted many years ago in the statistics of the Registrar General of England and Wales. Data published in the United States show similar trends, in that the standardized mortality ratio (SMR) for respiratory disease is markedly increased in certain occupations. Thus, the SMR for bronchitis and emphysema is much higher for manual laborers than it is for professional classes (10). A similar, but lesser, trend is present for lung cancer (table 1). When allowance is made for differences in smoking habits, it is evident that cigarette smoking alone probably cannot explain

TABLE 1

STANDARDIZED MORTALITY RATIOS FOR SELECTED RESPIRATORY DISEASES FOR CERTAIN OCCUPATIONAL GROUPS OF MEN 20 TO 64 YEARS OF AGE (10)

Occupation	Bronchitis, Emphysema, and Other Respiratory Diseases	Lung Cancer	Percentage of Smokers (Age-Corrected)
Laborers, except farm and mine	168	127	79
Operatives, including miners	158	107	81
Clerical workers	79	95	77
Managers, officials, and proprietors	58	94	77

the differences in SMR for lung diseases that occur in different occupations. It is reasonable to assume that some of the deaths in table 1 under the heading "Bronchitis, Emphysema, and Other Respiratory Diseases" are the result of industrial pulmonary disease, such as silicosis and CWP. Nevertheless, the fact that laborers not exposed to dust have a higher SMR for bronchitis and emphysema than do the operatives and miners indicates that the number of occupationally related deaths due to lung disease cannot be unduly great.

Enterline (8, 11), in a series of retrospective analyses, showed that the SMR for selected groups of U. S. coal miners was considerably increased above that for nonminers. Many of the excess deaths could be accounted for by trauma and accidents. When deaths due to these causes were excluded, a relationship between excess mortality and age emerged. This ranged from a 23 per cent excess between 20 and 24 years of age to a 122 per cent excess between 60 and 64 years of age. The excess at all ages was believed to represent the cumulative effects of environmental factors, some of which may be occupational, on the health of coal miners.

When the causes of this excess mortality were broken down, many were found to be respiratory. Although chronic bronchitis and emphysema accounted for much of the excess, the SMR for lung cancer and tuberculosis for U. S. miners was also greater than that of the general population (11). Although it is comparatively easy to postulate a cause-and-effect relationship among coal mining, bronchitis, and CWP, the same cannot be said of lung cancer and tuberculosis, especially when it is known that British coal miners have a rate that is less than the national average for lung cancer (12). Many of these confusing data can be attributed to lack of uniformity and reliability in death certification in the United States and to the great decrease in the number of U. S. coal miners during the period of observation. Thus, the work force has decreased from 800,000 persons in the 1920s to 120,000 persons in 1973. Moreover, prospective studies conducted by the Appalachian Laboratory for Occupational Respiratory Disease have shown that lung cancer occurs less often in U. S. bituminous miners than it does in the general population (13).

Recently, Liddell (14) studied the morbidity of a group of more than 29,000 British coal miners. He showed that miners lost more time from work than men of other occupations. This state of affairs prevailed even when mining was compared with other nonmining tasks of an arduous nature. Among underground miners as a whole, those who were paid the least had the greatest amount of time off work. Incapacity varied between coal fields and was related to the miner's financial status, to the category of pneumoconiosis, and to the depth of the mine. In an additional study published at the same time, Liddell (15) considered the mortality rates of British coal miners. He showed that miners generally had high death rates from accidents and pneumoconiosis, but low death rates from lung cancer. Surprisingly, death rates for face workers were lower than expected.

In the past 2 years, several studies from Britain and the United States have added greatly to the available knowledge concerning respiratory disease in coal miners. Unlike the earlier studies, the recent investigations relied on the follow-up of randomly selected cohorts of miners. In following the Rhondda Fach population for 20 years, Cochrane (16) showed that although complicated pneumoconiosis was associated with premature death, simple CWP had no effect on life expectancy. Ortmeyer and associates (17) followed for 10 years a cohort of Pennsylvania miners who had been awarded disability compensation for CWP. The sample was divided according to radiographic category, and also according to whether the ratio of forced expiratory volume in 1 sec (FEV_1) to forced vital capacity (FVC) was greater or less than 55 per cent. Excess deaths were found primarily in subjects with a reduced ventilatory capacity, and secondarily in subjects with complicated pneumoconiosis. In a further study, 2 randomly chosen cohorts consisting of 2,549 working miners and 1,177 ex-miners were followed by Ortmeyer and co-workers (18) for 10 years. For those who died, the cause of death was determined. Again, it was shown that whereas simple CWP had no effect on life expectancy, complicated pneumoconiosis led to an increased SMR. Cigarette smoking had a far greater effect on the SMR than did exposure to dust. Whereas the over-all SMR of the working miners was decreased, that of the retired miners was increased. Because the former represented a "survivor" group, and because the ex-miners in many instances had retired because of ill health, neither sample was believed to reflect the true life expectancy of coal miners. By considering both groups and calculating a combined SMR, it was shown that the life expectancy was almost exactly that of the general male U. S. population, thereby indicating that miners as a whole have a normal life expectancy.

A study of the death rate from lung cancer in the same 2 cohorts confirmed earlier British studies (13) showing that among coal miners, the death rate from this condition was lower than expected. The lower incidence of lung cancer in the United States is almost certainly related to the fact that miners smoke slightly fewer cigarettes than do nonminers. Deaths due to heart disease, in general, and coronary artery disease, in particular, were likewise shown to occur less frequently in coal miners (19). In conclusion, it is apparent that in both Britain and the United States at the present time, coal miners have a normal life expectancy, and that the excess deaths due to complicated pneumoconiosis are counterbalanced by the lower death rate from lung cancer and coronary artery disease. A final word of caution is necessary in that the British and U. S. studies come from large, unionized mines with low accident rates. Many smaller U. S. mines have appreciably higher death rates due to accidents and injuries.

Role of Silica in Coal Miner's Lung Disease

The discovery of x-rays by Roentgen in 1896 provided a powerful tool for the investigation of occupational lung diseases. Abnormal shadows were soon noted in the chest films of gold, silver, and iron miners, the appearance being similar regardless of the dust to which the miner had been exposed. Because of the more drastic effects of inhaled silica, silicosis received more attention. When, at a later date, coal miners were observed to have similar radiographic changes, it was assumed that the silica present in the coal dust was responsible for the radiographic abnormalities. To this day, certain persons persist in this view.

It was the occurrence of radiographic abnormalities in Welsh coal trimmers that first raised doubts concerning the silica theory. A coal trimmer was a type of stevedore who was responsible, in the early part of this century, for the loading and distribution of coal in the holds of ships. Mechanized loading has rendered the job of coal trimming extinct. The coal that was exported from Wales had been washed and the rock separated from it, so that the silica content was minimal. Collis and Gilchrist (20) showed that coal trimmers had radiographic changes in their chest films that were indistinguishable from those seen in classic silicosis. Post mortem, the trimmers' lungs were found to have a normal silica content (21). Later epidemiologic studies showed that the prevalence of CWP bore a poor relation to the silica content of the mine dust to which the miners were exposed. In contrast, the relation between coal content and radiographic category was shown to be close (22). Additional support for the concept that carbon alone may produce disease came after the demonstration of a type of pneumoconiosis in men exposed to pure carbon (23–25).

Many questions remain to be answered. There is little doubt that the macules seen in simple CWP have little, if any, relation to the silica content of the dust inhaled. Thus, similar macules without accompanying fibrosis may be seen in urban dwellers, in subjects with stannosis (26), and in workers exposed to pure carbon (23). On the other hand, if the macules are accompanied by some collagenous fibrosis (an uncommon but well-documented finding), then it is likely that the inhaled dust to which the miner has been exposed contained appreciable quantities of either silica or silicates (27).

Although there is some evidence that complicated pneumoconiosis can be produced by pure carbon (23), as far as coal miners are concerned, there is a fair amount of circumstantial evidence to incriminate silica as the etiologic agent responsible for the onset of progressive, massive fibrosis (PMF). It has been shown by Nagelschmidt (28) that, although the dust burden in the massive lesion of complicated pneumoconiosis or PMF is higher than it is in the rest of the lungs, the composition of the dust in the massive lesion and elsewhere in the lungs does not differ significantly in its quartz content. Pratt (29), however, recalculated the data of Nagelschmidt and suggested that when the total weight of silica, rather than the percentage of silica in the lung, is considered, there is an association between high silica values and the presence of PMF. A recent study conducted by the Institute of Occupational Medicine, Edinburgh, Scotland showed that although the development of PMF is not clearly related to dust exposure, when the percentage composition of affected and nonaffected portions of the lung is compared with that of mine dust to which the men are exposed, there is strong evidence for the differential retention of quartz in those who have developed PMF (30). Suffice it to say that at this time, the role of silica in the etiology of PMF remains uncertain.

Coal Worker's Pneumoconiosis
Radiology of CWP

Coal worker's pneumoconiosis is subdivided

into simple and complicated pneumoconiosis, according to the radiographic appearance of the chest film. Simple CWP is further classified into categories 1, 2, and 3 according to the profusion of small opacities in the lung fields. When the number of small opacities is insufficient to make a diagnosis of category 1, the film is classified as category 0. Although numerous classifications of pneumoconiosis have been used in the past, the Union Internationale Contra Cancre-International Labour Organization (UICC-ILO) classification is now most widely accepted (31).

To render more sensitive the reading of radiographic progression, Liddell and May (32) devised a 12-point elaboration of the old ILO classification. Each major category, including zero, was divided into 3 subcategories, so that in the full elaboration, there were 12 categories ranging from 0/- to 3/4. Thus, when an unknown film is being classified and the reader considers category 1, but eventually decides that the film is category 0, then the classification is 0/1. Thus, the numerator represents the category in which the film is placed, and the denominator represents the category that was also considered. The same situation applies to categories 1/2, 2/1, 2/3, 3/2, and 3/4. If, in contrast, the interpreter does not consider any other category but the one he places it in, then the film is read as 1/1, 2/2, or 3/3. Details of the complete description of the classification can be found in a paper by Jacobson and Lainhart (31).

Small opacities are subdivided according to whether they are regular or irregular. Those that are regular are further separated into p, q, and r-type opacities according to their size. The irregular opacities are divided into types s, t, and u. Although irregular opacities are common in asbestosis and certain other interstitial fibroses, they are infrequently seen in coal miners and, when present, appear to be related to cigarette smoking, rather than to dust retention (33).

Complicated pneumoconiosis or PMF is diagnosed when there is a large opacity 1 cm or more in diameter. It is classified as stage A, B, or C according to the size of the large opacity or opacities. When the chest radiograph has an opacity or opacities whose combined diameter is between 1 and 5 cm, it is classified as A. Should the opacity or opacities have a diameter greater than 5 cm, but less than one third of the lung, the chest film should be read as Stage B, whereas if the opacities occupy more than one third of the lung field, the film is classified as Stage C. PMF develops almost entirely on a background of Category 2 or 3 simple pneumoconiosis. It may appear after dust exposure has ceased and may progress in the absence of further exposure. There is an attack rate of about 1.5 to 2 per cent per annum in active miners with Category 2 or more simple CWP.

The radiographic diagnosis of CWP, like that of tuberculosis, is subject to both inter- and intraobserver variation (34, 35). In general, the variation found between readers is appreciably greater than that observed when the same reader interprets the same film on different occasions. Observer variation is more marked in simple CWP than it is in complicated CWP, but even in the latter, appreciable differences of opinion are frequent. These divergencies relate not so much to whether a large opacity is present, but to what condition is producing the large opacity, e.g., PMF, tuberculosis, atelectasis, or some other condition (34). Much can be done to lessen observer variation by insisting that readers compare the films they are classifying to the series of standard films distributed by the ILO. In addition, when a panel of readers is involved in classifying films for pneumoconiosis, the readers should be brought together at regular intervals to try to achieve a measure of consistency in interpretation and also to ensure that their reading habits do not change. Within these limitations, serial chest radiographs provide a useful means, and indeed the only means available, of measuring exposure to coal dust during life. Their usefulness in this regard is based on the close relationship that exists between the radiographic category of simple CWP and the coal dust content of the lungs.

Prevalence of CWP

The prevalence of CWP at any particular time is a reflection of the environmental conditions that have prevailed in the mines in the previous 20 to 30 years and may have little relevance to present working conditions. Although most major coal-producing nations have published prevalence data for CWP, different radiographic classifications often have been used, so that comparisons cannot be made. Prevalence rates are also influenced by the "reading habits" of those who interpret the films, and the reading of the same series of chest films by different observers may yield prevalence data that differ as much as 100 per cent (35). Similarly, liberalization of compensation laws may halve the prevalence rate in 3 to 4 years, because miners with

CWP are more likely to apply for and be awarded compensation and, hence, leave the industry. The extent of participation in any survey also influences prevalence rates.

Aside from the effects mentioned, prevalence rates are influenced by the dust levels to which the miners have been exposed in the preceding 30 to 40 years. Thus, CWP is much more common in face and transportation workers than in maintenance and surface workers (6, 36). Cutting machine and continuous miner operators and their helpers have the highest prevalence rates, and roof bolters, shuttlecar operators, and those who work on transportation are not far behind (36). Despite the general relationship between years spent underground and the dust levels to which the men have been exposed, there are marked regional differences in prevalence that cannot be explained by dust exposure alone (6, 36). It seems probable that the physical and chemical composition of the coal being mined is also important. Thus, certain coals may fragment more easily and produce more harmful particles of 1 to 2 μm, whereas others may tend to generate more particles of 4 to 6 μm. Similarly, the chemical composition or rank of coal appears to influence the prevalence of CWP (6, 37).

Data from the U. S. coal mines suggest that the present prevalence is 10.1 per cent, of which 0.4 per cent is PMF. These data are derived from medical examinations conducted by the U. S. Public Health Service second round of the Interagency Study (Popovich, P.: Personal communication, 1975). The first-round prevalence figures were much higher, and over-all rates of nearly 30 per cent were found (6). Comparisons, however, cannot be made between the first and second rounds for these reasons: (1) the panel of readers changed, and there is little doubt that the panel in the first round tended to over-read; (2) a large number of affected miners have applied for and have been granted compensation, and are therefore no longer included in the population survey.

Radiographic Progression of CWP and Its Relationship to Dust Levels

The only way of assessing the risk of developing CWP depends on comparing serial radiographs made at known intervals with the dust levels that have prevailed in the mines during the same period. There is seldom any point in comparing paired films, unless there is at least a 5-year interval between them; even then, progression is observed only in a minority of those most heavily exposed, i.e., face workers. Progression is often so slight that it is imperative to use the full 12-point scale devised by Liddell and May (32), and even then, there is usually only a 1- or 2-subcategory increment.

Paired films may be assessed for progression by placing them side by side with the chronologic sequence known to the reader (side-by-side method) or by reading each film independently, without any knowledge of its partner and with the dates unknown to the reader. Despite widespread acceptance of the side-by-side method, there is no doubt that a knowledge of the temporal sequence of the films introduces bias (38). This applies not only to CWP, but also to tuberculosis and sarcoidosis (39). If the position of each member of a pair of films that has previously been read as showing progression is then interchanged without the observer's knowledge, a marked reluctance to read regression becomes apparent (38, 39).

It has been argued by some that the side-by-side method allows the interpreter to compensate for disparities in film technique, e.g., over versus underexposed films. That such compensation is relatively minor has been demonstrated by Amandus and associates (40). There is no doubt that the side-by-side method reduces variability and lessens the chance of reading regression, but it does so at the expense of introducing appreciable bias related to the assumed chronologic sequence of the films. Nonetheless, most studies have shown that mines having a high progression index with the side-by-side method also have a high index with the independent method (40). It cannot be assumed that the independent method is free from bias, because it is known that film technique, the depth of the inspiration, and several other factors influence radiographic categorization of CWP (41, 42).

The only reliable long-term studies relating levels of respirable dust to radiographic progression come from Britain and West Germany (43, 44). The National Coal Board began its Pneumoconiosis Field Research (PFR) in 1952. Twenty-five collieries were selected, and the miners employed there have had serial chest radiographs taken at 5-year intervals. The PFR study was designed to answer the following questions. (1) Can radiographic progression be related to respirable dust measurements? (2) Does the risk of developing pneumoconiosis increase with increasing dust exposure; if so, is there a linear relationship? (3) What dust levels lead to pneumoconiosis and how quickly? (4) Does the composition of the dust affect the risk of developing CWP?

The findings of this study have appeared in a series of papers. The earliest was published in 1967 and summarized the findings obtained during the first 10 years (45). A radiographic index of progression for each mine was related to the mean coal face dust measurements as determined with the thermal precipitator. The relationship between particle counts and progression index was weak. Later, the National Coal Board changed to gravimetric sampling, and the clear-cut relationship between dust levels and radiographic progression became evident.

At a meeting in Luxembourg in 1972, Jacobsen (43) described the findings of the study up to 1971. He was able to show (1) a significant correlation between radiographic progression and exposure to airborne dust, and (2) that the disease in miners with early dust retention (category 0/1 and 1/0) is more likely to progress than that classified as category 0/0. Thus, in men who develop the disease sooner, it progresses more rapidly.

In addition, Jacobsen was able to construct curves correlating the probability of radiographic progression for various dust exposures; from them, he demonstrated that with a mean long-term dust exposure of 4.3 mg per m³, the likelihood of reaching category 2 or higher would be less than 3.4 per cent with 35 years of exposure (43). Assuming that these predictions are accurate, and there is every reason to accept them, the present U. S. standard of 2 mg per m³ should reduce the prevalence of simple CWP to a negligible level in the next 20 years.

Since 1960, Reisner (44) has been conducting a similar investigation of 17,000 German coal miners employed in the Ruhr Valley. The similarity of Reisner's results to those of the National Coal Board are remarkable in view of the different methods used for sampling respirable dust. Until recently, the Germans have used a tydalloscope; even so, their results closely coincide with those obtained by the National Coal Board.

Pathology of Simple CWP

Coal miners are exposed to dusts that are a mixture of coal, kaolin, mica, and silica in varying proportions, but only the dust deposited in the gas-exchanging portions of the lung leads to CWP. The first reaction of the body to the deposition of coal dust in the alveoli and respiratory bronchioles is to increase the number of macrophages, which, in turn, phagocytose the deposited particles and carry them to the terminal bronchioles, from which they are removed by the mucociliary escalator (46). If this dust load is excessive, the clearance mechanisms are slowly overwhelmed, and the macrophages begin to aggregate in the respiratory bronchioles and the alveoli that originate from them. Should this condition persist for any length of time, fibroblasts begin to appear, and a thin network of reticulin is laid down surrounding the stationary macrophages. If the macrophages contain silica, they undergo lysis more quickly; in doing so, they liberate enzymes that stimulate the fibroblasts to produce some collagen fibers as well. As a result, the respiratory bronchioles of the first, and more commonly, the second, division, together with the alveoli arising from them, become slowly engulfed in a mesh of dying macrophages, coal dust, and fibroblasts. This aggregation of debris and fibroblasts leads to the formation of the coal macule, this being the primary lesion of simple CWP. For the most part, such macules appear as blackish dots on a large lung section. Although they are fairly evenly distributed, they appear to have a predilection for the upper lobes and may be as large as 5 mm in diameter (figure 1). As the macules enlarge, the respiratory bronchiolar smooth muscle atrophies. The weakened bronchiole then dilates as a consequence of the stresses and strains to which it is subjected (47, 48). Whether the dilatation comes about as a result of extraluminal traction or as a consequence of increased intraluminal pressure is unknown. The end result, however, is known as focal emphysema; unlike the centrilobular and panacinar forms of this condition, it is not disabling.

The products of the degenerating macrophages are taken up by the lymphatics that drain from a sump at the level of the atria. The lymphatics and blood vessels in turn drain into the hila of the lungs. Every so often, the lymphatics can be seen to enter clusters of reticuloendothelial cells and later in their course, lymph glands. In some instances, such cells are situated around the arterioles at the level of the second-order bronchioles, which themselves are situated in the center of the secondary lobule (47, 49). The deposition of cellular debris and coal induces a fibroblastic response, with the production of a little reticulin and occasionally some collagen. The fibrosis sometimes encroaches on the arteriole and gradually occludes it. Despite the occasional obliteration of the lobular arterioles, no significant reduction of the capillary bed occurs.

Simple CWP has the same features the world over and appears to be uninfluenced by the rank of coal, whether anthracite or bituminous, or

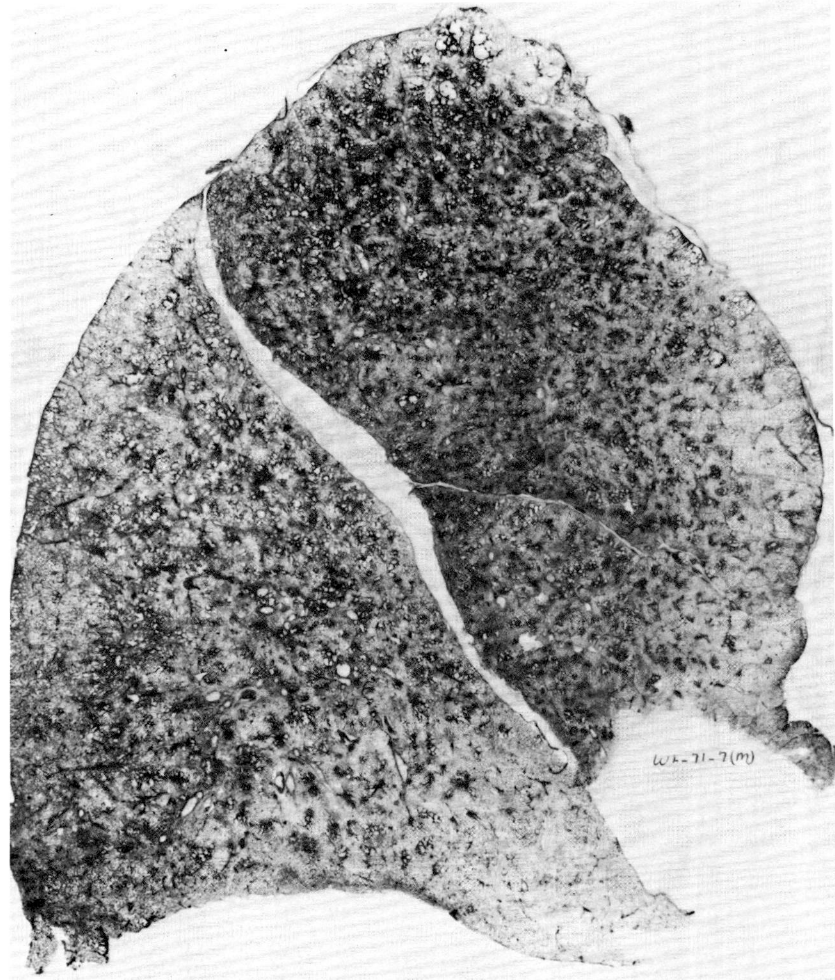

Fig. 1. Whole lung section from subject with simple pneumoconiosis. (Courtesy of Ms. Patsy Willard.)

by the coal field, whether in Britain, the United States, South Africa, or elsewhere (47). In coal miners whose lung residue contains 18 per cent mine quartz, the classic pathologic lesions of silicosis, rather than CWP, are observed.

Simple CWP does not affect the heart, unless there is coincident chronic bronchitis. Wells (50) has studied at autopsy the lungs and hearts of 388 Welsh coal miners. He showed that although there was a slight loss of the capillary bed, the effects on the pulmonary arterioles were negligible. The innocence of the findings in simple CWP contrast with the gross changes observed in subjects dying from PMF. Wells' findings have subsequently been confirmed by James and Thomas (51), who found that among 546 subjects dying with simple CWP, only 9 had pulmonary heart disease that seemed to be a consequence of simple CWP alone. Thus, it may be concluded that if simple CWP ever leads to the development of right heart failure, such an occurrence is exceptional.

Pathology of PMF

The pathologic lesions of PMF first appear mainly in the posterior segment of one or the other upper lobe, or in the superior segment of the lower lobe (52). There are those who believe that the radiographic separation of simple and complicated CWP is artificial and that the process that initiates the massive lesion starts long before the lesion is 1 cm in diameter (53).

Macroscopically, the lesions consist of large aggregates of black tissue that are often adherent to the chest wall. The masses tend to be rubbery in consistency and are usually ill defined. Unlike the conglomerate lesions of silicosis that can be seen to consist of matted aggregates of several silicotic nodules, the massive lesion of PMF is amorphous, irregular, and relatively homogeneous. Cavitation may occur from ischemic necrosis or secondary tuberculosis, but the latter is now relatively rare in Britain and the United States (54). Atypical acid-fast bacilli are often isolated from subjects with PMF (55).

The concept that the lesions of PMF are composed almost entirely of fibrous tissue has recently been challenged. Wagner and associates (56) have shown that although collagen is present in the capsules of the massive lesions, the center is replaced by insoluble protein that is probably stabilized by some form of cross linking. The protein complex accounts for one third of the weight of the lesions, the remaining two-thirds consisting of mineral dusts and calcium phosphate.

The lesions of PMF are composed of a capsule of dense, fibrous tissue often containing an

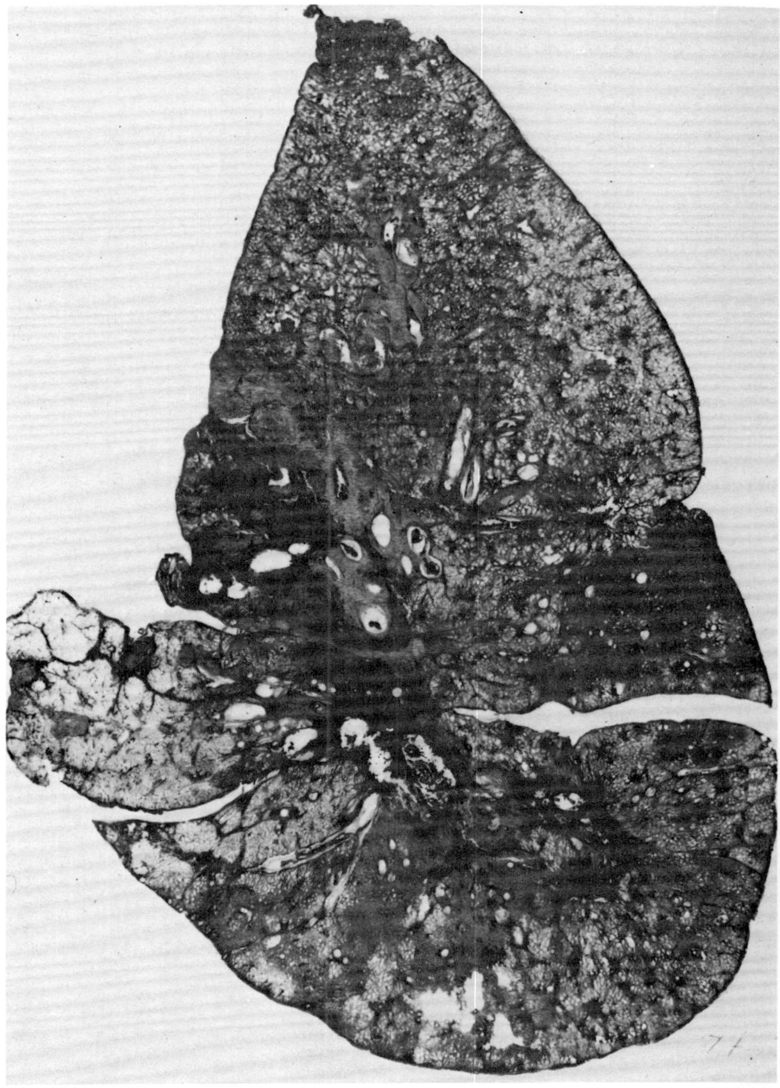

Fig. 2. Whole lung section of a subject with progressive, massive fibrosis, showing amorphous, black conglomerates. (Courtesy of Ms. Patsy Willard.)

amorphous black material. The masses encroach on blood vessels and the bronchi of the affected lobe and eventually destroy them (figure 2). In some instances, traces of the obliterated vessels persist in the fibrous masses; both large and small arteries, and also veins are encroached upon and obliterated. Uncommonly, massive thrombosis of a large pulmonary vessel takes place as a result of the pulmonary hypertension that results from advanced PMF. The adventitia and media of the muscular arteries are often infiltrated with dust-laden cells, and there is frequent evidence of endarteritis. These changes are clearly illustrated in the classic paper of Wells (50).

Symptoms and Signs of CWP

Simple CWP has neither signs nor symptoms. Although many miners with CWP complain of cough, shortness of breath, and black sputum, these symptoms are seen equally frequently in miners with clear chest films. The presence of severe shortness of breath in a coal miner with simple CWP is virtually always related to a nonoccupationally related disease, such as chronic bronchitis or emphysema, rather than to coal mining.

In stages B and C of complicated CWP, some degree of excessive exertional dyspnea is usually present. Cough and sputum are common, and melanoptysis may occur. The latter is characterized by the expectoration of several ounces of inky, black sputum. Pain and hemoptysis rarely, if ever, occur.

The signs of complicated CWP are those of consolidation and collapse of the affected area. In advanced PMF, signs of pulmonary hypertension and right ventricular hypertrophy may develop along with congestive failure. Clubbing is not seen.

Pulmonary Function in CWP

The extent and nature of cardiopulmonary functional impairment found among coal workers depends, to a large extent, on subject selection. Random selection of working miners for the most part yields a sample of asymptomatic, physically fit subjects. When studies are made of nonworking miners, the sample contains a significant number of the less fit, many having stopped working because of poor health. This out-migration of the less fit workers is particularly true in industries involving physical exertion, such as mining. Because this out-migration in the coal mining industry has not been quantified, and because the factors that influence it have not been entirely elucidated, it is desirable to study both working and nonworking miners to obtain a true picture of the functional impairments associated with coal mining.

This review of the functional abnormalities associated with coal mining has been arranged as follows: ventilatory capacity, lung volumes, diffusing capacity, gas exchange, hemodynamics, mechanics, and special studies. In each instance, we have indicated whether the findings were obtained in symptomatic, asymptomatic, or randomly selected samples.

Ventilatory Capacity

Several studies have demonstrated that miners have a slightly lower ventilatory capacity than nonminers, and that this reduction is related to the number of years spent underground. Pemberton (57) studied 242 working coal miners using the FEV_1 as his index of ventilatory function. He compared the mean FEV_1 of the miners to that of the 2 control groups, one a rural group and the other an urban group of factory workers. The miners had a slightly lower FEV_1 than did either of the control groups, despite the fact that the miners smoked somewhat less. The miners also had more respiratory symptoms, such as cough, sputum, and shortness of breath than the control groups; however, there was no relationship between the symptoms and the radiographic category of CWP.

Hyatt and co-workers (58) studied a random sample of bituminous coal miners and ex-miners between 45 and 58 years of age. Thirty-nine per cent of these had simple CWP, and a further 7 per cent had complicated CWP or PMF. Using the forced expiratory flow between 25 and 75 per cent of the forced expiratory volume ($FEF_{25\text{-}75}$) as their index of lung function, Hyatt and associates found a relationship between increasing impairment of ventilatory function, increasing prevalence of bronchitis, and the number of years worked underground. Only in category 3 simple CWP and complicated CWP were they able to demonstrate that CWP per se led to a reduction of ventilatory capacity; unfortunately, the values were not corrected for age.

Higgins and associates (59) studied randomly selected working and nonworking miners in 5 communities in northern West Virginia. They used the FEV_1 to assess functional status. They demonstrated that only in miners and ex-miners with 30 years or more of underground experience was the FEV_1 significantly decreased. In miners who had less than 30 years of underground exposure, the FEV_1 did not differ significantly from that of the nonminers from the same communities.

A random sample of nearly 3,500 working and nonworking miners was studied by the Public Health Service in 1962 to 1963 (60). Because adequate control groups were not available in each of the communities in which the study was carried out, the results were compared with predicted values. In this study, the FVC of the miners did not differ from predicted values. Among the older miners, the FEV_1 was slightly lower than the predicted figure. Both bronchitis and smoking were associated with a decrease in FEV_1. No relationship between increasing radiographic category and FEV_1 was apparent, except in PMF. Unfortunately, most of the data used in this study were not corrected for age.

Recently, data from the first round of the Interagency Study of the Public Health Service (61) have become available for more than 9,000 working U. S. coal miners. Again, because adequate control groups were not available in each of the communities in which the studies were carried out, the results were compared to predicted values (figure 3). The FVC and FEV_1 of anthracite miners were lower than those of the bituminous miners. Both the anthracite and bituminous miners had a mean FEV_1 that was lower than predicted, but the difference between observed and predicted values was greater in

the anthracite miners. There were variations in the difference between observed and predicted FEV_1 that were related to the geographic region in which the miners worked, and these differences could only partially be explained by ethnic origin and other nonoccupational factors. Some of these differences appeared to be related to differences in the physical or chemical characteristics of the coal mine dust to which the workers were exposed.

Among the miners with simple CWP, there was no clear-cut relationship between decrease in FEV_1 and increasing radiographic category. In contrast, regardless of the geographic region, complicated CWP was associated with significant decreases in FEV_1 and FEV_1/FVC (figures 4 and 5).

In virtually all of the studies cited, it has been clearly demonstrated that respiratory symptoms are associated with a decrease in ventilatory capacity, and that smoking is by far the most important factor in producing respiratory symptoms and a decrease in ventilatory function. The contributions of a simple CWP and years spent underground to decrease in ventilatory capacity are relatively slight by comparison.

Comparable studies have been carried out in Britain (62–65) and in Germany (66) with essentially similar findings.

Lung Volumes

Gilson and Hugh-Jones (67) systematically studied the lung volumes of a group of coal miners in Britain. They were unable to detect changes in the lung volumes that were related to the presence of radiographic category of simple pneumoconiosis. In an attempt to find a method of determining total lung capacity (TLC) and residual volume (RV) that could be applied to large-scale epidemiologic studies, O'Shea and associates (68) compared Barnhard's radiographic method to that of the body plethysmograph (Barnhard, H. J., Pierce, J. A., Joyce, J. W., and Bates, J. H.: Roentgenographic determination of total lung capacity, Am J Med, 1960, 28, 51.) They demonstrated that the radiographic method yielded essentially similar values for TLC in subjects with simple pneumoconiosis and with airway obstruction; however, in subjects with large, conglomerate shadows, the method was less accurate. The RV was calculated by subtracting the FVC determined by spirometry from radiographic TLC.

Morgan and associates (69, 70) reported on the radiographically determined RV and TLC

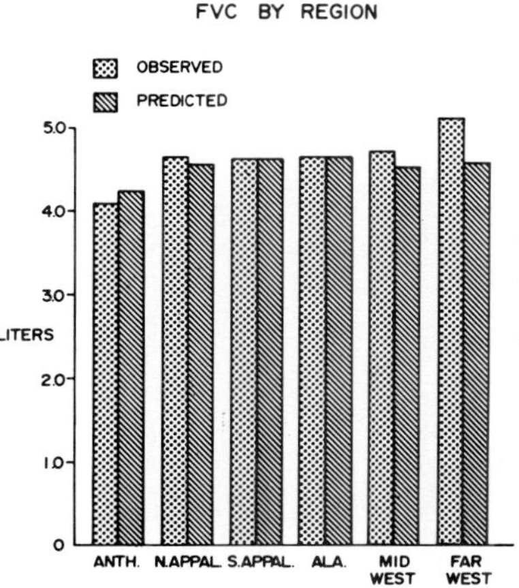

Fig. 3. Observed and predicted mean forced vital capacity (FVC) for 9,076 working U.S. miners, according to region. (From Morgan and co-workers [61]; reprinted by permission of publishers.) ANTH = anthracite; N. APPAL. = Northern Appalachia; S. APPAL. = Southern Appalachia; ALA. = Alabama.

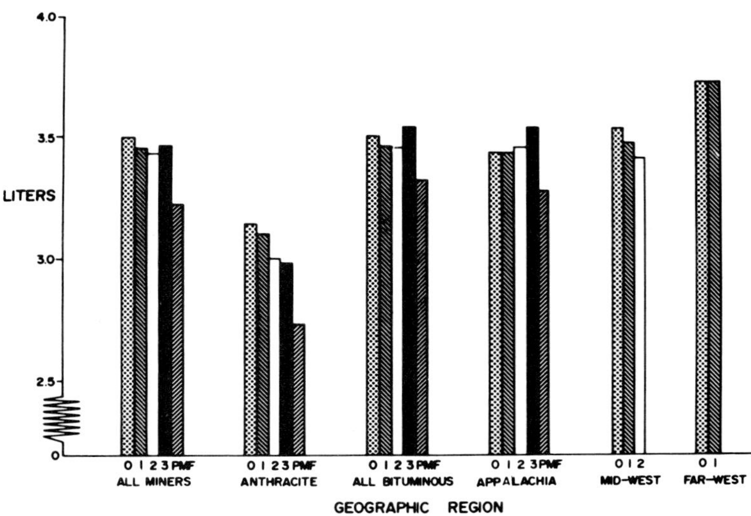

Fig. 4. Mean 1-sec forced expiratory volume (FEV_1) for 9,076 working miners for various radiographic categories, according to region. (From Morgan and co-workers [61]; reprinted by permission of publisher.)

of 1,455 working Pennsylvania coal miners. They compared these results to the predicted values for RV and TLC determined by Needham and co-workers (71) and also to the results in a small control group. The miners were divided into 2 main groups according to whether or not they had airway obstruction (FEV_1/FVC less than 70 per cent). These groups were further subdivided according to radiographic category of pneumoconiosis. Among the obstructed miners, the ratio of observed TLC to predicted TLC (TLC_o/TLC_p) was increased in each of the radiographic subcategories, including category 0. Among the obstructed miners, the increase in TLC did not appear to be related to the category of simple CWP; however, among the nonobstructed miners, the ratio of TLC_o/TLC_p showed a slight but significant increase between

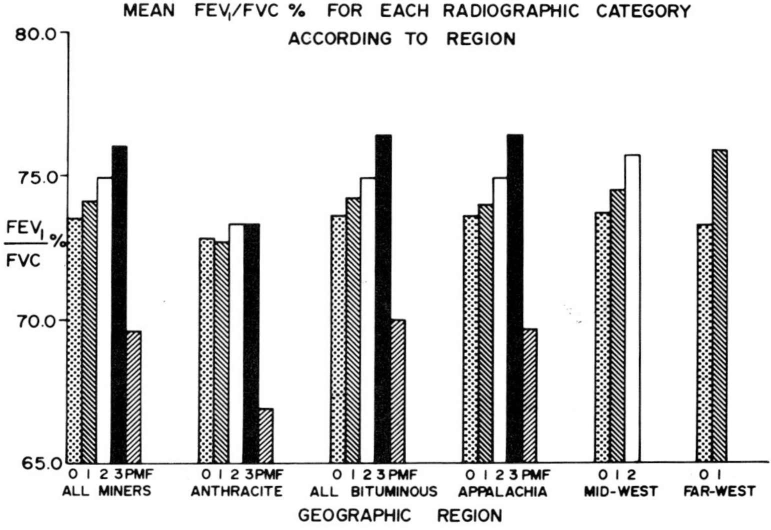

Fig. 5. Mean ratio of 1-sec forced expiratory volume (FEV_1) to forced vital capacity (FVC), expressed as per cent, for 9,076 working miners for various radiographic categories (see text). (From Morgan and co-workers [61]; reprinted by permission of publisher.) PMF = progressive massive fibrosis.

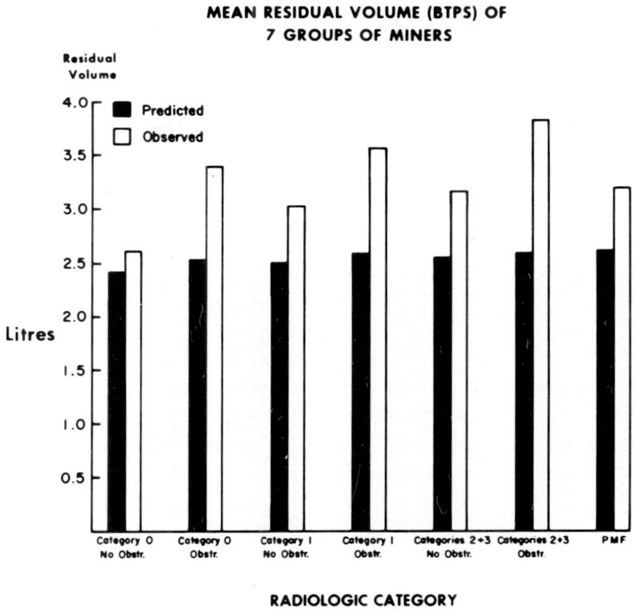

**MEAN RESIDUAL VOLUME (BTPS) OF
7 GROUPS OF MINERS**

Fig. 6. Mean observed and predicted residual volumes of 1,455 working Pennsylvania miners for various radiographic categories. (From Morgan and co-workers [69]; reprinted by permission of publisher.) Obstr. = obstruction.

category 0 and category 1. The slight additional increase in categories 2 and 3 of simple CWP was not significantly different from that of the non-obstructed subjects with category 1 CWP. When the observed RV (RV_o) was compared to the predicted RV (RV_p) for the various categories of simple pneumoconiosis, it was apparent that increasing radiographic category was associated with an increment in RV in both the obstructed and nonobstructed groups (figure 6). Using the index RV_o/RV_p, the nonobstructed miners with simple pneumoconiosis had significant increases when compared to nonobstructed miners with category 0 radiographs (figure 7). Morgan and associates (70) believed that their findings indicated that the lungs of nonobstructed miners with simple CWP were hyperinflated, and that the overdistension was, in a general way, related to the degree of dust retention indicated by the radiographs. The cause of the overdistension was believed to be either obstruction within small airways in the peripheral parts of the lungs that is not readily detected by conventional spirometry (72) or, alternatively, a loss of retractive forces due to focal emphysema. The latter was believed to be more likely, because the coal macule in simple pneumoconiosis is situated around the respiratory bronchiole. Further confirmation of this hyperinflation in nonobstruct-

ed coal miners with simple pneumoconiosis was obtained by Morgan and co-workers in nearly 10,000 working coal miners who participated in the Public Health Service's Interagency Study (61). In that study, the age- and height-adjusted

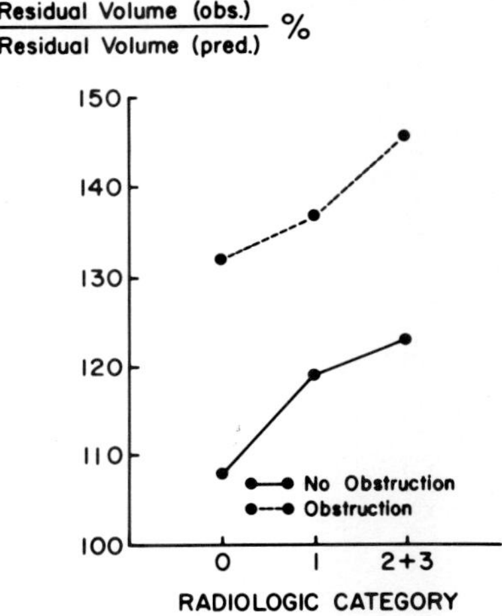

Fig. 7. Mean ratio of observed (obs.) residual volume to predicted (pred.) residual volume for 1,455 obstructed and nonobstructed Pennsylvania miners according to radiologic category. (From Morgan and co-workers [69]; reprinted by permission of publisher.)

mean RV was plotted versus radiographic category of pneumoconiosis for 4 groups of subjects according to obstruction, as previously defined, and smoking category. It was apparent from this study that both large airway obstruction and cigarette smoking had effects on RV; however, the nonsmoking, nonobstructed miners, in whom the effects of mining should be most evident, and in whom the other confounding influences were absent, showed a definite increase in RV with increasing radiographic category.

Diffusing Capacity

Relatively few measurements of the diffusing capacity of the lung for CO (D_{LCO}) had been carried out in American coal miners until recently. Gaensler and co-workers (73) reported a group of subjects, 2 of whom were American coal miners in whom a reduced single-breath and steady-state D_{LCO} were related to proved interstitial fibrosis and silicosis. Rasmussen and co-workers (74, 75) and Rasmussen (76, 77) reported that they frequently encountered low steady-state D_{LCO} in symptomatic coal miners from southern West Virginia; however, their studies also indicated marked reductions in the fractional uptake of CO associated with an increased ventilatory equivalent, suggesting that their findings may be accounted for by hyperventilation or, perhaps, faulty technique (78).

Seaton and colleagues (79) reported the single-breath D_{LCO} for 25 working, nonsmoking U. S. coal miners with category 2 or 3 simple CWP. All had values for D_{LCO} within the normal range, and the lung volumes and pulmonary mechanics in these subjects did not differ from those of miners with other small, regular opacities (figure 8); however, the mean value for D_{LCO}/TLC for the miners demonstrating the pinhead type of opacity (p) was significantly lower than the mean value for subjects demonstrating the q (or m) type of opacity. Cotes and associates (80) had previously reported differences in D_{LCO} between miners with simple pneumoconiosis of the p and m(q) variety in British coal miners. A survey of the literature by Lapp and Seaton (81) appeared to reveal that Sartorelli and co-workers (82) had first demonstrated this finding, without specifically commenting on it. Frans and co-workers (83) recently reviewed the entire subject and probably correctly attribute this discovery to Billiet and Ulburghs (84). Most studies reporting D_{LCO} in coal workers from Britain (80, 85–87) and from Europe (83, 84, 88, 89) appear to support the opinion that there is a difference in D_{LCO} between miners with the p type of opacity and those with other types of small opacity; the reduction has been attributed to mismatching of ventilation and perfusion. Nevertheless, 2 groups of investigators have been unable to find a difference in D_{LCO} between silicotic patients (90) or coal miners (91) with the p type of opacity and those with other types of small opacity.

Kibelstis (92) measured the steady-state D_{LCO} of 133 working, underground, bituminous

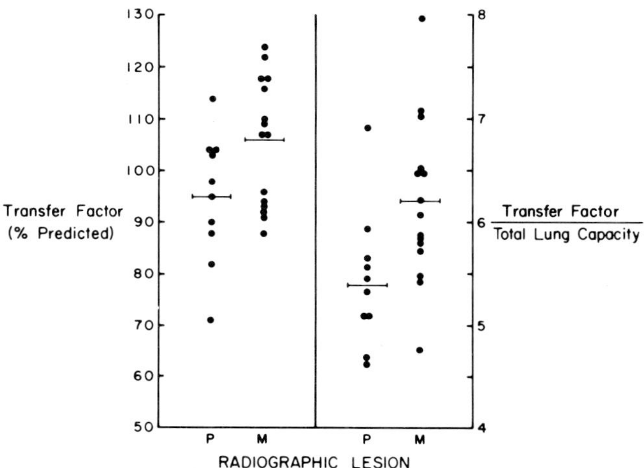

Fig. 8. Diffusing capacity for CO (transfer factor) for 25 nonsmoking, working miners with category 2 or 3 simple coal worker's pneumoconiosis. The sample was separated according to the type of small opacity present, i.e., p or m (q). (From Seaton and co-workers [79]; reprinted by permission of publisher.)

TABLE 2

STEADY-STATE DIFFUSING CAPACITY FOR CO IN SUBJECTS WITH
COMPLICATED COAL WORKER'S PNEUMOCONIOSIS

Stage	No. of Subjects		Age (years)	Height (cm)	FEV_1/FVC (%)	DL_{CO} (ml/min/mm Hg)		DL_{CO} (% pred)
						Predicted	Observed	
B	8	Mean	65	171	48	25	12	47
		SD	8	6	17	7	5	10
C	8	Mean	60	171	63	23	11	47
		SD	9	5	15	5	6	21

coal miners at rest and during moderate exercise. The subjects were divided into smokers and nonsmokers and were matched according to age and years in underground mining. The mean values for DL_{CO} both at rest and during exercise were within the normal range for the nonsmoking miners, regardless of age and years spent underground. On the other hand, the smoking miners had significantly lower DL_{CO} at rest and during exercise than the nonsmoking miners in all categories of underground exposure. There seems to be little doubt that simple CWP does not lead to a significant reduction in the steady-state DL_{CO}.

A recent study of Belgian coal miners using the single-breath DL_{CO} at rest and during exercise showed that the diffusion indices at rest were slightly decreased in simple CWP (83). This study demonstrated that during exercise, the DL_{CO} increased normally in most coal miners and that smoking decreased DL_{CO} more than did pneumoconiosis. These findings confirm those of Kibelstis (92).

In contrast to these findings in simple pneumoconiosis, complicated pneumoconiosis of stages B and C is often associated with a decrease in the DL_{CO}. Lapp and Seaton (81) studied 16 coal miners with complicated stage B or C pneumoconiosis, using the steady-state DL_{CO}. As usually occurs with the onset of complicated pneumoconiosis, their subjects had airway obstruction, as defined by FEV_1/FVC less than 70 per cent. The mean DL_{CO} was 47 per cent of the predicted normal for those with category B and 47 per cent of predicted for those with category C pneumoconiosis (table 2).

Gas Exchange

Reports of studies of gas exchange among U. S. coal miners have been relatively infrequent and limited, for the most part, to symptomatic subjects. Motley (93) and Motley and associates (94, 95) studied gas exchange among nonworking, symptomatic anthracite and bituminous coal miners. Most of these miners had obstructive airway disease, as indicated by increased RV/TLC. They also had decreased resting arterial Po_2 (Pa_{O_2}), increased resting alveolar-arterial Po_2 difference ($[A\text{-}a]Po_2$), and increased resting arterial Pco_2. These indices worsened on exercise. Motley and associates attributed these findings to unequal distribution of ventilation and perfusion in their subjects.

Ferris and Frank (96) studied 25 symptomatic, nonworking miners from Pennsylvania, West Virginia, and Ohio. Six subjects with complicated CWP showed the most striking abnormalities of lung volumes and air flow resistance. Eight subjects with category 2 or category 3 simple CWP showed the most abnormal blood gases, but a number of these also had bullous lesions on their radiographs, which may have contributed to this.

Lainhart and associates (60) studied the work capacity and some aspects of gas exchange in 5 groups of subjects as part of the U. S. Public Health Service prevalence study. They were unable to find any significant differences between miners and nonminers from the same community with regard to pulse rate, O_2 consumption, and minute ventilation at rest and during moderate exercise.

Two comprehensive studies of gas exchange in 51 symptomatic coal miners without evidence of airway obstruction, as defined by FEV_1/FVC greater than 70 per cent, have been reported (81, 97). Three of these subjects had category A complicated CWP, and the rest had disease ranging from 0 through all of the categories of simple CWP. The Pa_{O_2} values obtained at rest and during exercise in this group of miners are shown in figure 9. Subjects with categories 0 and 1 radiographs showed a mean Pa_{O_2} at rest that was slightly reduced, but that returned to normal on

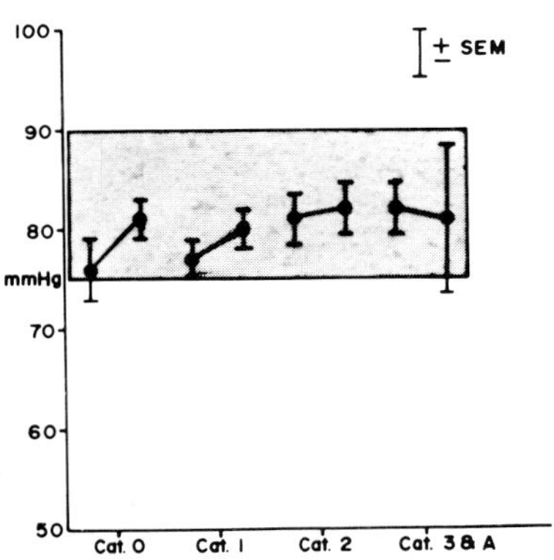

Fig. 9. Mean arterial P_{O_2} (mmHg) at rest and during exercise in 51 nonobstructed miners with various categories (Cat.) of coal worker's pneumoconiosis up to Stage A complicated. The shaded area represents the normal range; SEM = standard error of the mean. (Reprinted from Occupational Lung Diseases, chapter 10, by W. K. C. Morgan and A. Seaton, W. B. Saunders Company, Philadelphia, 1975.)

exercise. We also studied the (A-a)P_{O_2} at rest and during exercise for this same group of miners. The mean values for (A-a)P_{O_2} in category 0 were increased at rest and tended to remain increased during exercise. Category 1 subjects demonstrated mean values at rest and during exercise that tended to be high. Subjects with category 2 and category 3 or stage A pneumoconiosis showed high values at rest that tended to increase further on exercise. The ratio of dead space to tidal volume (V_D/V_T) was abnormally increased at rest in all groups, but returned toward the normal range on exercise in all except the group with category 3 and stage A complicated CWP (figure 10).

Fourteen additional symptomatic coal miners with stage B or C complicated CWP also underwent studies of gas exchange (table 3). In general, these subjects did demonstrate airway obstruction by spirometric tests. Their Pa_{O_2} values were low at rest and decreased further on exercise. They demonstrated an increased (A-a)P_{O_2} at rest that further increased on exercise; the V_D/V_T was increased at rest and did not return to the normal range on exercise.

That symptomatic coal miners, and especially nonworking miners seeking compensation or those who smoke, demonstrate abnormalities of gas exchange has been confirmed by studies in Europe (98–100). On the other hand, when coal miners with simple pneumoconiosis, but without airway obstruction, are studied, only slight alterations in Pa_{O_2}, (A-a)P_{O_2}, and V_D/V_T can be demonstrated (80, 83, 91).

Hemodynamics

In 1968, Rasmussen and associates (74) suggested, on the basis of abnormalities of gas exchange, that pulmonary hypertension might be frequent in U. S. coal miners. They demonstrated a high systolic pulmonary artery pressure in certain of the subjects they were investigating. This work was criticized in that systolic pressure, rather than mean pressure in the pulmonary artery, was recorded and that no measurements of pulmonary vascular resistance were made (101).

Lapp and associates (102, 103) studied hemodynamic indices in 47 Appalachian coal miners, all of whom professed respiratory symptoms and most of whom were seeking compensation. The mean pulmonary artery pressures at rest and during exercise in 23 of these miners who did not demonstrate airway obstruction are shown in figure 11. Only one of the subjects without obstruction, many of whom had abnormalities of gas exchange, had pulmonary hypertension at rest, whereas 3 additional subjects had slight to

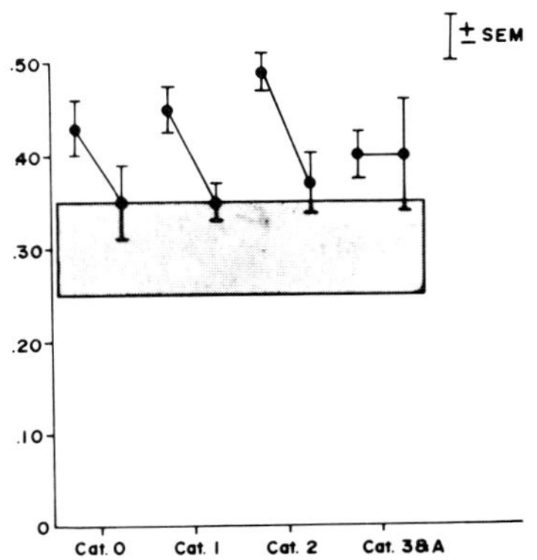

Fig. 10. Mean ratios of dead space to tidal volume at rest and during exercise in 51 nonobstructed miners with various categories (Cat.) of coal worker's pneumoconiosis up to Stage A complicated. The shaded area represents the normal range; SEM = standard error of the mean. (Reproduced from Occupational Lung Diseases, chapter 10, by W. K. C. Morgan and A. Seaton, W. B. Saunders Company, Philadelphia, 1975.)

TABLE 3

GAS EXCHANGE IN SUBJECTS WITH COMPLICATED COAL WORKER'S PNEUMOCONIOSIS

Radio-graphic Category	No. of Subjects		Age (years)	(A-a)PO$_2$ (mm Hg)		Pa$_{O_2}$ (mm Hg)		VD/VT		Minute Ventilation (liter/min/m^2)		O$_2$ Uptake (liter/min/m^2)		FEV$_1$/FVC (%)
				Rest	Exercise	Rest	Exercise	Rest	Exercise	Rest	Exercise	Rest	Exercise	
B	7	Mean	63	29	31	74	71	0.51	0.40	5.50	16.20	0.148	0.476	57
		SD	8.8	14.4	12.5	6.3	14.2	0.08	0.14	1.23	5.68	0.029	0.139	19.5
C	7	Mean	53	25	35	76	64	0.52	0.43	6.42	17.05	0.150	0.476	65
		SD	6.1	7.4	11.6	11.1	7.6	0.10	0.08	1.13	8.08	0.047	0.224	11.5

moderate increases in pulmonary artery pressure on exercise. All of these had the pinhead (p) type of radiographic opacity. Two gave a history of having been exposed to silica as well as coal dust. One of the subjects who demonstrated an increase in pulmonary artery pressure on exercise was markedly obese, and this may have contributed to his pulmonary hypertension. In figure 12, the mean pulmonary artery pressures at rest and during exercise are plotted versus Pa$_{O_2}$ at rest and during exercise for the 24 miners who had airway obstruction. All subjects who had pulmonary hypertension had either complicated pneumoconiosis or severe airway obstruction.

Seaton and co-workers (104) investigated the integrity of the pulmonary capillary bed in CWP by use of lung perfusion scans. Among 21 subjects with simple pneumoconiosis, they found only 2 minor abnormalities of perfusion scans. In contrast, they found areas of decreased to absent perfusion in all of 16 subjects with complicated pneumoconiosis. On comparison of the scans with the radiographs, these areas coincided with either the large opacities or the bullae.

The findings of Lapp and associates (102, 103) are consistent with previous studies in this country by Stoeckle and co-workers (105), who reported slight pulmonary hypertension in several of 17 disabled Appalachian miners. European investigators have also demonstrated that in miners with simple pneumoconiosis, hemodynamic alterations are relatively uncommon. Kremer and Lavenne (106) and Kremer and associates (107) showed that pulmonary artery pressure was related to airway resistance and that obstructed miners did not differ from obstructed nonmining control subjects. They did demonstrate a significant increase in pulmonary artery pressure in miners with category 2 and 3 pneumoconiosis compared to miners with category 0 and 1 or normal control subjects; however, none of their unobstructed subjects had an increased pulmonary artery pressure. In a later paper, Kremer (108) claimed that categories 2 and 3 were more often associated with increased mean pulmonary artery pressure on exercise; however, he failed to take into account the effect of age on pulmonary artery pressure. In contrast, Navratil and co-workers (109) found pulmonary hypertension in only one of 24 subjects with simple pneumoconiosis. They also found that 5 of 23 miners with complicated category B or C pneumoconiosis had pulmonary hypertension.

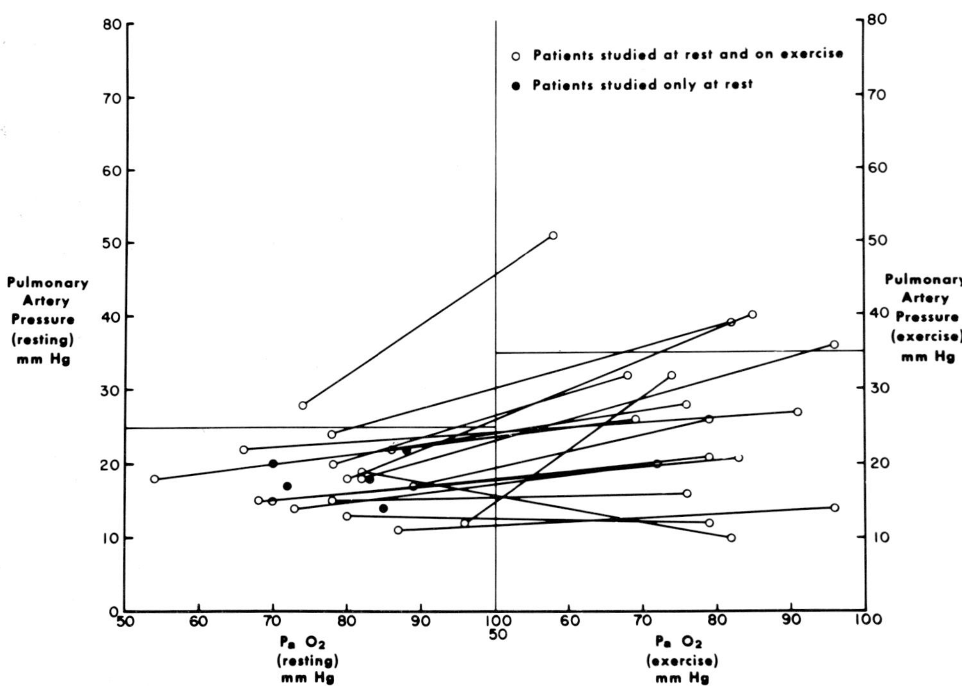

Fig. 11. Mean pulmonary artery pressure and arterial P_{O_2} (Pa_{O_2}) at rest and during exercise in 23 miners without airway obstruction. (Reproduced by permission from Inhaled Particles III, Unwin Brothers, Old Woking, Surrey, England, 1971.)

Mechanics

Ferris and Frank (96) investigated the mechanical properties of the lungs of 25 symptomatic Appalachian coal miners. Two of these subjects, both of whom had complicated pneumoconiosis, had reduced static lung compliance. Recently, the findings of a series of studies of respiratory mechanics in coal workers have been reported (110–112). The first report included 66 symptomatic, but unobstructed, coal miners of whom 22 had no evidence of pneumoconiosis: 24 had category 1, 15 had category 2, and 5 had either category 3 or complicated stage A pneumoconiosis. These studies revealed (figure 13) that in subjects with simple pneumoconiosis, static compliance was mostly in the normal range, whereas in complicated disease, it was often reduced. Dynamic compliance at quiet breathing frequencies tended to be low in all of these subjects. The coefficient of retraction (pulmonary recoil pressure at TLC divided by total lung capacity) was normal in most subjects or tended to be slightly reduced, except in subjects with stage B or C complicated disease, in whom this coefficient tended to be increased (figure 14).

A subgroup of 25 nonsmoking, working miners with category 2 and 3 simple pneumoconiosis were studied and compared with a group of 6 age-matched control subjects. None of the miners or control subjects had evidence of large airway obstruction. The static compliance of the miners and the control subjects was within the normal limit. The pulmonary recoil pressure at TLC was also within normal limits, except for 2 miners and one control subject. The dynamic compliance at differing respiratory rates is shown for the miners who complained of symptoms of bronchitis (10 of the 25) in figure 15. Of these, 6 showed definite frequency dependence of dynamic compliance. The dynamic compliance at various respiratory rates is shown for miners who had no symptoms of bronchitis in figure 16. Eleven of these 15 miners demonstrated definite frequency dependence of compliance. Inhalation of isoproterenol did not alter the frequency dependence of compliance in these miners. None of the control subjects demonstrated frequency dependence of dynamic compliance.

Lapp and Seaton (111) extended their observations in these subjects by relating maximal expiratory flow to static recoil pressures and lung

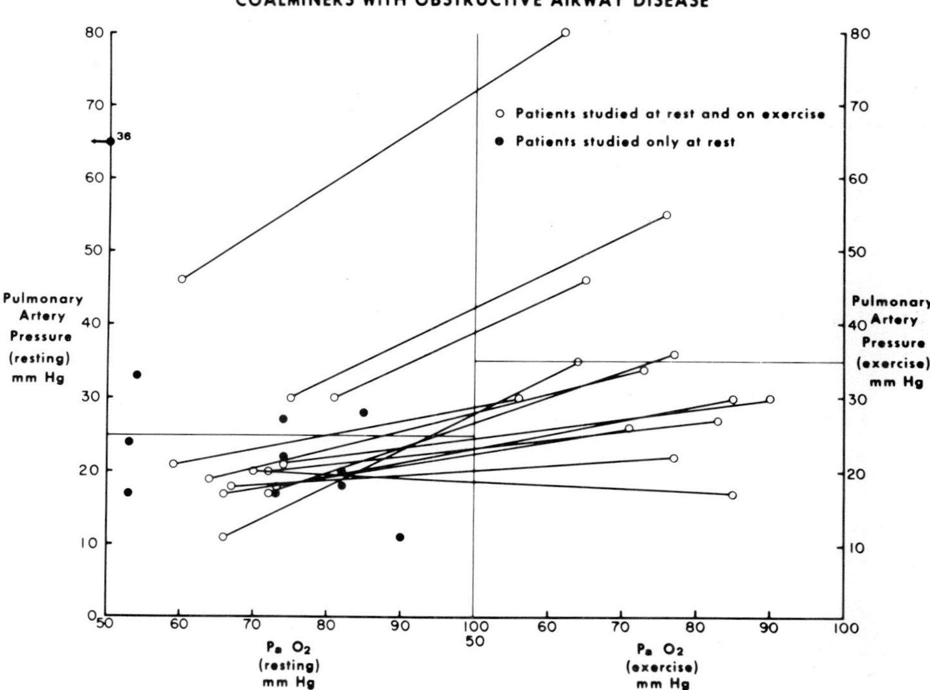

Fig. 12. Mean pulmonary artery pressures and arterial Po_2 (Pa_{O_2}) at rest and during exercise for 24 obstructed miners. (Reproduced by permission from Inhaled Particles III, Unwin Brothers, Old Woking, Surrey, England, 1971.)

volumes. The miners as a group achieved lower flows than did control subjects at comparable lung volumes and static recoil pressures. In the 17 miners who demonstrated frequency dependence of compliance, the reduced maximal expiratory flow appeared to be related to an increase in the resistance to air flow in small peripheral airways. The mechanism for the reduced maximal expiratory flows in the remaining 8 miners appeared to be related to a slight decrease in lung static recoil pressure. Lapp and Seaton (111) could not relate these alterations in lung mechanics to the type of radiographic

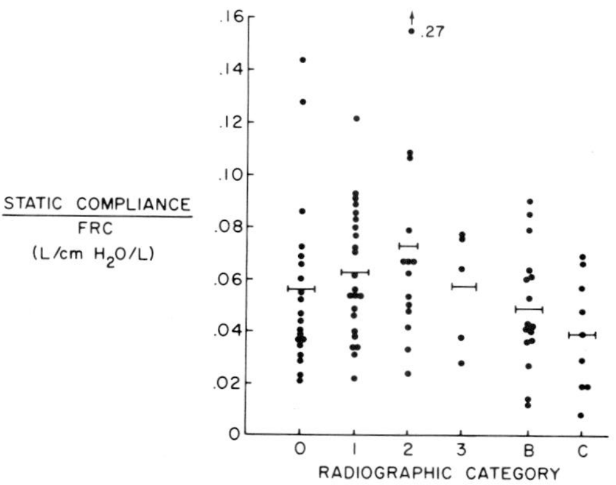

Fig. 13. Static compliance of miners and ex-miners with different radiographic categories of coal worker's pneumoconiosis. (From Seaton and co-workers [110]; reprinted by permission of publisher.) FRC = functional residual capacity.

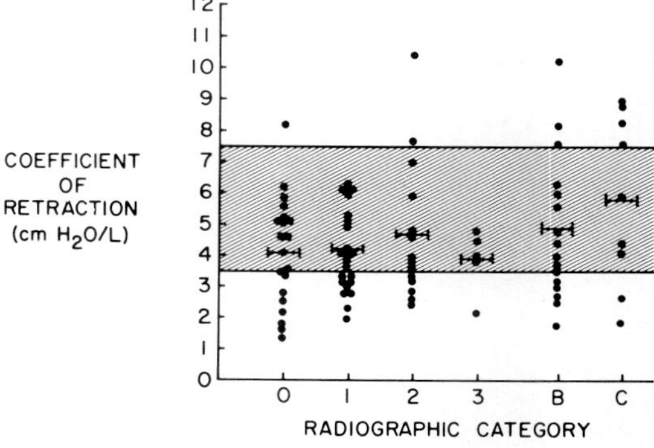

Fig. 14. Coefficient of retraction of miners and ex-miners with different radiographic categories of coal worker's pneumoconiosis. Shaded area = normal range. (From Seaton and co-workers [110]; reprinted by permission of publisher.)

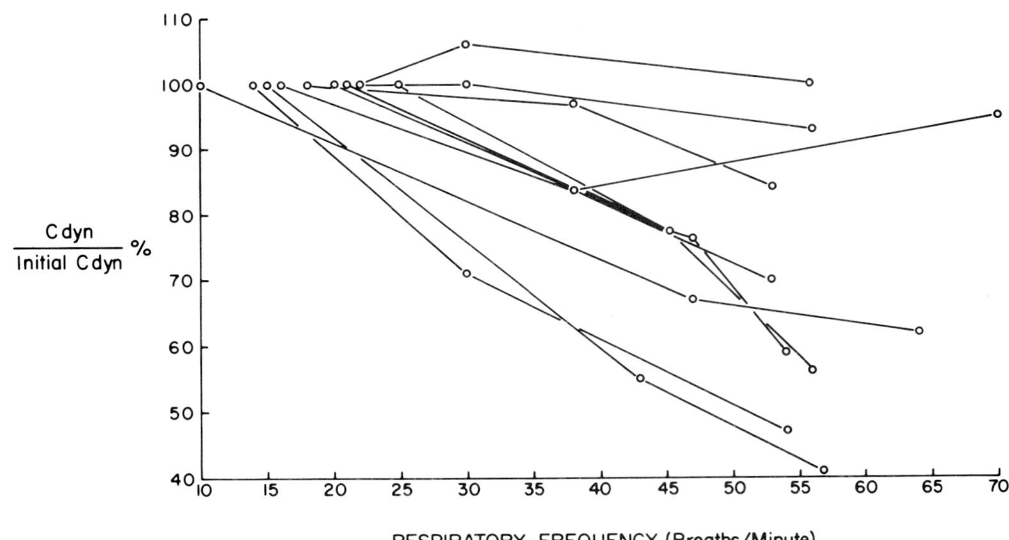

Fig. 15. Dynamic compliance (Cdyn) at different respiratory rates in bronchitic, but nonobstructed miners with categories 2 and 3 simple coal worker's pneumoconiosis (CWP). (From Seaton and co-workers [110]; reprinted by permission of publisher.)

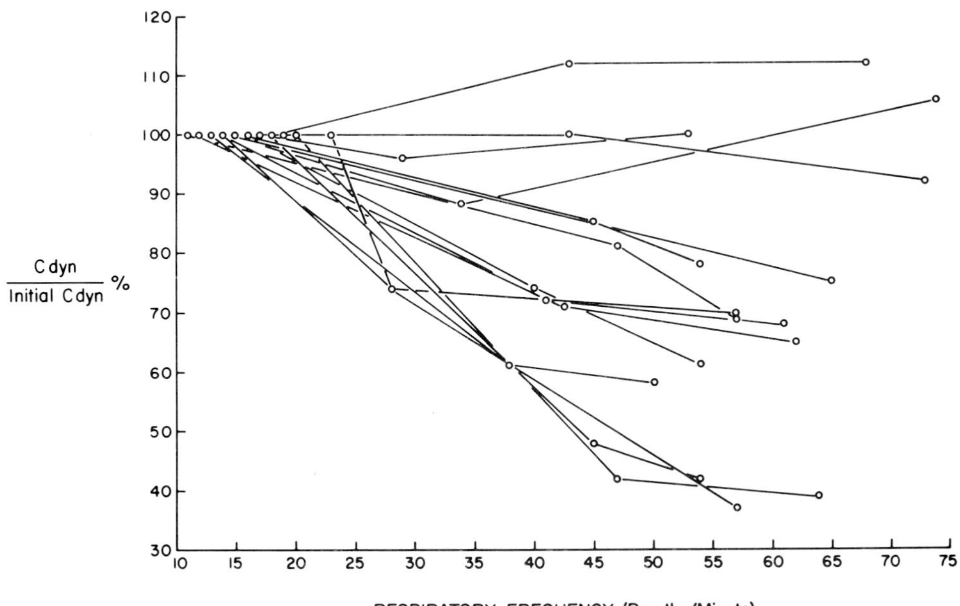

Fig. 16. Dynamic compliance (Cdyn) at different respiratory rates in nonbronchitic, nonobstructed miners with categories 2 and 3 simple coal worker's pneumoconiosis (CWP). (From Seaton and co-workers [110]; reprinted by permission of publisher.)

opacity (p or q) or to symptoms of bronchitis.

Morgan and associates (112) investigated miners with category 0 and 1 simple pneumoconiosis using the dynamic compliance at different respiratory frequencies. Whereas an occasional miner with category 1 disease showed a decrease in dynamic compliance at increased respiratory frequencies, none of the miners with category 0 disease showed this phenomenon. Interestingly, 2 of the younger and one older control subject also demonstrated frequency dependence at the faster respiratory frequencies.

Special Studies

Lapp and colleagues (113) studied the acute effects of exposure to coal dust in 93 miners of an underground shift and compared these results with those in an age-matched control group of 42 nonminers. They found small, but significant decreases in FEV_1, FVC, and forced expiratory flow at 75 per cent of vital capacity exhaled (FEF_{75}) during the course of the work shift in the miners (table 4). When viewed according to smoking status, all of these indices were decreased after the shift in the smoking miners, whereas among the nonsmoking miners, only the FEF_{75} decreased (table 5). These findings suggested that in smokers, both large and peripheral airways were affected, whereas in the nonsmoking miners, the effect was largely on the peripheral airways.

When the miners were divided into groups according to high, medium, and low exposure to dust on the basis of time spent at the working face, there was a general tendency for the high and medium groups to show decreases after the workshift, whereas the low group did not (table 6).

Lapp and associates (114) recently evaluated another index of peripheral airway obstruction, namely closing volume and closing capacity, determined by the single-breath N_2 method in 82 miners with various categories of CWP and 58 age-matched control subjects. The two groups did not differ with regard to the standard spirometric indices, such as FEV_1, FVC, or FEV_1/FVC.

TABLE 4

MEAN CHANGE* IN VENTILATORY FUNCTION IN MINERS AND NONMINERS AFTER WORK SHIFT

	Miners[†]	Nonminers
No. of subjects	93	42
FVC, liter	−2.5[†]	+1.5[†]
	(6.3)	(4.4)
FEV_1, liter	−2.9[†]	+3.8[†]
	(7.0)	(9.1)
Peak flow, liter/sec	−2.8	+0.2
	(13.6)	(8.8)
FEF_{50}, liter/sec	−4.8	+6.6[†]
	(29.5)	(18.6)
FEF_{75}, liter/sec	−16.7	+4.2[†]
	(38.0)	(35.4)

*Expressed as per cent of control value. In the table, values in parentheses, SD; direction of change from before-shift values, +, −.

[†] The probability, P, that a change of this magnitude could occur by chance was less than 0.05.

TABLE 5

MEAN CHANGE IN VENTILATORY FUNCTION RELATED TO SMOKING STATUS IN MINERS AND NONMINERS AFTER WORK SHIFT*

	Miners		Nonminers[†]	
	Smokers	Nonsmokers	Smokers	Nonsmokers
No. of subjects	50	43	13	29
FVC, liter	−3.5**	−1.4	+3.4**	+0.7
	(6.2)	(6.2)	(5.3)	(3.8)
FEV_1, liter	−4.2**	−1.3	+7.4	+2.2**
	(6.2)	(7.6)	(15.5)	(2.9)
Peak flow, liter/sec	−2.2	−3.4	+2.5	−0.9
	(13.6)	(13.7)	(11.2)	(7.5)
FEF_{50}, liter/sec	−4.0	−5.8	+5.9	+6.9**
	(31.9)	(26.9)	(25.9)	(14.7)
FEF_{75}, liter/sec	−17.4**	−15.8**	+4.7	+4.0
	(32.6)	(43.8)	(37.2)	(35.2)

*Expressed as per cent of control value.

[†] Values in parentheses, SD; direction of change from before-shift values, +, −.

**Probability that change of this magnitude could occur by chance (P < 0.05).

TABLE 6

MEAN CHANGE* IN VENTILATORY FUNCTION RELATED TO DUST EXPOSURE IN MINERS AFTER WORK SHIFT

	Dust Exposure		
	High	Medium	Low
No. of subjects	28	35	30
FVC, liter	$-3.6^{\dagger}$ (5.2)	$-3.2^{\dagger}$ (6.1)	-0.8 (7.1)
FEV_1, liter	$-3.6^{\dagger}$ (7.2)	$-2.7^{\dagger}$ (6.5)	-2.4 (7.5)
Peak flow, liter/sec	-1.0 (11.5)	$-4.9^{\dagger}$ (12.6)	-1.9 (16.2)
FEF_{50}, liter/sec	-6.7 (27.9)	$-11.3^{\dagger}$ (26.5)	-4.4 (32.8)
FEF_{75}, liter/sec	$-15.2^{\dagger}$ (31.9)	$-23.0^{\dagger}$ (36.7)	-10.7 (44.4)

*Expressed as per cent of control value. In the table, values in parentheses, SD; direction of change from before-shift values, −.

†The probability, P, that a change of this magnitude could occur by chance was < 0.05.

The forced expiratory flow at midvital capacity (FEF_{50}) adjusted for age, height, and smoking was significantly lower among the nonbronchitic miners than the nonbronchitic control subjects, but it did not distinguish between miners and control subjects when grouped according to smoking habits.

In contrast, the age- and height-adjusted closing capacities were consistently higher in the miners than in the control subjects, regardless of their smoking status. Age- and height-adjusted closing volume was less sensitive than closing capacity in detecting differences between miners and control subjects when they were grouped according to smoking habits. Only in the nonsmoking group was there a significant difference between the miners and the control subjects with regard to closing volume. Neither closing capacity nor closing volume was significantly different between miners with and without simple pneumoconiosis.

Finally, Hall and co-workers (115) were able to make follow-up measurements 4 years later in 17 of the original cohort of 25 nonsmoking, working coal miners and the age-matched control subjects studied by Seaton and associates (110). They also measured closing capacity and closing volume in the follow-up study. They found that compared with control subjects, miners showed a marked decreasé in maximal expiratory flow at midvital capacity (FEF_{50}) during the 4-year period that occurred without sig-

nificant change in the FEV_1. This decrease in FEF_{50} occurred regardless of whether the subjects in the original study showed frequency dependence of dynamic compliance in association with increased upstream airway resistance, or loss of lung recoil. They found abnormally increased closing capacities in 53 per cent and abnormally increased closing volumes in 23 per cent of the miners who returned for follow-up studies. None of the control subjects demonstrated abnormal closing capacity or closing volume. The presence of an abnormal closing capacity or closing volume on the follow-up study did not appear to be related to the type of mechanical abnormality present at the original study.

Immunology of CWP

Caplan's syndrome and the relationship of rheumatoid factors to CWP. In 1953, Caplan (116) described a syndrome characterized by the presence of certain peculiar appearances in the chest radiograph of miners that were associated with rheumatoid arthritis. The condition he described is now commonly referred to as Caplan's syndrome, or rheumatoid pneumoconiosis.

In contrast to those of PMF, the opacities that characterize Caplan's syndrome tend, for the most part, to be rounded and peripherally situated. They occur most often on a background of category 0 or 1 simple CWP, and may appear in the space of a few weeks. The nodules are usually 0.5 to 5 cm in diameter and most often develop concomitantly with the joint manifestations of rheumatoid arthritis. In a few subjects, they may precede the arthritis by several years. Fresh crops of nodules may appear at intervals and often portend an exacerbation of the arthritis. There is an association between the rheumatoid nodules found in the elbows and Achilles tendon and those that appear in the lungs.

The epidemiology of the condition was first studied by Miall and associates (117). Their studies showed that there was an increased prevalence of rheumatoid arthritis in Welsh miners with PMF, but that rheumatoid arthritis did not appear to be more common in miners and exminers compared to the normal population.

The pathology of the condition has been well described by Gough and co-workers (118). This group studied at autopsy the pathologic findings in 14 subjects who in life had had rheumatoid pneumoconiosis. They observed that cavitation occurred in the nodules and that in some subjects, evidence of "burnt out" tuberculosis was present. In a few instances, difficulties were experienced in differentiating the Caplan nodule not only from the ordinary collagenous nodule of pneumoconiosis, but also from PMF and the silicotuberculotic nodule. Histologically, the Caplan nodule was shown to be formed of necrotic tissue with varying amounts of collagen and dust present. Outside the necrotic area was a cellular zone that was often infiltrated with lymphocytes and plasma cells. Endarteritis was frequently observed. In many nodules, there was a peripheral zone of more active inflammation with polymorphonuclear leukocytic infiltration and what Gough and associates chose to refer to as the "rheumatoid zone." Caplan nodules were often observed to be present in lungs that showed relatively little dust retention.

Since the original studies, Caplan and co-workers (119) have shown that the prevalence of rheumatoid factors is increased in miners with the r type of small, rounded opacity and also in subjects with irregular, large opacities. They also showed that many miners without overt rheumatoid arthritis had positive serologic findings for rheumatoid factor when the type of radiographic abnormalities described were present.

Recently, Wagner and McCormick (53) related the presence of rheumatoid factors to the clinical and radiographic status of several groups of miners. They were able to show that rheumatoid factor was present in 70 per cent of their subjects with Caplan's syndrome. Approximately 30 to 40 per cent of their subjects with PMF also had a positive test for rheumatoid factor. There was a further decrease in the prevalence of rheumatoid factor in subjects with simple CWP, and only 2 per cent of the control subjects were positive. These workers also examined fresh lung tissue by means of immunohistologic techniques designed to demonstrate the presence of rheumatoid factor in the tissues. As a result of their findings, they suggested that PMF exists in 2 forms, namely, PMF associated with vasculitis, which is related to the rheumatoid diathesis, and nonspecific PMF. The latter was believed by them to differ histologically from PMF associated with vasculitis, and rheumatoid factors were absent from tissue and serum.

At a later date, Lippman and co-workers (120) examined the sera of 156 U. S. underground miners for the presence of rheumatoid factor and antinuclear antibody. A relationship between humoral autoimmune activity and the type of radiographic capacity was sought. They divided their subjects into 4 groups: subjects with PMF, subjects with simple CWP, subjects with clear chest films, and subjects whose films suggested or were diagnostic of Caplan's syndrome.

Only subjects with a classic appearance of Caplan's syndrome were found to have rheumatoid factor in their serum. Rheumatoid factor was not observed to be present more often in either simple CWP or PMF than in the group with category 0 pneumoconiosis. None of the sera from miners with clear chest films showed either rheumatoid or antinuclear activity. In contrast, antinuclear antibody was present in 55 per cent of the sera of anthracite miners, as opposed to 21 per cent of the sera of bituminous miners. Among anthracite miners with PMF, no less than 74 per cent had evidence of antinuclear activity. There seemed to be a relation between antinuclear activity and the presence of CWP; regions with the highest prevalence of CWP showed the greatest prevalence of sera with antinuclear activity. With the exception of subjects whose films strongly suggested Caplan's syndrome, the type of nodular opacity appeared to be unrelated to humoral autoimmune activity. The findings of Lippman and associates (120) in Appalachian miners do not support Wagner and McCormick's (53) theory that the development of PMF in a significant proportion of coal miners is related to the rheumatoid diathesis.

Lung Autoantibodies in CWP

In a comprehensive review of the immunologic aspects of CWP, Burrell (121) has demonstrated that lung reactive antibodies are often present in the sera of miners and that they are derived from globulin-reactive materials. The major antigenic targets of the immune response are the connective tissue components of the lung (collagen, elastin, and reticulin). Both types of IgA, secretory and humoral, are involved in the immune response, and the antibodies can be demonstrated in pneumoconiotic nodules and in the alveolar septa. Nonetheless, the role of the antibodies in the etiology and progression of pneumoconiosis remains uncertain.

Recently, Burrell and colleagues (122) have been able to demonstrate the development of lung autoantibodies in laboratory animals exposed to coal dust. Rats and mice exposed to approximately 2 mg of respirable coal dust per m^3 have been shown to develop lung autoantibodies similar to those seen in coal miners.

Industrial Bronchitis

Most, but not all, studies of coal miners have shown that they have a greater prevalence of cough and sputum and a slightly lower ventilatory capacity than do comparable control groups of nonminers. Although Stages B and C PMF lead to a definite decrement in ventilatory capacity as detected by the commonly used tests of this function (FEV$_1$ and FVC), no comparable decrement in ventilatory capacity is evident with increasing category of simple pneumoconiosis. This finding is somewhat surprising in view of the well-established relation between radiographic category of simple CWP and the coal content of the lung, a relation that has on repeated occasions shown that the higher the category, the greater the amount of coal dust retained in the lungs. In interpreting these anomalous findings, 2 hypotheses should be considered. (1) Differential migration is responsible, in that only the fitter miners with better pulmonary function work long enough to develop CWP. Thus, men who eventually develop CWP originally had ventilatory capacities that were better than average, but long exposure to dust and the development of CWP caused their function to decrease to that of the general work force. (2) A form of industrial bronchitis exists that affects the lung function of all miners to a limited extent and is not associated with radiographic evidence of dust retention.

Although the second hypothesis seems more probable, it is only in the last few years that evidence to confirm the existence of industrial bronchitis has become available.

In 1966, the Medical Research Council of Great Britain produced a report on the role of occupation in the etiology of chronic bronchitis (123). The Council concluded that the intensity of dust exposure did not appear to play a significant role in determining the prevalence of bronchitis and airway obstruction in workers exposed to dust. Their reasons for this were related partly to the difficulty in demonstrating a significant reduction in ventilatory capacity in the groups exposed to the most dust, and also to the fact that chronic bronchitis, as diagnosed by the presence of cough and sputum, was observed to occur more frequently in the wives of coal miners than in the wives of other workers. Nonetheless, it was observed that the wives of coal miners did not demonstrate a concomitant reduction in ventilatory capacity, and in this, differed from their husbands.

Since the Medical Research Council reports, several studies have related the prevalence of bronchitis to dust exposure. Reichel and Ulmer (124), Minnette (125), and Lowe and Khosla (126) have all been able to demonstrate that bronchitis becomes more prevalent as exposure to coal dust increases. Kibelstis and co-workers (9) studied the frequency of bronchitis and airway obstruction in more than 8,000 working U. S. coal miners. They divided their work force into 4 groups according to the degree of dust exposure, i.e., face workers, transportation workers, maintenance workers, and surface workers. Bronchitis was most common in the group exposed to the most dust, namely, the face workers, and decreased with increasing distance from the coal face, being least common in surface workers. In contrast, the effect of increasing exposure to dust on ventilatory capacity was minimal and significant only when the nonsmoking face workers were compared with the nonsmoking surface workers. Even then, difference was minimal, in that the mean FEV$_1$ values of the face and surface workers were, respectively, 98 and 102 per cent of the predicted values. With regard to airway obstruction, cigarette smoking had 5 to 6 times the effect of exposure to dust.

Recently, the medical staff of the National Coal Board of Great Britain were able to demonstrate a reduction in ventilatory capacity with increasing exposure to dust (127). The presence of simple CWP, however, was not associated with any further decrement in FEV$_1$ over and above that associated with lifetime exposure to dust. The final confirmation that the decrease in ventilatory capacity that is seen in miners is a consequence of industrial bronchitis is to be found in a paper by Hankinson and associates (128). These investigators studied the effects of age, smoking, bronchitis, radiographic category, and years spent underground on the forced expiratory flows of a sample of 6,014 working miners. As expected, age and cigarette smoking had profound effects on flows at all lung volumes. Years underground affected peak flow and flow at high lung volumes to a limited extent; in contrast, flows at lower lung volumes were not affected. These observations indicate that the process responsible for the decreased flows is to be located in the larger bronchi, rather than the smaller airways. Like Rogan and associates (127), Hankinson and co-workers (128) were not able to demonstrate that increasing radiographic category had an effect over and above that due to years spent underground.

Industrial bronchitis has been observed in

South African gold miners (129), in cotton mill workers (130), and in asbestos miners (131). At the present time, the evidence suggests that the inhalation of most mineral and some vegetable dusts can lead to an increased prevalence of cough and sputum. If such exposure is prolonged and severe, a small decrease in ventilatory capacity develops in some of the exposed workers. Industrial bronchitis, for the most part, affects the larger airways and can be assumed to be due to the deposition of larger particles (nonrespirable particles larger than 6 μm) in the trachea and bronchi from whence they are removed by the mucociliary escalator, leaving no radiographic stigmata.

Relationship of Emphysema to Coal Mining

Although focal emphysema is a frequent accompaniment of the higher degrees of simple CWP and may lead to minor abnormalities in the distribution of expired gas, as manifested by slight increases in $(A\text{-}a)P_{O_2}$ and V_D/V_T, and by a minimal decrease in the diffusing capacity, it does not affect ventilatory capacity. Were focal emphysema to have an effect on the bellows function of the lungs, the FEV_1 and FVC would decrease with increasing category of simple CWP, because it has been observed that the higher the category of simple CWP, the more probable is focal emphysema (132). That this cannot be demonstrated in life is well accepted, but a minority maintain that disabling emphysema is more common in coal miners. The evidence for this assertion comes from postmortem studies in which the presence of emphysema in deceased coal miners was compared to that in comparable control groups. Ryder and co-workers (133) were able to demonstrate in their autopsy series of 247 miners that the FEV_1 decreased as the emphysema count increased. They were able to show a relation between radiographic category of the p, or puntiform, type of simple pneumoconiosis and the FEV_1. This study has been criticized on several grounds. First, the miners who subsequently came to autopsy had previously been awarded compensation; therefore, they probably represented a biased group. Second, much of the decrease in FEV_1 that was observed to be related to the emphysema count can be explained by the inclusion of a significant number of subjects with PMF. Because PMF itself leads to a decrease in the FEV_1, and because an appreciable number of subjects with PMF was included in the autopsy series, the association between the decrement in FEV_1 and emphysema is partially spurious (134). Next, the p type of opacity has not been shown to be associated with decreased survival; indeed, the reverse is true (135). Finally, it has been shown that no significant difference could be demonstrated in the FEV_1, RV, or any other index of pulmonary function other than the diffusing capacity when a working population of miners with simple CWP was broken down into groups according to the type of small opacity (p, q, or r) present in the chest film (79). Thus, it can be concluded at the present time that there is no evidence that simple CWP or coal mining per se leads to the development of disabling emphysema in the absence of PMF.

Silicosis

Both simple and complicated silicosis are occasionally seen in coal miners, but only in roof bolters and miners who have worked for long periods on transportation. The onset of simple silicosis usually is delayed in coal mining, compared to other industries, and is seldom seen without at least 20 years of exposure. It cannot be differentiated radiographically from CWP unless eggshell calcification is present in the hilar nodes. Simple silicosis causes little in the way of symptoms and signs, but the conglomerate lesions destroy the alveolocapillary bed and adjacent parenchyma. A detailed description of this condition is inappropriate in this review, and the reader is referred to appropriate texts elsewhere.

References

1. Gregory, J. C.: Case of peculiar black infiltration of the whole lungs, resembling melanosis, Edin Med J, 1831, *36*, 389.
2. Laennec, R. T. H.: Traite de l'auscultation médiate, ed. 4, Paris, 1819.
3. Meiklejohn, A.: History of lung disease of coal miners in Great Britain, Part I, 1800–1875, Br J Ind Med, 1951, *8*, 127.
4. Meiklejohn, A.: History of lung disease of coal miners in Great Britain, Part II, 1875–1920, Br J Ind Med, 1952, *9*, 93.
5. Meiklejohn, A.: History of lung disease of coal miners in Great Britain, Part III, 1920–1952, Br J Ind Med, 1952, *9*, 208.
6. Morgan, W. K. C., Burgess, D. B., Jacobson, G., O'Brien, R. J., Pendergrass, E. P., Reger, R. B., and Shoub, E. P.: The prevalence of coal workers' pneumoconiosis in U. S. coal mines, Arch Environ Health, 1973, *27*, 221.
7. Doyle, H. N.: Dust concentrations in the mines, Proceedings of Symposium on Respirable Coal Mine Dust, Bureau of Mines Information Circular, No. 8458, Washington, D. C., 1970.

8. Enterline, P. E.: Mortality rates among coal miners, Am J Public Health, 1966, *54*, 758.

9. Kibelstis, J. A., Morgan, E. J., Reger, R. .B., Lapp, N. L., Seaton, A., and Morgan, W. K. C.: Prevalence of bronchitis and airway obstruction in American bituminous coal miners, Am Rev Respir Dis, 1973, *108*, 886.

10. Guralick, L.: Mortality by occupation and causes of death in United States, 1950, Vital Statistics, Special Reports, Vol. 53, No. 3, Department of H.E.W., September 1963.

11. Enterline, P.: A review of mortality data for American coal miners, Ann N Y Acad Sci, 1972, *400*, 260.

12. Goldmann, K. P.: Mortality of coal miners from carcinoma of the lung, Br J Ind Med, 1965, *22*, 72.

13. Costello, J., Ortmeyer, C. E., and Morgan, W. K. C.: Mortality from lung cancer in U. S. coal miners, Am J Public Health, 1974, *64*, 222.

14. Liddell, F. D. K.: Mortality of British coal miners in 1961–1962, Br J Ind Med, 1973, *30*, 1.

15. Liddell, F. D. K.: Mortality of British coal miners in 1961, Br J Ind Med, 1973, *30*, 15.

16. Cochrane, A. L.: Relation between radiographic categories of pneumoconiosis and expectation of life, Br Med J, 1973, *2*, 532.

17. Ortmeyer, C. E., Baier, E. J., and Crawford, G. M.: Life expectancy of Pennsylvania coal miners compensated for disability as affected by pneumoconiosis and ventilatory impairment, Arch Environ Health, 1973, *27*, 227.

18. Ortmeyer, C. E., Costello, J., Morgan, W. K. C., Swecker, S., and Petersen, M.: The mortality of Appalachian coal miners, 1963–1971, Arch Environ Health, 1974, *29*, 67.

19. Costello, J., Ortmeyer, C. E., and Morgan, W. K. C.: Mortality from heart disease in coal miners, Chest, 1975, *67*, 417.

20. Collis, E. L., and Gilchrist, J. C.: Effect of dust on coal trimmers, J Ind Hyg, 1928, *10*, 101.

21. Gough, J.: Pneumoconiosis of coal trimmers, J Pathol Bacteriol, 1940, *51*, 277.

22. Rivers, D., Wise, M. E., King, E. J., and Nagelschmidt, G.: Dust content, radiology, and pathology in simple pneumoconiosis of coal workers, Br J Ind Med, 1960, *17*, 87.

23. Watson, A. J., Black, J., Doig, A. T., and Nagelschmidt, G.: Pneumoconiosis in carbon electrode workers, Br J Ind Med, 1959, *16*, 274.

24. Gaensler, E. A., Cadigan, J. B., Sasahara, A. A., Fox, E. O., and MacMahon, H. E.: Graphite pneumoconiosis of electrotypers, Am J Med, 1966, *41*, 864.

25. Rüttner, J. R., Bovet, P., and Aufdermaur, F.: Graphite, carborund, staublunge, Dtsch Med Wochenschr, 1952, *77*, 1413.

26. Morgan, W. K. C., and Seaton, A.: Occupational Lung Diseases, W. B. Saunders Company, Philadelphia, 1975, p. 241.

27. Spink, R., and Nagelschmidt, G.: Dust fibrosis in the lungs of coal workers from the Wigan area of Lancashire, Br J Ind Med, 1963, *20*, 818.

28. Nagelschmidt, G.: The study of lung dust in pneumoconiosis, Am Ind Hyg Assoc J, 1965, *26*, 1.

29. Pratt, P. C.: The role of silica in progressive massive fibrosis, Arch Environ Health, 1968, *16*, 734.

30. Walton, W. H., Dodgson, J., Hadden, G. G., and Jacobsen, M.: The effect of quartz and other non-coal dusts in coal workers' pneumoconiosis, Paper presented at the Fourth International Congress of Inhaled Particles and Vapours, Edinburgh, Scotland, September 1975.

31. Jacobson, G., and Lainhart, W. S.: ILO/UC 1971 International Classification of Radiographs of the Pneumoconioses, Med Radiogr Photogr, 1972, *48*, 67.

32. Liddell, F. D. K., and May, J. D.: Assessing the Radiological Progression of Simple Pneumoconiosis, National Coal Board Medical Service, 1966, London.

33. Amandus, H. E., Lapp, N. L., Jacobson, G., anf Reger, R. B.: Significance of irregular small opacities in the radiographs of U. S. coal miners, Br J Ind Med, 1976, *33*, 13.

34. Reger, R. B., and Morgan, W. K. C.: On the factors influencing consistency in the radiologic diagnosis of pneumoconiosis, Am Rev Respir Dis, 1970, *102*, 905.

35. Reger, R. B., Amandus, H. E., and Morgan, W. K. C.: On the diagnosis of coal workers' pneumoconiosis: Anglo-American disharmony, Am Rev Respir Dis, 1973, *108*, 1186.

36. Lainhart, W. S., and Morgan, W. K. C.: Extent and distribution of respiration effects in pulmonary reaction to coal dust, M. M. Key, L. E. Kerr, and M. Bundy, ed., Academic Press, New York, 1972, pp. 29–56.

37. Morgan, W. K. C.: Prevalence of coal workers' pneumoconiosis, Am Rev Respir Dis, 1968, *98*, 306.

38. Reger, R. B., Butcher, D. F., and Morgan, W. K. C.: Assessing changes in the pneumoconioses using serial radiographs: Sources and quantifications of bias, Am J Epidemiol, 1973, *98*, 243.

39. Reger, R. B., Petersen, M. R., and Morgan, W. K. C.: Variation in the interpretation of radiographic change in pulmonary diseases, Lancet, 1974, *1*, 111.

40. Amandus, H. E., Reger, R. B., Pendergrass, E. P., Dennis, J. M., and Morgan, W. K. C.: The pneumoconioses: Methods of measuring progression, Chest, 1973, *63*, 236.

41. Liddell, F. D. K.: Assessment of radiological progression of simple pneumoconiosis in individual miners, Br J Ind Med, 1974, *31*, 185.

42. Reger, R. B., Smith, C. R., Kibelstis, J. A., and

Morgan, W. K. C.: The effect of film quality and other factors on the roentgenographic categorization of coal workers' pneumoconiosis, Am J Roentgenol Radium Ther Nucl Med, 1972, *115*, 462.

43. Jacobsen, M.: Progression of coal workers' pneumoconiosis in Britain in relation to environmental conditions underground, Proceedings of Conference on Technical Measures of Dust Prevention and Suppression in Mines, European Iron and Steel Community, Luxembourg, October 1972, p. 77.

44. Reisner, M. T. R.: Results of epidemiological studies of pneumoconiosis in W. German coal miners, in *Inhaled Particles III*, vol. 2, W. H. Walton, ed., Unwin Brothers, 1970, p. 921.

45. Rogan, J. M., Rae, S., and Walton, W. H.: The National Coal Board's pneumoconiosis field research, in *Inhaled Particles and Vapours II*, C. N. Davis, ed., Pergamon Press, Oxford, 1967, p. 493.

46. Seal, M. R. E., and Wagner, J. C.: Pathological reactions of the lungs to dust, in *Occupational Lung Diseases*, W. K. C. Morgan, and A. Seaton, ed., W. B. Saunders Company, Philadelphia, 1975, pp. 51–58.

47. Heppleston, A. G.: The essential lesion of pneumokoniosis in Welsh coal workers, J Pathol Bacteriol, 1947, *59*, 453.

48. Heppleston, A. G.: The pathogenesis of simple pneumokoniosis in coal workers, J Pathol Bacteriol, 1954, *67*, 51.

49. Kleinerman, J.: The pathology of some familiar pneumoconioses, Semin Roentgenol, 1967, *2*, 244.

50. Wells, A. L.: Pulmonary vascular changes in coal workers' pneumoconiosis, J Pathol Bacteriol, 1954, *68*, 573.

51. James, W. R. L., and Thomas, A. J.: Cardiac hypertrophy in coal workers' pneumoconiosis, Br J Ind Med, 1956, *13*, 24.

52. James, W. R. L.: The relationship of tuberculosis to the development of massive pneumoconiosis in coal workers, Br J Tuberc Respir Dis, 1954, *48*, 89.

53. Wagner, J. C., and McCormick, J. N.: Immunological investigations of coal workers' disease, J R Coll Physicians Lond, 1967, *2*, 49.

54. Kilpatrick, G. S., Heppleston, A. G., and Fletcher, C. M.: Cavitation in the massive fibrosis of coal workers' pneumoconiosis, Thorax, 1954, *9*, 260.

55. Seaton, A.: Infectious diseases, in *Occupational Lung Diseases*, W. K. C. Morgan, and A. Seaton, ed., W. B. Saunders Company, Philadelphia, 1975, pp. 348-349.

56. Wagner, J. C., Wusteman, F. S., Edwards, J. H., and Hill, R. J.: The composition of massive lesions in coal miners, Thorax, 1975, *30*, 382.

57. Pemberton, J.: Chronic bronchitis, emphysema, and bronchial spasm in bituminous coal workers, Arch Ind Health, 1956, *13*, 529.

58. Hyatt, R. E., Kistin, A. D., and Mahan, T. K.: Respiratory disease in southern West Virginia coalminers, Am Rev Respir Dis, 1964, *89*, 387.

59. Higgins, I. T. T., Higgins, M. W., Lockshin, M. D., and Canale, N.: Chronic respiratory disease in mining communities in Marion County, West Virginia, Br J Ind Med, 1968, *25*, 165.

60. Lainhart, W. S., Doyle, H. M., Enterline, P. E., Henschel, A., and Kendrick, M. A.: Pneumoconiosis in Appalachian Bituminous Coal Miners, U. S. Department of Health, Education, and Welfare, Washington, D. C., U. S. Government Printing Office, 1969, pp. 77–111.

61. Morgan, W. K. C., Handelsman, L., Kibelstis, J., Lapp, N. L., and Reger, R. B.: Ventilatory capacity and lung volumes of U. S. coal miners, Arch Environ Health, 1974, *28*, 182.

62. Cochrane, A. L., and Higgins, I. T. T.: Pulmonary ventilatory function of coal-miners in various areas in relation to the x-ray category of pneumoconiosis, Br J Prev Soc Med, 1961, *15*, 1.

63. Ashford, J. R., Brown, S., Morgan, D. C., and Rae, S.: The pulmonary ventilatory function of coal miners in the United Kingdom, Am Rev Respir Dis, 1968, *97*, 810.

64. Higgins, I. T. T., and Oldham, P. D.: Ventilatory capacity in miners, Br J Ind Med, 1962, *19*, 65.

65. Muir, D. C. F.: Pulmonary function in miners working in British collieries: Epidemiological investigations by the National Coal Board, Bull Physiopathol Respir (Nancy), 1975, *11*, 403.

66. Ulmer, W. T., and Reichel, G.: Functional impairment in coal workers' pneumoconiosis, Ann N Y Acad Sci, 1972, *200*, 405.

67. Gilson, J. C., and Hugh-Jones, P.: Lung Function in Coal Workers' Penumoconiosis, Med Res Counc Spec Rep Ser (Lond), No. 290, H. M. Stationery Office, 1955.

68. O'Shea, J., Lapp, N. L., Russakoff, A. D., Reger, R. B., and Morgan, W. K. C.: Determination of lung volumes from chest films, Thorax, 1970, *25*, 544.

69. Morgan, W. K. C., Burgess, D. B., Lapp, N. L., Seaton, A., and Reger, R. B.: Hyperinflation of the lungs in coal miners, Thorax, 1971, *26*, 585.

70. Morgan, W. K. C., Seaton, A., Burgess, D. B., Lapp, N. L., and Reger, R. B.: Lung volumes in working coal miners, Ann N Y Acad Sci, 1972, *200*, 478.

71. Needham, C. D., Rogan, M. C., and McDonald, I.: Normal standards for lung volumes, intrapulmonary gas-mixing, and maximal breathing capacity, Thorax, 1954, *9*, 313.

72. Mead, J.: The lung's "quiet zone", N Engl J Med, 1970, *282*, 1318.

73. Gaensler, E. A., Hoffman, L., and Ellicott, M. F.: Troubles de la diffusion et fibrose inter-

stitielle dans la silicose, Poumon Coeur, 1960, *16*, 1137.

74. Rasmussen, D. L., Laquer, W. A., Futterman, P., Warren, D. H., and Nelson, C. W.: Pulmonary impairment in southern West Virginia coal miners, Am Rev Respir Dis, 1968, *98*, 658.

75. Rasmussen, D. L., and Nelson, C. W.: Respiratory function in southern Appalachian coal miners, Am Rev Respir Dis. 1971, *103*, 240.

76. Rasmussen, D. L.: Impairment of oxygen transfer in dyspneic, nonsmoking soft coal miners, J Occup Med, 1971, *13*, 300.

77. Rasmussen, D. L.: Patterns of physiological impairment in coal workers' pneumoconiosis, Ann N Y Acad Sci, 1972, *200*, 455.

78. Gaensler, E. A.: Discussion, Ann N Y Acad Sci, 1972, *200*, 463.

79. Seaton, A., Lapp, N. L., and Morgan, W. K. C.: The relationship of pulmonary impairment in simple coal workers' pneumoconiosis to type of radiographic opacity, Br J Ind Med, 1972, *29*, 50.

80. Cotes, J. E., Deivanayagam, C. N., Field, G. B., and Billiet, L.: Relation between type of simple pneumoconiosis (p or m) and lung function, in *Inhaled Particles III*, vol. 2, W. H. Walton, ed., Unwin Brothers, Old Woking, 1971, p. 633.

81. Lapp, N. L., and Seaton, A.: Pulmonary function, in *Pulmonary Reactions to Coal Dust*: A Review of United States Experience, M. M. Key, L. E. Kerr, and M. Bundy, ed., Academic Press, New York and London, 1971, p. 215.

82. Sartorelli, E., Baraldi, V., Grieco, A., and Zedda, S.: La capacita di diAusione polmonare dei gas nei silicoti, Med Lav, 1963, *54*, 191.

83. Frans, A., Veriter, C., and Brasseur, L.: Pulmonary diffusing capacity for carbon monoxide in simple coal workers' pneumoconiosis, Bull Physiopathol Respir (Nancy), 1975, *11*, 479.

84. Billiet, L., and Ulburghs, M.: Alveolo-capillair bloc door kleinvlekkige silicose: Commentaar big 4 gevallen, Acta Tuberc Pneumol Belg, 1966, *57*, 151.

85. Cotes, J. E., and Field, G. B.: Lung gas exchange in simple pneumoconiosis of coal workers, Br J Ind Med, 1972, *29*, 268.

86. Cotes, J. E., and Rivers, D.: Relation entre la fonction alveolo-capillaire, le pronostic et les decouvertes d'autopsie dans les pneumopathies chroniques, Poumon Coeur, 1960, *16*, 1121.

87. Lyons, J. P., Ryder, R., Campbell, H., and Gough, J.: Pulmonary disability in coal workers' pneumoconiosis, Br Med J, 1972, *1*, 713.

88. Englert, M., and DeCoster, A.: La capacité de diffusion pulmonaire dans l'anthracosilicose micronodulaire, J Fr Med Chir Thorac, 1965, *19*, 159.

89. Kanagami, H., Katsura, T., Shiroishi, K., Baba, K., and Ebina, T.: Studies on the pulmonary diffusing capacity by the carbon monoxide breath-holding technique. II. Patients with various pulmonary diseases, Acta Med Scand, 1961, *169*, 595.

90. Teculescu, D., Muica, N., and Preda, N.: Impairment of pulmonary mixing in simple and complicated silicosis, Bull Physiopathol Respir (Nancy), 1975, *11*, 447.

91. Pivoteau, C., and Dechoux, J.: Le retentissement fonctionnel des pneumoconioses a opacités fines des mineurs de charbon sans troubles ventilatoires, Respiration, 1972, *29*, 161.

92. Kibelstis, J. A.: Diffusing capacity in bituminous coal miners, Chest, 1973, *63*, 501.

93. Motley, H. L.: Pulmonary function studies in bituminous coal miners, W. Va Med J, 1950, *46*, 8.

94. Motley, H. L, Lang, L. P., and Gordon, B.: Pulmonary emphysema and ventilation measurement in one hundred anthracite coal miners with respiratory complaints, Am Rev Tuberc, 1949, *59*, 270.

95. Motley, H. L., Lang, L. P., and Gordon, B.: Studies on the respiration gas exchange in one hundred anthracite coal miners with pulmonary complaints, Am Rev Tuberc, 1950, *61*, 201.

96. Ferris, B. G., and Frank, N. R.: Pulmonary function in coal miners, J Occup Med, 1962, *4*, 274.

97. Lapp, N. L., and Morgan, W. K. C.: Cardiorespiratory function in United States coal workers, Bull Physiopathol Respir (Nancy), 1975, *11*, 527.

98. Brasseur, L.: L'Exploration Fonctionelle Pulmonaire dans la Pneumoconiose des Houilleurs, Arscia, Brussells, 1963.

99. Worth, G., Gasthaus, L., Muysers, K., and Siehoff, F.: Neuere Ergebnisse atemphysiologischer Untersuchungen von Kohlenbergarbeitern unter Berucksichtigung von Silikose, Bronchitis und Emphysem. III. Mitteilung, Alveolo-arterielle Sauerstoff-und Kohlensauere druck differenzen, Arch Gewerbepath Gewerbehyg, 1961, *18*, 581.

100. Stanek, V., Widimsky, J., Kasalicky, J., Navratil, M., Daum, S., and Levinsky, L.: The pulmonary gas exchange during exercise in patients with pulmonary fibrosis, Scand J Respir Dis, 1967, *48*, 11.

101. Stanescu, D.: Pulmonary impairment in coal miners, Am Rev Respir Dis, 1969, *100*, 106.

102. Lapp, N. L., Seaton, A., Kaplan, K. C., Hunsaker, M. R., and Morgan, W. K. C.: Pulmonary hemodynamics in symptomatic coal miners, Am Rev Respir Dis, 1971, *104*, 418.

103. Lapp, N. L., Seaton, A., Kaplan, K. C., Hunsaker, M. R., and Morgan, W. K. C.: Pulmonary hemodynamics in coal workers' pneumoconiosis, in *Inhaled Particles III*, W. H. Walton, ed., Unwin Brothers, Old Woking, 1971, pp. 645–656.

104. Seaton, A., Lapp, N. L., and Chang, C. H. J.:

Lung perfusion scanning in coal workers' pneumoconiosis, Am Rev Respir Dis, 1971, *103*, 338.

105. Stoeckle, J. D., Hardy, H. L., King, W. B., Jr., and Nemiah, J. C.: Respiratory disease in U. S. soft coal miners: Clinical and etiological considerations, J Chronic Dis, 1962, *15*, 887.

106. Kremer, R., and Lavenne, L.: La circulation pulmonaire dans les pneumoconioses, Poumon Coeur, 1966, *22*, 767.

107. Kremer, R., Timmerman, G., Baudrez, J., and Lambrecht, P.: Hemodynamique pulmonaire dans les pneumoconioses des houilleurs, Rev Inst Hyg Mines, 1967, *22*, 3.

108. Kremer, R.: Pulmonary hemodynamics in coal workers' pneumoconiosis, Ann N Y Acad Sci, 1972, *200*, 413.

109. Navratil, M., Widimsky, J., and Kasalicky, J.: Relationships of pulmonary hemodynamics and ventilation and distribution in silicosis, Bull Physiopathol Respir (Nancy), 1968, *4*, 349.

110. Seaton, A., Lapp, N. L., and Morgan, W. K. C.: Lung mechanics and frequency dependence of compliance in coal miners, J Clin Invest, 1972, *51*, 1203.

111. Lapp, N. L., and Seaton, A.: Lung mechanics in coal workers' pneumoconiosis, Ann N Y Acad Sci, 1972, *200*, 433.

112. Morgan, W. K. C., Lapp, N. L., and Morgan, E. J.: The early detection of occupational lung disease, Br J Dis Chest, 1974, *68*, 75.

113. Lapp, N. L., Hankinson, J. L., Burgess, D. B., and O'Brien, R.: Changes in ventilatory function in coal miners after a work shift, Arch Environ Health, 1972, *24*, 204.

114. Lapp, N. L., Block, J., Boehlecke, B., Lippmann, M., Morgan, W. K. C., and Reger, R. B.: Closing volume in coal miners, Am Rev Respir Dis, 1976, *113*, 155.

115. Hall, D. R., Lapp, N. L., Reger, R., and Seaton, A.: Small airways disease in coal miners: A longitudinal study, Bull Physiopathol Respir (Nancy), 1975, *11*, 863.

116. Caplan, A.: Certain unusual appearances in the chest film of miners suffering from pneumoconiosis, Thorax, 1953, *8*, 29.

117. Miall, W. E., Caplan, A., Cochrane, A. L., Kilpatrick, G. S., and Oldham, P.: An epidemiological study of rheumatoid arthritis associated characteristic chest x-ray appearances in coal workers, Br Med J, 1953, *2*, 1231.

118. Gough, J., Rivers, D., and Seal, R. M. E.: Pathological studies of modified pneumoconiosis in coal miners with rheumatoid arthritis, Thorax, 1955, *10*, 9.

119. Caplan, A., Payne, R. B., and Withey, J. L.: A broader concept of Caplan's syndrome related to rheumatoid factors, Thorax, 1962, *17*, 205.

120. Lippman, M., Eckert, H. L., Hahon, W., and Morgan, W. K. C.: The presence of circulating antinuclear and rheumatoid factors in United States coal miners, Ann Intern Med, 1973, *79*, 807.

121. Burrell, R.: Immunological aspects of coal workers' pneumoconiosis, Ann N Y Acad Sci, 1972, *200*, 94.

122. Burrell, R., Flaherty, D. K., and Schreiber, J. E.: Immunological studies of experimental coal workers' pneumoconiosis, Presented at the Fourth International Conference on Inhaled Particles, Edinburgh, September 1975.

123. Medical Research Council: Statement on Chronic Bronchitis and Occupation, Br Med J, 1966, *1*, 101.

124. Reichel, G., and Ulmer, W. T.: The interrelationship of coal miners pneumoconiosis and bronchitis in *Inhaled Particles III*, W. H. Walton, ed., vol. 2, 1971, Unwin Brothers, London, p. 897.

125. Minnette, A.: Role de empoussierage professionnel dans la production des bronchites chronique des mineurs de charbon in *Inhaled Particles III*, vol. 2, W. H. Walton, ed., 1971, Unwin Brothers, London, p. 873.

126. Lowe, C. R., and Khosla, T.: Chronic bronchitis in ex-coal miners working in the steel industry, Br J Ind Med, 1972, *29*, 45.

127. Rogan, J. M., Attfield, M. D., Jacobsen, M., Rae, S., Walker, D. D., and Walton, W. H.: Role of dust in working environment in development of chronic bronchitis in British coal miners, Br J Ind Med, 1973, *30*, 217.

128. Hankinson, J. L., Reger, R. B., Fairman, R. P., Lapp, N. L., and Morgan, W. K. C.: Factors influencing expiratory flow rates in coal miners, Presented at the Fourth International Conference on Inhaled Particles, Edinburgh, Scotland, September 1975.

129. Sluis-Cremer, G. K., Walters, L. G., and Sichel, H. S.: Chronic bronchitis in miners and nonminers: An epidemiological survey of a community in the gold area of Transvaal, Br J Ind Med, 1967, *24*, 1.

130. Merchant, J. A., Kilburn, K. H., O'Fallon, W. M., Hamilton, J. D., and Lumsden, J. C.: Byssinosis and chronic bronchitis among textile workers, Ann Intern Med, 1972, *76*, 423.

131. McDonald, J. C., Becklake, M. R., Fournier-Massey, G., and Rossiter, C. E.: Respiratory symptoms in chrysotile asbestos mines and mill workers of Quebec, Arch Environ Health, 1972, *24*, 358.

132. Heppleston, A. G., and Leopold, J. G.: Chronic pulmonary emphysema, Am J Med, 1961, *31*, 179.

133. Ryder, R., Lyons, J. P., Campbell, H., and Gough, J.: Emphysema in coal workers' pneumoconiosis, Br Med J, 1970, *3*, 481.

134. Gilson, J. C., and Oldham, P. D.: Coal workers' pneumoconiosis, Br Med J, 1970, *4*, 305.

135. Wates, W. E., Cochrane, A. L., and Moore, F.: Mortality in punctiform type of coal workers' pneumoconiosis, Br J Ind Med, 1974, *31*, 196.

Asbestos-Related Diseases of the Lung and Other Organs: Their Epidemiology and Implications for Clinical Practice[1,2]

MARGARET R. BECKLAKE[3]

Contents

____

[1] From the Departments of Epidemiology and Health, and of Experimental Medicine, McGill University, and from the Department of Medicine, Royal Victoria Hospital, Montreal, Quebec, Canada.

[2] Requests for reprints should be addressed to Department of Epidemiology and Health, McGill University, 3775 University Street, Montreal, Quebec, Canada.

[3] Associate of the Medical Research Council of Canada.

Introduction

Although the fire-resistant qualities of asbestos have been recognized since ancient times (1, 2), its commercial exploitation was modest until the latter part of the nineteenth century, when as a result of the industrial revolution, the need arose to develop the means of insulating the steam engine (2). The discovery in 1877 and subsequent development in the 1880s of the extensive chrysotile deposits in eastern Quebec was followed by further exploitation of the already known and extensive deposits in the Ural mountains in Russia and of the more limited deposits in Italy and Cyprus (2, 3). The existence of blue asbestos deposits in the Cape (South Africa) was recorded in the early nineteenth century, but large scale mining only began in the past decade. Amosite, discovered in the Transvaal in 1907, was first commercially extracted in 1908 (2). Milling of the fiber to release it from the ore is usually done at the mine-head, and the fiber is then bagged and exported to the factories of the industrialized world, in particular Britain, other European countries, and the United States.

The world sources of production and use of this mineral are shown in figure 1 in a way that underlines the need for worldwide appreciation of its potential threat to health; figure 2 traces the history of medical recognition of its health effects in relation to the commercial exploitation of the mineral. Thus, adverse effects on health were observed in the early 1900s and first reported in 1907 (1), and it is now recognized that exposure to asbestos may lead to the pathologic conditions listed in table 1. These include fibrosis of varying degrees and virulence of the lungs and pleura; and neoplasms of the lung, pleura, peritoneum, gastrointestinal tract (5–9), and, possibly, the larynx (11–14), ovary (15), and breast (16). Despite legislative action aimed at controlling the health effects in Europe and North America (Gilson, 5, p. 696), deleterious effects on health continued to be reported. Indeed, asbestos-related lung disease has been called "the occupation illness of the 60s," a description that also reflects the extent of current public concern for this health hazard (1).

Although recognition of the association between asbestos exposure and the various health effects listed in table 1 was made initially by shrewd clinical, pathologic, and epidemiologic observation, exploration of the nature of the association with asbestos exposure has subsequently been made by epidemiologic studies. Results of such studies are frequently found in journals of epidemiology, public health, and environmental health, rather than in clinical journals, and in reports of international conferences not covered by the usual clinical reference systems, such as the Cumulative Index (5–9). The published proceedings of these conferences, all internationally supported, in keeping with the international nature of asbestos use, provide excellent source material to which extensive reference is made in this review. For this reason, the proceedings of each conference are cited only once, in references 5 to 9. Individual presentations are subsequently identified in the text by the name of the first author and page number.

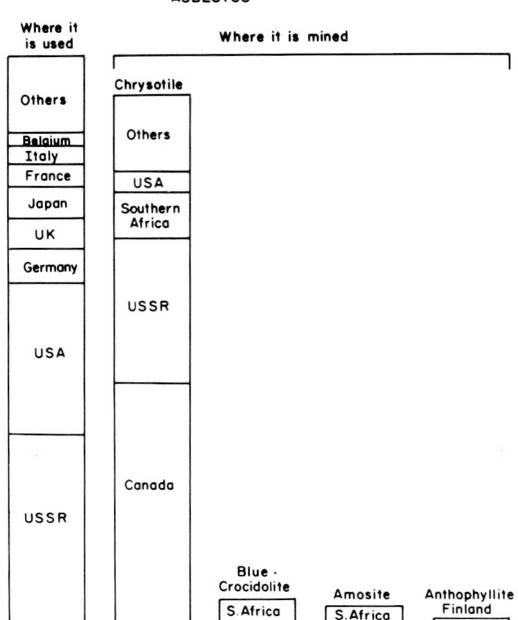

Fig. 1. [From Smither (4); reprinted by permission of publisher.] Asbestos: where it is mined and where it is used. This figure was based on world consumption for 1970, estimated at 3,000,000 tons. The figure for 1974 is estimated at 5,100,000 tons, with Russian production now surpassing the production of the western world.

Nevertheless, the practicing physician is often the first source of medical help for the exposed person whose health is affected, particularly if the exposure is related to the use, rather than production of, asbestos products, or if exposure is nonoccupational, i.e., by neighborhood or household contact.

It has been said by Weiss (17) that "the clinician sees the sick patient against his memories of individuals with a similar constellation of abnormalities half-buried in his apperceptive background and in relation to what he recalls from the literature, usually written by peers with the same small field of vision" and that he "founders into erroneous conclusions because he looks only at the people directly in front of him." By contrast, the epidemiologist sees "the sick patient as an impersonal unit in relation to a populational universe" and "misses a truth because it is buried in a mass of data." Perhaps these remarks apply only to the bad clinician and the bad epidemiologist. Nevertheless, the differences in approach seem to be sufficient to merit a review that attempts to bridge the gap; thus, the

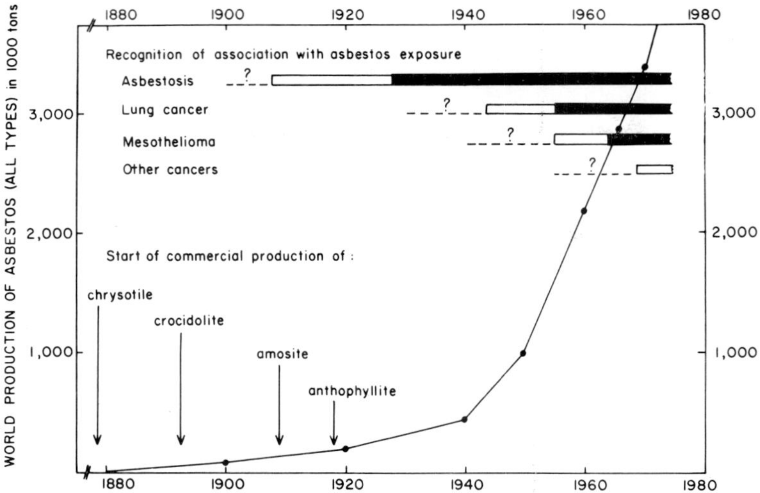

Fig. 2. Diagrammatic representation of the growth of the asbestos industry and the recognition of the associated biologic effects. The following symbols indicate the association with asbestos: ? = suspected; ☐ = probable; ■ = established.

purpose of the present review is to evaluate current information, particularly that obtained from epidemiologic studies, in light of the implications of this knowledge for clinical practice.

The Asbestos Minerals

Physical Characteristics and Fiber Types

The physician may well question the relevance of the physics and chemistry of the asbestos minerals to the state of his art. The answer is contained in Gilson's summary of the 1964 New York Conference on the "Biological Effects of Asbestos" (5), in which he identified one of the

questions requiring further investigation: "Is the type of asbestos an important factor in the risk of asbestosis, bronchial carcinoma, mesothelioma, and other tumors?" Because subsequent observations have suggested that this is so (see later in this review), knowledge of the type of asbestos to which a person has been exposed should guide the practicing physician in establishing a diagnosis and estimating a prognosis.

Asbestos is the general term given to a group of minerals that are fibrous in character and resistant to high temperatures, the two qualities on which their industrial use depends. The most important commercial fibers (shown in table

TABLE 1

PATHOLOGIC EFFECTS OF ASBESTOS EXPOSURE IN MAN

Organ	Effect	Association with Asbestos Exposure*	Reference
Skin	Asbestos corns	Established	5–9
Larynx	Carcinoma	Possible	11–14
Lungs	"Asbestos" bodies and/or fibers	Established	5–9
	Diffuse interstitial fibrosis (asbestosis)	Established	5–9
	Carcinoma (bronchial)	Cofactor with cigarettes	5–9
Pleura	Hyaline plaques and calcification	Established	5–9
	Malignant mesothelioma	Established†	5–9
	Pleural effusion	Possible	10
Peritoneum	Malignant mesothelioma	Established†	5–9
Gastrointestinal tract	Neoplasia	Established	5–9
Ovary	Carcinoma	Remotely possible	15
Breast	Carcinoma	Remotely possible	16

*Association thought to be causal, except where indicated.
†Association, not cause, established.

2) are chrysotile (a white, usually long, silky fiber), crocidolite (a harsher blue fiber), amosite (brown and harsh), and anthophyllite, chiefly mined and used in Finland. In addition, some of these fibrous minerals also occur in the bearer rock of mines developed primarily for the exploitation of other minerals, such as talc, mica (18), and iron, as, for example, in the iron mines at the head of Lake Superior and in Labrador.

Differences in the physical properties of the various fibers determine their particular commercial usefulness. Thus, for example, chrysotile, which consists of long, mainly pliable fibers that split progressively into finer fibrils, lends itself to incorporation into textiles, whereas crocidolite and amosite, which are more acid resistant, are of particular value for marine insulation. Certain asbestos cement products may be made from blends of chrysotile and amosite and/or crocidolite. These differences in the physical properties of the fibers (and in consequence, in their aerodynamic behavior) may account for differences in the health effects of exposure; indeed, it has been argued that "only by relating experimental biologic evidence with the variations in physical size and form . . . can we ultimately arrive at valid medical conclusions" (18). This question is discussed in a later section of the present review.

Uses of Asbestos: Occupations at Risk

World production and use of asbestos have grown greatly since the late nineteenth century; between 1877 and 1967, asbestos production and use increased from 50 tons to 4,000,000 tons per year, an 80,000-fold increase. For industrialized countries, such as Britain and the United States, the increase in asbestos use between 1910 and 1970 was 7-fold (18, 19). This reflects increases in volume of manufactured goods as well as in the variety of uses developed for the material. These are outlined broadly in table 2.

Appreciation of the wide variety of uses of asbestos is important to the physician and serves as an indicator of the many occupations potentially at risk from exposure (table 3). These occupations include asbestos mining, milling, and handling in preparation for its use, either directly (as, for instance, in spraying when mixed with oil) or for its incorporation into the manufacture of a great variety of asbestos-containing products. The latter may be classified broadly into textiles, asbestos cement and other construction products, paper products, friction materials, and insulation products. It is also used in the chemical and plastics industries, where its binding properties (in particular, the positive charge of chrysotile) enhances its union with filler and pigment (Lindell, 7, p. 323).

Once incorporated into manufactured items, the fiber is relatively well bound and is therefore less likely to pose a health hazard to the many workers who use the newly manufactured products (see Secondary Uses, table 2), so long as the product is not sawn, disrupted, or cut in any way; however, asbestos fibers are virtually indestructible. Thompson, 5, p. 196) aptly describes this as a "half-life of an infinity of years." The fibers may be released into the atmosphere again when the original product is removed, replaced, or destroyed, as may occur in the construction and shipbuilding industries, in connection with demolition, repair, and/ or refitting. Exposures of this sort, particularly if they occur in a contained environment, such as the hold of a ship undergoing refitting, may involve workers whose primary job has nothing to do with asbestos, e.g., welders or masons. Indeed, failure to appreciate these sources of exposure in both construction and shipbuilding industries (19, 20) probably accounts for the re-emergence of asbestos-related disease in the 1960s. There appears to be no direct information on the numbers of workers at risk in different countries, other than an estimate of 250,000 persons for the United States in 1972 (21).

The reason for including the information on the occupations at risk (table 3) in a clinical review is to offer the physician an overview of the uses of the mineral, so that when faced with an individual with an illness that may be asbestos related, he can formulate a systematic enquiry into the person's occupational history. The physician should thus cover possible exposures in mining, milling, and manufacturing, as well as in the application of manufactured products containing asbestos, directly, or at the time of demolition or replacement (19, 20, 22–26). The physician must not only seek the details of the patient's own jobs, past and present, but must also ascertain whether this work was carried out at the side of other workers whose jobs involved the handling of asbestos products or materials, particularly if in a closed or poorly ventilated environment.

TABLE 2

VARIETIES OF ASBESTOS: PROPERTIES, SOURCES, AND USAGE*

Mineral Type	Serpentine	Amphiboles				
Chemistry, approximate	$Mg_3Si_2O_5(OH)_4$	$X_{2-3}Y_5(Si,A1)_8O_{22}(OH)_2$ with X,Y representing different elements				
Fiber type	Chrysotile (White)	Crocidolite (Blue)	Ambosite (Brown)	Anthophyllite	Tremolite	Actinolite
Main elements determining specific composition	Mg	Na, Fe^{2+}, Fe^{3+}	Fe^{2+}, Mg	Similar to amosite, but more Fe^{2+}, less Mg	Ca, Mg	Like tremolite, but contains Fe^{2+}
Physical properties						
Tensile strength, 1,000 psi	350–450	500	175–350	240	< 75	
Flexibility	Very good	Good	Poor	Fair to brittle	Brittle	Brittle
Acid resistance	Poor	Good	Good	Fair to good	Fair	Very good
Texture	Silky to harsh	Harsh	Coarse	Harsh to soft	Harsh to soft	Harsh
Heat resistance	500° C	200° C	200° C	200° C	Fair to good	Very good
Major sources, present and past	Canada (Quebec, B. C., Yukon, Newfoundland, Ontario) Russia (Urals, Siberia) S. Rhodesia Botswana Swaziland Australia (NSW) Cyprus Italy United States (Vt.,† Ariz., Calif.)	S. Africa (N. W. Cape, Transvaal) Bolivia W. Australia†	S. Africa (Tvl)	Finland United States (Georgia† Carolinas)	Italy	Not usually commercially exploited
World use, approximate %	93	3.5	2.5	< 1	< 1	
Industrial uses	Textiles Cement products Friction materials Insulation** "Paper" products	Textiles Pressure pipes Cement products Felts for plastics	Cement Plastic reinforcement Refractory tiles Pressure pipes	Cement (limited) Chemical industry	Chemical industry (as fillers and filters) Talc fillers	

*Information collected by Dr. Graham Gibbs from the following reference sources: Zussman (3), Speil and Leineweber (18), N. W. Hendry, in (5), p. 12; R. Gaze, in (5), p. 23; K. V. Lindell, in (7), p. 323.

†No longer in operation.

**Being phased out.

TABLE 3

OCCUPATIONS AT RISK FOR ASBESTOS EXPOSURE IN MINING,
MILLING, MANUFACTURING, AND SECONDARY USES*

Process	Products Made or Used	Jobs Potentially at Risk
Production		
Mining		Rock mining, loading, trucking
Milling		Crushing, milling
Handling		Transport workers, dockers, loaders, those who unpack jute sacks (recently replaced with sacks that do not permit fibers to escape)
Primary uses in		
Spray insulation	Spray of fiber mixed with oil	Spray insulators (construction, ship-building)
Filler and grouting		
Manufacturing of		
Textiles	Cloth, curtains, lagging, protective clothing, mailbags, padding, conveyor belts	Blending, carding, spinning, twisting, winding, braiding, weaving, slurry mixing, laminating, moulding, drying
Cement products	Sheets, pipes, roofing shingles, gutters, ventilation shafts, flower pots	Blending, slurry preparation, rolling, pressing, pipe cutting
"Paper" products	Millboard, roofing felt, fine quality electrical papers, flooring felt, fillers	
Friction materials	Automotive products: gaskets, clutch plates, brake linings	
Insulation products	Pipe and boiler insulation, bulkhead linings for ships	
Application		
Construction		
New construction	Boards and tiles; putties, caulk, paints, joint fillers; cement products (tiles, pipes, siding, shingles) Insulation materials	Directly, carpenters, laggers, painters, tile layers, insulation workers, sheet metal and heating equipment workers, masons; indirectly all other workers on construction sites, such as plumbers, welders, electricians
Repair, demolition		Demolition workers for all of these
Shipbuilding		
Construction	Insulation materials (boards, mattresses, cloth) for engines, hull, decks, lagging of ventilation and water pipes, cables	Laggers, refitters, strippers, steam fitters, sailmakers, joiners, ship-wrights, engine fitters, masons, painters, welders, caulkers
Repair, refits	Insulation materials, as described for "construction"	Directly, all above jobs on refits, dry dock, and other repairs operations Indirectly, maintenance fitters and repair men, electricians, plumbers, welders, carpenters
Automotive industry		
Manufacture	Gaskets, brake linings, undercoating	Installation of brake linings, gaskets, and so on
Repair	Gaskets, brake linings, undercoating	Service men, brake repairmen, body repairmen, auto mechanics

*Information collated by Dr. Graham Gibbs from references 2, 3, 18–20, and 22–26.

Indirect Exposure (Domestic, Neighborhood, Environmental)

Exposure to asbestos fiber is not confined to the place of work (27); the search for exposure in the background of patients with mesothelioma (10, 28–31) has brought to light several forms of indirect nonoccupational exposure. The occurrence of mesothelioma in the family members of asbestos workers led to the recognition of indirect domestic exposure; the source here is presumed to be the dust brought home in the worker's overalls (10, 31). Likewise, the association between residence near a mine, mill, or factory and the occurrence of mesothelioma brought to light the importance of neighborhood exposures (27). Such neighborhood exposure is also presumed to account for occurrence of pleural plaques and/or calcification in residents of the mining area of Finland (32). Pleural plaques have also been described in agricultural populations (33–35); in some instances, they have been attributed to the working of soil that contains asbestos fibers, e.g., in Bulgaria (33, 34).

The surprisingly high prevalence of asbestos bodies (as evidence of exposure) in routine autopsies indicates an environmental exposure for the residents of most of the larger cities of the world; however, the amounts in the general atmosphere are small (36), and these autopsy findings should probably be regarded more as an index of exposure rather than of disease potential. The Advisory Committee report that followed the Lyon Conference (7) concluded that "there is at present no evidence of lung damage by asbestos to the general public," and "the amount of asbestos in the lungs of members of the general public is very small compared to those occupationally exposed."

Finally, attention has recently been directed toward the widespread occurrence of asbestos fibers in certain natural water sources (37–40). An event that brought this to the notice of the general public was the discharge of mine tailings containing fiber into Lake Superior, a source of drinking water to many cities in the center of the North American continent (38). It is now also recognized that fibers also occur in many natural waters, particularly in mining regions; however, the Advisory Committee report emanating from the Lyon Conference (7) judged there to be no evidence at present of "an increased cancer risk resulting from asbestos fibers present in water, beverages or food or in the fluids used for the administration of drugs." The question must, however, remain under close scrutiny.

The Fate and Biologic Effects of Inhaled Asbestos Particles

Deposition in the Lung

Whether or not inhaled asbestos fibers will be deposited in the lung depends on the aerodynamic behavior of the particles, the dimensions of the respiratory tract they enter, and the pattern of breathing that carries the particles. The aerodynamic behavior of particles is a function mainly of diameter, but also of size, shape, and density. The varying characteristics of commercially used asbestos fibers make it obvious that the environment to which asbestos workers are exposed will contain particles having great variation in size and composition. These include fibers (so-called if their length is at least 3 times their diameter), which may be long (as long as 200 μm) or short. In addition, a working environment is likely to include a range of smaller particles and/or fibers released from the breakdown and disruption of the primary fiber, as well as those due to any other nonasbestos particles added by the mining or industrial process.

Inhaled asbestos particles follow the moving airstreams with each inspiration, and, once they make contact with any part of the surface of the airways or airspaces, are not resuspended in the expiratory airstreams (41, 42). Deposition of the larger inhaled particles (more than 5 μm in diameter) occurs mainly in the nose (assuming nose breathing) and major airways, owing to inertial impaction and sedimentation. Because of Brownian movement, deposition of the smaller particles (less than 1 μm in diameter) occurs mainly in the more peripheral airways and airspaces. This deposition profile is summarized in figure 3.

Deposition patterns can be profoundly modified by breathing patterns; nose breathing causes a high retention rate, even of small fibers, within the nose (41, 42). However, under working conditions, including heat and exertional stress, most workers resort to mouth breathing. Deeper, slower respirations favor a more even distribution of inspired air, and, thus, a more even distribution of inhaled particles. Lung volume also influences distribution and, possibly, retention patterns, particularly if breathing occurs at less than the normal functional residual capacity (FRC) in the range of airway closure (43, p. 98). Likewise, there is some evidence that the state of the airways in smokers is such that inhaled particles will penetrate less deeply into the bronchial tree and thus tend to be deposited more centrally than in nonsmokers (44).

Pulmonary Clearance

Clearance of particles deposited on the mucous blanket is brisk, with half-times of minutes

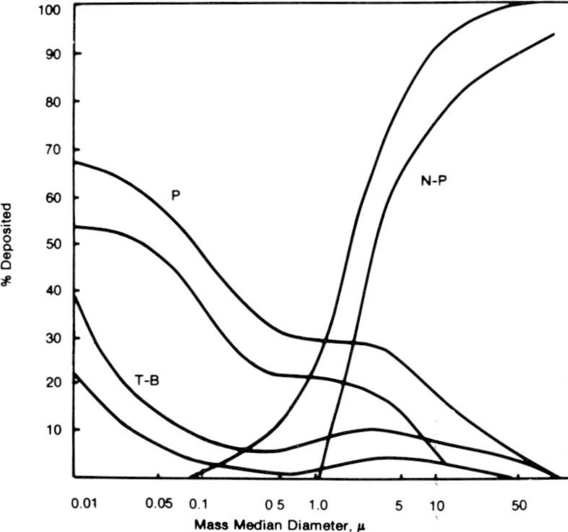

Fig. 3. [From Brain and Valberg (42); reprinted by permission of publisher; copyright 1974, American Medical Association.] Aerosol deposition in respiratory tract. The percentage aerosol deposited was calculated from the assumptions in the model referred to above for a tidal volume of 1,450 ml and a frequency of 15 breaths per min. The profile of deposition of an aerosol is influenced by its effective aerodynamic behavior that (since the distribution of mass for many aerosols is log-normal) may be described by the mass median diameter of the aerosol and its geometric standard deviation. In this figure, per cent aerosol deposited is related directly to the mass median diameter, whereas the 2 lines referring to each lung zone (i.e., N-P, T-B, and P, respectively) indicate the differences in per cent deposition that would result if the geometric standard deviation of the mass median diameter varied from 1.2 to 4.5 μ. N-P = nasopharyngeal surface; T-B = ciliated tracheobronchial surface; P = nonciliated pulmonary surface.

to hours. Mucus and cells from nonciliated airways bearing ingested particles from the major airways are cleared to the pharynx; the material trapped in the nose is also cleared to the pharynx. Here, pulmonary and nasal debris mix with saliva and are swallowed or expectorated (42). This phase of clearance does not appear to be affected by the presence of asbestos lung disease (45) and, under certain circumstances, the effects of smoking in producing bronchitis may even speed this phase of clearance (46, 47).

Particles deposited in the nonciliated regions may be cleared relatively rapidly if they remain on the surface (with a half-time of 24 hours), but once they penetrate fixed tissues, clearance is slowed, with half-times ranging from days to thousands of days (42). It has also been suggested that macrophages decrease the likelihood of fibers penetrating the alveolar walls (42), and

that a system of macrophage recruitment meets onslaughts of free fibers and/or particles. Short fibers (< 5 μm) appear to be readily and completely phagocytosed, but long fibers are not, even when attacked by more than one macrophage, which may lead to cell fusion (Allison, 7, p. 89). Clearance of inhaled particles by these mechanisms is believed to be more than 98 per cent effective for most deposited particles (48).

Penetration, Retention, Distribution, and Mobilization of Uncoated Asbestos Particles within the Lung

The use of electron microscopy has revealed the presence of many, many submicroscopic, uncoated asbestos fibers and fibrils in the lung substance of the exposed worker, far more than was ever imagined when the lung fiber population was evaluated by light microscopy alone (49–51). It is also now evident that the proportion of uncoated to coated fibers (i.e., those that form the core of an asbestos body) is very large, of the order of 75 per cent (49), an observation that suggests a very high penetration and retention rate for the submicroscopic particles released into the working environment. Alternatively, these small fibers and/or particles might represent the breakdown products of what were initially larger fibers that had penetrated the alveolar parts of the lung. A second reason for underestimation of the amount of asbestos fiber retained in the lung is the difficulty encountered in its recovery from lungs at autopsy, compared to that of other pneumoconiosis-producing dusts (Nagelschmidt, 5, p. 64). The difficulty in recovery applies more to chrysotile than to other fibers, presumably because of its greater solubility (magnesium, in particular, tends to be leached out) and, hence, its tendency to break down chemically and physically after prolonged residence (51).

Within the lung, there appears to be a tendency for fibers to accumulate in the peripheral regions of the lower zones as indicated by the early appearance of fibrotic reactions in these areas. This distribution has been attributed to posture and gravity effects (Thomson, 9, p. 138).

Most uncoated particles that have penetrated the lung tissue appear likely to remain where they are, particularly if they are intracellular. Some clearance does occur via lymph channels to hilar and mediastinal nodes, where coated and uncoated particles are seen (Hourihane, 5, p. 647), although this appears to be less than in the case of other fibrogenic dusts, such as silica. This difference in clearance attributed to the greater cytotoxic effect of silica, which tends, therefore, to maintain an extracellular position (50), may explain why hilar node enlargement is a more consistent finding in association with silica exposure than in association with asbestos exposure (52).

Less is known about the penetration of ingested fibers through the wall of the gastrointestinal tract, although animal studies suggest that this does not occur (53), except in the face of a heavy load delivered directly into the stomach (40). What relevance this has to human disease, such as peritoneal mesothelioma, remains to be determined.

Once it has penetrated the lung, the dust appears to remain fixed, but may be remobilized, apparently even from dust macules or scars, the operative mechanism perhaps being episodes of pulmonary edema and/or infection (48). It is believed that such remobilization of dust may result in its excretion, a phenomenon that might explain the rare event of apparent regression of radiologic changes in the worker removed from exposure (Manfreda, Y.: Unpublished data). Alternatively, it may become resequestered and contribute to the extension of disease in the face of no further exposure.

Despite the fact that pleural reactions (effusion, fibrosis, and/or calcification and neoplasm) are common manifestations of asbestos exposure, there is little direct evidence as to how the asbestos gains access to the pleura, which presumably must happen to explain the pleural reactions. Asbestos bodies are rarely seen in the visceral pleura and have never been reported in plaques located in the parietal pleura of exposed persons, even though they may be readily found in the interstitial tissue of the same lung (54). By contrast, asbestos fragments have been found in mesotheliomas even without evidence of asbestosis or coated fibers in the lung (Hourihane, 5, p. 647). This has led to the suggestion that fibers that become coated in the lung are less mobile and less susceptible to lymphatic clearance than uncoated fibers. Thus, electron microscopic studies may reveal many more uncoated fibers in the pleura than anticipated from the scarcity of coated fibers. Alternatively, any fibers that are cleared to subpleural lymphatics may undergo dissolution more readily here than elsewhere in the lung. In any event, information that would shed light on this paradox might well lead to improved understanding of the factors underlying the pathogenesis of mesothelioma.

Coated Asbestos Fibers (Asbestos Bodies)

The coated asbestos fiber was recognized early in the 1900s, because of its characteristic appearance under light microscopy (55). It is usually a rod-shaped structure with clubbed ends, often beaded along its length, is yellow to brown in color, ranges in length from 10 to 30 μm and in thickness from 1 to 6 μm, and has a central, paler core. The coating, consisting of ferritin granules and an amorphous material, probably protein, varies in thickness from very thin to 5 μm (55–57).

On the basis of animal studies, coating is now believed to be an intracellular process and follows the engulfing of particles by macrophages to which they adhere (56). Several macrophages may fuse to engulf large fibers. It is while the fibers are surrounded by partially fused macrophages that coating begins (58). The fiber then becomes incorporated into intracytoplasmic vacuoles, and the first coating material appears to be some form of acid mucopolysaccharide (56). Iron in the form of hemosiderin then accumulates in the cytoplasm of the macrophage. Iron micelles, possibly derived from breakdown of hemoglobin, become subsequently incorporated into the phagosomes, and tend to concentrate around the fiber; eventually, there is clearing of ground substance (57). It is of interest that the process appears to be a progressive one, with the coating increasing with time and uncoated fibers becoming coated months or years after instillation (56); however, because the proportion of uncoated to coated fibers in human lungs appears to remain constant with time (49, 59), there must also be a parallel process of aging and dissolution of the coated fiber. There is some evidence that the coating of a fiber renders it nonfibrogenic. Why some particles become coated and others do not is not understood; however, size may be important, with the typical asbestos body developing only on large particles (greater than 5 μm) that cannot be completely engulfed by one macrophage (58).

It must also be emphasized that not all coated fibers seen in the lung have an asbestos core, and the process of coating is apparently used by the lung in response to a variety of other fibers encountered in the environment. These include glass and cotton fibers, diatomaceous earth, talc, graphite, and carborundum particles (10, 55).

For this reason, the noncommittal term, "ferruginous" body (60), has been suggested as a more exact description in the absence of positive identification of the fiber core. Although accurate identification is now possible using techniques like the electron beam, laser microprobes, ultrasonic disintegration, and mass spectroscopy (55), these techniques are expensive in time and money and will remain research tools for a while (Langer, 7, p. 119). As such, however, they have brought to light certain interesting facts. For instance, it has been shown that although all fiber types may become coated in the laboratory animal (56), in man it is the amphibole fiber that is found more frequently as the core of a ferruginous body than the chrysotile fiber (49, 59), even when both types of uncoated fiber are seen in the lung (Pooley 7, p. 222). The significance of this observation remains to be determined; it may simply represent the relatively high solubility of chrysotile in relation to the other asbestos fibers.

Cellular Effects

Neither the original theory that the fibrogenic effect of asbestos fibers and particles was due to physical irritation nor the solubility theory, attributing their action to leached-out metal ions and/or silicic acid, can satisfactorily explain all of the experimental and clinical observations (Wagner, 5, p. 691). This leads to the hypothesis that host factors, in particular the immune system, might be important, either because of the production or localization of abnormal globulins in alveolar phagocytes or fibroblasts, or because of autoantibodies developing in response to lysis of phagocytes.

The use of tissue and cell culture techniques has further increased understanding of the biologic effects of asbestos at the cellular level (Allison, 7, p. 89). Potential target cells in man are the macrophages (which are responsible for phagocytosis), mesothelial cells, alveolar epithelial cells (which may undergo malignant transformation), and fibroblasts (which participate in the fibrogenic reaction). Two types of cytogenic effects have been detected, an early one attributed to the interaction of asbestos with the cellular membrane, increasing permeability (a reaction that is inhibited by serum and other biologic macromolecules), and a late reaction attributed to inter-reaction of the already ingested particles with the membranes around the secondary lysosomes. Because of the findings of similar direct cytotoxic effects on

macrophages and mesothelial cells, but much less often on the fibroblast, it is believed that fibrogenesis may therefore be evoked through the macrophage response. In addition, there are differences between the various asbestos types in their cytotoxic effects, chrysotile showing more potent cytoxicity and capacity for hemolysis than amosite and crocidolite.

Effects at the organ level are presumed to result from the numbers of cells involved, the sites of their accumulation (e.g., the tendency for macrophages to aggregate in peribronchiolar locations), and the cumulative effects of continued assault from inhaled fibers and particles. It is not known whether the development of such changes is determined primarily by the amount of dust accumulated in the lung (to be discussed in detail under Dose Relationship) or whether it depends to an important extent on a person's biologic susceptibility. Experiments in animals and epidemiologic data in man suggest that both are important. The relevant evidence will be considered separately under the various asbestos-related lung diseases.

Dose Relationship of Biological Responses to Asbestos Exposure

The concept of a dose relationship of response to stimulus, already familiar in pharmacology, was introduced by Hatch (61) in an effort to throw light on the nature of the apparent variation in the biologic response to inhaled dust. (Why is one person affected and not the man who works beside him?) Its importance is obvious, not only as a tool for explaining variations in biologic response, but for the very practical reason that inherent in a dose relationship lies the information for a logical and scientific basis on which to establish the criteria for environmental control. Moreover, without such a relationship, the association between dose and response is probably not causal.

Hatch's concept (61), illustrated in figure 4, takes into account the possibility of differences in responsiveness between persons (or between populations) by introducing the third dimension. The implication is that a given dose-response curve can be developed for a given person (or population), but that it will be applicable only to another person (or population) of the same "susceptibility." In this context, susceptibility might be related to any of several biologic characteristics, for instance, the efficiency of clearance mechanisms in the lung, the anatomic characteristics of the lung/airway sys-

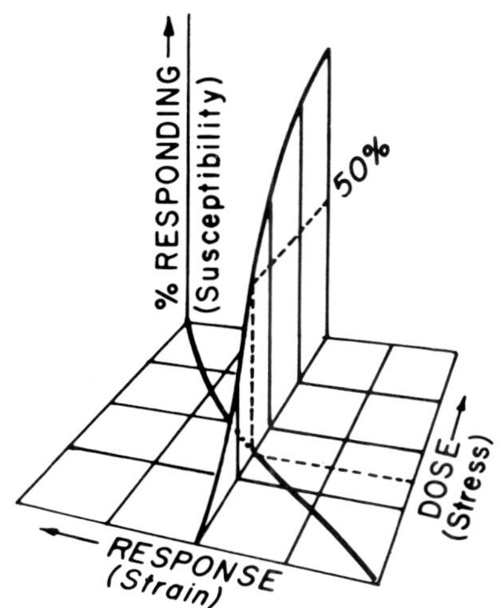

Fig. 4. [Modified from Hatch (61); reprinted by permission of publisher; copyright 1968, American Medical Association.] Dose response for a population. The curve on the horizontal plane portrays the dose-response relationship for a population of susceptibility such that 50 per cent respond to the dose indicated by the dotted line. If only 25 per cent were responsive to that dose, the curve would be proportionately displaced downward toward the dose axis; if 75 per cent were responsive, it would be appropriately displaced upward.

tem, or the physical fitness of the person (less fit persons ventilate more for a given work load). Alternatively, susceptibility might be considered in the immunologic sense.

A major problem, however, in applying the dose-response concept to the study of asbestos-related disease in animals and man lies in the measurement of dose. Presumably, the relevant dose (in Hatch's terms, the dose delivered at the critical site in the body) is the amount of asbestos dust and fiber retained in the lung, i.e., the amount inhaled less the amount exhaled and/or cleared from the lung. Although estimates of the amount inhaled can be derived from direct measurements of dust and fiber in the working environment and from ventilation volume, there is no practical way to measure the amount of dust exhaled and/or cleared from the lung, either in the laboratory animal or in man. Thus, at best, it is possible to measure (or estimate) only the first one half of the dose equation, i.e., the concentration and amount of dust inspired (in Hatch's terms, the magnitude of exposure to external conditions that give rise to stress).

This shortcoming is perhaps less crucial under experimental conditions in which animals can be raised throughout life in environments with different, but known and constant, dust concentrations. Such studies have, in general, shown dose relationships for amount of fibrosis and cancer risk (62). In addition, it seems possible that mathematical computation, taking into account intermittency and pulse exposures (42), may enable future studies to make even better estimates of dose.

In epidemiologic studies, estimates of dose have had to be much more crude, being based on the number of years of service in an industry (63–68); the number of years since first exposure (63, 69, 70); or the total years of exposure, together with an estimate of the dustiness of a worker's job (71–79); or cumulative dust exposure calculated from dust concentrations for given jobs. Doses may be calculated for each individual worker on the basis of his or her work history (80–95), or for groups of workers in given jobs in a given industry (96–98). In all of these studies, there has been the problem of calculating the dose for workers whose exposure usually extended into the remote past, with information about dust concentrations being at best scanty and incomplete and in most instances nonexistent.

Despite the shortcomings of the methods for estimating dose, a relationship of estimated dose to response has, nevertheless, been a consistent finding (table 4). This consistency has been true with exposures encountered in mining, manufacturing, and secondary usage, including removal of old asbestos insulation. Furthermore, it applied to all of the responses examined, i.e., lung fibrosis, as reflected by symptoms (64, 77, 92), lung function (64, 78, 84, 87) and radiographic changes (65, 69, 88, 95), and lung cancer, as reflected in mortality statistics (63, 66–68, 71, 74, 77, 79–83, 85, 93). For mesothelioma, in which much less exposure seems to be capable of producing a response in certain circumstances (see neighborhood and domestic exposure), there is also some evidence for a dose effect using fiber counts in the lungs at autopsy as a measure of exposure. A more complete discussion of dose-response relationships follows in the sections devoted to various asbestos-related lung diseases.

It must be pointed out that although dose-response relationships are evident to a greater or lesser extent for all responses, the degree of correlation is surprisingly low, perhaps because one seldom, if ever, finds more than a 50 per cent response rate, even in those exposed to the heaviest doses. In addition, the response is usually the result of past, rather than current, exposures. This poor correlation has led to the current interest in "susceptibility," i.e., factors accounting for between-subject differences in response.

The concept of the dose-response relationship, insofar as it applies to exposed workers, can be explored only by studies that use epidemiologic techniques and consider all of those at risk. Of what relevance is the concept of dose-response to a physician dealing with the health problems of an individual patient? In the first place, knowledge of dose-response relationships may provide the answer to why a particular patient was at risk; second, this information may alert the physician to the potential risk to other workers; third, it may have importance in establishing prognosis and determining management. Thus, in the detailed descriptions of the various asbestos-related lung diseases that follow, their relationship to exposure dose, and

possible differences in the dose-response relationships of the various fiber types will be discussed and summarized in the final section in terms of the implications to the physician.

Significance of Coated and Uncoated Fibers in Clinical Material

The presence of ferruginous bodies (so called in this section because positive identification of the fiber core has been undertaken in only a few of the more recent studies) or coated fibers in biologic material derived from persons who are occupationally exposed to asbestos has long been recognized as a hallmark of exposure (55). Their presence in routine autopsy material, first reported from Cape Town, South Africa (99), has subsequently been confirmed in many countries, in urban and rural communities, in all parts of the world, in fact, whenever sought (table 5). Prevalence tends to increase with the vigor of the search and depends on the amount

TABLE 4

LISTING OF STUDIES* THAT SHOW A DOSE RELATIONSHIP
BETWEEN ESTIMATED EXPOSURE† TO ASBESTOS AND BIOLOGIC RESPONSE

Dose as Measured by \ Response	Fibrosis		Cancer	
	Lung	Pleura	Lung	Pleura
Years of exposure	Bader et al (65) Sluis-Cremer (66) Zedda et al (72)		Knox et al (67) Doll (68) Meurman et al (77)	
Years since first exposure	Selikoff et al (64) Regan et al (70)	Selikoff et al (64)	Selikoff et al (64) Selikoff et al (64)	

Occupation	Harries et al (75)
	Sheers and
	  Templeton (76)
		Harries et al (75)
		Sheers and
		  Templeton (76)		

Occupation and duration	Meurman et al (77)
	Balaam and
	  McCullagh (78)
			Newhouse et al (30)
			Newhouse (29, 71)
			Berry et al (73)
			Maneuso and
			  El-Attar (74)
			Meurman et al (77)
			Enterline and
			  Kendrick (79)
			Enterline (80)
			Enterline and
			  Henderson (81)
				Newhouse (71)

Cumulative dust exposure	Jodoin et al (84) McDonald et al (86) Becklake et al (87) Rossiter et al (88) Weill et al (94, 95)	Rossiter et al (88)	Enterline et al (82, 83) McDonald et al (85)	
Fiber count in pathologic material (electron microscopy)			Pooley, F D. (7), p. 222	

* Identified by reference number in parentheses.
†Mining (66), mining and milling (84–88, 92), manufacturing (29, 30, 64, 94, 95), and secondary use including removal of old asbestos insulation (64, 65, 75, 76).

TABLE 5

PREVALENCE OF FERRUGINOUS BODIES IN ROUTINE AUTOPSY MATERIAL

Location	No.[*]	Prevalence (%)	Men/Women	Method	Year[†]	Reference
Perugia, Italy	109	1.0	1.5	Smears	1969	100
Schwerin, E. Germany	234	9.0	1.4		1971	Quoted in 101
Ann Arbor, USA	100	18.0	1.9		1969	102
Newcastle, England	311	20.3	2.4	Scrapings	1968	103
Glasgow, Scotland	100	23.0	?	Smears	1967	105
Jerusalem, Israel	100	26.0	1.3	Smears	1968	106
Cape Town, S. Africa	500	26.4	1.5	Smears	1963	99
Miami, USA	500	27.2	1.6	Smears	1966	98
London, England	394	36.8	1.4	Sections: left lower lobe	1975	16
Sarajevo, Jugoslavia	100	38.0	2.5	Smears	1971	Quoted in 101
Belfast, N. Ireland	200	40.5	—	Smears	1965	104
Pittsburg, USA	100	41.0	1.4	Smears	1965	107
Dresden, E. Germany	250	43.2	—	Smears	1967	Quoted in 101
Melbourne, Australia	200	43.5	1.0		1969	108
Johannesburg, S. Africa		47.0		Smears, scraping	1965	109
Montreal, Canada	100	48.0	1.7	Scrapings	1966	110
Malmo, Sweden	97	48.4	1.4	Smears	1967	101
Milan, Italy	100	51.0	1.2		—	111
New York, USA	100	53.0	1.2	Ashed sections	1934	9, p. 99
	100	60.0	1.0		1967	9, p. 99
	1,975	47.7	1.3	Smears	1966	9, p. 99
London, England	127	0.0		Sections	1936	112
	100	3.0	4.9	Sections	1946	112
	100	14.0	1.3	Sections	1956	112
	100	20.0	0.8	Sections	1966	112

*Number of autopsies in which a search for ferruginous bodies was made.

†Year of publication was usually within 1 to 2 years of the year in which the study was carried out. Note that for New York and London data at the end of the table, the actual year of the study is given.

of tissue examined (99), or if lung juice is examined, the vigor with which it is extracted. When digested lung tissue is examined, prevalence approaches 100 per cent (113, 114). It is not likely that these figures have been much influenced by the presence of overt asbestos-related lung disease, which was usually specifically excluded from the autopsy series examined (16) or was found to be minimal, perhaps a small single area of basal fibrosis (98, 99).

Despite the fact that ferruginous bodies may not contain an asbestos core, it is probable that most of those found in the lungs of many city dwellers do (Planteydt, 7, p. 80). Thus, prevalence of ferruginous bodies may reasonably be regarded as a reflection of community exposure. In keeping with this is the rural-urban gradient, evident in table 5, which lists the data by increasing prevalence. Thus, rural areas and small cities fall at the beginning of the table; large industrialized urban centers, at the end. A similar rural-urban gradient was seen in another series in which counting methods were standardized (Oldham, 7, p. 231). Prevalence was also consistently higher among men than women. In addition, it increased with age (16, 111), and when within-city distribution was examined, as in the study of London, England, higher prevalences were found among those who lived closest to the docks and/or the industrial heart of east London, among those engaged in heavy manual work, and among those whose occupations were in shipping, transport, and engineering (16). In addition, there is the interesting observation that prevalence increased with time (1936 to 1966) in London, England, but not in New York (see table 5).

Ferruginous bodies have been found on rare occasions in the hilar nodes in persons believed to have been heavily exposed (120), and more rarely, beyond the limits of the thoracic cavity, e.g., in spleen, sinuses; tonsils (54), and hyaline liver plaques (59). Further, in autopsy material obtained from cases with asbestos-related lung disease, fiber count appeared to be some reflection of dose (54, 59, 120).

As already mentioned, the ratio of coated to uncoated fibers within the lung appears to be fairly constant at 10 to 30 per cent (49, 59). Thus, although a count of coated fibers underrepresents the total fiber content of the lung, it should, nevertheless, reflect reasonably accurately trends with respect to age, sex, residence, and occupation.

From the clinician's point of view, this information, based on epidemiologic studies, carries the clear message that the presence of asbestos fibers, coated or uncoated, in biopsy material, autopsy material, or, for that matter, sputum (117–119), which after all, only reflects the lungs' effluent, is an indication of past or current exposure to asbestos (provided the fiber is positively identified). If the fiber is not positively identified, exposure to asbestos remains the likely, but not the only, explanation. Given a history of occupational exposure to asbestos, the physician is unlikely to require positive fiber identification for any clinical purposes. In the absence of history of asbestos exposure, such identification might be useful, but of more importance would be an exhaustive review of all of the patient's previous occupations for however brief a period of time, as well as investigation of the possibility of nonoccupational exposure.

Pleural Plaques, Hyaline or Calcified (Fibrotic Thickening of the Parietal Pleura)

Two types of pleural reaction are seen in association with asbestos exposure: (*1*) an exudative reaction, usually widespread, involving both parietal and visceral pleura and usually, the lung parenchyma, with obliteration of the pleural space; and (*2*) a discrete reaction, involving the parietal pleura, usually in more than one location, and referred to as a pleural plaque (120). The first is associated with symptoms and affects function (121) and will be considered later in this review together with pulmonary fibrosis. The second, usually a radiographic diagnosis in an otherwise healthy person, will be considered in the present section. Both reactions may, of course, occur together in the same person; however, the clinical presentation is likely to be dominated by the extent of the exudative reaction.

Pathology

Macroscopic appearances. Pleural plaques occur as discrete, raised, grey-white lesions on the inner surface of the rib cage and on the diaphragm. In a series of patients who had pleural plaques described at thoracoscopy, Mattson and Ringqvist (121) commented that "despite the confusion of different sizes and shapes, sometimes suggesting an archipelago, the pattern of the plaques is nevertheless monotonous: a flat or slightly uneven surface, white and shiny like synovia or mother-of-pearl, steep edges rising abruptly from the surrounding normal pleura, here and there rounded mounds with overhanging edges. The consistency was that of cartilage." The distribution of pleural plaques is irregular; they tend to be more marked over the lower ribs, may follow or cross rib lines, may be concentrated in the posterior, lateral, or anterior surfaces, but not the cartilaginous portions (54). The diaphragm is usually involved, frequently in the area of the central tendon (54). They do not occur in the costophrenic angles or over the apices. Mediastinal plaques have not been observed (120), but the pleural surface of the pericardium is not infrequently involved, particularly in the advanced case (54).

Plaque formation appears to occur in areas free of adhesions, and the same person might have unilateral obliteration of the pleura in one hemithorax and abundant plaques in the other, with unfused pleural surfaces (54). Alternatively, plaques might involve one part of the hemithorax; adhesions, another part. Occasionally, plaques are found under adhesions (54). Their thickness varies greatly. Calcification appears to be more common in plaques situated in relation to the anterolateral portion of the upper ribs; it does not appear to relate in any way to the thickness of a plaque (54).

Microscopic appearances. The plaques consist of collagenous connective tissue, cell-poor, with few fibrocytic nuclei, arranged in undulating fashion in a coarse, basket-weave pattern, and containing only few thin-walled capillaries (54, 121). Elastic staining shows intact lamellae beneath the plaque in continuity with the surrounding normal parietal pleural connective tissue, suggesting that plaques are extrapleural and develop between the latter and its covering layer of mesothelial cells (54). Some calcium deposition is present in a high proportion of plaques, and occurs as granules along the course of the collagen fibers, ceasing abruptly where the connective tissue changes into normal pleural tissue (54). Cuboidal mesothelial cells may occur at the edge of the plaque (54), occasionally with metaplastic changes (121, 122). Association with bronchial cancer is discussed subsequently.

Although coated asbestos fibers have not been reported in relation to pleural plaques, even in the extensive series of 172 sections examined by Meurman (54) under polarized light, examination of ashed tissue has revealed the presence of uncoated fibers in many cases

(123, 124). With electron microscopy, it is apparent that most plaques contain many small, submicroscopic fibers. It is of interest that these are more concentrated in the calcified zones than in the fibrous zones (Le Bouffant, 7, p. 249).

Epidemiology and Pathogenesis

The association between pleural plaques and asbestos exposure, originally suspected on clinical and epidemiologic grounds, has been amply confirmed by population studies, whether exposure was occupational or nonoccupational. In occupationally exposed groups, such as miners (88) and shipyard workers (75, 76), the prevalence of pleural changes on the chest radiograph has been shown to increase in relation to estimated dose of asbestos, although it is difficult to disentangle age and exposure effects. All varieties of fiber have been implicated, the highest rates occurring with anthophyllite (Jones, 7, p. 243). In addition, factors associated with the site and nature of the deposit appear to be important; for instance, in Quebec, prevalences of calcification differed by as much as 13-fold in 2 adjacent mining areas, working the same fiber in the same geologic deposit (88).

In those not occupationally exposed, particularly in Finland, there is some evidence to suggest that prevalence relates to the proximity of place of residence to mining areas (33, 54). Similarly, there is an increase in the prevalence of pleural changes on the radiograph in some agricultural populations in which the soil contains asbestiform mineral (33, 34).

Given this association between exposure and pleural plaques, however, no satisfactory theory has been developed to explain how parietal pleural reactions develop in response to the inhalation of fibers and particles and their deposition in the lung, which may itself show no reaction to the dust. Furthermore, until recently, the presumed causative agent, namely, the asbestos fiber or particle, had only rarely been detected at the site of the reaction, that is, in the pleural plaque using electron microscopy as indicated above.

One hypothesis is that pleural plaques result from traumatization of the parietal pleura during breathing by sharp asbestos spicules penetrating the pleura. This trauma is believed to produce hemorrhage and subsequent organization of the blood clot in a manner comparable to the process seen in large hemothoraces (33, 123). Against this theory is the failure to demonstrate inflammatory exudates, and the conspicuous absence of adhesions in association with pleural plaques. Also, intracellular transportation via pulmonary lymphatics and then retrograde spread via the chest wall lymphatics due to the massaging action of the respiratory muscles does not seem likely in the absence of hilar and/or mediastinal lymph node enlargement, neither of which has been found in association with pleural plaques (124, 125). The disproportion between the marked parietal pleural response and the small amount of etiologic agent led to speculation about individual sensitivity as a factor, a hypothesis for which there is support in some studies, but not in others. Asbestos-exposed workers with plaques have higher concentrations of gammaglobin (126), but similar concentrations of circulating rheumatoid factor and antinuclear antibodies (127), compared to persons not exposed to asbestos.

Thomson (9, p. 138) suggests the following sequence of events: Fibers, particularly long ones, tend to move toward the lung periphery; some leave the lung and reach the parietal pleura and/or the diaphragm, and those that are held up by the ribs or tendinous part of the diaphragm elicit a reaction in the submesothelial tissues that eventually leads to the formation of a pleural plaque. Calcification, when it occurs, is essentially of a dystrophic type in acellular and degenerated collagen.

It is probably more realistic, however, to accept the conclusion of Jones and Sheers (7, p. 243) that the pathogenesis of pleural plaques that occur in association with asbestos exposure is unknown. For this reason, and because the dose relationship only partly explains the observations, any further light that could be thrown on the pathogenesis of pleural plaques might make an important contribution to the understanding of how asbestos produces its biologic effects, and eventually, how they might be controlled.

Clinical and Radiologic Manifestations

Pleural plaques, hyaline or calcified, in the absence of obliterative pleural lesions and pulmonary fibrosis, are rarely associated with respiratory symptoms, including dyspnea (128). This is in keeping with the fact that their effect on function, although detectable in population studies (128), is modest and is mainly seen as small reductions in lung volumes (129).

By contrast, radiologic changes may be very striking, particularly in the presence of calcifi-

cation. Hyaline plaques, however, may be difficult to see without special oblique views, and will be detected best by high kV techniques, i.e., 110 to 140 kV, whereas calcified plaques are better demonstrated by lower kV techniques (60 to 80 kV) (Bohlig and Gilson, 7, p. 25).

Calcified plaques are usually seen on the posteroanterior film as irregular outlines of uneven density; they can easily be missed in overpenetrated films, particularly if they overlie the coastal cartilages (10). Noncalcified plaques, usually only seen on the posteroanterior film if they lie in the lateral costal regions, i.e., at right angles to the X-ray beam, appear as ill-defined opacities along the costal margins. Oblique films will be necessary to visualize plaques that are located anteriorly or posteriorly. Routine radiography, however, can apparently detect only a small proportion of plaques identified at autopsy; in one series, only 15 per cent were detected, and detection was confined to the most heavily calcified plaques (124).

The most usual clinical presentation is as an incidental radiologic finding in an asymptomatic patient. This should alert the physician to the possibility of exposure if this is not already known; in the absence of occupational exposure, neighborhood or domestic exposure should be sought.

Although the presence of hyaline pleural plaques alone does not appear to cause symptoms of disability, there is some evidence that they affect prognosis. Thus, in some series (130), they were associated with a higher-than-expected incidence of bronchial carcinoma (Smith, 8, p. 277), whereas in Quebec chrysotile miners and millers, this was not so (92). Malignant mesothelioma has also been reported as developing in the mesothelial cells at the edge of the plaque (122).

Pleural Effusion (Benign)

Exudative pleural reactions, which may occur in association with all of the asbestos-related lung diseases, may also occur as the primary, or at least the most prominent, clinical manifestation (131–135), presenting as an "idiopathic pleural effusion" (131); hence, the justification for considering this diagnosis separately in a clinical review of the asbestos-related lung diseases. The present description is based on the 30 cases so far published (134); however, pleural effusion may well be a more frequent manifestation of asbestos exposure than this modest number suggests, particularly if it were subsequently shown to be a phase in the development of other pleural changes.

Pathology. On macroscopic examination at thoracotomy, the pleural surfaces show an active exudative process, characterized by increased vascularity and symphysis. Associated pleural plaques do not appear to be a feature. Microscopic examination shows variable pleural thickening, with "pleural drift of carbon and other dusts and iron-positive granules" (131). Other features include regenerating mesothelium and extensive collateral circulation (131), and there is one report of a granuloma (134). The underlying lung tissue shows varying degrees of interstitial pneumonitis, from mild, low grade inflammation to organized interstitial fibrosis, in which asbestos bodies and fibers are usually, but not invariably, found. Electron microscopic analysis for uncoated fibers has not been reported in this type of case, but it can be assumed that these would be found.

Clinical features. The usual presentation is one of recurring pleural effusion of unknown cause, associated with chest pain (131). The effusion may be unilateral, bilateral, or one side may follow the other in sequence. The presentation may be acute, with fever, leukocytosis, and an increased sedimentation rate, or chronic, with minimal systemic reaction. The pleural fluid is frequently blood stained (red blood cell counts ranging from 5,000 to 50,000 cells per mm^3) and, in most cases, is an exudate. The clinical course varies from that of a benign and self-limiting illness (132, 133) to the development of chronic pleural thickening that requires decortication (131). The patient's association with asbestos may be current, or more often may have been brief and in the remote past (131).

Differential diagnosis. The diagnosis of a benign asbestos pleural effusion should be considered a diagnosis only by exclusion. The chief alternative to be excluded is malignant mesothelioma, one of the manifestations of asbestos exposure that may not develop until many years after the first exposure. The pleural effusions that commonly complicate the latter tumor may precede by months or years the definitive diagnosis of the tumor. Indeed, one could argue against accepting the diagnosis of benign asbestos pleural effusion until all of the present reported cases are followed to death, and death is shown to be attributable neither to carcinoma of the lung nor to mesothelioma. However, as follow-up becomes longer (134), the justifica-

tion for this diagnosis increases, and asbestos exposure can reasonably be added to the long list of causes of benign, recurrent pleural effusion.

Diffuse Interstitial Pulmonary Fibrosis (Asbestosis)

Definition

Diffuse interstitial fibrosis of the lung associated with asbestos exposure was recognized in the early years of the twentieth century, the first asbestos-related disease to be so recognized (1); however, the term "asbestosis" to describe this pneumoconiosis was not suggested until 1927, when Cooke (136) used it to describe the case of a female asbestos textile worker. It is usual to include fibrosis of the associated visceral pleura under this term, but not that of the parietal pleura (10). There is merit in maintaining this specific usage in line with the widely accepted use of the term pneumoconiosis (137), rather than to use the term "asbestosis" in a generic sense to describe all asbestos-related diseases of the lung and pleura, even neoplasms (10).

Pathology

Macroscopic appearances. The main pathologic features that had been described with care by the 1930s in individual case reports (138, 139) were reviewed by Hourihane and McCaughey (116) in the light of their own pathologic material, based on 69 cases of clinical asbestosis examined at the London Hospital. Macroscopic changes ranged from small areas of basal fibrosis (if sufficiently localized, these may escape recognition by the naked eye) to the fully developed case of a diffuse, fine fibrosis affecting both lungs. Lung size tends to reflect the extent of the fibrosis; when this is diffuse, the lungs tend to be small. Cut surface shows the fine, grey-colored fibrosis that generally appears to affect subpleural areas first, often quite extensively, before advancing into other lobes with the extension of the disease process. Lower lobes tend to be affected first, then middle lobes, and eventually, upper lobes (10, 116, 140). Small honeycomb cysts may be seen, in the lower lobes particularly, and fibrosis and honeycombing also tend to be concentrated subpleurally (140). Emphysema, centrilobular or bullous, is frequently found, with characteristics essentially the same as in emphysema not associated with asbestosis (140, 141). The pleural surface in relation to the fibrosis is invariably involved in the fibrotic process, either mildly, giving the appearance of a milky covering to the fibrosis, or with widespread fibrosis and symphysis (116, 140). The hilar lymph nodes are not usually enlarged or otherwise affected (10, 142).

Conglomerate lesions of massive fibrosis, comparable to the progressive massive fibrosis of coal workers, occur in the absence of tuberculosis (Gough, 5, p. 368), but are rare, unless the exposure has been to mixed dust including talc (10, 143) or silica (142, 144). In addition, these lesions appear to have a predilection for the lower lobes (142, 144), unlike other forms of progressive massive fibrosis. The occasional solitary fibrotic lesion is seen, for which the term asbestoma has been used (145). Necrobiotic nodules associated with rheumatoid disease (similar to those seen with Caplans' disease in coal workers) are seen (146–149), but only rarely (10).

Microscopic appearances. In animal studies, early dust reactions include a desquamative alveolar response (Webster, 9, p. 117), a reaction that may have its counterpart in man (144, 150). In addition, there is one case report of desquamative interstitial pneumonia with asbestos bodies in the lung (150), and the view has been expressed that this is one end of a spectrum that ends with fibrosing alveolitis (151). An idea of the abnormalities in the early stages of fibrosis comes from examination of biopsy material, usually sought to establish a diagnosis of asbestosis (131, 145). The early reaction in the interstitial tissue resembles that of other forms of interstitial pneumonia, with mixed leukocyte infiltration of the alveolar walls, moderate numbers of phagocytes in the alveoli, and varying degrees of organization with fibrosis (131, 145). In some cases, the early changes are concentrated at the level of the respiratory bronchiole, where reticulin fibers, macrophages, and dust particles collect (10, 116), leading subsequently to what has been termed the basic lesion of asbestosis, namely, a peribronchiolar fibrosis (116). From here, the process extends outward to involve the surrounding alveoli, leading to diffuse alveolar wall thickening, with peribronchiolar and perivascular fibrosis (116). In an occasional case, the fibrosis remains almost exclusively peribronchiolar (144, figure 5), but the more usual picture is that of a diffuse fibrosis, involving the interstitium, frequently associated with areas of solid fibrosis, where laminated collagen may replace the entire parenchyma. Such areas may also show alveolar cell hyperplasia and sclerosis of vessel

walls (116). The presence of ferruginous bodies is to be expected, and electron microscopy is likely to reveal very large numbers of uncoated and very fine particles and fibers (152). The pathologic findings in workers exposed to amosite and crocidolite have been shown to be essentially similar to those associated with chrysotile exposure (Wagner, 8, p. 373).

Pathogenesis

Reactions at the cell level have already been discussed, and at the organ level are presumed to relate to the number of cells reacting, which in turn is believed to relate to the retained "dose" of asbestos dust and/or fiber. This appears to be true for mild and moderate fibrosis, respectively, in animals (62) as well as in man, in whom the response has been related to "dose" retained, as reflected by concentration of coated and uncoated particles in the lung tissue at autopsy (49); however, there does not appear to be further progression from moderate to severe fibrosis associated with an increase in dose (49, 62). It is, therefore, postulated that the progression from moderate to severe fibrosis is due to other factors, e.g., nonspecific inflammation, as suggested by Ashcroft and Heppleston (49) or possibly to self-perpetuating host responses, as suggested by Turner-Warwick (144). Thus, based on her observations that non–organic-specific autoantibodies, especially antinuclear antibodies (ANA), occur with only slightly greater frequency in exposed, compared to nonexposed, persons in the general population, and within exposed populations, with greater frequency in those with clinical disease than those without (153–155), Turner-Warwick proposes that ANA acts as an accelerator once the fibrosis has been initiated by a separate agent (Turner-Warwick, 7, p. 258). Such an explanation would fit the clinical observation that asbestosis may appear for the first time and progress long after exposure to dust has ceased. The possibility that genetic factors influence the response to exposure is suggested in one study in which the HL-A B27 occurred with greater frequency in asbestosis cases compared to the general population (156). There is also a progressive decrease in the total lymphocyte count with advancing fibrosis, and the suggestion has been made that the cellular immune mechanism is disturbed in asbestosis (157).

The progression from diffuse interstitial fibrosis to conglomerate fibrosis may, in the past, have been associated with tuberculosis (125), but this is rare today in the United States (Enterline, 5, p. 156) and in Britain (Smither, 5, p. 166). Nor does such progression appear to relate to a "rheumatoid" diathesis (90). On the other hand, rheumatoid disease developing in the asbestos worker is liable to be associated with the appearance of lung changes of unusual and rather marked character.

The relationship of emphysema to asbestos dust exposure remains to be elucidated. Physiologic studies suggest that airway obstruction is common; in the presence of fibrosis, particularly if this is peribronchiolar in location, it would seem reasonable to ascribe it to the dust load. In the absence of dust fibrosis, and given the importance of the smoking habit, it is more difficult to determine the role of a dust load in the development of emphysema. To date, there has been no systematic autopsy study in which the prevalence of emphysema and/or chronic bronchitis in workers exposed to asbestos was compared with the prevalence in nonexposed persons, such as that of Ryder and associates (158) in coal workers, a study that clearly showed the excess of emphysema in coal miners. An open mind should be kept on the subject until further evidence is available.

Clinical Features

The symptoms and signs of diffuse interstitial fibrosis due to asbestos exposure are no different from those of all other forms of diffuse interstitial fibrosis. Thus, the most prominent symptom is breathlessness, first noted under the stress of effort, then at rest, as the large working reserve of the lung becomes progressively reduced. Cough, either dry or with sputum, not as consistently present as dypsnea, may be severe, with distressing paroxysms (10). Although generally attributed to airway, rather than to interstitial, lung disease, this symptom occurs with greater frequency in the asbestos-exposed worker than in his nonexposed counterpart (96, 97, 118) and often cannot be attributed to differences in smoking habits, suggesting that this symptom also relates to asbestos exposure. Chest pain, not a frequent complaint, has been attributed to muscle aches, because it appears to be present only when dyspnea is severe (10).

The most characteristic physical sign is the presence of crepitations, which are described as having a "crisp, clean, quality" and occurring late in inspiration, usually over the lower or middle lung zones (10). A deep inspiration may be necessary to elicit them. As fibrosis progresses, they become more widespread and occupy a greater part of inspiration. They are attributed to the "sudden opening of airways in deflated territories of the lung" (159), an explanation supported by the fact that they shift to the gravitationally lower lobes with changes in posture (128) and have been shown to be consistently detectable at a given transpulmonary pressure (160). Other adventitious sounds, such as wheezes and rhonchi, are less common. Air entry and chest expansion are likely to be affected in proportion to associated pleural changes.

Clubbing of the fingers and toes is said to be present in most cases (10), although by no means is this always true (161). This sign does not necessarily indicate advanced disease, because it is also reported in men who are still able to work (96, 119). The lack of correlation with severity of fibrosis is seen particularly when the clubbing is evaluated systematically from casts of digits to allow measurement of the hyponychial angle (118, 119) by the method of Regan and associates (162). It is of interest that smoking also appears to play a part in the development of this sign (Harries, 7, p. 19), an association detected in epidemiologic studies, the significance of which is unknown.

Radiographic Changes

In considering the chest radiograph of the individual case for diagnostic purposes (10, 163), evaluation of the pulmonary parenchyma should be based on the following features: small, irregular, and/or round opacities, scored for size or length, profusion, and number of zones affected; hairline ring (honeycomb) shadows; a diffuse haze or ground-glass appearance not obviously due to pleural shadows; short horizontal septal lines or Kerley B-lines, believed to represent lymphatic obstruction (144), and occasional longer hairline shadows. Pleural changes are likely to be present as well (in more than one half of the cases in one series of compensation board material), whereas in 20 per cent of cases, they were present without parenchymal changes (163). Rounded opacities are more evident when the occupational exposure has included silica (95). These findings are in general agreement with previous reports (163–166). Thus, it can be seen that the radiologic features of asbestosis are no different from those of all other forms of interstitial fibrosis, except for the prominence of associated pleural changes, in particular, calcification, which should always call attention to the possible association with asbestos exposure.

A systematic classification of the radiologic changes associated with asbestos exposure embodying most of the features described, together with the pleural changes, was developed for epidemiologic purposes, first as the UICC/Cincinnati classification (167), later adopted as the ILO U/C classification (168). Its features include a reading sheet, an extended 12-point scale to grade parenchymal changes, and standard films to assist in the evaluation of pleural and parenchymal changes (obtainable from the International Labour Office, Occupational Safety and Health Branch, CH 1211 Geneva 22, Switzerland. Price: Sw Francs 250.–) The use of this classification, by improving precision and probably also comparability between studies, has enhanced the value of the X-ray as an epidemiologic tool (169). Thus, it enables a better placement of the film in the multidimensional "continuum which extends from complete 'normality' at one end to the most severe degree of abnormality at the higher" (Bohlig 7, p. 25). In particular, it has permitted the exploration of the exposure-dose relationships (using the chest radiograph to measure response) in working populations. In addition, this classification has been adopted by compensation boards in several countries to improve consistency in the reading of the chest radiograph and should be used whenever the evaluation of a person's films must be considered relative to those of others. It must be emphasized, however, that this classification is descriptive and not diagnostic; furthermore, although radiologic changes so described relate reasonably well to lung function changes in population studies (87, 95), their relationship to disability, which is likely to vary considerably from subject to subject, has not been widely studied.

Lung Function

Lung function tests have been applied to the study of asbestosis since their general introduction to clinical medicine in the 1940s. In general, there are 4 clinical areas of application (10): first, for diagnosis and assessment of disability; second, for following the evolution of disease with time; third, for the surveillance of healthy workers, with a view to detecting early changes; and fourth, for preemployment examination to screen the "susceptible" person.

In addition, information gained from epidemiologic studies using pulmonary function testing to determine exposure-response relationships has permitted inferences to be drawn about early effects of asbestos on the lung, information that may ultimately have considerable practical value in terms of the worker's health.

Diagnosis. Interstitial fibrosis associated with exposure to asbestos is generally believed to be associated with the restrictive and "alveolar capillary" block patterns of pulmonary function, similar to that seen with the interstitial fibrosis from other causes (Becklake, 7, p. 3). Characteristic features of the established case (with clinical and/or radiographic evidence of disease) are: general restriction of lung volumes, particularly vital capacity (VC), with less effect on residual volume; decrease in flows, such as 1-sec forced expiratory volume (FEV_1), in proportion to the decrease in VC, so that the ratio of FEV_1 to forced vital capacity (FVC) is relatively well preserved; decrease in diffusing capacity, attributable in part to the decreased lung volume (170), although decreased membrane transfer and inhomogeneity of regional ventilation-perfusion relationships within the lung undoubtedly contribute to the impaired gas transfer (43, p. 379). Impairment of gas exchange capability, reflected by arterial desaturation, increased alveolar-arterial Po_2 gradient, and hyperventilation, may at first be evident only under the stress of exercise, but later occurs at rest. The CO_2 exchange is not usually affected, and arterial CO_2 retention is not usually a feature of the established case.

Although there is no evidence to suggest that asbestosis due to chrysotile is any different from that due to other fibers, one epidemiologic study suggests that there may be greater decrease in function for equivalent estimated exposure to crocidolite compared to chrysotile (94), a difference that could be explained by greater retention of crocidolite compared to chrysotile for equivalent estimated exposure; however, in the light of the potential and, indeed, inevitable inaccuracies that beset all efforts to evaluate remote past dust exposure, in amount and/or nature of the fiber, this interesting observation requires further confirmation before it is assumed that different fibers have different fibrogenic potential in man.

It is usually claimed that airway obstruction is not a feature of asbestosis (10, 170–172); however, a review of 375 published cases (173), most with unequivocal parenchymal radiologic changes, indicated that a considerable number of patients had airway obstruction (11 per cent compared to 39 per cent with a restrictive pattern), whereas in 18 per cent, the function impairment suggested a mixed picture of obstruction and restriction. In addition, scrutiny of epidemiologic studies in working populations (i.e., studies that, by their nature, exclude the disabled and all but a few of those with radiologic disease) invariably shows a sizeable number of persons with evidence of airway obstruction (64, 72, 170, 174–176). However, there is no clear evidence showing an excess of airway obstruction in asbestos-exposed populations compared to those not so exposed (96, 172), and there is no clear evidence that within exposed populations, the prevalence of obstruction increases with increasing exposure (172). The restrictive patterns of lung function also does not show an increased prevalence in relation to exposure (172).

To this time, therefore, epidemiologic studies of lung function have not been able to elucidate the relationship between airway obstruction and asbestos exposure, or the part played by the cigarette habit (additive or synergistic). In consequence, even in the presence of radiologic changes, there is usually hesitation in attributing the obstructive component of a worker's disease to asbestosis, despite the fact that decreased conductance has been shown in other forms of interstitial lung disease (177). Without radiologic changes, there is even greater reluctance to attribute the obstruction to asbestos exposure. Nevertheless, there is enough indirect evidence to suggest that in response to asbestos exposure, the character of the function impairment may be obstructive in a certain number of cases (173); until further evidence is available, an open mind should be kept in this regard.

Assessment of disability. The relationships between *organ malfunction* (as reflected in what may be called descriptive measurements of the lung, i.e., its size or lung volumes, and in the measurements related to its mechanical properties), *organ failure,* generally considered to be present only when gas exchange function is impaired (43, p. 442), and *disability* (diminution of performance as perceived by the subject himself) are not straightforward. Thus, considerable amounts of organ malfunction (i.e., abnormalities of lung function tests) can be present without organ failure (i.e., abnormal blood gases), even under the stress of effort. Likewise, disability in the form of unusual breathlessness may be perceived by the subject

early or late in the development of his disease. This discrepancy between function and symptoms is also found in some epidemiologic studies (172, 178, 179), but not others (96, 97). The important conclusion for clinical practice is that in the individual case, disability cannot be predicted with reliability from symptoms, function, or radiographic changes. It should therefore be evaluated by appropriate exercise tests, if necessary at more than one load, for each case individually (Becklake, 7, p. 3).

Evaluation of changes with time. Serial measurements of lung function in individual cases of asbestosis with time suggest that deterioration is most closely reflected in VC (64, 78, 180) and, possibly, maximal voluntary ventilation. The diffusing capacity of the lung for CO ($D_{L_{CO}}$), originally proposed on theoretic grounds as well as on the basis of some limited observations (176), may not be as useful (128).

Support for these conclusions also comes from epidemiologic studies of exposed working populations in which decrease in VC, in particular the IC component of VC, showed a closer relationship to estimated dust exposure than did $D_{L_{CO}}$, measured either by the single-breath or the steady-state technique (87, 94). Other tests that showed a relationship to exposure were FEV_1 (87) and maximal mid-expiratory flow (94); however, serial studies of an epidemiologic nature (i.e., following changes in a whole working population, rather than in a few selected subjects) would provide more precise information on this point.

Early detection. This implies detection of dust effects in a person before he or she perceives them as symptoms. Persons showing these early changes are more likely to be found in a working population than in a clinic population, because clinic attendance presupposes symptoms. Furthermore, within a working population, it is reasonable to suppose that symptoms will occur more frequently in those with heavier exposures. In one epidemiologic study confined to exposed persons without clinical or radiologic evidence of disease, and with normal routine lung function, it was possible to detect changes in the lungs' mechanical properties (specifically, a decrease in compliance and an increase in calculated upstream resistance) in those with heavier dust exposure (84). These changes suggesting a dust effect at the small airway level would be compatible with peribronchiolar fibrosis (116). Similar results were obtained in a subsequent study of a larger number of subjects, reported in preliminary form (181), using the closing volume test. At present, these observations have no practical significance, because it remains to be shown (*1*) that what is detected is, in fact, the beginning of a process that will ultimately lead to asbestosis, and (*2*) that any intervention, such as removal from exposure, would prevent the ultimate development of disease. From what has been said about pathogenesis, however, it appears that in its earlier stages of development, the fibrosis of asbestosis appears to be related to dust accumulated, and therefore, by implication, removal from exposure by preventing further accumulation might slow the process. These findings, therefore, have potential application in the future.

Function versus radiographic methods in the early detection of asbestosis. Several early clinical studies, some based on small numbers of subjects, suggested that in asbestosis changes in function preceded radiographic changes (64, 128, 176). The changes in function identified were in VC (64, 128) and $D_{L_{CO}}$ (176). Subsequent epidemiologic studies suggest that at least as far as these two tests of function were concerned, they were no more sensitive than radiologic changes (87, 94, 95). It must be emphasized that the latter conclusions were based on between-group comparisons of subjects classified by dust exposure, for which identification of appropriate "normal" standards is unnecessary. Detecting abnormality in the individual case with certainty is another matter, because this requires reference to standards of normality, which for both radiographic studies and tests of function have fairly wide ranges. Periodic comparative chest radiographs or function tests, are likely to improve the chance of detecting early abnormalities in a given person. It must be borne in mind, however, that the radiologic changes are invariably of a nonspecific nature, similar to those occurring with aging or the cigarette habit (182); hence, the opinion that in an individual case they reflect early fibrosis should be guarded.

Diagnosis

The criteria for diagnosis of asbestosis depend on the purpose for which diagnosis will be used, and the degree of certainty required. A working clinical diagnosis can be reached on the basis of an exposure history (present, past, or remote past) and the presence of one or more of the following: effort dyspnea, basal crepitations, radiographic changes of parenchymal and/or pleural disease, and lung function impairment of any sort (10, 96, 97, 172). If all 5 criteria are present, the diagnosis would generally be considered established for most compensation boards. With fewer criteria, there is less certainty.

In the absence of an exposure history, or if the exposure history is considered too short to account for the amount of disease present, a tissue diagnosis may be called for, particularly in compensation cases for which attributability is in doubt. In such situations, an open lung biopsy (145) is preferable to a needle biopsy (183), particularly if radiographic changes are minimal. Biopsy material should be critically examined by light microscopy for pathologic features, including presence of coated fibers, and by electron microscopy for the presence of uncoated fibers, using appropriate extraction procedures (Pooley, 7, p. 50). Also, occasionally, the presence of asbestos bodies in the sputum (117–119) may alert the physician to the possibility of exposure and result in an appropriately exhaustive enquiry to reveal the source of exposure. Coated fibers are, of course, commonly found under conditions of heavy and current exposure.

Prognosis, Complications, and Medical Management

The outlook for the person with asbestosis has undoubtedly improved considerably during the past 20 years, both in Europe (67) and in North America (63), with age at death, years of exposure until diagnosis, and years of survival after diagnosis increasing conspicuously in most countries. Also, risk of premature death due to other respiratory diseases seems to be confined to those with high dust exposures (McDonald, 7, pp. 155–179).

Perhaps because of the longer survival period, workers with asbestosis are now surviving into the lung cancer age (63), and deaths from this cause are assuming a much greater importance (McDonald, 7, pp. 189–217). In addition, it should be noted that lung cancer is becoming a more common cause of death in the general population.

Medical management of asbestosis is restricted to the symptomatic care given to subjects with interstitial fibrosis, whatever the cause. The use of corticosteroids is not advocated, because the agent, asbestos, is, as far as is known, fixed in the lung tissue. Appropriate treatment of intercurrent infections may be particularly important in view of the suggestion that nonspecific inflammation may contribute to progression of fibrosis (Ashcroft, 7, p. 236). There is no real evidence to suggest that the only possible effective therapeutic intervention, namely, to remove the person from exposure, has any real influence on the outcome of the case. One assumes that removal might halt further progression, a hypothesis for which there is some evidence (62). It is also known, however, that disease can both appear and progress many years after removal from exposure (63); thus, research should be directed at possible ways of determining what factors determine this future progression and whether it is possible to define the stage or level of exposure at which removal might be an effective preventive measure.

Pre-employment evaluation of lung function to screen out high-risk persons is, in theory, the most important area of future health protection; yet, this is also the area in which there is no systematic evidence to indicate what type of person to screen in or screen out. Attention has been directed toward the pre-employment detection of obstructive lung disease, acute or chronic, on the assumption that such persons are at high-risk of developing asbestosis (Hunt, 5, p. 406). The smoking habit, certainly the greatest risk factor for bronchogenic cancer, does not usually constitute grounds for refusing a recruit. Its role in the development of fibrosis is less clear, there being some evidence to suggest a synergistic effect with dust (185), and some evidence to the contrary.

An interesting possibility, as yet completely unexplored, is that certain physiologic characteristics, for instance, the relative size of airways to air spaces (184), may constitute risk factors and might, for example, be the basis for exclusion of certain types from dust hazard. Finally, it is possible that pre-employment and annual measurements of lung function, particularly FVC, might also prove to be a useful tool in the health care of the worker (87); however, this, too, should be introduced only in a way that permits a critical evaluation of the effectiveness of such a procedure.

Malignant Mesothelioma of the Pleura and Peritoneum

Primary malignant mesotheliomas arise from the pluripotential mesothelial cells (of the pleura, peritoneum, and pericardium) and in consequence, may present with widely varying histologic features. Nevertheless, they have been considered a pathologic entity (10, 185), albeit rare, for some time; their association with asbestos exposure was mentioned as early as 1946 in an individual case report (10). This association was dramatically brought to the attention of the medical public by Wagner and colleagues (27) in a report of 33 cases with occupational and/or environmental and/or domestic exposure in the crocidolite mining area of the Northwest Cape, South Africa. The association with asbestos exposure has now been confirmed from many parts of the world (table 6).

Pathology

A characteristic feature of the macroscopic appearance of the malignant variety is the tendency to spread along serosal membranes (186), encasing the lung by a bulky, lobulated mass that usually invades the fissures. Areas of necrosis within the tumor may give rise to cystic spaces filled with glutinous fluid, a distinctive feature of this tumor, although not necessarily a specific one, because it is also seen in adenocarcinoma (10). Local metastases to chest wall, mediastinum, and pericardium, rather than remote metastases, declare malignancy of the tumor; however, metastases to hilar and abdominal lymph nodes are not uncommon, and, occasionally, more distant sites, such as liver, thyroid, adrenals, bone, and brain are involved (10, 186). It has been emphasized, however, that the diagnosis is one of exclusion, and that all potential sites for primary growth (particularly lung, pancreas, intestine, and ovary) must be examined; consideration must also be given to the possibility that the primary tumor has already been removed (McCaughey, 5, p. 603). The peritoneal tumors present a similar appearance, but do not tend to engulf the abdominal organs to the same extent as the pleural tumors. Glutinous ascitic fluid, however, is a common feature (10). Primary pericardial tumors do not appear to be associated with asbestos exposure.

Microscopically, 4 varieties are recognized according to the dominant cell types (186, 187). *Epithelial*, or tubulopapillary, tumors are characterized by branching acini, lined by columnar or cuboidal cells, often containing mucin and having a tendency to spread. *Mesenchymal*, or sarcomatous, tumors range in appearance from cellular fasciculated fibrosarcoma to myxoma, with the amount of associated collagen in the tumor varying considerably. The *undifferen-*

TABLE 6

ASSOCIATION BETWEEN MESOTHELIOMA* AND ASBESTOS EXPOSURE†

Country	Years Reviewed	Cases of Mesothelioma		Control Subjects		Main Source of Exposure, Occupation, and/or Fiber	Reference
		No.	Per Cent Exposed	No.	Per Cent Exposed		
Uncontrolled case studies							
South Africa	1956–1960	33	97			Crocidolite mining	Wagner et al (27)
	1956–1971	252	82			area in N-W Cape	Webster** (8, p. 195)
UK: Liverpool	1955–1970	52	80			Shipyard occupations	Whitwell and Rawciffe (187)
France: Rouen, LeHavre	?	14***	86			Textile manufacture	Fondimare et al†† (188)
Germany: Hamburg	1958–1968	98	58			Shipyard and manufacture	Bohlig et al (189)
Holland: Walcheren	1962–1968	25	88			Shipyard occupations	Stumphius (117)
USA: Harrisburg, Pa.	1958–1963	42	74			Textile insulation manufacture	Lieben and Pistawka (190)
Chicago, Ill.	c. 1969	77	86			Various industrial exposures	Godwin and Jagatic (191)
Somerville, N.J.	1948–1970	72	83			Mainly chrysotile textiles	Borow et al (192)
Australia: Victoria	1962–1968	15	87			Crocidolite or mixed	Milne (193)
Case-control studies							
UK: London	1917–1967	76	53	76	12	Factory processing crocidolite	Newhouse and Thompson††† (28)
Scotland	1950–1967	80	67	80	32	Shipyard occupations	McEwen et al†† (194)
Belfast	1950–1964	42***	76	42	21	Shipyard occupations and insulation	Elmes et al (195)
Newcastle	1948–1969	41	95	56	41	Shipyard occupations	Ashcroft (196)
Italy: Piedmont	1960–1970	50	18	50	2	Various manufacturing processes	Rubino et al (197)
Sweden: Malmo	1957–1966	34	53	34	12	Textiles, insulation, shipyards	Hägerstrand et al (198)
Germany: Hamburg	1958–1968	150	71	104	24	Shipyard and manufacture	Hain et al (199)
Holland: Walcheren	Not stated	67	72	67	18	Shipyard occupations	Zielhaus et al (200)
Canada: all provinces	1960–1972	190	26	182	7	Production more than mining	McDonald†††(201)
USA: all states	1972	99	48	86	20	Production and manufacturing	McDonald†††(201)

*Usual source was hospital autopsy records; pleural and peritoneal included, except for references 195 and 201.

†Exposure was established by interview, except where stated; includes occupational and domestic exposures, possible as well as definite.

**Includes Wagner's cases.

††Exposure deduced from presence of coated or uncoated fibers.

***Pleural tumors only.

†††Men only.

tiated, or polygonal, type is usually composed of solid sheets of cells with abundant eosinophilic cytoplasm, which may look remarkably benign. The *mixed* type comprises all of the characteristics previously described. Some believe that all tumors would turn out to be of the mixed variety if a sufficient number of sections were taken (Planteydt, 5, p. 80). A surprising and not uncommon finding is the presence of only one tumor element in the metastases (10).

Although ferruginous bodies are usually found in the lungs in cases of asbestos-associated mesothelioma (Hourihane, 5, p. 647), it is unusual to find parenchymal fibrosis (i.e., asbestosis) of any degree when the tumor arises in the pleura; on the other hand, in peritoneal tumors, pulmonary fibrosis may be a prominent feature, giving rise to the hypothesis of obstruction to the thoracic lymphatic drainage and retrograde lymphatic spread of the asbestos fiber to the abdominal lymphatic system. Peritoneal tumors, representing perhaps 10 per cent of cases, appear to occur more frequently in some series (30) than in others (201), and one study shows a sex difference in the preponderant tumor site, peritoneal tumors being more frequent in women (30); however, peritoneal tumors predominate in some all-male series (Selikoff, 7, p. 209).

Epidemiology: Association with Asbestos Exposure

Despite their being rare tumors, estimated to have an incidence of the order of 1 per 1,000,000 per annum in the general population, the association of mesothelioma with asbestos exposure has been consistent in all parts of the world (table 6). Although all commercial fibers except anthophyllite (77), but including talc, have been implicated, there are important between-fiber differences in mesothelioma risk, being greatest with crocidolite, less with amosite, and apparently even less with chrysotile. With amosite and chrysotile, there appears to be a higher risk in manufacturing than in mining and milling. These were the conclusions reached by the Advisory Committee on Asbestos Cancers at the Lyon meeting (7, p. 341) and are based on published epidemiologic studies, including prospective and retrospective mortality studies. In addition, mesothelioma rates seem, in general, to be increased in cities that have ship building or ship repair industries (202), and in some working populations may approach 10 per cent, particularly if exposed to crocidolite

(Newhouse, M. L.: Personal communication). Unlike bronchial cancer, smoking does not play a synergistic role in the development of mesotheliomas.

The most disconcerting aspect of the relationship between malignant mesothelioma and asbestos exposure is its documented association with apparently low levels of exposure, for relatively brief periods in the remote past from neighborhood or domestic sources described (27, 30, 31). The commonest documented neighborhood exposure is that of children playing in the streets within one-half mile of a factory or mine, usually for several years in early childhood, although one cannot usually be certain that they did not also play in the waste and/or the tailings. However, neighborhood exposures seem certain to have been less than those to which workers themselves were exposed, implying lack of a dose relationship to exposure. On the other hand, in certain other occupational groups, such as the workers in the London asbestos textile factory studied by Newhouse and associates (30), a dose effect on risk can be discerned. Furthermore, when dose is measured by number of asbestos bodies and/or fibers in pathologic material (187, 188, 197), this is found to be higher than in the general population, although lower than usually seen in relation to pulmonary fibrosis.

Pathogenesis

Animal experiments indicate that, when given intrapleurally, all types of asbestos fiber, as well as certain types of glass fiber, are capable of producing malignant mesothelial tumors, and risk appears to increase with dose (Wagner, 7, p. 285). Inhalation experiments, on the other hand, tend to produce cancers. This has led to the hypothesis that all types of fiber, once they reach the pleura, exercise "biologic activity." There is some evidence, however, that this activity is size dependent, fibers less than 2.5 μm in diameter or between 10 and 80 μm in length being particularly effective at inciting mesothelial growths (Stanton, 7, p. 289). For these reasons, opinion is moving away from the view that the gradient of biologic activity shown in man, at least with regard to risk of developing mesothelial tumors, is due to chemical differences between fibers, and toward the view that it is due to physical differences between fibers. Thus, it is believed that the determinants of pathogenicity of a fiber are the degree to which it penetrates and settles in deep lung spaces, and this, in turn, is controlled by its aerodynamic properties (Timbrell, 7, p. 295).

In addition, it must be pointed out that malignant mesothelioma is not uniquely associated with asbestos exposure, and a small number of cases without such a history are seen in all series; this proportion is usually small, but has reached over 80 per cent (197). Mesothelial tumors arising in the pericardium have not been linked to asbestos.

Despite the now accepted association of malignant mesothelioma with asbestos exposure in man, the pathogenesis of this tumor is far from clear. Presumably, it is only by sustained research, using animal models, and looking for risk factors in exposed populations, that an understanding will eventually be reached of the mechanisms underlying its development. Indeed, some believe elucidation of the relationship of this tumor to exposure to be the most important area for future research, and the key to understanding the mechanism by which exposure to asbestos produces its effects in man (202).

Clinical Features

Pleural tumors invariably present with dull chest or shoulder pain, of insidious onset, but slowly becoming persistent enough to interfere with sleep (Elmes, 7, p. 267). In some cases, however, the pain may be severe and pleuritic. Breathlessness, usually related to accumulation of pleural fluid, weight loss, tiredness, and cough follow. As mentioned previously, there may also be a history of previous pleural effusions (203). The presumed sequence of events is as follows: serous effusion, perhaps developing in association with plaques, possibly clearing later, to recur with blood staining, increasing in amount as the tumor develops; invasion and thickening of parietal and visceral pleura, eventually leading to the lung's becoming imprisoned, with retraction and immobilization of the chest cage on the affected side (117). The presenting symptom of a peritoneal tumor is also usually dull pain, later followed by swelling and weight loss.

The physical signs will depend on the stage at which the patient first presents; usually, pain precedes systemic symptoms and the presence of clear physical signs by weeks or months. Apart from the clinical signs of the effusion and/or pleural invasion, clubbing of the fingers is common; acute arthropathy which may also be a feature of associated asbestosis (204) has been reported, with regression and reappearance, after surgical removal and recurrence of the tumor, respectively (Elmes, 7, p. 267). There is only one report of hypoglycemia in association with pleural mesothelioma (204); the association may therefore be taken as incidental. The presenting signs of abdominal tumors are invariably fluid and swelling; complications include partial or complete intestinal obstruction.

The clinical course is usually one of rapid progression; for pleural tumors, the average survival time from onset of symptoms is approximately 6 months; for peritoneal tumors, 13 to 14 months. This varies, however, and in one series, 17 per cent were alive after 3 years (187). Nevertheless, the more benign the course, the more likely that the pathologic classification should be revised to benign mesothelioma (205).

Diagnosis and Treatment

The diagnosis can be definitely made only by tissue examination. There are a number of reasons why it is difficult to make a positive diagnosis of this tumor during life, even when adequate biopsy material is available. These include the wide variety of cell types within a single tumor, especially those of the mixed type, and the need to exclude primary tumors elsewhere. Nevertheless, it is claimed that diagnosis on biopsy material can be accurate in most cases (Hourihane, 5, p. 647). In addition, there is the difficulty of obtaining agreement between pathologists on histologic characteristics (McCaughey, 7, p. 58), a difficulty reflected by the relatively modest number of cases, less than 50 per cent in some series (206), subsequently confirmed by mesothelioma review panels. This difficulty may be less important in clinical medicine, in which the important distinction is between a benign and a malignant tumor, than in epidemiologic studies that seek to investigate the association with a history of asbestos exposure, in which consistency of diagnostic criteria in exposed and unexposed groups is all important.

Because of the between-tumor and within-tumor histologic variation mentioned previously, and the not infrequent development of the growth in the track of the biopsy needle, other methods of examination have been used to increase the certainty of diagnosis. Thus, the presence of hyaluronic acid in the pleural fluid (207) or its demonstration in tumor tissue by histochemical techniques (208) may be of some value in distinguishing between mesothelioma and secondary carcinoma, but is not the definitive test it was originally believed to be (207). Cytologic examination of pleural fluids, by light and electron microscopy, may offer useful contributory evidence. A series of papers under the general title "Assessment of Methods Used in the Studies of the Biological Effect of Asbestos to Pathology" (7, pp. 58–81) provides a most convenient and up-to-date summary of these methods, their precision, and general applicability.

The radiologic appearances vary according to the stage to which the disease has progressed. Common features are the presence of a pleural effusion, lobulated tumor masses that may be visible only after removal of the pleural fluid, chest wall masses, satellite lung lesions, and, occasionally, hydropneumothorax (209).

In a review of treatments (13, p. 277) Elmes pointed out that there is no effective curative treatment, although surgical excision, local and/or systemic cytotoxic therapy, and radiotherapy have all been tried. He also pointed out several features that suggest a considerable contribution of the body's defense mechanism, both in the formation of abnormal tissue and in the shaping of its clinical course. Relative to the first point is the apparently low dose of exposure capable of eliciting a response; relative to the second is the not infrequent occurrence of chest injuries and/or infections at the onset of the clinical course, and the sometimes rapid dissemination, apparently provoked by treatments, such as radiation or cytotoxic drugs. For these reasons, he believes that this tumor may eventually turn out to be controllable through improving body defenses. Thus, it is not surprising that the use of BCG vaccine in treatment is a matter of great current interest, with, as yet, no definitive evidence on which to base clinical action.

Meanwhile, therapy is symptomatic, and diagnostic measures should be kept to a minimum. Removal of fluid for diagnostic examination and to relieve breathlessness should be done as infrequently as possible. Indeed, as Elmes notes, the establishment of a precise diagnosis in life, given the absence of a potentially curative treatment, is an academic, rather than a clinically useful, exercise.

Carcinoma of the Lung Associated with Asbestos Exposure

An association between asbestosis and bronchial carcinoma, suspected in the 1930s on the basis of individual case reports (210), was subsequently confirmed in two British reports, one by the Chief Inspector of Factories, issued in 1947, and the second, an analysis of autopsy material from more than 1,000 cases of pneumoconiosis published in 1951 (211). From these, it appeared that asbestosis was associated with a much higher lung cancer risk than other pneumoconiosis, with 15 to 20 per cent of men recorded as having asbestosis dying from this cause. This risk was reported to have further increased considerably in Britain by 1963 (10), and a similar increase in lung cancer risk during the same decades has been reported from Germany (Jacob, 5, p. 536). The emergence of lung cancer as an important threat to the health of asbestos workers is attributed to the improvement in dust conditions, with less mortality from asbestosis occurring after longer periods of exposure and, therefore, survival of workers through the long latent period of lung cancer (63).

Subsequent epidemiologic studies have amply confirmed the association between asbestos exposure and lung cancer, mortality experience being the chief method of study (63, 67, 82); however, table 7 indicates that despite the consistently increased relative risk in these reports, there are considerable between-study differences as to its degree. Some of these differences must certainly be ascribed to between-study differences in the methods used to calculate risk (217), particularly in such factors as composition of the risk group (in terms of age, years of exposure, and length of follow-up), and the nature of the control or reference group, which could be either a low-exposure group within the working population, or an appropriate reference population derived from national statistics. In addition, most studies deal with relatively small numbers of deaths (less than 100 in all but 2 of the studies), so that calculation would inevitably be influenced by the addition or loss of one case. Finally, differences in exposure dose and smoking habits are other relevant factors for which standardization is seldom possible. As Wagner and associates point out, however, "an additional lesson to be learnt from the apparent conflict of evidence is the need to pay more attention to the type of asbestos and to the physical state of the respirable faction of the dust" (218), and the evidence that there are real differences in risk associated with the different fiber types, as well as the different types of exposure to the same fiber, is becoming more convincing. Such differences, however, have a greater significance in the field of environmental control and safety standards than in the practice of clinical medicine.

The interaction of cigarettes and asbestos exposure as risk factors, clarified to some extent by epidemiologic studies, is, however, of very real importance in clinical practice. Carcinoma of the lung appears to develop only very rarely in the nonsmoker exposed to asbestos (63, 73) whereas the risk associated with exposure to both is considerably more than additive, and probably multiplicative (63, 73, 219).

It was originally believed that the tumor was a scar cancer, because of its common location in the lower lobes, where fibrosis tends to be most marked (220). Animal experiments support this hypothesis (62). However, although usually found in lungs, which are the seat of fibrosis (67, 221), this is not always so (220). Cases have also been reported in association with relatively mild fibrosis, and occasionally in the absence of fibrosis (220). Similarly, although cases occur almost exclusively in smokers (63, 219), there is some evidence to suggest that the distribution of cell types is different from that seen in smokers without exposure, namely, a greater preponderance of adenocarcinoma (222). This has led to the hypothesis that the carcinogens in cigarette smoke may have been delivered to the more peripheral regions of the bronchial tree by the fibers and dust particles (222). Not all series show this greater preponderance of adenocarcinoma, however, and the question remains open. In one series, the presence of pleural plaques appeared to be associated with a higher risk for developing cancer (130), but it also seems possible that the presence of plaques may also merely reflect a higher exposure dose. Multiple primary tumors, sometimes of different cell types, have also been described in relation to asbestos exposure (223).

The clinical picture, prognosis, and treatment are no different from those seen in the person not exposed to asbestos, except that the associated fibrosis may limit the treatment options. Advice to, and help in, quitting smoking are clearly even more important for the worker exposed to asbestos than his or her unexposed companion, and a concerted effort at worker education might prove worthwhile.

Another practical problem concerns compensation, in particular, the question of attributability of lung cancer to exposure in the absence of significant fibrosis. Some compensation boards, acting on the dose-relationship information, award the benefit of the doubt if exposure has been considerable in a nonsmoker.

Finally, as has been emphasized elsewhere (220, 223), the "occupational history may not seem important in patients with carcinoma and is often not diligently pursued." The epidemiologic evidence summarized here underlines the importance of establishing this association.

Other Asbestos-Related Cancers

In most mortality studies of asbestos workers, there is a greater-than-expected risk for all cancers (table 7). Lung cancer shows the greatest relative risk, followed by cancers of the gastrointestinal tract. The excess of gastrointestinal cancers is evident in all series, whatever the reference population used to calculate expected number of deaths, with one exception, namely, workers exposed in anthophyllite mining (77). This presumably is further evidence of the difference in the biologic effects of the different fiber types. There is also some evidence to suggest that environmental exposures may be of importance in gastrointestinal cancer (16).

In addition to lung cancer, there is increasing evidence that asbestos exposure is associated with cancer of the larynx (11–14). Like lung cancer, this cancer also has a long latent period (13). and cigarette smoking is a well-recognized associated risk factor. Indeed, it is surprising that its association with asbestos has only recently been recognized, but this is perhaps because it is less common than lung cancer.

An association between asbestos exposure and ovarian cancer, suggested originally on the basis of both clinical (10) and animal studies (15), has not, in the view of the Advisory Committee on Asbestos Cancers (7, p. 342), been confirmed in the first large mortality survey of women asbestos workers (7, p. 203). It is believed that the clinical cases originally believed to be ovarian tumors were malignant mesothelioma of the peritoneum (10, 186).

An association of asbestos exposure (as reflected in the lung count of asbestos bodies) and carcinoma of the breast in women has been reported in one study from London, England (16), a study that, paradoxically, did not show the same thing for carcinoma of the bronchus. Other cancers with suspected, but unsubstantiated, associations with asbestos exposure are leukemia, multiple myeloma, and Waldenström's macroglobulinemia (10). They are mentioned here, not to alarm physicians or their patients, but to underline the strength of the association between asbestos and many human cancers. For certain cancers this association calls for clinical action, even though it remains to be proved whether asbestos itself is the

TABLE 7

RELATIVE RISK OF CANCER FOR MALE ASBESTOS WORKERS

Occupation and Country	Fiber	Population Studied			Deaths		Relative Risk of Cancer*			Reference
		No.	Minimal Exposure	Years of Follow-Up	Total No.	No. Due to Lung Cancer	All Others	Lung	G-1	
Mining and milling										
Canada	Chrysotile	5,958	5 years	6	187	12	—	1.5	—	Braun and Trauen (212)
	Chrysotile	9,692	1 month	ave., 25	3,270	135	—	1.4	—	McDonald (7, p. 155)
	Chrysotile		1 month	ave., 25	3,270	134	1.4†	3.1†	1.6†	McDonald (7, p. 155)**
Finland	Anthophyllite	1,041	3 months	2–33	248	21	—	1.6	0.5	Meurman *et al* (77)
	Anthophyllite	?	10 years	2–33				3.3	0.9	Meurman *et al* (77)
Production: Secondary use										
UK										
Textiles	Mainly chrysotile	113	20 years (pre 1933)	≥ 20	39	11	4.8	13.7	1.7	Doll (68)
Textiles	Mainly chrysotile	674	10 years (post 1933)	ave., 17	69	8	0.6	1.0	—	Knox *et al* (67)
Insulation production	Mainly chrysotile	1,024	6 months	15	133	7	1.1	2.3	—	Elwood and Cochrane (213)
Mainly textiles	Mainly crocidolite	1,834	1 month	1	180	46	—	4.8	—	Berry *et al* (73)
	Mainly crocidolite	1,304	2 years	10–25	114	36	3.6	5.6	—	Newhouse (71)
Insulators; pipecovers	Chrysotile, crocidolite, amosite	165	Not stated	26	98	28††	6.7	17.6	—	Elmes and Simpson (214)
USA										
All types of production	Not stated	529	Not stated	3	41	10	1.4	3.2	—	Dunn and Weir (215)
All types of production	Not stated	1,265	Not stated	20	330	35	3.1†	3.3†	3.1†	Mancuso and El-Atar (74)
All types of production	Little amosite or crocidolite	1,026	3 years	Retirees from age 65 on	568	29	1.2	1.7	1.1	Enterline *et al* (83)
Maintenance	Includes amosite and crocidolite	438	3 years	Retirees from age 65 on	254	30	2.1	4.3	1.7	Enterline *et al* (83)
Insulation production	Amosite	933	1 year	ave., 26	484	73	5.1	6.4	2.0	Selikoff *et al* (216)
Insulation workers***	Mainly chrysotile	623	20 years†††	28	421	84	4.0	8.3	3.1	Selikoff (7, p. 209)
Insluation workers***		5,118	20 years†††	4	881	191	3.5	5.1	2.1	Selikoff (7, p. 209)

*Comparisons were made with appropriate national statistics, except where indicated. Relative risk = observed/expected number of deaths.

†Internal comparison of low- and high-exposure groups.

**Best estimate of relative risk for lung cancer was 5.0 using other methods.

††Includes cancer of the pleura and larynx.

***Engaged in a wide variety of jobs.

†††Years since first exposure.

human carcinogen, or a cocarcinogen, and/or potentiator of cigarette smoke and/or other factors.

The Influence of Fiber Type and the Nature of Exposure on Biological Response

After the 1964 New York Conference (5), the UICC working group on cancer urged study of "the relationship of dust dosage (including concentration and duration of exposure) and the composition and physical state of the dust to the incidence of asbestosis, carcinoma of the lung, mesothelioma and other cancers." In other words, 2 areas were identified for urgent future research: (1) to establish whether dose-response relationships exist between exposure and biologic response, and (2) to establish whether the composition and physical state of the dust affects these dose-response relationships.

In the ensuing 11 years, health scientists throughout the world have gathered data in support of the first hypothesis, namely, that a dose-response relationship exists for all of the responses listed (asbestosis, carcinoma of the lung, other cancers, and, probably, mesothelioma). Furthermore, this holds for all types of fiber and for all types of exposure investigated. The evidence has been already summarized in table 4.

It has proved more difficult to investigate the second hypothesis, that composition and physical state of the dust influence the responses, because this requires the comparison of dose-response curves for different fibers, or for the same fiber under different exposure conditions, e.g., mining and milling compared to manufacturing. Even animal studies in which exposure can be relatively well controlled are inconclusive about the relative fibrogenicity of different fiber types (62, 224) although differences in carcinogenic potential have been shown (224). Epidemiologic studies in man in different occupationally exposed groups suggest differences between fibers, and between exposures, in terms of their carcinogenic potential both for lung cancer (table 6) and for mesothelioma (224); however, it is usually impossible to establish to what extent these can be explained by differences in exposure levels and associated factors, such as cigarettes and other co-carcinogens. Furthermore, exposures to one fiber type only are rare (usually in mining), and most production workers have mixed exposures (224). For instance, table 8 summarizes data collected in Quebec asbestos workers, exposed only to chrysotile fibers. Even in these results,

which show a dose effect for all responses, there are between-area differences, particularly for radiologic changes, for men of the same stock and working the same geologic deposit, and with exposure calculated using the same type of index. Given these between-area differences, to what extent, if any, are these dose-response curves applicable to other working populations?

Criteria for comparability require that both the dose and the response be measured in a similar fashion and that the populations compared have equivalent susceptibility. Enough has already been said to indicate that even if the first 2 criteria were met, virtually nothing is known about the factors accounting for susceptibility, much less whether it is possible to measure them in practice. The only comparison attempted was inconclusive, because mortality was assessed by fundamentally different techniques (figure 5). Thus, it is not possible to deduce from this comparison whether, indeed, there is greater risk for production workers compared to miners (figure 5, upper panel) attributable to differences in the nature of the exposure, an interpretation for which there is little scientific justification, or whether the risk is comparable for both groups, but the scaling (figure 5, lower panel) requires appropriate adjustment.

Despite the difficulties in making between-study comparisons, a consensus has emerged, outlined in a carefully reasoned paper by Kleinfeld (224), and in the conclusion of the Advisory Committee on Asbestos Cancers (7, p. 341). It is believed that there are gradients in the mesothelioma-producing potential, related to fiber type (greatest with crocidolite, less with amosite and with chrysotile, least with anthophyllite) and to occupation (e.g., for amosite, greatest in insulation workers compared to miners). Gradients in fibrogenic capability of the different fibers, less clear, may also be present, with crocidolite leading chrysotile, whereas gradients in lung cancer risk may be more closely related to the nature of the exposure, with production leading mining, at least for chrysotile.

To date, the best explanation of these gradients in biologic potential is that developed by Timbrell (7, p. 295), namely, that biologic activity relates to the degree of penetration and deposition in the lung (see also figure 6). Thus, the greater mesothelioma potential of crocidolite compared to amosite, anthophyllite, and chrysotile, could be due to its smaller fiber size and its other aerodynamic properties, which permit greater penetration and deposition. Similar-

TABLE 8

EXPOSURE-RESPONSE RELATIONSHIPS IN QUEBEC CHRYSOTILE ASBESTOS MINERS AND MILLERS

Dust Index*	<10	10–	100–	200–	400–	800–	Source	Reference
Death rate/1,000 persons[†] from								
Respiratory cancer	10	13	13	16	21	32	Cohort of	85, 92
Pneumoconiosis	2	2	1	5	5	24	11,107	
Abdominal cancer	18	14	19	12	26	29	men born	
Other respiratory causes	12	18	24	19	16	25	1891–1920)	
Circulatory causes	123	119	118	116	118	135		
Prevalence of radiologic changes in men 56–65 years, %**								
Small, irregular opacities (1/0 or +)							Study of chest	88, 92
Thetford area	—	7	10	13	21	34	radiographs of	
Asbestos area	10	6	17	23	15	20	13,021 past	
Any pleural changes							and present	
Thetford area	23	20	33	29	34	39	employees	
Asbestos area	5	15	18	14	15	24		
Prevalence, %[††]								
Dyspnea	7	18	23	26	30	37	(1,015 current	86, 92
Decrease in lung function, %***							workers)	
VC	0	−4	−9	−11	−14	−15	(1,015 current	87, 92
FEV$_1$	0	−4	−7	−10	−13	−14	workers)	
Steady-state DL$_{CO}$, at rest	0	−3	−6	−5	−9	−11		

*Million particles per foot^3 per year (91).

[†]Age corrected; followed up to 1969.

**Standardized for age and years of employment.

[††]Age standardized.

***Age and height standardized.

ly, the greater mesothelioma and, possibly, cancer potential of amosite in manufacturing processes, compared to mining, could be attributed to the smaller particle size for the fiber released in a production plant compared to that at the mine head.

At the practical level of environmental control, regulations proposed for chrysotile in 1968 (225) by the British Occupational Hygiene Society were at a level (2 fibers per cm³ averaged over 3 months) that, it was hoped, would allow no more than 1 per cent risk of disease (specifically, asbestosis) in a 50-year working life. Evidence suggests that this would also re-

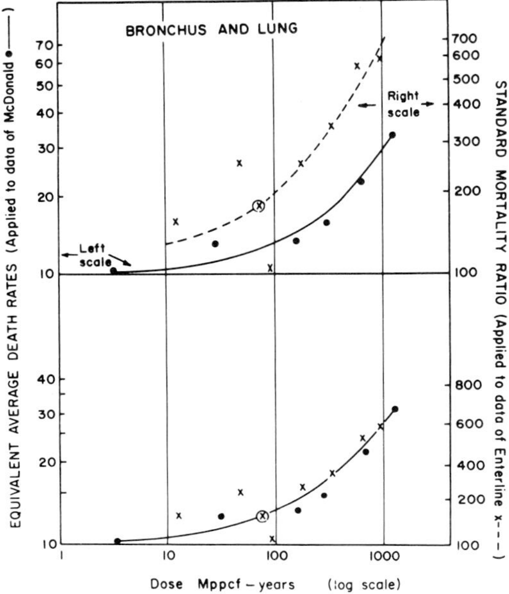

Fig. 5. [From Schneiderman (93); reprinted by permission of publisher.] Dose-response relationship for cancer of the bronchus and lung. The data shown are those of McDonald (7, p. 189), describing chrysotile asbestos miners (*left* scale), and those of Enterline and associates (82, 83), describing production workers (*right* scale). In McDonald's data, mortality was expressed as equivalent average death rates (85, 92) to enable a within-population comparison between men with low and higher dust exposure. The data of Enterline and associates were reported as standardized mortality ratios, which used for comparison the most appropriate general population statistics. Dust exposure in both studies was calculated in similar fashion and expressed in million particles per foot³-years (82, 83, 91). The vertical scales are drawn so that an equivalent average death rate of 20 is equated with a standardized mortality ratio of 200 in the top panel and 400 in the bottom panel, which results in both sets of data falling on the same curve.

duce risk of bronchogenic cancer. At the time, the British Occupational Hygiene Society was uncertain that standards for other fibers should follow "by analogy." They subsequently proposed the same standards for amosite (226), but a standard 10 times more stringent for crocidolite (227) was promulgated by government regulation. Furthermore, because all standards should be regarded as no more than an expression of the "best available hypothesis" of levels adequate to protect human health, they should always be reviewed in the light of subsequent evidence. This was done in 1973 for chrysotile, and no change was recommended (228). In the United States, the Occupational Health and Safety Administration (OSHA) promulgated a standard of 5 fibers per cm³ in 1972, to be reduced to 2 fibers per cm³ in 1976 (229), and there was a recent proposal to lower further the standard to 0.5 fibers per cm³ (230). These standards apply to all fiber types.

Research should continue in an attempt to identify more precisely the reasons for between-fiber differences in biologic effect, because a better understanding of what determines the biologic responses of this mineral can only result in its human use being conducted under conditions that more effectively protect the health of the exposed worker.

Clinical Implications of the Epidemiologic Findings

Faced with a patient in whom the diagnosis of one of the described diseases has been made, i.e., fibrosis of the lungs and/or pleura, or cancer of the lungs and/or pleura, it may be important to establish whether, in this particular case, the disease is asbestos related. If the patient is currently known to be exposed, this rarely presents a problem. If not, a systematic history is called for, and should include all his or her previous occupations (including short-term jobs, summer jobs, and so on), as well as those of his or her work colleagues and family members. In addition, places of residence should be noted, particularly if the diagnosis is mesothelioma and/or pleural plaques. The discovery of asbestos fibers, coated or uncoated, in biologic material (sputum or biopsy or surgical material) requires explanation, if not already evident from the history. Establishment of an association with asbestos has importance if attributability is questioned (in cases of compensation), as well as for other workers if the risk had not previously been recognized.

The dose relationship, particularly of fibrosis,

CROCIDOLITE AMOSITE

ANTHOPHYLLITE CHRYSOTILE

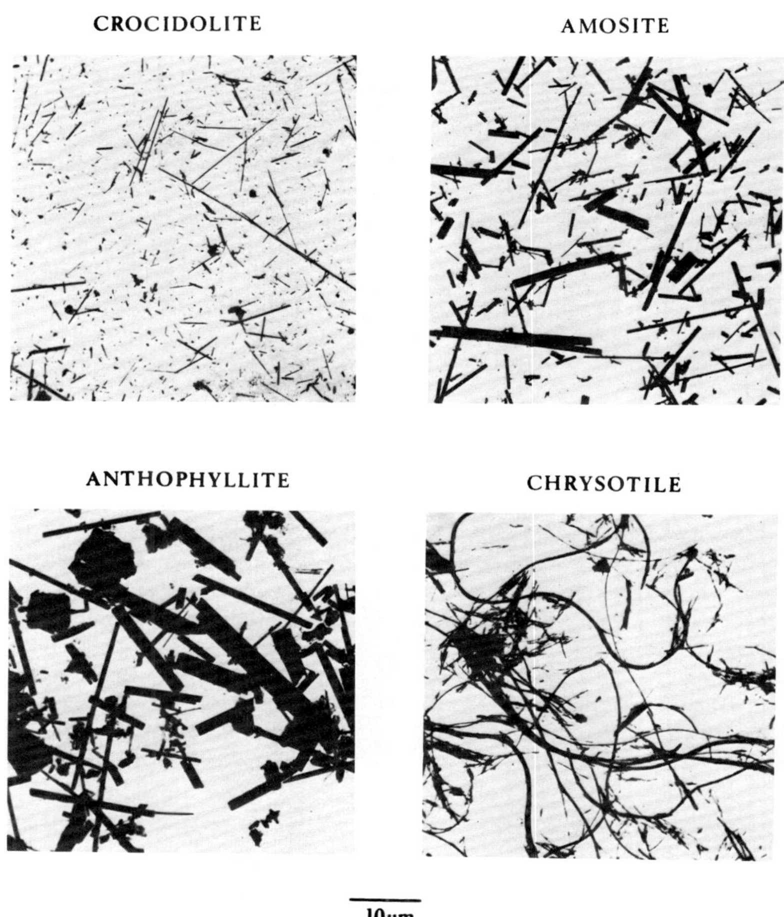

Fig. 6. [From Timbrell, V.: Physical factors as, etiologic mechanisms, in *Biological Effects of Asbestos*, IARC Scientific Publication No. 8, Lyon, 1973, p. 295; reprinted by permission of publisher.] Electron micrographs of crocidolite (north-western Cape Province), amosite (Transvaal), anthophyllite (Finland), chrysotile (Canada) at the same magnification (× 1700). Features to note are (*1*) the rectilinear shape of the amphibole fibers compared with the curved and twisted morphology of chrysotile fibers; (*2*) the order of the diameters of the amphibole fibers, suggested by numerous electron micrographic examinations of these fibers from the 3 geographical areas, crocidolite < amosite < anthophyllite; (*3*) the longitudinal fragmentation of the chrysotile fibers and the small diameter (about 0.03 μm) of the ultimate fibrils.

to exposure should always be borne in mind, and the patient in whom disease develops after a relatively short period (for example, less than 25 years) must be taken as an indicator of unsatisfactory past and/or present working conditions, requiring forceful corrective action. The same attitude should be taken toward the person in whom fibrosis is believed to be present in its early stages or development, either on clinical, radiologic, or functional evidence. Any claim that this is not so because the "environmental levels" to which the person was exposed were "safe" is incorrect; levels were clearly not

"safe" for the particular person concerned, either because of greater-than-suspected dose, or greater-than-average susceptibility.

It must be emphasized that the clinician's job is not only to recognize the case of asbestos-related disease, but also to see that it is brought to the attention of the appropriate executive authority (in many areas, the Workmen's Compensation Committee, which informs the company concerned). This recognition and referral has social implications at 2 levels. For the person, the implication is appropriate compensation, society's fumbling best to make up for his or her loss of health. At the second level the occurrence of an asbestos-related illness is approached as a failure of control measures, and one seeks to identify the point of failure so that appropriate action can be taken to protect the health of the new generation of workers (the children and younger colleagues of today's victims), who may be currently entering the industry.

Nowhere is this more evident than with the finding of a patient with malignant mesothelioma whose only possible contact with asbestos is indirect, through neighborhood and/or domestic exposure. Given a history of neighborhood exposure, should one advise the family to move for the sake of its other members? Probably not, because the long time lag of this tumor makes it most likely that they have already received any exposure relevant to the future development of mesothelioma. Should new families moving into the district be advised against this, unless there has been appropriate action for environmental control over the previous years? An unanswerable question. Given a history of domestic exposure, the clinician should at least be able to assure the new families that work practice codes now insist that dusty work clothes are not taken home to be cleaned.

Faced with a person with a known exposure risk, what medical measures can be taken to protect his or her health? Sadly, it must be admitted that there are none, because effective health protection lies in effective environmental control, and medical surveillance is, probably correctly, considered a form of biologic monitoring supplementary to environmental monitoring (231). Thus, good work practices and quitting or refraining from smoking are the best "medical measures" for the individual worker; however, the examination implied by medical surveillance can provide other services, including case detection and other forms of health care. As knowledge improves, it is possible that medical surveillance will be able to fulfill its hoped-for role, namely, the detection of health effects in a person at a stage when some action (for instance, removal from exposure) might prevent eventual disablement.

Given the "imperfect" state of the art, it is, at present, believed that medical surveillance should include a clinical examination (emphasis on basal crepitations), an annual chest radiograph, and a measurement of lung function, probably the most useful being the forced expiratory volume test, and possibly the diffusing capacity. At what point in time changes in one or more of these methods of examination call for action remains to be established.

For the currently exposed worker, research in this area certainly has the most relevance, in particular, methods of identifying the persons in whom the disease will progress, whether or not exposure continues. Animal work suggests that withdrawal from exposure may slow progression (62), and in the absence of definitive data, this must also be assumed to occur in man. With regard to the future worker, it remains to be determined whether the person at high risk can be identified before entry into the industry. Meanwhile, there seems to be merit in deploying energy into maintaining currently proposed standards. Three times in the twentieth century, levels have been set, because the asbestos worker's health became a matter of public concern. Had the standards been more systematically adhered to, it is likely that the asbestos-related diseases would not have re-emerged as the "occupational illness of the 60s," a testimony to the working conditions of the previous decade. It is to be hoped that current concern is translated into effective action for the workforce currently entering the industry.

Acknowledgment

The writer wishes to express her very sincere appreciation to Dr. S. Hurwitz of the University of the Witwatersrand, Johannesburg, South Africa, for able help in the literature search behind this review; to Dr. J. C. McDonald, director, and all members of the McGill University group engaged in research into the health effects of asbestos exposure since 1964, in recognition of their stimulating collaboration during this period, experience that forms the basis of the present review; to Dr. R. Oseasohn, Chairman, and Prof. F. D. K. Liddell, Dr. G. Gibbs, and Dr. M. Arhirii of the Department of Epidemiology and Health, McGill University, and Dr. M. Newhouse of the London School of Tropical Medicine and Hygiene for valuable editorial comment; to Dr. M. Pelnar, of the Institute of Occupational and Environmental Health, Quebec Asbestos Mining Association, for access to the Institute's extensive library of reprints and for his editorial comment; and to Diane L. Cloutier, Jane Ross, Arlette Maurus, and Thea Hopkinson for their willing help in preparation of the manuscript.

References

1. Hamilton, A., and Hardy, H.: Industrial Toxicology, ed. 3, Publishing Sciences Group Inc., Acton, Mass., 1974, p. 421.
2. Gilson, J. C.: Asbestos cancer: Past and future

hazards, Proc R Soc Med, 1973, *66*, 395.

3. Zussman, J.: Asbestos: Nature and history, Rev Ciba-Geigy, 1972, *2*, 3.

4. Smither, W. J.: Asbestos and asbestosis, Ann Occup Hyg, 1970, *13*, 3.

5. Biological effects of asbestos, I. J. Selikoff, and J. Churg, co-chairmen, Proceedings of a conference held at the New York Academy of Sciences, Oct. 19–21, 1964, Ann N Y Acad Sci, 1965, *132*, pp. 1–766.

6. Biological effects of asbestos, M. Anspach, Chairman, Deutsches Zentralinstitut fur Arbeitsmedizin: Gesellschaft fur Arbeitshygiene und Arbeitsschutz in der DDR, Dresden, April 22–25, 1968, pp. 1–312.

7. Biological effects of asbestos, P. Bogovski, J. G. Gilson, V. Timbrell, and J. C. Wagner, ed. Proceedings of a working conference at IARC, Lyon, October 2–6, 1972, IARC Scientific Publications, No. 8, Lyon, 1973, pp. 1–341.

8. Proceedings of the Pneumoconiosis Conference, Johannesburg, South Africa, February 1959, A. J. Orenstein, ed., J. and A. Churchill Ltd., London, 1960, pp. 1–629.

9. Pneumoconiosis, H. A. Shapiro, ed., Proceedings of the International Conference, Johannesburg, South Africa, 1969, Oxford University Press, Cape Town, 1970, pp. 3–645.

10. Parkes, W. R.: Asbestos-related disorders, Br J Dis Chest, 1973, *67*, 261.

11. Stell, P. M., and McGill, T.: Asbestos and laryngeal carcinoma, Lancet, 1973, *2*, 416.

12. Newhouse, M. L., and Berry, G.: Asbestos and laryngeal carcinoma, Lancet, 1973, *2*, 615.

13. Libshitz, H. I., Wershba, M. S., Atkinson, G. W., and Southard, M. E.: Asbestos and carcinoma of the larynx, JAMA, 1974, *228*, 1571.

14. Guidotti, T. L., Abraham, J. L., and DeNee, P. B.: Asbestos exposure and cancer of the larynx, West J Med, 1975, *122*, 75.

15. Graham, J., and Graham, R.: Ovarian cancer and asbestos, Environ Res, 1967, *1*, 115.

16. Doniach, I., Swettenham, K. V., and Hathorn, M. K. S.: Prevalence of asbestos bodies in a necropsy series in East London: Association with disease, occupation, and domiciliary address, Br J Ind Med, 1975, *32*, 16.

17. Weiss, W.: Clinical epidemiology, Arch Environ Health, 1970, *20*, 5.

18. Speil, S., and Leineweber, J. P.: Asbestos minerals in modern technology, Environ Res, 1969, *2*, 166.

19. Wright, G. W.: Asbestos and health in 1969, Am Rev Respir Dis, 1969, *100*, 467.

20. Harries, P. G.: Asbestos dust concentrations in ship repairing: A practical approach to improving asbestos hygiene in naval dockyards, Ann Occup Hyg, 1971, *14*, 241.

21. Respiratory Diseases: Task Force Report on Problems, Research Approaches, Needs, The Lung Program, National Heart and Lung Institute, October 1972, U. S. Department of Health, Education and Welfare.

22. Lee, G. L., and Smith, D. J.: Steelwork insulated with sprayed crocidolite asbestos: Controlling a potential hazard, Ann Occup Hyg, 1974, *17*, 49.

23. Byrom, J. C., Hodgson, A. A., and Homes, S.: A dust survey carried out in buildings incorporating asbestos based materials in their construction, Ann Occup Hyg, 1969, *12*, 171.

24. Greenburg, M.: Asbestos release from battery boxes, Ann Occup Hyg, 1970, *13*, 79.

25. Hickish, D. E., and Knight, K. L.: Exposure to asbestos during brake maintenance, Ann Occup Hyg, 1970, *13*, 17.

26. Murphy, R. L. H., Levine, B. W., Albazzaz, F. J., Lynch, J. J., and Burgess, W. A.: Floor tile installation as a source of asbestos exposure, Am Rev Respir Dis, 1971, *104*, 576.

27. Wagner, J. C., Sleggs, C. A., and Marchand, P: Diffuse pleural mesothelioma and asbestos exposure in the North-West Cape Province, Br J Ind Med, 1960, *17*, 260.

28. Newhouse, M. L., and Thompson, H.: Mesothelioma of pleura and peritoneum following exposure to asbestos in the London area, Br J Ind Med, 1965, *22*, 61.

29. Newhouse, M. L.: A study of the mortality of workers in an asbestos factory, Br J Ind Med, 1969, *26*, 294.

30. Newhouse, M. L., Berry, G., Wagner, J. C., and Turok, M. E.: A study of the mortality of female asbestos workers, Br J Ind Med, 1972, *29*, 134.

31. Champion, P.: Two cases of malignant mesothelioma after exposure to asbestos, Am Rev Dis, 1971, *103*, 821.

32. Kiviluoto, R.: Pleural calcification as a roentgenologic sign of non-occupational endemic anthophyllite asbestosis, Acta Radiol (Stockh), 1960, *194*, (Supplement, p. 1).

33. Zolov, C., Burilkov, T., and Babadjov, L.: Pleural asbestosis in agricultural workers, Environ Res, 1967, *1*, 287.

34. Burilkov, T., and Michailova, L.: Asbestos content of the soil and endemic pleural asbestosis, Environ Res, 1970, *3*, 443.

35. Rous, V., and Studeny, J.: Aetiology of pleural plaques, Thorax, 1970, *25*, 270.

36. Selikoff, I. J., Nicholson, W. J., and Langer, A. M.: Asbestos air pollution, Arch Environ Health, 1972, *25*, 1.

37. Cook, P. M., Glass, G. E., and Tucker, J. H.: Asbestiform amphibole minerals: Dectection and measurement of high concentration in municipal water supplies, Science, 1974, *185*, 853.

38. Round the world: Asbestos in water, Lancet, 1973, *2*, 1256.

39. Masson, T. J., McKay, F. W., and Miller, R. W.:

Asbestos-like fibers in Duluth water supply: Relation to cancer mortality, JAMA, 1974, *228*, 1019.

40. Pontefract, R., and Cunningham, H. M.: Penetration of asbestos through the digestive tracts of rats, Nature, 1973, *243*, 352.

41. Muir, D. E. F.: Deposition and clearance of inhaled particles, in *Clinical Aspects of Inhaled Particles*, D. C. F. Muir, ed., William Heinemann Medical Books Ltd., London, 1972, p. 1.

42. Brain, J. D., and Valberg, P. A.: Models of lung retention based on ICRP Task Group Report, Arch Environ Health, 1974, *28*, 1.

43. Bates, D. V., Macklem, P. T., and Christie, R. V.: Respiratory Function in Disease, ed. 2, W. B. Saunders Co., Philadelphia, 1971,

44. Sanchis, J., Dolovich, M., Chalmers, R., and Newhouse, M. T.: Regional distribution and lung clearance mechanisms in smokers and non-smokers, in *Inhaled Particles III*, W. Walton, ed., Unwin Bros. Ltd., Old Woking, England, 1970, p. 183.

45. Thomson, M. L., and Short, M. D.: Mucociliary function in health, chronic obstructive airway disease, and asbestosis, J Appl Physiol, 1969, *26*, 535.

46. Thomson, M. L., and Pavia, D.: Particle penetration and clearance in the human lung, Arch Environ Health, 1975, *29*, 214.

47. Albert, R. E., Peterson, H. T., Bohning, D. E., and Lippmann M.: Short term effects of cigarette smoking on bronchial clearance in humans, Arch Environ Health, 1975, *30*, 361.

48. Gross, P., and DeTreville, R. T. P.: The lung as an embattled domain against inanimate pollutants, Am Rev Respir Dis, 1972, *106*, 684.

49. Ashcroft, T., and Heppelston, A. G.: The optical and electron microscopic determination of pulmonary asbestos fibre concentration and its relation to human pathological reaction, J Clin Pathol, 1973, *26*, 224.

50. Pooley, F. D.: Electronmicroscope characteristics of inhaled chrysotile asbestos fibre, Br J Ind Med, 1972, *29*, 146.

51. Langer, A. M., Selikoff, I. J., and Sastre, A.: Chrysotile asbestos in the lungs of persons in New York City, Arch Environ Health, 1971, *22*, 348.

52. Gross, P., Davis, J. M. G., Harley, R. A., and DeTreville, R. T. P.: Lymphatic transport of fibrous dust from the lungs, J Occup Med, 1973, *15*, 186.

53. Gross, P., Harley, R. A., Swinburne, L. M., Davis, J. M. G., and Greene, W. B.: Ingested mineral fibers: Do they penetrate tissue or cause cancer, Arch Environ Health, 1974, *29*, 341.

54. Meurman, L.: Asbestos bodies and pleural plaques in a Finnish series of autopsy cases, Acta Pathol Microbiol Scand, 1966, (Supplement 181, p. 8).

55. Gaensler, E. A., and Addington, W. W.: Asbestos or ferruginous bodies, N Engl J Med, 1969, *280*, 488.

56. Suzuki, Y., and Churg, J.: Formation of the asbestos body: A comparative study with three types of asbestos, Environ Res, 1969, *3*, 107.

57. Suzuki, Y., and Churg, J.: Structure and development of the asbestos body, Amer J Pathol, 1969, *55*, 79.

58. Davis, J. M.: Further observations on the ultrastructure and chemistry of the formation of asbestos bodies, Exp Mol Pathol, 1970, *13*, 346.

59. Fondimare, A., and Desbordes, J.: Asbestos bodies and fibers in lung tissues, Environ Health Perspect, 1974, *9*, 147.

60. Gross, P., DeTreville, R. T. P., and Haller, M. N.: Pulmonary ferruginous bodies in city dwellers, Arch Environ Health, 1969, *19*, 186.

61. Hatch, T. F.: Significant dimensions of the dose-response relationship, Arch Environ Health, 1968, *16*, 571.

62. Wagner, J. C., Berry, G., Skidmore, J. W., and Timbrell, V.: The effects of the inhalation of asbestos in rats, Br J Cancer, 1974, *29*, 252.

63. Selikoff, I. J., Bader, R. A., Bader, M. E., Churg, J., and Hammond, E. C.: Asbestosis and neoplasia, Am J Med, 1967, *42*, 487.

64. Bader, M. E., Bader, R. A., Tierstein, A. S., Miller, A., and Selikoff, I. J.: Pulmonary function and radiographic changes in 598 workers with varying duration of exposure to asbestos, J Mt Sinai Hosp, 1970, *37*, 492.

65. Sluis-Cremer, G. K.: Asbestosis in South African asbestos miners, Environ Res, 1970, *3*, 310.

66. Knox, J. F., Holmes, S., Doll, R., and Hill, I. D.: Mortality from lung cancer and other causes amongst workers in an asbestos textile factory, Br J Ind Med, 1968, *25*, 293.

67. Doll, R.: Mortality from lung cancer in asbestos workers, Br J Ind Med, 1955, *12*, 81.

68. Kleinfeld, M., Messite, J., and Kooyman, O.: Mortality experience in a group of asbestos workers, Arch Environ Health, 1967, *15*, 177.

69. McDonald, J. C., Gibbs, G. W., Manfreda, J., and White, F. M. M.: Storage as a factor in disease due to mineral dusts, in *Multiple Factors in the Causation of Environmentally Induced Diseases*, D. H. K. Lee and P. Kotin, ed., Academic Press, New York, 1972, p. 185.

70. Regan, G. M., Tagg, B., and Walford, J., and Thomson, M. L.: The relative importance of clinical, radiological and pulmonary function variables in evaluating asbestosis and chronic obstructive airways disease in asbestos workers, Clin Sci, 1971, *41*, 569.

71. Newhouse, M. L.: Asbestos in the workplace and the community, Ann Occup Hyg, 1973, *16*, 97.

72. Zedda, S., Aresini, G., Ghezzi, I., and Sartonelli, E.: Lung function in relation to radiographic

changes in asbestos workers, Respiration, 1973, *30*, 132.

73. Berry, G., Newhouse, M. L., and Turok, M.: Combined effects of asbestos exposure and smoking on mortality from lung cancer in factory workers, Lancet, 1972, *2*, 476.

74. Mancuso, T., El-Attar, A. A.: Mortality pattern in a cohort of asbestos workers, J Occup Med, 1967, *9*, 147.

75. Harries, P. G., Mackenzie, F. A. F., Sheers, G., Kemp, J. H., Oliver, T. P., and Wright, D. S.: Radiological survey of men exposed to asbestos in naval dockyards, Br J Ind Med, 1972, *29*, 274.

76. Sheers, G., and Templeton, A. R.: Effects of asbestos in dockyard workers, Br Med J, 1968, *3*, 574.

77. Meurman, L. O., Kiviluoto, R., and Hakama, M.: Mortality and morbidity among the working population of anthophyllite asbestos miners in Finland, Br J Ind Med, 1974, *31*, 105.

78. Balaam, L. N., and McCullagh, S. F.: Vital capacity and one-second forced expiratory volume in Australian male asbestos cement workers, Ann Occup Hyg, 1975, *18*, 133.

79. Enterline, P. E., and Kendrick, M. A.: Asbestos-dust exposures at various levels and mortality, Arch Environ Health, 1967, *15*, 181.

80. Enterline, P. E.: Mortality among asbestos product workers in the United States, Ann N Y Acad Sci, 1965, *132*, 156.

81. Enterline, P. E., and Henderson, V.: Type of asbestos and respiratory cancer in the asbestos industry, Arch Environ Health, 1973, *27*, 312.

82. Enterline, P. E., Decoufle, P., and Henderson, V.: Respiratory cancer in relation to occupational exposures among retired asbestos workers, Br J Ind Med, 1973, *30*, 162.

83. Enterline, P. E., Decoufle, P., and Henderson, V.: Mortality in relation to occupational exposure in the asbestos industry, J Occup Med, 1972, *14*, 897.

84. Jodoin, G., Gibbs, G. W., Macklem, P. T., McDonald, J. C., and Becklake, M. R.: Early effects of asbestos exposure on lung function, Am Rev Respir Dis, 1971, *104*, 525.

85. McDonald, J. C., McDonald, A. D., Gibbs, G. W., Siemiatycki, J., and Rossiter, C. E.: Mortality in the chrysotile asbestos mines and mills of Quebec, Arch Environ Health, 1971, *22*, 677.

86. McDonald, J. C., Becklake, M. R., Fournier-Massey, G., and Rossiter, C. E.: Respiratory symptoms in chrysotile asbestos mine and mill workers of Quebec, Arch Environ Health, 1972, *24*, 358.

87. Becklake, M. R., Fournier-Massey, G., Rossiter, C. E., and McDonald, J. C.: Lung function in chrysotile asbestos mine amd mill workers of Quebec, Arch Environ Health, 1972, *24*, 401.

88. Rossiter, C. E., Bristol, L. J., Cartier, P. H., Gilson, J. G., Grainger, T. R., Sluis-Cremer, G. K., and McDonald, J. C.: Radiographic changes in chrysotile asbestos mine and mill workers of Quebec, Arch Environ Health, 1972, *24*, 388.

89. Gibbs, G. W., and Lachance, M.: Dust exposure in the chrysotile asbestos mines and mills of Quebec, Arch Environ Health, 1972, *24*, 189.

90. White, F. M., Swift, J., and Becklake, M. R.: Rheumatic complaints and pulmonary response to chrysotile dust inhalation in the mines and mills of Quebec, Can Med Assoc J, 1974, *11*, 533.

91. Gibbs, G. W., and Lachance, M.: Dust-fiber relationships in the Quebec chrysotile industry, Arch Environ Health, 1974, *28*, 69.

92. McDonald, J. C., Becklake, M. R., Gibbs, G. W., McDonald, A. D., and Rossiter, C. E.: The health of chrysotile asbestos mine and mill workers of Quebec, Arch Environ Health, 1974, *28*, 61.

93. Schneiderman, M. A.: Digestive system cancer among persons subjected to occupational inhalation of asbestos particles: A literature review with emphasis on dose response, Environ Health Perspect, 1974, *9*, 307.

94. Weill, H., Ziskind, M. M., Waggenspack, C., and Rossiter, C. E.: Lung function consequences of dust exposure in asbestos cement manufacturing plants, Arch Environ Health, 1975, *30*, 88.

95. Weill, H., Waggenspack, C., and Bailey, W.: Radiographic and physiologic patterns amongst workers engaged in manufacture of asbestos cement products, J Occup Med, 1973, *15*, 248.

96. Murphy, R. L. H., Ferris, B. G., Burgess, W. A., Worcester, J., and Gaenster, E. A.: Effects of low concentrations of asbestos: Clinical, environmental, radiologic and epidemiologic observations in shipyard pipe coverers and controls, N Engl J Med, 1971, *285*, 1271.

97. Ferris, B. G., Ranadive, M. V., Peters, J. M., Murphy, R. L. H., Burgess, W. A, and Pendergrass, H. P.: Prevalence of chronic respiratory disease: Asbestosis in ship repair workers, Arch Environ Health, 1971, *23*, 220.

98. Thomson, J. G., and Graves, W. M., Jr.: Asbestos as an urban air contaminant, Arch Pathol, 1966, *81*, 458.

99. Thomson, J. G., Kaschula, R. O. C., and MacDonald, R. R.: Asbestos as a modern urban hazard, S Afr Med J, 1963, *37*, 77.

100. Peacock, P. R., Biancifiori, C., and Bucciarelli, E.: Examination of lung smears for asbestos bodies in 109 consecutive necropsies in Perugia, Eur J Cancer, 1969, *5*, 155.

101. Hägerstrand, I., and Seifert, B.: Asbestos bodies and pleural plaques in human lungs at necropsy, Acta Pathol Microbiol Scand [A], 1973, *81A*, 457.

102. Dicke, T. E., and Naylor, B.: Prevalence of as-

bestos bodies in human lungs at necropsy, Dis Chest, 1969, *56*, 122.

103. Ashcroft, T.: Asbestos bodies in routine necropsies on Tyneside: A pathological and social study, Br Med J, 1968, *1*, 614.

104. Elmes, P. C., McCaughey, W. T. E., and Wade, O. L.: Diffuse mesothelioma of the pleura and asbestos, Br Med J, 1965, *1*, 350.

105. Roberts, G. H.: Asbestos bodies in lungs at necropsy, J Clin Pathol, 1967, *20*, 570.

106. Polliack, A., and Sacks, M. I.: Prevalence of asbestos bodies in basal lung smears, Isr J Med Sci, 1968, *4*, 223.

107. Cauna, D., Totten, R. S., and Gross, P.: Asbestos bodies in human lungs at autopsy, JAMA, 1965, *192*, 371.

108. Xipell, J. M., and Bhathal, P. S.: Asbestos bodies in lungs: An Australian report, Pathology, 1969, *1*, 327.

109. Pneumoconiosis Research Unit: Council for Scientific and Industrial Research, Annual Report, 1963/64, PRU Report No. 2164, Johannesburg, S. Africa.

110. Anjilvel, L., and Thurlbeck, W. M.: The incidence of asbestos bodies in the lungs at random necropsies in Montreal, Can Med Assoc J, 1966, *95*, 1179.

111. Ghezzi, I., Molteni, G., and Puccett, U.: Asbestos bodies in the lungs of inhabitants of Milan, Med Lavoro, 1967, *58*, 223.

112. Um, C-H.: Study of the secular trend in asbestos bodies in lungs in London 1936–66, Br Med J, 1971, *2*, 248.

113. Utidjian, M. D., Gross, P., and DeTreville, R. T. P.: Ferruginous bodies in human lungs, Arch Environ Health, 1968, *17*, 327.

114. Bignon, J., Goni, J., Bonnard, G., Jaurand, M. C., Dufour, G., and Pinchon, M. C.: Incidence of pulmonary ferruginous bodies in France, Environ Res, 1970, *3*, 430.

115. Plamenac, P., Pikula, B., Kahvic, M., Markovic, Z., Selak, I., and Zeger-Vidovic, Z.: Incidence of asbestos bodies in basal lung smear, Acta Med Iugosl, 1971, *25*, 325.

116. Hourihane, D. O'B., and McCaughey, W. T. E.: Pathological aspects of asbestosis, Postgrad Med J, 1966, *42*, 613.

117. Stumphius, J.: Epidemiology of mesothelioma on Walcheren Island, Br J Ind Med, 1971, *28*, 59.

118. Wallace, W. F. M., and Langlands, J.: Insulation workers in Belfast. 1. Comparison of a random sample with a control population, Br J Ind Med, 1971, *28*, 211.

119. Langlands, J. H. M., Wallace, W. F. M., and Simpson, M. J. C.: Insulation workers in Belfast. 2. Morbidity in men still at work, Br J Ind Med, 1971, *28*, 217.

120. Navratil, M., and Dobias, J.: Development of pleural hyalinosis in longterm studies of persons exposed to asbestos dust, Environ Res, 1973, *6*, 455.

121. Mattson, S. B., and Ringqvist, T.: Pleural plaques and exposure to asbestos, Scand J Respir Dis, 1970 (Supplement 75, p. 4).

122. Lewinsohn, H. C.: Early malignant changes in pleural plaques due to asbestos exposure: A case report, Br J Dis Chest, 1974, *68*, 121.

123. Roberts, G. H.: The pathology of parietal pleural plaques, J Clin Pathol, 1971, *24*, 348.

124. Hourihane, D. O'B., Lessof, L., and Richardson, P. C.: Hyaline and calcified pleural plaques as an index of exposure to asbestos: A study of radiological and pathological features of 100 cases with a consideration of epidemiology, Br Med J, 1966, *1*, 1069.

125. Knox, J. F., and Beattie, J.: Mineral content of the lungs after exposure to asbestos dust, Arch Ind Hyg, 1954, *10*, 23.

126. Navratil, M.: Pleural calcifications due to asbestos exposure compared with relevant findings in the non-exposed populations, in *Inhaled Particles and Vapours III*, W. H. Walton, ed., Proceedings of the British Occupational Hygiene Society Symposium, London, 1970, Unwin, Old Woking, p. 695.

127. Stansfield, D., and Edge, J. R.: Circulating rheumatoid factor and antinuclear antibodies in shipyard asbestos workers with pleural plaques, Br J Dis Chest, 1974, *68*, 166.

128. Leathart, G. L.: Pulmonary function tests in asbestos workers, Trans Soc Occup Med, 1968, *18*, 49.

129. Becklake, M. R., Fournier-Massey, G. G., McDonald, J. C., Siemiatycki, J., and Rossiter, C. E.: Lung function in relation to chest radiographic changes in Quebec asbestos workers, Bull Physiopathol Respir (Nancy), 1970, *6*, 637.

130. Fletcher, D. E.: A mortality study of shipyard workers with pleural plaques, Br J Ind Med, 1972, *29*, 142.

131. Gaensler, E. A., and Kaplan, A. I.: Asbestos pleural effusion, Ann Intern Med, 1971, *74*, 178.

132. Eisenstadt, H. B.: Benign asbestos pleurisy, JAMA, 1965, *192*, 419.

133. Eisenstadt, H. B.: Pleural effusions in asbestosis, N Engl J Med, 1974, *290*, 1025.

134. Chahinian, P., Hirsch, A., Bignon, J., Chofel, D., Pariente, R., Brouet, G., and Chrétien, J.: Les pleurésies asbestotiques nontumorales, Rev Fr Mal Respir, 1973, *1*, 5.

135. Leménager, J., Rousselot, P., and Le Bouffant, L.: Pleurésies asbestotiques non-tumorales: A propos de 4 observations, La Nouvelle Presse Med, 1975, *4*, 1134.

136. Cooke, W. E.: Pulmonary asbestosis, Br Med J, 1927, *2*, 1024.

137. Becklake, M. R.: Respiratory disease: Section 7: Physical and chemical irritants, in *Cecil-Loeb*

Textbook of Medicine, ed. 14, W. Saunders, Philadelphia, 1972, p. 854.

138. Gloyne, S. R.: Morbid anatomy and histology of asbestosis, Tubercle, 1933, *14*, 445.

139. Egbert, D. S.: Pulmonary asbestosis, Am Rev Tuberc, 1935, *31*, 25.

140. Heard, B. E., and Williams, R.: The pathology of asbestosis with reference to lung function, Thorax, 1961, *16*, 264.

141. Cartier, P.: Contribution a l'étude de l'amiantose, Arch Mal Prof, 1949, *10*, 38.

142. Solomon, A., Goldstein, B., Webster, I., and Sluis-Cremer, G. K.: Massive fibrosis in asbestosis, Environ Res, 1971, *4*, 430.

143. Green, R. A., and Dimcheff, D. G.: Massive bilateral upper lobe fibrosis secondary to asbestos exposure, Chest, 1974, *65*, 52.

144. Turner-Warwick, M.: A perspective view on widespread pulmonary fibrosis, Br Med J, 1974, *2*, 371.

145. Gaensler, E. A., Carrington, C. B., Coutu, R. E., Tomasian, A., Hoffman, L., and Smith, A. A.: Pathological, physiological, and radiological correlations in the pneumoconioses, Ann N Y Acad Sci, 1972, *200*, 574.

146. Rickards, A. G., and Barrett, G. M.: Rheumatoid lung changes associated with asbestosis, Thorax, 1958, *13*, 185.

147. Telleson, W. G.: Rheumatoid pneumoconiosis (Caplan's syndrome) in asbestos workers, Thorax, 1961, *16*, 372.

148. Morgan, W. K. C.: Rheumatoid pneumoconiosis in association with asbestosis, Thorax, 1964, *19*, 433.

149. Mattson, S. B.: Caplan's syndrome in association with asbestosis, Scand J Respir Dis, 1971, *52*, 153.

150. Corrin, B., and Price, A. B.: Electron microscopic studies in desquamative interstitial pneumonia associated with asbestos, Thorax, 1972, *27*, 324.

151. Scadding, J. G., and Hinson, K. F. W.: Diffuse fibrosing alveolitis (diffuse interstitial fibrosis of the lungs), Thorax, 1967, *22*, 291.

152. Miller, A., Langer, A. M., Tierstein, A. S., and Selikoff, I. J.: "Non-specific" interstitial pulmonary fibrosis: Association with asbestos fibers detected by electron microscopy, N Engl J Med, 1975, *292*, 91.

153. Turner-Warwick, M., and Haslam, P.: Antibodies in some chronic fibrosing lung diseases. I. Non-organic specific autoantibodies, Clin Allergy, 1971, *1*, 83.

154. Turner-Warwick, M., Haslam, P., and Weeks, J.: Antibodies in some chronic fibrosing lung diseases. II. Immunofluorescent studies, Clin Allergy, 1971, *1*, 209.

155. Turner-Warwick, M., and Parkes, R.: Circulating rheumatoid and antinuclear factors in asbestos workers, Br Med J, 1970, *3*, 492.

156. Merchant, J. A., Klouda, P. T., Soutar, C. A., Parkes, W. R., Lawler, S. D., and Turner-Warwick, M.: The HL-A system in asbestos workers, Br Med J, 1975, *1*, 189.

157. Kang, K-Y., Sera, Y., Okuchi, T., and Yamamura, Y.: T-lymphocytes in asbestosis, N Engl J Med, 1974, *291*, 735.

158. Ryder, R., Lyons, J. P., Campbell, H., and Gough, J.: Emphysema in coalworkers' pneumoconiosis, Br Med J, 1970, *3*, 481.

159. Forgacs, A. R.: Lung sounds, Br J Dis Chest, 1969, *63*, 1.

160. Nath, A. R., and Capel, L. H.: Inspiratory crackles and mechanical events of breathing, Thorax, 1974, *29*, 695.

161. Chew, P. K., Chia, M., Chew, S. F., Supramaniam, J. M. J., Chan, W., Chew, C. H., Ng, Y. K., and Gandevia, B.: Asbestos workers in Singapore: A clinical, functional and radiological survey, Arch Environ Health, 1973, *26*, 290.

162. Reagan, G. M., Tagg, B., and Thomson, M. L.: Subjective assessment and objective measurement of finger-clubbing, Lancet, 1967, *1*, 530.

163. Soutar, C. A., Simon, G., and Turner-Warwick, M.: The radiology of asbestos-induced disease of the lungs, Br J Dis Chest, 1974, *68*, 235.

164. Solomon, A.: The radiology of asbestosis, S Afr Med J, 1969, *43*, 847.

165. Hurwitz, M.: Roentgenologic aspects of asbestosis, Am J Roentgenol, 1961, *85*, 256.

166. Leathart, G. L.: Clinical, bronchographic, radiological and physiological observations in ten cases of asbestosis, Br J Ind Med, 1960, *17*, 213.

167. UICC/Cincinnati classification of the radiographic appearances of pneumoconiosis, Chest, 1970, *58*, 57.

168. International Labour Office: ILO U/C classification of radiographs of the pneumoconioses 1971, Occupational Health and Safety Series, No. 22, International Labour Office, Geneva, 1972.

169. Weill, H.: The chest roentgenogram as an epidemiologic tool: Report of a Workshop sponsored by the Division of Lung Diseases, National Heart and Lung Institute, Arch Environ Health, 1975, *30*, 435.

170. Becklake, M. R.: Pneumoconioses, in *Handbook of physiology,* sec. 3, *Respiration,* vol. II, W. O. Fenn and H. Rahn, ed., American Physiological Society, Washington, D.C., 1965.

171. Woitowitz, H. J.: Berufliche Asbeststaubexposition und obstruktive ventilationsstorungen, Int Arch Arbeitsmed, 1970, *27*, 244.

172. Murphy, R. L. H., Gaensler, E. A., Redding, R. A., Belleau, R., Keelan, P. J, Smith, A. A., Goff, A. M., and Ferris, B. G.: Low exposure to asbestos: Gas exchange in ship pipe coverers and controls, Arch Environ Health, 1972, *25*, 253.

173. Fournier-Massey, G., and Becklake, M. R.: Pul-

monary function profiles in Quebec asbestos workers, Bull Physiopathol Respir (Nancy), 1975, *11*, 429.

174. Muldoon, B. C., and Turner-Warwick, M.: Lung function studies in asbestos workers, Br J Dis Chest, 1972, *66*, 121.

175. Pilat, L., Rafaila, E., Craciun, O., Teculescu, D., Georgescu, A. M., and Apostolescu, R.: Contribution à l'étude des corrélations entre les aspects radiologiques, cliniques, et fonctionnels respiratoires de l'asbestose, Med Lavoro, 1971, *62*, 495.

176. Williams, R., and Hugh-Jones, P.: The significance of lung function changes in asbestosis, Thorax, 1960, *15*, 109.

177. Ostrow, D., and Cherniak, R. M.: Resistance to airflow in patients with diffuse interstitial lung disease, Am Rev Respir Dis, 1973, *108*, 205.

178. Kleinfeld, M., Messite, J., Kooyman, O., and Sarfaty, J.: Effect of asbestos dust inhalation on lung function, Arch Environ Health, 1966, *12*, 741.

179. Kleinfeld, M., Messite, J., and Shapiro, J.: Clinical, radiological and physiological findings in asbestosis, Arch Intern Med, 1966, *117*, 813.

180. Gandevia, B.: Pulmonary function in asbestos workers: A three year follow-up study, Am Rev Respir Dis, 1967, *96*, 420.

181. Peress, L., Hoag, H., White, F., and Becklake, M. R.: The relationship between closing volume, smoking and asbestos dust exposure (abstract), Clin Res, 1975, *23*, 647A.

182. Weiss, W.: Cigarette smoking and pulmonary fibrosis: A preliminary report, Arch Environ Health, 1967, *14*, 564.

183. Scott, J. K., and Hunt, R.: The diagnosis of asbestosis, Br J Dis Chest, 1975, *69*, 51.

184. Green, M., Mead, J., and Turner, J. M.: Variability of maximum expiratory flow-volume curves, J Appl Physiol, 1974, *37*, 67.

185. Weiss, W.: Cigarette smoking, asbestos, and pulmonary fibrosis, Am Rev Respir Dis, 1971, *104*, 223.

186. McCaughey, W. T. E.: Primary tumours of the pleura, J Pathol Bacteriol, 1958, *76*, 517.

187. Whitwell, F., and Rawcliffe, R. M.: Diffuse malignant pleural mesothelioma and asbestos exposure, Thorax, 1971, *26*, 6.

188. Fondimare, A., Desbordes, J., Perrotey, J., Tayot, J., and Ernoult, J-L.: Etude semi-quantitative de l'empoussiérage par l'amiante dans 14 observations de mésothéliomes pleuraux, Arch Anat Pathol (Paris), 1974, *22*, 55.

189. Bohlig, H., Dabbert, A. F., Dalquen, P., Hain, E., and Hinz, I.: Epidemiology of malignant mesothelioma in Hamburg, Environ Res, 1970, *3*, 365.

190. Lieben, J., and Pistawka, H.: Mesothelioma and asbestos exposure, Arch Environ Health, 1967, *14*, 559.

191. Godwin, M. C., and Jagatic, J.: Asbestos and mesotheliomas, Environ Res, 1970, *3*, 391.

192. Borow, M., Conston, A., Livornese, L., and Schalet, N.: Mesothelioma following exposure to asbestos: A review of 72 cases, Chest, 1973, *64*, 641.

193. Milne, J.: Fifteen cases of pleural mesothelioma associated with occupational exposure to asbestos in Victoria, Med J Aust, 1969, *2*, 669.

194. McEwen, J., Finlayson, J. A., Mair, A., and Gibson, A. A. M.: Mesothelioma in Scotland, Br Med J, 1970, *4*, 575.

195. Elmes, P. C., McCaughey, W. T. E., and Wade, O. L.: Diffuse mesothelioma of the pleura and asbestos, Br Med J, 1965, *1*, 350.

196. Ashcroft, T.: Epidemiological and quantitative relationships between mesothelioma and asbestos on Tyneside, J Clin Pathol, 1973, *26*, 832.

197. Rubino, G. F., Scansetti, G., Donna, A., and Palestro, G.: Epidemiology of pleural mesothelioma in North-western Italy (Piedmont), Br J Ind Med, 1972, *29*, 436.

198. Hägerstrand, I., Meurman, L., and Odlund, B.: Asbestos bodies in the lungs and mesothelioma (a retrospective examination of a 10-year autopsy material), Acta Pathol Microbiol Scand, 1968, *72*, 177.

199. Hain, E., Dalquen, P., Bohlig, H., Dabbert, A., and Hinz, I.: Katamnesticha untersuchungen zur genese des mesothelioms, Int Arch Arbeitsmed, 1974, *33*, 15.

200. Zielhaus, R. L., Versteeg, J. P. J., and Planteijdt, H. T.: Pleural mesothelioma and exposure to asbestos: A retrospective case control study in the Netherlands, Int Arch Occup Environ Health, 1975, *36*, 1.

201. McDonald, A. D., and McDonald, J. C.: Epidemiologic surveillance of mesothelioma in Canada, Can Med Assoc J, 1973, *109*, 359.

202. McDonald, A. D.: Etudes epidémiologiques sur les maladies dues a l'amiante au Canada, La Revue de l'Appareil Respiratoire, in press.

203. Roberts, G. H.: Diffuse pleural mesothelioma: A clinical and pathological study, Br J Dis Chest, 1970, *64*, 201.

204. Belleau, R., and Gaensler, E. A.: Mesothelioma and asbestosis, Respiration, 1968, *25*, 67.

205. Jordanoglou, J., Lymbaratos, K., and Arapakis, G.: An unusual case of mesothelioma of the pleura, Am Rev Respir Dis, 1971, *103*, 418.

206. Magner, D., and McDonald, A. D: Malignant mesothelial tumours: Histologic type and asbestos exposure, N Engl J Med, 1972, *287*, 570.

207. Harrington, J. S., Wagner, J. C., and Smith, M.: The detection of hyaluronic acid in pleural fluids of cases with diffuse pleural mesotheliomas, Br J Exp Pathol, 1963, *44*, 81.

208. Aria, H., Endo, M., Sasai, Y., Yokosawa, A., Sato, H., Motoniya, M., and Konno, K.: Histochemical demonstration of hyaluronic acid in

a case of pleural mesothelioma, Am Rev Respir Dis, 1975, *111*, 699.

209. Solomon, A.: Radiological features of mesothelioma, Environ Res, 1970, *3*, 330.

210. Egbert, D. S., and Geiger, A. J.: Pulmonary asbestosis and carcinoma, Am Rev Tuberc, 1936, *34*, 143.

211. Gloyne, S. R.: Pneumoconiosis: A histological survey of necropsy material in 1205 cases, Lancet, 1951, *1*, 810.

212. Braun, D. C., and Traun, T. D.: An epidemiologic study of lung cancer in asbestos miners, Arch Ind Health, 1958, *17*, 634.

213. Elwood, P. C., and Cochrane, A. L.: A follow-up study of workers from an asbestos factory, Br J Ind Med, 1964, *21*, 304.

214. Elmes, P. C., and Simpson, M. J. C.: Insulation workers in Belfast. 3. Mortality 1940–1966, Br J Ind Med, 1971, *28*, 226.

215. Dunn, J. E., and Weir, J. M.: Cancer experience of several occupational groups followed prospectively, Am J Public Health, 1965, *55*, 1367.

216. Selikoff, I. J., Hammond, E. C., and Churg, J.: Carcinogenicity of amosite asbestos, Arch Environ Health, 1972, *25*, 183.

217. Enterline, P. E.: Estimating health risks in studies of the health effects of asbestos, Am Rev Respir Dis, 1976, *113*, 175.

218. Wagner, J. C., Gilson, J. C., Berry, G., and Timbrell, V.: Epidemiology of asbestos cancers, Br Med Bull, 1971, *27*, 71.

219. Selikoff, I. J., Hammond, E. C., and Churg, J.: Asbestos exposure, smoking and neoplasia, JAMA, 1968, *204*, 104.

220. Kannerstein, M., and Churg, J.: Pathology of carcinoma of the lung associated with asbestos exposure, Cancer, 1972, *30*, 14.

221. Newhouse, M. L., and Wagner, J. C.: Validation of death certificates in asbestos workers, Br J Ind Med, 1969, *26*, 302.

222. Whitwell, F., Newhouse, M. L., and Bennett, D. R.: A study of the histological cell types of lung cancer in workers suffering from asbestosis in the United Kingdom, Br J Ind Med, 1974, *31*, 298.

223. Dohner, V. A., Beegle, R. G., and Miller, W. T.: Asbestos exposure and multiple primary tumors, Am Rev Respir Dis, 1975, *112*, 181.

224. Kleinfeld, M.: Biologic response to kind and amount of asbestos, J Occup Med, 1973, *15*, 296.

225. British Occupational Hygiene Society: Committee on Hygiene Standards: Hygiene standards for chrysotile asbestos dust, Ann Occup Hyg, 1968, *11*, 47.

226. British Occupational Hygiene Society: Committee on Hygiene Standards: Hygiene standards for airborne amosite asbestos dust, Ann Occup Hyg, 1973, *16*, 1.

227. The Asbestos Regulations (1969) S.I. 1969 No. 690, HMSO London.

228. British Occupational Hygiene Society: Committee on Hygiene Standards: Review of the hygiene standard for chrysotile asbestos dust, Ann Occup Hyg, 1973, *16*, 7.

229. U. S. Department of Labor: Federal Register, 1972, *37*, 11318.

230. U. S. Department of Labor: Federal Register, 1975, *40*, 47652.

231. Schilling, R. F.: Occupational Health Practice, Butterworths, London, 1973, pp. 408–420.

State of the Art

Expression of Immune Mechanisms in the Lung[1,2]

H. BENFER KALTREIDER

Contents

1 From the Respiratory Care Section, Department of Medicine, San Francisco Veterans Administration Hospital, the Cardiovascular Research Institute and Department of Medicine, School of Medicine, University of California, San Francisco, Calif. 94143.

2 Supported by U. S. Public Health Service Grant AI–12296. Veterans Administration MRIS No. 4823.

Introduction

The immune response is critical to the defense of the host against potentially harmful antigenic materials inhaled into the respiratory tract.

There is evidence that immunologic mechanisms contribute to the pathogenesis of pulmonary disease by tissue-damaging reactions of hypersensitivity. To understand the immunologic derangements pertinent to the pathogenesis of lung diseases, recent investigations have attempted to elucidate the mechanisms by which both humoral and cellular immune phenomena are expressed in the respiratory tract. Whereas a great deal is known about the fundamentals of immune responses in systemic lymphoid tissue, little of this information has been related directly to the lung. It is not clear whether the respiratory tract functions autonomously as an immunologically competent organ, whether it is simply a passive framework upon which systemically generated immune reactions occur, or whether there is some degree of interdependence between the local and systemic immune apparatus. Resolution of this fundamental question is essential to any definition of a local immune system unique to the lung.

It appears that the lymphatic tissue of the respiratory tract is not homogeneous; rather, it is a composite of multiple subpopulations of lymphoid cells that, in all likelihood, differ in their functional capabilities, immune competence, and degree of interaction with systemic lymphoid tissue. Our knowledge is not sufficiently well developed to allow a clear definition or detailed integration of these various components. At present, only a fragmented and incomplete description of the expression of immunity in the respiratory tract can be presented. This paper will attempt to review the "State of the Art" with respect to the mode of expression of immune reactions in the respiratory tract in order to provide the basis for an understanding of the role of these mechanisms in the defense of the lung and in the pathogenesis of immunologically mediated lung diseases.

Fundamental Concepts of Immunobiology

During the past 3 decades, investigative effort has produced an enormous amount of fundamental information regarding the mechanisms of induction and expression of immune responses (1). The vast majority of this knowledge has been derived from studies of immune phenomena as manifested in organized systemic lymphoid tissue, such as spleen and lymph nodes. Concepts derived from such studies have been extrapolated to the lung by analogy, because only recently has lymphatic tissue derived from the respiratory tract been studied directly. This section will review briefly selected modern concepts of the functional and structural organization of systemic lymphatic tissue as a background for review of the current knowledge of the expression of immune reactions in the lung. This fundamental information has been recently reviewed in several texts (2–6).

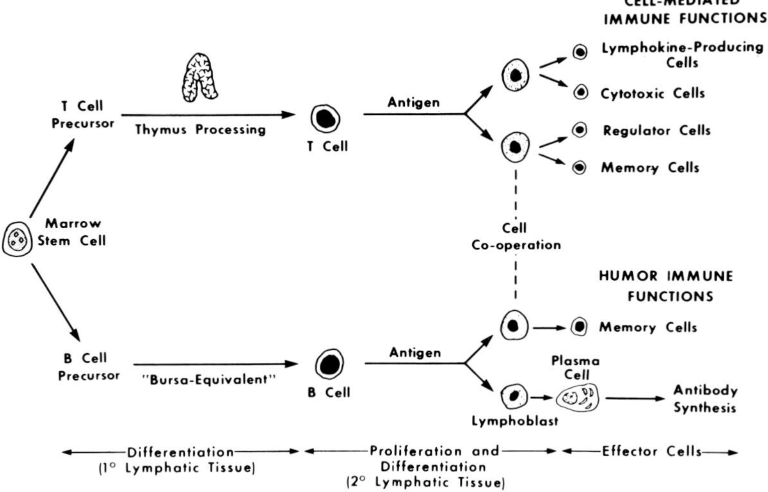

Fig. 1. Diagrammatic representation of the differentiation, proliferation, and effector functions of thymus-dependent lymphocytes (T cells) and bone marrow-derived lymphocytes (B cells). After antigenic stimulation, T cells effect cell-mediated immune functions, and B cells carry out humoral immunity (1° = primary; 2° = secondary).

Functional Organization of Systemic Lymphatic Tissue

The immune system may be divided functionally into two major effector systems: humoral, or antibody-mediated immunity, and cell-mediated immunity (CMI). Lymphatic tissue is responsible for expression of both types of immune reactions. There are two major subpopulations of lymphocytes whose biologic functions parallel those of the two effector systems (figure 1.) The two types of lymphocytes can be distinguished on the basis of their mode of differentiation, surface membrane characteristics, and functional properties. Thymus-dependent lymphocytes (T cells) arise from stem cells in the bone marrow, differentiate in or under the influence of the thymus gland (primary lymphatic tissue), populate the periarterial lymphatic sheath in the spleen and interfollicular regions of lymph nodes (secondary lymphatic tissue), and carry out the functions of CMI. Bone marrow-derived lymphocytes (B cells) differentiate in the bursa of Fabricius in avian species, or the "bursa equivalent" in mammals, concentrate in lymphoid follicles of lymph nodes and spleen (secondary lymphatic tissues), and serve as precursors for antibody-forming cells that effect humoral immunity.

The T cells constitute a mobile population of lymphocytes that continuously recirculate. They migrate from the peripheral blood through postcapillary venules into secondary lymphatic tissue (lymph nodes, spleen, and respiratory and gut submucosa), where they remain for a variable period of time before entering efferent lymphatic vessels, the thoracic duct, and, again, peripheral blood (7). The recirculation of lymphocytes theoretically provides a pathway for the migration of sensitized T cells from lymphatic tissue to the site of antigen deposition (e.g., tuberculin skin test). By contrast, B cells are relatively sessile and migrate slowly within lymphatic tissues. After antigenic stimulation, they differentiate into plasma cells *in situ* and synthesize and secrete soluble antibody that is disseminated via the circulating blood and mucosal secretions (figure 1).

Although they are indistinguishable morphologically (figure 2), T and B cells may be identified and quantified on the basis of their distinctive surface membrane receptors and functional characteristics (table 1). The presence of a distinctive surface-membrane antigen (theta) and the characteristic adherence of sheep erythrocytes to their surfaces *in vitro* (sheep cell rosettes) identify T cells. By contrast, B cells possess easily detectable surface-membrane immunoglobulin and receptors for complement and for immunoglobulin (8). Functionally, T cells can be identified by their proliferative response to certain

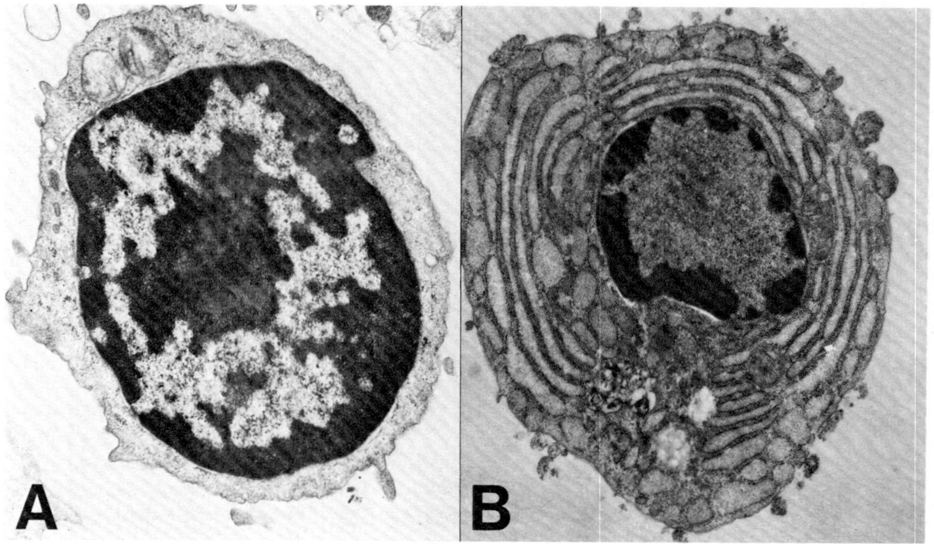

Fig. 2. A. An electron micrograph of a typical small "resting" lymphocyte (original magnification: ×11,000). At this stage of development, T and B cells are not distinguishable morphologically. B. An electron micrograph of a plasma cell (original magnification: × 8,000). Plasma cells are fully differentiated, antibody-producing B cells. (From Kaltreider and co-workers [43].)

TABLE 1

IDENTIFICATION OF SUBPOPULATIONS OF LYMPHOCYTES

	T Cells	B Cells
Surface membrane characteristics	Theta, Ly alloantigens	Surface immunoglobulin
	Sheep erythrocyte rosettes	Receptor for complement
		Receptor for immunoglobulin
Functional characterisitcs	Proliferative response to phytohemmaglutinin, concanavalin A	Synthesis and secretion of immunoglobulin (antibody)
	Synthesis of lymphokines	Effectors of humoral immunity
	Effectors of cell-mediated immunity	

mitogens, such as phytohemagglutinin and concanavalin-A, and by their elaboration and secretion of soluble mediator substances (lymphokines) when exposed to specific antigen. Synthesis of immunoglobulin (antibody) is the characteristic feature of B cells.

Biology of the Immune Response

The fundamental characteristics that define the immune response include: (*1*) the exquisite specificity of antibodies or of sensitized cells for the immunizing antigen that is recognized as foreign or "non-self"; (*2*) the capacity for quantitative amplification of the resident population of antigen-reactive lymphoid cells and hence of their effector products; (*3*) the phenomenon of memory, or the recall characteristic of the secondary, or anamnestic, response to rechallenge of a sensitized host with antigen. The physiology of immune responses, both cell mediated and humoral, may be divided arbitrarily into 3 functional limbs (figure 3). The afferent limb includes processes involved in the transport of antigen to lymphatic tissue. The central limb encompasses the biologic processes occurring among immunocompetent cells, culminating in the generation of effector lymphocytes (antibody-producing B cells or sensitized T cells). The efferent limb includes processes occurring between the generation of effector lymphocytes and their ultimate action on the original antigen.

Antigens and phagocytic cells—the afferent limb. Antigens, or immunogens, are substances that, when introduced into a host, give rise to specific antibodies or specifically sensitized T cells. Antigenic determinants are the portions of an antigen toward which a specific immune response is directed. Most antigens are composed of a macromolecular carrier portion, toward which T cell specificity is directed, and a hapten, or a low molecular weight chemical group, which determines the specificity of the humoral antibody response (figure 3). Under physiologic conditions, the respiratory tract is likely to be exposed to highly complex, naturally occurring antigens, such as bacteria, viruses, fungal spores, and various dusts and fumes. These materials are composed of a vast array of incompletely defined antigenic determinants. Experimentally, well-defined synthetic or purified natural antigens (proteins or polysaccharides) have been used extensively. Synthetic immunogens offer the advantage that the antigenic determinant is chemically defined and constitutes a precise experimental probe for dissection of the events occurring during the immune response. A major difficulty in the study of the fate and immuno-

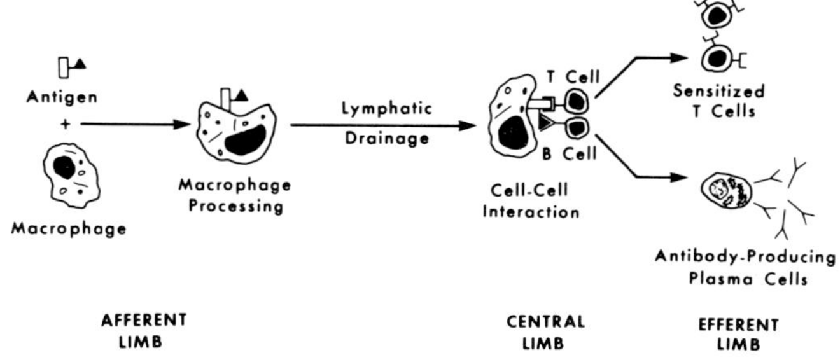

Fig. 3. A diagrammatic representation of the cellular interactions that may occur during the generation of an immune response to a carrier (⊏⊐) —hapten (▲) antigen complex. The over-all process of the immune response has been divided functionally into afferent, central, and efferent limbs.

logic consequence of the inhalation of complex natural antigens, either normally or in human allergic lung disease, is the heterogeneity of the component antigenic determinants and the difficulty in identifying the antigen relevant to production of the disease process. New experimental models of immunologically mediated lung disease should use chemically defined, homogeneous preparations of antigens.

The route of administration of an antigen determines, to a large extent, the distribution of the lymphatic tissue participating in the immune response. Intravenously administered material is distributed widely by the vascular system. The antigen concentrates in multiple organs, including the liver, spleen, lymph nodes, bone marrow, and the lung (9, 10). Subcutaneously administered antigen drains both via lymphatics to the regional lymph nodes, and via blood to systemic lymphatic tissue. Quantitatively, the most important physiologic route for the entry of antigens is through the respiratory and gastrointestinal tracts; however, the exact fate of antigen applied directly to gut, to respiratory mucosa, or to alveolar surfaces has not been determined (see below).

After entry into the body, antigen is taken up by mononuclear phagocytes (macrophages) of the reticuloendothelial system, particularly those lining sinusoids and lymphatic channels in lymphoid tissues (9). Particulate antigens are cleared far more efficiently by the reticuloendothelial system than are soluble antigens. After phagocytosis, most antigen is degraded and excreted in low molecular weight form. The remainder is processed into an enhanced immunogenic form and is retained at or near the surface membrane of the macrophage. The altered antigen is presented to immunocompetent lymphocytes for the efficient initiation of an immune response (figure 3) (11–13).

Generation of immune effector cells—the central limb. The interaction of antigen with organized lymphatic tissue usually results in the generation of both cell-mediated and antibody-mediated effector mechanisms. The magnitude of stimulation of each effector system depends on the physicochemical properties of the immunizing antigen. Interaction among immunocompetent cells, cellular proliferation, and differentiation characterize the central limb of the immune response (figures 1 and 3). It is generally thought that anatomically organized lymphatic tissues (lymph nodes and spleen) contain a full complement of antigen-reactive cells, T and B

cells, each of which is precommitted and available to recognize and interact with foreign antigenic determinants. The interaction of antigen-reactive cells with antigen processed by macrophages stimulates a rapid proliferation and differentiation of both T and B cells, resulting in an amplified or expanded pool of precursor cells destined to become effector lymphocytes (12, 13).

In cell-mediated immune mechanisms, antigen stimulation of precommitted T cells produces a proliferative wave of lymphoblasts, which differentiate into multiple subsets of sensitized T cells, each performing specific functions (figure 1). These include cells secreting mediators of CMI (lymphokines), cytotoxic cells, regulator ("helper" and "suppressor") cells, and memory cells important in the anamnestic response.

The response of B cells to antigenic stimulation usually requires specific "helper" T cells (T-dependent antigens) to culminate successfully in the generation of antibody-producing plasma cells (figure 2B) and memory B cells (figure 1); however, certain natural (pneumococcal polysaccharide) and synthetic antigens do not require "helper" T cells for the generation of a B cell response (T-independent antigens). Recent evidence suggests that the interaction of at least 3 different cell types (T cells, B cells, and macrophages) is required for optimal expression of antibody-mediated immunity against complex natural antigens (11–13). The successful generation of a humoral response requires the presentation of antigen by macrophages to antigen-reactive cells of both T and B cell types (figure 3). Although the intimate details of the mechanisms of the cellular interactions are complex and incompletely understood, both "helper" and "suppressor" T cells interact with B cells at several steps along their path of differentiation and serve to regulate both the magnitude and the duration of antibody production.

When considering data obtained from studies of immune reactions in the respiratory tract, it is important to bear in mind the complexity of the cellular interactions required for the generation of immune responses. It is probable that events of such complexity require a high degree of organization of lymphatic tissue to effect immune responses efficiently.

Expression of immunity—the efferent limb. Sensitized T cells generated in the central limb of the immune response recirculate through blood and lymph and accumulate at the site of deposition of the sensitizing antigen (7). The interaction of antigen in tissues with the appropriate receptors on sensitized T cells results in the expression of at least two major cell-mediated effector mechanisms: (*1*) inflammatory reactions mediated by soluble products (lymphokines) released by sensitized T cells; (*2*) direct T cell-mediated cytotoxicity.

The B cells that have been stimulated by antigen to differentiate into plasma cells synthesize and secrete antibody that is immunochemically specific for the sensitizing antigen. Antibody is distributed throughout the body in blood, lymph, and mucosal secretions. The interaction of soluble antibody with the original sensitizing antigen and the ensuing biologic consequences constitute the effector mechanism for humoral immunity.

Biologic Significance of Antibody-mediated Immune Reactions

Immune responses play a protective role against pathogenic or potentially toxic antigenic materials. These biologic functions are carried out by both humoral and cell-mediated immune mechanisms, which, acting in concert, comprise an important and integral component of the over-all mechanism for the defense of the host (14).

Structure and function of antibody. Antibody-mediated immune mechanisms are effected by immunoglobulin molecules (figure 4). The prototype of the immunoglobulin molecule consists of 4 polypeptide chains (2 heavy and 2 light) covalently linked by disulfide bonds. The molecule may be cleaved enzymatically to produce two Fab (<u>F</u>ragment, <u>antib</u>ody) portions and one Fc (<u>F</u>ragment, <u>c</u>rystallizable) portion. The amino acid sequence at the N-terminal end of the Fab is variable, and this variability allows for the development of the specificity of the antibody for the antigenic determinant. The Fc portion is relatively constant in its amino acid sequence within each class of immunoglobulin (i.e., IgG, IgA, and so on), and this portion determines the biologic property of the antibody (e.g., complement-fixing, precipitating, opsonizing, heterocytotropic, or cytophilic) (table 2). Several classes and subclasses of immunoglobulins are distinguishable on the bases of their physicochemical structure and biologic functions (table 2). Antigenic stimulation leads to the elaboration of specific antibody within any or all of these classes, depending on the nature of the sensitizing antigen. For example, ragweed

pollen efficiently stimulates IgE antibodies, whereas spores of thermophilic actinomycetes result predominantly, but not exclusively, in IgM and IgG antibodies.

The major biologic functions of antibodies are in the defense against microbial organisms (bacteria and certain viruses) and in the clearance of inanimate particles (14). The activities of antibodies include agglutination of bacteria and other particulates, precipitation of foreign proteins, neutralization of bacterial exotoxins, enhancement of phagocytosis through opsonization, activation of the complement sequence, complement-dependent lysis of gram-negative bacteria, and neutralization of a wide variety of viruses.

Measurement of antibody activity. The effect of antigenic stimulation on the humoral immune system can be measured in several ways. Various biologic functions of the antibody itself can be assayed *in vitro* using techniques of hemagglutination, complement fixation, viral neutralization, precipitation, or antibody-dependent cytolysis. These assays measure a secondary effect, or consequence of the antigen-antibody interaction, and are usually expressed as a titer. Assays designed to quantify the primary antigen-binding capacity are more direct measures of antibody activity. These assays generally measure the amount of radiolabeled antigen bound by antibody in a sample. Comparisons of antibody titer or antigen-binding capacity between serum and respiratory secretions are of questionable reliability, because the class-specific immunoglobulin composition and the absolute concentrations of immunoglobulin differ enormously in the two

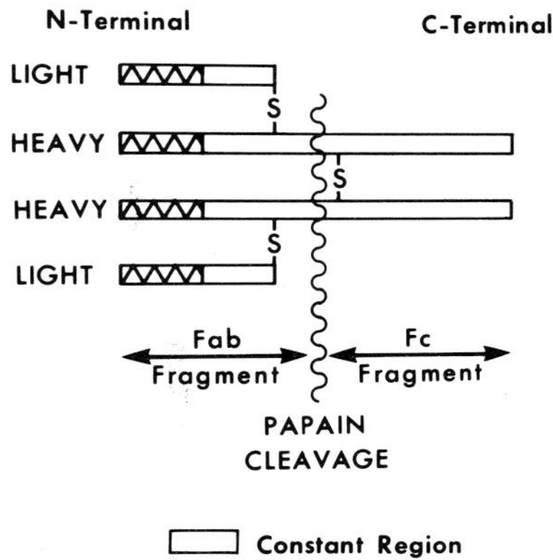

Fig. 4. Diagram depicting a monomeric unit of an immunoglobulin molecule. Enzymatic digestion with papain results in the generation of one crystallizable fragment (Fc) and 2 antibody fragments (Fab).

TABLE 2

PROPERTIES OF MAJOR HUMAN SERUM AND SECRETORY
IMMUNOGLOBULIN CLASSES

	IgG*	IgA	S-IgA†	IgM	IgD	IgE**
Sedimentation coefficient, S	7S	7S††	11S	19S	7S	8S
Molecular weight (x 10^3), daltons	150	160††	390	900	185	200
No. of Ig monomers	1	1††	2	5	1	1
Heavy chain	γ	α	α	μ	δ	ϵ
Concentration in normal serum, mg/ml	8–16	1.4–4	–	0.5–2	0.03	0.0001
Complement fixation	+	–	–	+	?	–
Prominent in mucous secretions	±	+	+	–	–	+
Fix to mast cells (heterocytotropic)	–	–	–	–	–	+
Fix to Macrophages (cytophilic)	+	?	?	–	?	?

*Made up of the 4 subclasses, IgG-1, IgG-2, IgG-3, and IgG-4.

†Dimeric, secretory IgA containing additional "secretory component" and "J-chair."
This is the predominant immunoglobulin species in external secretions.

**Serum and secretory IgE appear to be physiochemically identical.

††Monomeric form; polymers of various sizes exist normally in serum.

fluids. Valid comparisons between serum and secretions can be made only if differences in class-specific and total immunoglobulin concentrations are taken into account. Many studies have failed in this regard.

The lymphoid cells themselves may be assayed for their ability to secrete specific antibody with the hemolytic-plaque technique of Jerne and associates (15). This method detects and quantifies individual antibody-producing cells among suspensions of lymphocytes with a high degree of sensitivity and accuracy. Lymphoid populations obtained from the respiratory tract can be compared directly to those derived from the systemic immune apparatus, because the assay determines concentrations of individual antibody-forming cells in the respective populations, rather than their secretory products.

Biologic Significance of Cell-mediated Immune Reactions

It is generally accepted that sensitized T cells are responsible for cell-mediated immune reactions. As currently understood, CMI is expressed biologically by soluble products (lymphokines) elaborated by sensitized T cells and by T cell-mediated cytotoxicity. Several subsets of T cells have been defined recently, each of which appears to effect one of these biologic functions. The role of CMI in the defense of the host and in the pathogenesis of disease is less well defined than that of humoral immunity, owing primarily to the lack of a reproducible, rapidly performed, and quantitative assay for CMI *in vitro* or *in vivo*.

The delayed-type hypersensitivity cutaneous reaction constitutes the classic and only *in vivo* assay for assessing the integrity of the presence and normal expression of CMI in the intact host. This reaction consists of localized induration, edema, and a mononuclear cell infiltration arising 24 to 48 hours after the intradermal injection of an antigen to which the recipient possesses sensitized T cells. In assessing the status of T cell-mediated functions, the cutaneous reaction suffers from two drawbacks: it is difficult to quantify, and cutaneous reactivity may not be pertinent to events occurring elsewhere, such as in the respiratory tract. Certain metabolic derangements, such as renal failure, hepatic failure, and debilitation, may interfere with the expression of cell-mediated immunity without necessarily indicating a defect in T cells themselves (16).

In attempts to quantify cell-mediated immune reactions better, a variety of *in vitro* assays have been developed (17). Each of these assays possesses certain inherent disadvantages, and each has been criticized as not necessarily reflecting CMI events occurring *in vivo;* however, the assays do represent partially defined systems suitable for laboratory investigation of the functions of sensitized lymphoid cells *in vitro*.

Lymphokine-mediated reactions. Lymphokines are soluble substances secreted by sensitized lymphocytes on interaction with antigen. They are defined by the nature of the *in vitro* assay system used for their characterization (table 3). It is assumed, but not proved, that *in vivo,* these soluble factors mediate the cellular and inflammatory reactions characteristic of delayed hypersensitivity. To measure the production of lymphokines, suspensions of lymphocytes are incubated in the presence of a specific antigen. The interaction of antigen with the sensitized lymphocytes in the population stimulates the release of soluble mediators into the culture medium. The culture supernatants are then assayed for their ability to perform the appropriate biologic function (e.g., migration inhibition, macrophage activation, and chemotaxis) (table 3).

The lymphokine most extensively characterized is the migration inhibition factor (MIF). To date, this is the only factor that has been demonstrated to be elaborated by lymphatic tissue associated with the respiratory tract. In this assay, supernatants are tested for their ability to impede the migration of a test macrophage out of a capillary tube. It is believed that *in vivo,* this factor may play an important role in the accumulation of the mononuclear phagocytes typical of a delayed hypersensitivity immune reaction. Another soluble lymphokine, macrophage activation factor (MAF), may be important in the defense of the host against intracellular parasites, such as *Mycobacterium tuberculosis* or *Listeria monocytogenes* (18, 19). This material appears to activate macrophages, enhancing their properties of phagocytosis and bacterial killing. Additional alterations include increased motility and glass adherence, increased numbers of mitochondria and lysosomes, and increased metabolic rate and enzyme content. Activated macrophages then become superior defenders against a wide variety of infectious organisms. Whereas the synthesis and release of MAF are immunologically specific, requiring antigen and specifically sensitized T cells, once activated the macrophages appear to be nonspecific in their effector function, namely, they display enhanced phagocytosis and bactericidal ability against a wide range of intracellular pathogens.

Cytotoxic reactions. Cell-mediated cytotoxicity involves a subset of specifically sensitized T cells ("killer" lymphocytes) that interact directly with foreign cells bearing alloantigens and render them nonviable (20). The reaction does not depend on lymphokines, immunoglobulin, or complement. This particular cell-mediated reaction is important in the rejection of transplanted tissues, the graft versus host reaction, and in the immune surveillance against neoplasia (20, 21). Cell-mediated cytotoxicity can be measured *in vitro* by incubating suspensions of sensitized lymphocytes with target cells labeled with chromium-51 that bear the sensitizing alloantigen. Release of free chromium into the supernatant is a measure of the number of "killer" lymphocytes present.

Hypersensitivity Immune Reactions

Immune reactions usually serve a host-defense function. Under certain circumstances, allergic or hypersensitivity immune reactions lead to tissue injury. It is beyond the scope of this review to discuss these immunopathogenic mechanisms in detail. A brief summary of hypersensitivity or

TABLE 3

PARTIAL LIST OF SOLUBLE PRODUCTS RELEASED *IN VITRO*
BY SENSITIZED LYMPHOCYTES

Product	Effect *in Vitro*
Migration inhibition factor	Inhibits migration of mononuclear phagocytes from a capillary tube.
Macrophage activation factor	Enhances metabolic and functional capacities of macrophages.
Lymphotoxin	Displays cytotoxicity toward cultured cell lines (e.g., fibroblasts).
Chemotactic factor	Attracts the migration of polymorphonuclear and mononuclear leukocytes.
Mitogenic factor	Induces blastogenesis and cell division of lymphocytes.

TABLE 4

CLASSIFICATION OF ALLERGIC LUNG DISEASES

Reaction Type	Reaction Time	Immunologic Mediator	Mechanism	Example of Disease
Type I	Immediate (10–20 min)	IgE (Reagin)	Antigen: IgE-induced release of pharmacologic mediators from mast cells	Asthma; hay fever
Type II	Variable	IgM, IgG	"Autoantibodies" ± complement lyse host's tissues	Goodpasture's disease
Type III	Intermediate (6–18 hours)	IgM, IgG	Precipitating antigen-antibody complex and complement produce an Arthus reaction	Hypersensitivity pneumonitis; allergic alveolitis
Type IV	Delayed (48 hours)	T-lymphocytes (cell-mediated)	Sensitized thymus-dependent lymphocytes plus antigen lead to release of lymphokines or cellular cytotoxicity	Granulomatous disease, e.g., sarcoid, tuberculosis

allergic mechanisms as they apply to the lung is presented for completeness (22–24).

Hypersensitivity or allergic immune mechanisms have been classified by Gell and Coombs (25) into types I through IV (table 4). Type I, immediate hypersensitivity, is mediated by IgE and is pertinent to the pathogenesis of hay fever and asthma. The type II hypersensitivity reactions refer to cytotoxic antibodies produced by the host against his own tissues (autoantibodies), and this mechanism appears to be responsible for Goodpasture's disease. Type III, or intermediate hypersensitivity, involves tissue damage and destruction secondary to the formation of immune complexes and is postulated to be the major mechanism for the pathogenesis of hypersensitivity pneumonitis or allergic alveolitis. Type IV hypersensitivity is exemplified by the familiar delayed hypersensitivity cutaneous reaction to tuberculin and is probably important in granuloma formation. The relationship between delayed hypersensitivity as manifested by skin reactivity and cell-mediated immunity as manifested by resistance to infection is highly controversial and has been discussed recently (26–28).

Immune Apparatus of the Respiratory Tract

Lymphoid Apparatus of the Lung

The normal anatomy of the lymphatic drainage and the distribution of lymphoid tissue throughout the respiratory tract has been reviewed in detail (29, 30). A brief discussion of pulmonary lymphatic tissue will be presented here as it relates to the expression of immune responses in the lung.

Lymphatic tissue. Lymphoid tissue is present throughout the respiratory tract, extending from nasopharynx to respiratory bronchioles and alveolar ducts (figure 5). At least 3 levels of lymphoid tissue organization exist in the lung: (1) lymph nodes; (2) lymphoid nodules; (3) lymphoid aggregates and infiltrates (29). The degree of structural organization of lymphatic tissue decreases progressively from proximal airways to peripheral air spaces. Typical lymph nodes with afferent and efferent channels, a limiting capsule, well-developed follicles, and germinal centers are limited to the region of the trachea and around major bronchi (tracheobronchial and hilar lymph nodes). These serve as the regional lymph nodes for the lung, receiving lymphatic drainage from most of the respiratory tract (29, 31).

Lymphoid nodules contain follicles, but lack capsules. They occur in aggregates in the walls of large- and medium-sized bronchi, particularly at points of branching, and extend from subepithelium through submucosa to the peribronchial connective tissue (29, 32). The nodules are covered on their air side by a single layer of flattened, nonciliated epithelium that is infiltrated by lymphocytes (lymphoepithelium). Attention has been drawn to the morphologic similarity between bronchial lymphoid nodules and similar structures in the gastrointestinal tract (32). Ultrastructural analyses of bronchial lymphoid nodules in rats demonstrate an abundance of lymphatic channels and blood vessels within the follicles. These studies also provide morphologic evidence for both transvascular and transepithelial migration of lymphocytes (33), providing potential pathways for interchange of

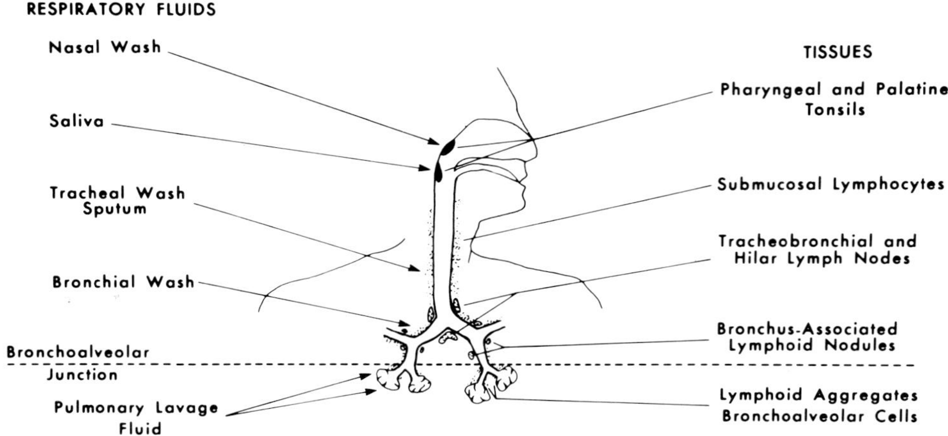

Fig. 5. Schematic representation of the various fluids and lymphatic tissues associated with the respiratory tract that have been studied experimentally. The bronchoalveolar junction arbitrarily demarcates the upper from the lower respiratory tract.

lymphoid cells among vascular, interstitial, and intra-alveolar compartments.

Lymphocytes are present diffusely throughout peripheral lung tissue (figure 5). Nodules, aggregates, and diffuse collections of lymphocytes and phagocytes are distributed along the entire submucosa and lamina propria of airways and throughout lobular and subpleural interstitial tissue, and are closely approximated to both lymphatic and blood vessels (29, 30). Particularly prominent in respiratory bronchioles are discrete aggregates of densely packed lymphatic tissue subjacent to morphologically specialized lymphoepithelium. These structures, termed "lymphoepithelial organs" by von Hayek (30), bring into close approximation respiratory epithelium, lymphatic tissue, blood vessels, and the blind-pocket origin of lymphatic channels. Macklin (34) has suggested that such structures serve as filters for dust and as functional pathways for the removal of alveolar fluids and particulates from airways to lymphatics ("pulmonary sumps"). If true, this would serve as a potential mechanism for the initial interaction of inhaled antigens with lymphoid tissue or as a pathway for antigen transit from distal airways to hilar lymph nodes (31).

The foregoing has been a morphologic description of lymphoid tissue associated with the respiratory tract. These studies define the immune apparatus potentially available to the lung, but provide no information about the functional capacity or role of any of these tissues or their cellular components. Although the gross and light microscopic description of pulmonary lymphoid tissue is relatively complete, a great deal more ultrastructural analysis is now required to provide morphologic clues to the role of these tissues in immune responses to antigenic stimulation.

Lymphatic vessels. The lungs are richly endowed with lymphatic vessels that are closely associated with all lymphatic tissue of the bronchial tree and pulmonary vasculature (29, 30, 35). Lymphatic capillaries arise as blind pouches within lymphoid aggregates (e.g., lymphoepithelial organ) near respiratory bronchioles and small blood vessels. Most workers agree that interalveolar septa are devoid of lymphatics (31, 36). Although the exact details of the route of lymphatic flow are not fully delineated and vary among species, it is evident that most pulmonary lymphatic channels drain ultimately into the hilar and tracheobronchial lymph nodes. Materials gaining access to lymphatic channels in peripheral lung encounter multiple collections of phagocytes and lymphocytes en route to the hilar lymph node complex (31).

Definitions of Upper and Lower Respiratory Tracts

The entire air-tissue interface of the respiratory tract, extending from the nasopharynx proximally to the alveolar spaces distally, is lined with epithelial cells (29, 30). Ciliated epithelium of gradually diminishing thickness lines the airways from trachea to terminal bronchioles. At the junction of terminal and respiratory bronchioles (bronchoalveolar junction), the ciliated epithelium gives way abruptly to a single layer of nonciliated, flattened epithelial cells that cover distal air spaces.

Because structural and functional differences exist between airways above and below the bronchoalveolar junction, it is convenient to use this anatomic site to demarcate arbitrarily the upper from the lower respiratory tract. It is useful to consider mucosal immunity of the upper respiratory tract separately from immune reactions occurring distal to the bronchoalveolar junction (lower respiratory tract), recognizing that this distinction is arbitrary. In the remainder of this review, these operational definitions will be used.

Samples of Respiratory Fluids and Lymphoid Tissues

It is evident from the above that the degree of organization of lymphatic tissue and the anatomic relationship of this tissue to pulmonary airways and vessels varies greatly throughout different regions of the respiratory tract. The most serious and major obstacle to the investigation of pulmonary immune reactions has been the technical difficulty of obtaining lymphoid tissues and secretions from anatomically defined regions of the lung in quantities sufficient for the requisite studies. Thus far, it has been impossible to characterize reliably the cellular composition and immune functions of the various anatomically defined lymphatic tissues in the lung (figure 5).

Respiratory fluids that have been studied frequently include nasal washes, saliva (natural or stimulated), tracheal washes, expectorated sputum, bronchial washes, and fluid obtained by pulmonary lavage of peripheral lung segments.

Tissues that have been studied include nasopharyngeal tonsils (37), slices of tracheal or bronchial tissue (38), minced fragments of pulmonary parenchyma (38), teased suspensions of submucosal lymphoid nodules (39), bronchoalveolar cells obtained by pulmonary lavage (40–43), and hilar lymph nodes (43, 44). In general, the yield of lymphoid cells with these techniques is quite low, and the exact anatomic derivation of the cells is difficult to identify. It is important to realize that many of these techniques sample multiple anatomic and functional subpopulations of lymphoid cells, the interrelationships of which are yet to be defined. Major advances in this field will largely depend on the development of techniques for isolation and separation of anatomically defined lymphoid populations from various regions of the lung.

Fate of Antigenic Materials Deposited in the Respiratory Tract

Clearance of Inhaled Particles

The clearance of inhaled particulate materials from the respiratory tract is the subject of intensive investigation and has been reviewed recently (29, 31, 45–48). Mucociliary and bronchoalveolar clearance mechanisms are briefly summarized here as the basis for a discussion of the fate of antigens applied to respiratory surfaces.

Mucociliary clearance. Tightly packed, ciliated epithelial cells line the air-tissue interface of the respiratory tract from the trachea to the terminal bronchioles (29, 30). Air spaces distal to the bronchoalveolar junction possess nonciliated epithelium. Approximately 90 per cent of inhaled particles with diameters greater than 2 to 3 μm are deposited on the mucus overlying ciliated epithelium (45). These particles are carried from the terminal bronchioles to the trachea by the flow of mucus propelled along the surface of airways by the wavelike motion of beating cilia. Mucociliary transport is rapid, with 90 per cent of the particles being cleared in the first hour after deposition.

The fate of antigen applied to mucosal surfaces depends on its ability to resist enzymatic degradation and penetrate cellular, physical, chemical, and immunologic barriers of the mucosa (49). Most particulates are eliminated by the mucociliary blanket and by reflex cough mechanisms (48); however, microbial organisms may infect the respiratory epithelium, destroy the integrity of the mucosa, and penetrate to submucosal structures (49). Some soluble molecules appear to escape enzymatic degradation and to enter the submucosa in immunogenic form. The fate of antigens penetrating mucosal surfaces is incompletely defined. Such materials may be taken up by phagocytes associated with local lymphatic tissue, may enter blood vessels and be distributed systemically, or may drain via lymphatic channels to regional lymph nodes (figure 6). Current evidence indicates that any or all of these mechanisms may occur under a given set of conditions, the predominant route being determined by the characteristics of the individual antigen. The ultimate outcome of any interaction of an immunogen with respiratory mucosa is not entirely predictable from current knowledge. Each antigen must be characterized individually for its ability to reach immunocompetent tissue and to evoke immune responses

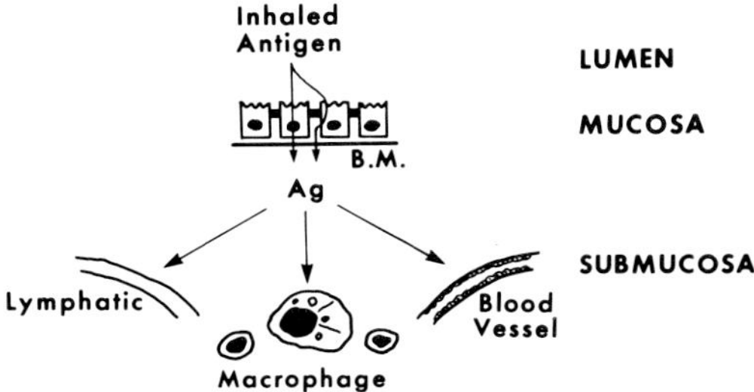

Fig 6. A diagrammatic representation of the possible routes of entry and the fate of antigen (Ag) penetrating the mucosa and basement membrane (B.M.) of the respiratory tract. Antigen reaching the submucosa may enter lymphatic channels or blood vessels, or be ingested locally by phagocytic cells. The nature and anatomic distribution of the resultant immune response may be largely determined by the exact fate of the antigen.

(49). This is an area in need of intensive investigation.

It is possible that specialized structures exist at mucosal surfaces that facilitate the transport of antigenic materials. The flattened, nonciliated lymphoepithelium overlying lymphoid nodules of large- and medium-sized bronchi presents a potential portal of entry of antigens into submucosa, thereby bypassing the mucociliary blanket (32). Recent evidence suggests that this may occur in similar nodules of the gastrointestinal tract (50, 51). Such a portal of entry would be important not only in the efficient transport of antigens to mucosal lymphatic tissue, but also might help to explain how allergens appear to gain access to submucosal mast cells rapidly in such conditions as hay fever and asthma (47, 52).

Bronchoalveolar clearance. Approximately 90 per cent of inhaled particles with diameters of 0.5 to 3.0 μm will be deposited on the nonciliated epithelial surface of the lower respiratory tract distal to terminal bronchioles (45). The clearance of particles from distal segments of the lung is poorly understood and occurs during a period of days to years (46, 47).

The ultimate fate of particles deposited in distal air spaces depends on the dose and the physicochemical properties of the material (31, 45). If the exposure is light, nontoxic, and avirulent, most particles remain localized to the air-fluid interface and are gradually eliminated by a number of mechanisms (31, 45–47). Some particles may be carried by alveolar fluid to the ciliated epithelium of terminal bronchioles, where they gain access to the mucociliary transport mechanism. Some enter interstitial spaces, are ingested by tissue macrophages (histiocytes), and are retained for prolonged periods in subpleural, perivascular, and interstitial lymphatic storage depots. Most particles are ingested by alveolar macrophages and are transported either directly or via interstitial pathways to the bronchoalveolar junction and exit via the mucous blanket (46). The specialized lymphoepithelial structures near respiratory bronchioles have been proposed to be both a filter for free particles from alveolar fluid (34) and a portal of exit for particle-laden macrophages that have migrated through interstitial pathways (46). These two functions may not be mutually exclusive.

After massive exposure to noxious particles, virulent organisms, or liquid suspensions of particulates, acute inflammatory reactions occur, and the normal clearance mechanisms are overwhelmed (45). Under these conditions, particulate materials gain access to interstitial spaces. A major controversy exists as to whether alveolar macrophages that have ingested intra-alveolar particles are capable of re-entering interstitial spaces, or whether particulates must penetrate bronchoalveolar epithelium as naked particles, which are then ingested by interstitial phagocytes (45, 53, 54). Whichever proves to be correct, inflammatory lesions (infective or toxic) of the lower respiratory tract clearly allow absorption of particulate antigens that might be excluded under noninflammatory conditions. In general, particles absorbed from the lower respiratory tract into the interstitium are cleared by lymphatic channels to local lymphoid nodules and subsequently to the hilar and tracheobronchial lymph nodes (31). In contrast to particulates, soluble substances appear to enter blood vessels and are distributed systemically (29, 31, 44).

Although considerable investigation has been directed toward defining the mechanisms by which particles are cleared from upper and lower respiratory surfaces, little work has attempted to correlate the site and mode of particle deposition with the consequent immune responses in lymphatic tissues associated with the respiratory tract. In one such study, inflammatory doses of a complex organic particulate antigen (sheep erythrocytes) instilled into bronchoalveolar spaces of dog lungs resulted in pulmonary consolidation, rapid ingestion and degradation of the particles by phagocytes, and an antibody-mediated immune response that occurred in the hilar lymph nodes, but not in systemic lymphoid tissue (55, 56). These results suggest that under the experimental conditions used, particles bypassed bronchoalveolar barriers, gained access to interstitial lymphatics, but not blood vessels, and generated an immune response in the regional hilar lymph nodes.

Alveolar Macrophages and Inhaled Antigens

Alveolar macrophages play a critical role in the clearance of particles from bronchoalveolar spaces of the lower respiratory tract (31, 45–48, 53, 54, 57). This effective mechanism of phagocytosis and digestion of bacteria (54, 58) and other particulate antigens maintains cleanliness and sterility of air spaces. The degree to which the ingested material is degraded within macrophages depends on its susceptibility to intracellular hydrolytic enzymes (11, 59). The elimination of most particle-laden macrophages appears to be via the mucociliary clearance mechanism (45–47). Controversy exists as to whether or not some macrophages with ingested particles are capable of transalveolar migration into interstitial spaces (53).

The role of the alveolar macrophage in the induction (afferent limb) of immune responses has not been defined. Systemic macrophages (peritoneal and splenic) appear to engulf and "process" both soluble and particulate antigens, rendering them highly immunogenic (11, 12). The presentation of such material to the appropriate antigen-reactive T and B cells enhances the induction of immune responses (11–13). There is no direct evidence that alveolar macrophages perform a similar function in the lower respiratory tract. Indeed, their efficiency in clearing inhaled particles argues just the opposite, namely, that alveolar macrophages function to shield lymphoid tissue from antigenic insults, as has been suggested by some (19).

Thus, a major fundamental question with respect to the immunologic function of the alveolar macrophage remains to be answered. Does the alveolar macrophage function to protect immunocompetent tissue from interaction with inhaled antigenic materials, or does it process inhaled antigens and serve to enhance the immune response of regional lymphoid tissue? Because populations of alveolar macrophages are undoubtedly functionally heterogeneous, these two possibilities are not necessarily mutually exclusive; however, more information on this point is essential to the understanding of the expression of immunity against inhaled antigens by the lower respiratory tract.

Humoral Immune Functions of Pulmonary Lymphoid Tissue

The variety of lymphoid populations associated with the respiratory tract, as defined anatomically, suggests that functional subpopulations of immunocompetent cells exist as well. The presence of such diverse populations of immunocytes requires a definition of the inherent immunocompetence of each, the relationships among the various subpopulations, and the interaction of these with circulating lymphocytes and systemic lymphoid tissue. The remainder of this paper will review the current state of knowledge of immune phenomena as they occur in various regions of the lung. In this section, information pertinent to humoral immunity occurring at mucosal surfaces and in other pulmonary lymphoid populations will be summarized. In the subsequent section, cell-mediated immune reactions occurring in the lung will be reviewed. Because knowledge of these subjects is sparse, consideration of this material will be arbitrary and incompletely integrated.

Humoral Immunity at Mucosal Surfaces

Most work on the immune reactions occurring in the respiratory tract has focused on the immunoglobulin composition of respiratory fluids and on the secretory antibody response to infection or antigenic stimulation of the mucous membranes of the upper respiratory tract (reviewed in 49, 60–66). These studies have defined the composition of secretory immunoglobulins, partially delineated the origin and mechanisms for their secretion, and described the kinetics of the appearance of specific antibodies. The function and the role of secretory antibody in the defense of the host are subjects of current investigation.

Secretory immunoglobulins. The mucosa of the upper respiratory tract consists of an epithelial lining, a basement membrane, and organized submucosal structures, including mucous and serous glands and lymphoid nodules. In addition to mucus, respiratory secretions contain numerous proteins, including several classes of immunoglobulins (IgG, IgA, IgM, and IgE) (reviewed in 60–66). The relative concentrations of each immunoglobulin class in mucosal secretions differ markedly from those in serum. As in most other mammalian external secretions, secretory IgA is the predominant species of immunoglobulin in upper respiratory fluids (saliva, nasopharyngeal, and tracheobronchial secretions). By contrast, serum contains predominantly IgG. Lavage fluids obtained from the lower respiratory tract have contents of IgA and IgG intermediate between those of upper airway secretions and serum, as illustrated in table 5 (42, 67). In general, IgA, IgE, and IgM are present in respiratory secretions in amounts greater than can be explained on the basis of transudation from serum alone, suggesting that at least part of these are produced locally.

Secretory IgA differs from serum IgA in that most (90 per cent) is dimeric (molecular weight, 390,000 daltons), consisting of two IgA monomers joined by a polypeptide ("J-chain," molecular weight: 23,000 daltons) (68) and containing a glycoprotein moiety termed secretory component (SC) (molecular weight: 60,000 daltons). Approximately 10 per cent of IgA in secretions is identical to that in serum, being monomeric and lacking both SC and J-chains. The physicochemical properties of secreted IgG and IgE are identical to those of the homologous immunoglobulins in serum (60–65, 69). A major proportion of secretory IgM is covalently bound to SC, in this respect differing from serum IgM (61, 62, 65).

There are two major sources of the immunoglobulins in respiratory secretions: local synthesis, and transudation or active transport from serum (60–62). All classes of immunoglobulins may be synthesized locally by collections of lymphocytes in the submucosa and lamina propria. The evidence for local synthesis comes from immunofluorescence studies of the lymphoid tissue in the submucosa of airways demonstrating that cells are present that contain each of the known classes of immunoglobulin (70–73). In addition, synthesis of immunoglobulins *in vitro* by tissue obtained from various levels of the respiratory tract has been shown (37, 38, 62). Although these studies demonstrate that the capacity to synthesize the various immunoglobulin classes is present in the respiratory tract, they do not define the mechanism by which antigenic stimulation leads to generation of specific secretory antibodies. A portion of each class of immunoglobulin is derived from the serum by transudation and, perhaps, selective transport (60–62). In the absence of inflammation, diffusion of immunoglobulins into airways is governed by the usual physicochemical constraints involved in the passive transport of macromolecules across semipermeable membranes (74). Inflammation of the mucous membranes results in enhanced exudation of all serum proteins, including immunoglobulins into the respiratory tract (62, 64, 75). Direct evidence for the derivation of immunoglobulins from serum has come primarily from radiotracer studies in which radiolabeled immunoglobulin infused intravenously has been detected in respiratory secretions (76). Although the relative proportions of immunoglobulin derived from either local synthesis or from the serum varies for each class, the bulk of evidence indicates that both mechanisms contribute to the total pool of each. Biologically, this implies that whereas there is a degree of local regulation of antibody synthesis, a strict separation between the local and systemic humoral immune systems cannot be made for mucosal surfaces of the upper respiratory tract.

Biologic function of secretory immunoglobulin classes. In an attempt to understand the role of each immunoglobulin class in the defense of the host against virulent organisms, secretory immunoglobulins with specific antibody activity have been investigated. To date, a unified and comprehensive formulation of the biologic function of the various classes and subclasses has not emerged.

TABLE 5

CONTENT OF CLASS-SPECIFIC IMMUNOGLOBULINS IN SAMPLES
FROM THE CANINE RESPIRATORY TRACT AND IN SERUM*

Fluid	N	Mean Per Cent of the Total Immunoglobulin Concentration			Ratio of Concentrations
		IgG	IgA	IgM	$\frac{IgG}{IgA}$
Stimulated saliva	5	6.3 ± 0.9[†]	83.4 ± 1.4	10.3 ± 0.9	0.1 ± 0.01**
Tracheal wash	7	52.7 ± 6.2	33.5 ± 6.2	13.8 ± 3.8	2.1 ± 0.6
Bronchial wash	10	75.0 ± 2.0	19.3 ± 1.9	5.6 ± 0.9	4.1 ± 0.6
Serum	15	77.6 ± 2.7	3.9 ± 0.3	18.6 ± 2.8	23.2 ± 3.0

*Data from Kaltreider and Chan (67).
[†]Mean $\pm$ SEM.
**Mean of the ratios of immunoglobulin concentrations present in each sample $\pm$ SEM.

IgG

Although IgG is not the predominant immunoglobulin in secretions of the upper airways, it is present in substantial quantities and occurs in relatively high concentrations in the lower respiratory tract (42, 49, 67, 70, 77; table 5). A fraction of the IgG normally present in secretions appears to originate from serum by transudation (63, 64, 76). The remainder, perhaps the majority, may be synthesized locally (39, 62, 70, 77–80) in both upper and lower respiratory tracts. There is enhanced exudation or transudation of IgG into the respiratory tract during allergic and inflammatory diseases of the lung, such as asthma (81), bronchitis, and cystic fibrosis (70). Specific antibody-forming cells of the IgG class appear in the respiratory tract after infection (38) or immunization (82–84). Regardless of its absolute concentration in respiratory fluids, IgG antibody is exceedingly active biologically. Serum IgG efficiently agglutinates particulates, opsonizes bacteria, activates complement, neutralizes bacterial exotoxins and viruses, and lyses gram-negative bacteria in the presence of complement. Because serum IgG has access to respiratory secretions, one might expect that these biologic functions of IgG would be expressed in the lung.

Secretory IgG antibody obtained from the respiratory tract has, in fact, been demonstrated to agglutinate and to opsonize pseudomonas organisms for phagocytosis by alveolar macrophages in humans (85) and rabbits (86, 87); IgG is more effective in these respects than secretory IgA antibody. Recent evidence suggests that human alveolar macrophages have surface receptors for the Fc fragment of IgG and complement, but not for those of IgA and IgM (88). If the Fc receptor on macrophages is critical for phagocytosis, then this evidence suggests that IgG in respiratory secretions is essential for optimal phagocytosis of some inhaled bacteria, such as *Pseudomonas aeruginosa*. It is impossible to know the relative quantities of transudated, as opposed to locally synthesized, IgG antibody in these studies. Lymphoid cells obtained from specific locations in the respiratory tract itself have been shown *in vitro* to synthesize IgG antibody to diphtheria toxin (79), *L. monocytogenes* (38), and complement-dependent hemolysis of heterologous red blood cells (82, 83). The relative importance of these biologic functions of secretory IgG in the over-all integrated defense against microbial organisms is not known.

IgM

Owing to its high molecular weight, more than 75 per cent of IgM is intravascular. Hence, little appears in respiratory fluids as a result of passive diffusion (60–64, 74). The relatively large quantities of IgM in saliva (67, 89, 90; table 5) plus the presence of J-chain in secretory IgM (61, 62) argues strongly for local synthesis or selective transport of IgM into respiratory secretions (62). The remainder of respiratory fluids contain IgM in low absolute and relative concentrations (49, 60, 63, 64, 67; table 5). Its presence in human bronchial secretions has been disputed by some (42, 85). Secretion of IgM into the respiratory tract is enhanced during acute inflammation (64). Cells containing IgM by immunofluorescent staining are present in normal human bronchial mucosa (70) and are abundant in peribronchial spaces of hamsters infected with *Mycoplasma pneumoniae* (77). The synthesis *in vitro* of IgM by tonsillar lymphocytes (37) and by fragments of rabbit lungs (38) demonstrates that the capability to produce IgM resides in respiratory tissue. Because of its low concentration in respiratory fluids, the biologic function of secretory IgM has not been characterized. Specific antibody-forming cells of the IgM class have been obtained by lavage from the lungs of rabbits (83, 91) and dogs (82). This IgM antibody is capable of complement-dependent lysis of heterologous erythrocytes. From a knowledge about serum IgM, it would be expected that the secretory immunoglobulin efficiently agglutinates particulate antigens, fixes complement, and lyses certain bacteria. The increase in IgM in secretions of persons with selective IgA deficiency (90, 92, 93) may be compensatory. The evidence taken together suggests an important biologic role for secretory IgM in the defense of the respiratory tract. Despite its presence in low concentrations, secretory IgM is worthy of more study.

IgE

The biologic role of IgE in immediate hypersensitivity (Type I) has been studied extensively (reviewed in 94–97). It is necessary for the specific interaction of inhaled extrinsic allergens with mediator-containing mast cells. Specific antibody of the IgE class combines with the surface of mast cells and basophilic leukocytes through its Fc fragment, leaving the Fab portion free to combine with the sensitizing allergen. After interaction of IgE and allergen, a cascade of intracellular metabolic processes is triggered, resulting in the synthesis and release of the mediators (98, 99) responsible for the clinical syndromes of allergic rhinitis, conjunctivitis, and asthma. In atopic persons, both the serum and the secretory concentrations of IgE are increased 3- to 10-fold, particularly during periods of allergic disease activity (69, 81, 94–96). The etiologic defect in atopic states is unknown. There is no direct evidence that an abnormality in the IgE system per se is at fault. It is of interest that the IgE antibody response to a specific allergen appears to be under genetic control (100).

Secretory IgE appearing in the respiratory tract appears to be synthesized locally (62, 71, 101), resembles serum IgE physicochemically and lacks SC (69), and is increased in concentration in atopic states (69, 81, 94). There appears to be a poor correlation between serum and secretory IgE concentrations. In humans and monkeys, lymphoid cells containing IgE are relatively rich in the bronchial and gastrointestinal mucosa, the hilar and mesenteric lymph node complexes, and pharyngeal tonsils (71), being relatively sparse in spleen and peripheral lymph nodes. The generation of specific antibody activity in IgE appears to be under genetic control, requires the participation of both T and B cells, and may be suppressed by IgG and IgM antibody (95). The latter observation may be pertinent to the mechanism of immunotherapy in hay fever. The role of IgE in the defense of the host is obscure. It appears to be related to resistance to parasitic infestation, particularly by nematodes (95). It may be that IgE-mediated reactions control or modulate the manifestations of other immune phenomena by regulating vascular (membrane) permeability and the availability of IgM and IgG antibody and mediator substances (95). It is unlikely that IgE antibody subserves only an allergic role. Investigative effort should be directed to elucidating protective or controlling functions of this class of immunoglobulin.

Secretory IgA

Secretory IgA is the predominant class of immunoglobulin in mammalian external secretions, including those of the upper respiratory tract. The elegant studies of Tomasi (60–63) and many others have elucidated the physicochemical features, the metabolism, and the immunologic reactivity of this unique molecular species (additional references 64, 65, 93). Despite inten-

sive investigation, the precise biologic function of IgA in the integrated system of host defenses is not fully understood.

Immunofluorescence studies demonstrate IgA-producing cells in the lamina propria and submucosa of the entire respiratory tract (60–63, 70, 72). Most secretory IgA is synthesized locally by these lymphoid cells (61–63). It is secreted from plasma cells as a dimer linked by J-chain. At this stage, the IgA dimer lacks secretory component. A similar formulation pertains to locally synthesized IgM. The released dimeric IgA (or IgM) binds to secretory component, which constitutes a receptor on the surface membrane of mucosal epithelial cells (65). The immunoglobulin molecules enter the epithelial cells and covalently combine with secretory component; the newly assembled secretory IgA (IgM) is secreted onto the mucosal surface. The addition of secretory component to the IgA dimer appears to render it relatively resistant to enzymatic digestion by proteolytic enzymes present at mucosal surfaces (102). As with the other immunoglobulins, there is increased secretion of IgA into the respiratory tract during inflammation (64, 103).

Approximately 10 per cent of secretory IgA is monomeric, lacking both J-chain and secretory component. Monomeric IgA arises in submucosal lymphoid cells and may either enter secretions or gain access to the blood. Much of serum IgA may be derived from mucosal surfaces by this mechanism (74), and some may originate in the bone marrow (65). Secretory component is synthesized in epithelial cells and may enter secretions in free form, especially in such states as selective IgA deficiency and agammaglobulinemia.

It is clear that specific antibody activity can be induced to appear in secretory IgA after antigenic stimulation (vida infra); however, the function of IgA antibody is not entirely clear. Several biologic activities of IgA antibodies have been defined. These include inhibition of microbial growth, agglutination of particles, neutralization of toxins, and blocking the entry of antigen. The complement-independent neutralization of a wide variety of respiratory viruses and some bacteria (86) constitutes the best-studied and clearest biologic activity of IgA antibody (reviewed in 48, 49, 60–66). Because secretory IgA is dimeric, it possesses 4 Fab combining sites and hence is a very efficient agglutinator of microbes (61); via this activity, it may enhance mucociliary clearance of particles. The exotoxin of *Vibrio cholera* is effectively neutralized at the gut mucosa surface by secretory IgA (61), and this activity may confer protection if appropriate antibodies are available at the time and site of infection.

Various "blocking" functions of secretory IgA may prove to be of critical importance in defense of the host. The absorption of soluble, potentially immunogenic macromolecules through mucosal surfaces may be impeded by secretory IgA (104). Persons with IgA deficiency frequently have circulating antibodies to food antigens, such as milk proteins, that have been absorbed through the gut mucosa (105, 106). It is postulated that normally, secretory IgA antibodies form nonabsorbable complexes with potential antigens and thereby play an important regulatory role in their absorption. Whether a similar phenomenon occurs at respiratory surfaces is unknown. Anti-ragweed antibodies of the IgA class have been detected in secretions of atopic persons, raising the possibility that they function to block the entry of pollen through respiratory mucosa (107, 108). In fact, selective IgA deficiency is significantly increased among allergic persons, strengthening the argument that IgA inhibits entry of inhaled allergens (62, 64). Secretory IgA derived from saliva specifically inhibits the adherence of bacteria to respiratory epithelial cells, thereby inhibiting bacterial colonization of the mucosa (109, 110). This may be a potent mechanism for the disposal of inhaled bacterial antigens. Hence, the function of regulation of antigen entry may be a major biologic property of secretory IgA.

Immunoglobulin A differs functionally from IgG and IgM in its relative inability to opsonize bacteria for effective phagocytosis (61, 62, 64) and its inability to activate complement in the usual manner (61, 62). Whether or not it can activate complement by an alternate pathway remains to be definitely established. In respiratory secretions, the necessary components of complement appear to be present only in very low concentrations (42, 86). These observations, taken together, cast some doubt on the importance of IgA in defense against bacterial infections in the lung. Although some patients with selective IgA deficiency have increased sinopulmonary infections (111, 112) this is not consistent, and many are perfectly normal (113), suggesting that, at least for common pathogens, secretory IgA plays a contributory, but not a critical, role in defense of the respiratory tract.

Secretory IgA antibody against viruses. The previous section discussed the various classes of immunoglobulins (IgG, IgA, IgM, and IgE) normally present in respiratory secretions, their demonstrated antibody activities, and some of their proposed functions. This section will review, in general, the massive bulk of information about specific antibody activity appearing in secretory IgA after antigenic stimulation of nasopharyngeal and upper respiratory mucosa. In attempting to understand the immune response in respiratory tissue, several questions should be considered. Does antigen penetrate locally? If so, what is its fate? Is the full complement of immunocompetent cells (phagocytes, antigen-reactive B cells, and T cells) required for an immune response present locally, or are such cells recruited from the systemic circulation? Is all the specific secretory antibody produced locally, or is it derived by transudation from the plasma? The answers to these questions will ultimately define the limits and capabilities of local immunity.

There is abundant and convincing evidence that viral antigens applied locally to the upper respiratory tract result in the local appearance of specific secretory antibody, most of which is dimeric IgA (reviewed in 48, 49, 60–65, 114). Because of the efficacy of mucosal barriers (mucus, mucociliary transport, enzymes, antibodies, phagocytes, and respiratory epithelium), most inert particles, killed viruses, and relatively insoluble substances do not gain access to the submucosal lymphoid tissue and hence fail to evoke an antibody response (49, 62). By contrast, natural or attenuated living viruses and some soluble substances effectively penetrate mucosal barriers, gain access to the submucosa, and, if viremia occurs, systemic lymphoid tissue. The resulting antibody response may be detectable only in secretory IgA if the virus remains localized. If viremia occurs, circulating antibody of all classes will appear (60–62). It may require 2 to 3 weeks for specific secretory IgA antibody to appear after exposure of the mucosa to a new virus (49). The details of the required cellular interactions and their kinetics are not fully known. It is clear that a population of T cells is required for normal expression of IgA-mediated immunity (61, 62). Anamnestic IgA responses may occur when a replicating antigen persists for prolonged periods in the mucosa; however, these are usually difficult to demonstrate (62, 64).

After viral infection, there are at least two general patterns of local and systemic humoral immune responses (60–62). These appear to reflect the biologic properties of the viruses themselves. Rhinovirus, respiratory syncytial virus, myxovirus (e.g., influenza), and some adenoviruses replicate and remain localized superficially in the mucosa. The specific antibody response to such infections is predominantly local and restricted to IgA. Little, if any, systemic antibody is detectable in the circulation. Hence, local sequestration (mucosal epithelium) evokes only a local response. By the same token, experimental studies show that local immunization (nasopharyngeal) with attenuated vaccines derived from this group of viruses stimulates a local secretory IgA antibody response that may confer resistance to subsequent reinfection with the homologous virulent organism.

The second pattern is exemplified by most adenoviruses and polio, ECHO, and measles viruses. Infection with these organisms results in penetration of the mucosa, passage through submucosa, and systemic dissemination (viremia). In addition to local antibody formation, circulating antibodies of all major classes appear in the blood owing to viremia. Protection against this group of viruses is generally most efficient with systemic vaccination, because the manifestations of the disease are primarily due to the effects of viremia; however, initial infection of the mucosa may be also prevented locally if sufficient quantities of specific IgA antibodies are present at the time and site of the infection.

These formulations are an oversimplification of complex situations, but serve to emphasize that it is critical to have antibody present at the site where organisms produce disease. When considering mucosal antibody responses, the characteristics of each antigen and the response to the antigen must be considered individually, and results from one system should not be extrapolated to those of others.

Response to naturally occurring viral infections. The early course of an initial viral infection of the upper respiratory tract is characterized by an enhanced exudation of nasopharyngeal secretions (rhinorrhea). The secretions are composed of exudated serum proteins of all types, as well as locally synthesized immunoglobulins, including, predominantly, IgA; however, in the absence of prior sensitization by contact with the same or a cross-reacting virus, the enhanced secretion of immunoglobulin does not contain antibody specific for the infecting organism. The exudate is nonspecific in that it represents an "out-pouring of previous immune experience" (49). Specific secretory IgA (and some IgG) antibody appears 2 to 3 weeks after initial infection. Specific antibody usually appears after resolution of the clinical syndrome and best correlates temporally with the decline in viral shedding. Symptomatic improvement actually occurs in conjunction with the local appearance of interferon (4 to 7 days) (115, 116). Thus, although natural or iatrogenic infection of the upper respiratory tract with a new virus is an exceedingly potent stimulus to local (and sometimes systemic) production of specific antibody, the exact role of the antibody in control of the naturally occurring infection is not entirely clear.

By contrast, infection of the upper respiratory tract with a virus with which the host has had previous experience (e.g., prior immunization or infection with a closely related strain) results in an initial outpouring of preformed specific antibody (both secretory IgA and IgG) from the submucosa onto the mucous membranes and serves to abort or prevent clinical illness (49, 66, 114). The resistance to infection is dependent on the presence of immunocytes in the submucosa that are actively synthesizing specific antibody at the time of infection. As noted previously, it has been difficult to demonstrate a secondary anamnestic response in the IgA system. Antibody production to reinfection tends to follow the kinetics of a second primary immune response. Whether or not the same holds for specific antibody in the IgG class that appears at mucosal surfaces is not known.

Vaccination of the upper respiratory tract. The response of mucosal surfaces to viral antigens has important clinical implications with respect to the route of administration of vaccines. From the foregoing discussion, it might be expected that the ideal route of vaccination against any given virus would be easily predictable from a knowledge of the biologic behavior of the organism. Namely, topical or local vaccination should confer protection against superficial viruses through locally produced secretory IgA. Systemic (subcutaneous) vaccination should produce resistance to disease produced by penetrating viruses through circulating antibodies. In fact, clinical immunization trials comparing local (nose drops, nasopharyngeal aerosols) with subcutaneous vaccination against a variety of respiratory viruses have produced conflicting results (reviewed in 14, 49, 60–63, 66). The discrepancies among the various studies are attributable to many factors, such as the difference between killed and attenuated live vaccines, the differences among types and strains of viruses, the differences in experimental design among these studies, and the rapid mutation rate of many viral strains.

There is no question that local vaccination with live viruses produces a secretory antibody response and that the secretory antibody does, indeed, modify subsequent clinical illness due to both superficially and deeply penetrating viruses if the immunizing and infecting antigenic determinants possess sufficient mutual cross reactivity. One difficulty is that most respiratory viruses mutate rapidly, develop novel, antigenic determinants, and become nonsusceptible to the preformed antibody (117). In addition, many locally applied vaccines produce a systemic antibody response as well. Conversely, subcutaneous vaccination results predominantly in circulating antibody that might not reach mucosal surfaces. In fact, however, if the immunizing dose is sufficiently great, antibody does appear in secretions and is protective. This route is a more convenient mode of vaccine administration. In addition, the subcutaneous route allows the use of killed vaccines; however, Mills has shown that inactivated respiratory syncytial virus administered parenterally to children may result in Arthus-type injury to the lungs during respiratory infection with the virus (66). Thus, there are advantages and disadvantages to both modes of vaccination, and the ideal program for each virus remains to be established.

Generation of mucosal antibodies. Although a great deal of information exists regarding the source, synthesis, assembly, and secretion of immunoglobulins at mucosal surfaces, little is known about the intimate details of the induction and expression of specific antibody responses locally in the respiratory tract. The exact fate of antigens penetrating to the submucosa is not known. Are they taken up by local phagocytes, or drained by lymphatics to the regional nodes? What is the nature of the local cell-cell interaction? Are the genetically appropriate antigen-reactive T and B cells present and organized in such a way as to initiate a primary immune response *in situ,* or do new cells appear by differentiation of local precursors or by recruitment of circulating immunocytes? It is certainly likely that antibody specificity in the secretory IgA system is locally and autonomously generated after initial contact with antigen. If true, then by inference, all of the cellular ingredients necessary for generation of humoral immunity

must be available to the mucosa of the upper respiratory tract. Rigorous proof of such a scheme is lacking, however. Such questions should be addressed in future investigations.

Tonsils

The palatine, lingual, and pharyngeal tonsils are oval-shaped bodies consisting of organized lymphatic tissue closely approximated to mucosal surfaces of the upper respiratory tract (figure 5). They consist of dense accumulations of lymphoid tissue organized into well-defined germinal centers, follicles, and perifollicular regions. The structures protrude into upper airways and are penetrated by deep crypts extending from mucosal surfaces to perifollicular areas, providing a potential anatomic pathway for the close approximation of inhaled antigens and organized lymphatic tissue. Their structure and location have raised the possibility that tonsils function to recruit, generate, and serve as a reservoir for antigen-reactive precursor cells to populate the lamina propria of mucosal surfaces with specific IgA antibody-forming cells (49). Peyer's patches appear to serve such a function for the gut (118).

The immunologic function of tonsils has received recent attention. Tonsillectomy results in a modest reduction in secretory antibody titer against polio virus in previously immunized children (114, 119). Children undergoing tonsillectomy before vaccination respond less well to a primary local immunization with live, attenuated polio virus than do control subjects (114, 120). These studies suggest a role for the tonsils in both the initiation and perpetuation of mucosal secretory immune responses in the upper respiratory tract.

The issue of the immunocompetence of tonsils has been confronted directly. Immunoglobulin-containing plasma cells of all major classes can be demonstrated in tonsils by immunofluorescence studies (62, 71). The T cells, B cells, and phagocytes are present in suspensions of cells obtained from human tonsils (37). Studies have further demonstrated a primary immune response *in vitro* by these lymphocytes against a protein-hapten complex. An optimal immune response occurred only in the presence of all 3 cell types (37). By these criteria, tonsils appear to be fully immunocompetent and to represent structures capable of a local immune response. In a similar experimental system, a secondary immune response *in vitro* to diptheria toxoid has been demonstrated by tonsils of children previously parenterally vaccinated (79). The antitoxin synthesized *in vitro* consisted of both IgG and dimeric IgA. These studies suggest that memory cells for diphtheria toxin persisted in tonsillar tissue after primary parenteral immunization. Whether or not tonsillar lymphocytes serve as a precursor pool for immunoglobulin-secreting cells in respiratory mucosa during either the primary or the secondary response remains an unanswered question.

Bronchus-associated Lymphoid Tissue

Anatomically organized lymphoid tissue in direct contact with the respiratory mucosa of bronchi has recently been described and studied by Bienenstock and colleagues (32, 39, 121–124). This bronchus-associated lymphoid tissue (BALT) consists anatomically of follicles containing small- and medium-sized lymphocytes, but lacking capsules, germinal centers, and plasma cells typical of lymph nodes (32). The nodules are covered by a single layer of flattened, nonciliated, surface epithelium infiltrated with lymphocytes (lymphoepithelium). The lymphoid nodules are distributed along the mucosal surface of large- and medium-sized bronchi, being particularly concentrated at points of bifurcation and being present in a variety of animal species (32). The relationship of this tissue to less well organized collections and aggregates of lymphoid cells occurring throughout the lung is not clear. The morphologic appearance of BALT bears a resemblance to that of Peyer's patches and other gut-associated lymphoid tissue (GALT).

The functional characteristics of BALT are incompletely understood. Cells bearing a surface marker for T cells appear to make up less than 20 per cent of this population (122). Plasma cells and lymphocytes staining positively for intracytoplasmic immunoglobulin are absent (32). Specific antibody-forming cells do not seem to appear after local immunization (39, 121). These findings suggest that BALT lacks B cells that are sufficiently differentiated to synthesize immunoglobulin and indicate that this tissue may participate only indirectly in mucosal immune responses.

Gut-associated lymphoid tissue contains lymphocytes lacking intracytoplasmic immunoglobulin, and these function as precursors for IgA-producing cells in the lamina propria of the gastrointestinal tract (118). The surface membrane characteristics of GALT and BALT are similar (122). In addition, BALT cells may repopulate the lamina propria of both gut and lung mucosa with IgA-producing cells after lethal irradiation of recipient animals (123). These studies suggest a functional similarity between GALT and BALT, indicate that BALT is composed of B cell precursors of IgA-producing cells, and raise the possibility that BALT serves as a cellular reservoir for immunocytes contributing to a common mucosal system for both the respiratory and gastrointestinal tracts. The results raise the possibility of the existence of migratory pathways between GALT, BALT, and lamina propria that may have clinical implications with respect to oral immunization against respiratory infections. While these studies do not define the functional relationship between BALT and the secretory immune mechanism, they represent an important advance in the anatomic and functional characterization of one of presumably many subpopulations of lymphoid cells subserving immunity in the respiratory tract.

Bronchoalveolar Cells

Definition and retrieval of bronchoalveolar cells. Bronchoalveolar cells (BAC) are defined operationally as the population of nucleated cells obtained from lung tissue by pulmonary lavage (40–43, 78, 82, 125). The cellular composition of BAC varies among animal species, but generally consists predominantly of alveolar macrophages, moderate proportions of lymphocytes and plasma cells, and a minor fraction of neutrophilic and eosinophilic granulocytes (table 6). The exact anatomic derivation of these cells is unclear, but it is postulated that they originate from cells populating distal air spaces and from subepithelial aggregates of lymphocytes infiltrating the lamina propria of terminal and respiratory bronchioles (29, 30, 34). The validity of lavage as a method of sampling lymphoid tissue present in the lower respiratory tract rests on the assumptions that the cells obtained are a representative sample of lymphoid tissue existing *in situ,* and that they are derived from distal air spaces (bronchioles and alveoli), and not from large airways.

In large mammalian species (e.g., dog, monkey, and human) the lavage catheter or bronchoscope is wedged into airways 3 to 4 mm in diameter. Under gentle conditions, in a living subject, the retrieved cells contain few, if any, erythrocytes, lending support to the notion that the BAC are derived from distal air spaces of the lung from the air side of the pulmonary vascular bed (43, 78, 82). In smaller animals (e.g.,

TABLE 6

REPRESENTATIVE VALUES FOR THE COMPOSITION OF
BRONCHOALVEOLAR CELLS FROM VARIOUS SPECIES

Species	Lymphocytes (%)	Macrophages (%)	Reference
Human			
Normal subjects	18.0 ± 2.2*	78.4 ± 3.1	Reynolds *et al.* (85)
Smokers	7.2 ± 1.8	89.8 ± 4.2	Reynolds *et al.* (85)
Rabbit	16†	84	Ford and Kuhn (83)
	2 – 10	90 – 98	Holub and Hauser (91)
	< 10	> 90	Galindo and Myrvik (136)
Dog	39 ± 12**	60 ± 11	Kaltreider *et al.* (43)
Guinea pig	20 – 30	70 – 80	Nash and Holle (138)
	30†	70	Waldman and Henney (137)
	38	62	Spencer *et al.* (143)

*Mean ± SEM.
†Mean value.
**Mean ± SD.

rabbit, rat, mouse, and guinea pig), the lung is usually lavaged *in toto* after or during sacrifice of the animal (40). The anatomic derivation of these cells is more difficult to define, because the entire length of the bronchial tree is subjected to the lavage procedure, and the retrieved population of cells contains numerous erythrocytes, suggesting significant contamination by peripheral blood. Despite limitations in defining anatomically the origin of BAC, this population is important, because it is virtually the only lymphoid population that is readily sampled from the lower respiratory tract during life. Hence, the BAC population offers the possibility for morphologic, metabolic, and functional studies directed toward understanding the etiology and pathogenesis of human lung disease.

Characterization of bronchoalveolar cells. The yield and composition of bronchoalveolar cells obtained from several species have been studied recently (table 6). Variations among species is characteristic. Chronic irritation (cigarette smoking) and acute and chronic inflammation (bronchitis) increase the total number of retrievable cells and alter the composition of the BAC. For example, chronic cigarette smoking by humans increases the total number, percentage, and metabolic activity of human alveolar macrophages (42, 53, 88, 126). The per cent of lymphocytes among BAC appears to serve as a useful guide in assessing the activity of human interstitial lung disease (127); however, monitoring yields and compositions of BAC populations will probably prove to be too insensitive to be a generally useful technique. Characterization of their functional properties

holds more promise for understanding pathogenesis.

The content of B and T cells among bronchoalveolar lymphocytes has been characterized in normal dogs (78) and humans (128). In dogs, B cells were identified by demonstrating synthesis of IgG *in vitro;* T cells, by their blastogenic response to phytohemagglutinin (figure 7). By these criteria, B cells predominated; T cells were normally absent and could be recruited by local immunization (78), and the BAC population clearly differed in lymphocyte subsets from blood, spleen (figure 7), and hilar lymph nodes (43), which possess both B and T cells. It is possible that precursor T cells are present in the BAC that are unable to respond to phytohemagglutinin. Alternatively, pulmo-

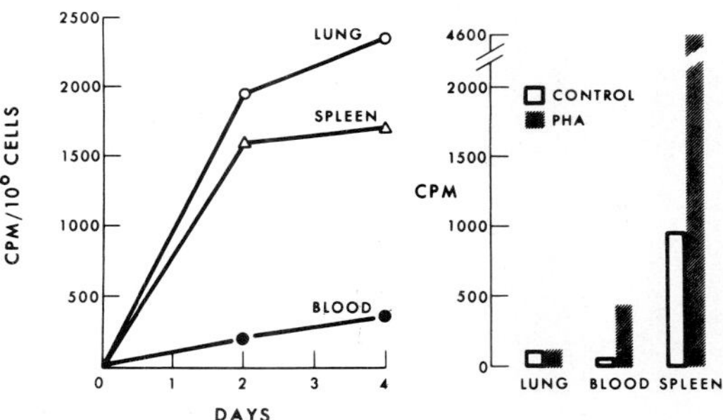

Fig. 7. Comparison of IgG synthetic capacities of lung (bronchoalveolar cells), blood and spleen leukocytes *(left)* with the blastogenic response to phytohemagglutinin of aliquots of the same cell populations *(right)*. The differences in the functional capacities of the lymphocytes in each population of cells is evident. (From Kaltreider and Salmon [78]; reprinted by permission of publisher.) CPM = counts per min.

nary lavage may sample lymphatic tissue that is neither fully organized nor immunocompetent in the usual sense. The recruitment of T cells after immunization is consistent with the migratory behavior of T cells (7), and suggests a route for the traffic of lymphocytes from blood into bronchoalveolar spaces.

Normal human bronchoalveolar lymphocytes have been characterized on the basis of surface membrane markers (table 7) (128). By these criteria, there were 47 per cent T cells (sheep erythrocyte receptors), 16 to 19 per cent B cells (complement receptors and surface immunoglobulin), and 34 per cent null cells (no detectable surface markers). The ratios of B cells to T cells for bronchoalveolar and peripheral blood lymphocytes were equal. These data suggest that the populations of lymphocytes in the vascular and the bronchoalveolar spaces are in equilibrium and raise the possibility that rapid exchange of immunocytes may occur between these two compartments. Whether or not such exchange occurs physiologically is a critical question.

The differences between the results of studies performed in dogs and in humans may reflect species variation or the differences in techniques used. The results of the two studies are not mutually exclusive (78, 128). Samples of BAC in each were obtained at a single point in time. Hence, the composition of lymphocytes may be a static reflection of the dynamic processes of current or previous antigenic experience, exchange rates of B and T cells from other lymphoid compartments, or the degree of maturation of the cells present. Recent improvements in the technology for classifying subsets of lym-

TABLE 7

LYMPHOCYTE SUBSETS IN HUMAN
BRONCHOALVEOLAR CELLS AND
PERIPHERAL BLOOD LEUKOCYTES*

	Lung (% ±SEM)	Peripheral Blood (% ±SEM)
T cells[†]	47 ± 5.6	67 ± 3.5
B cells**	19 ± 1.2	25 ± 1.6
Null cells[††]	34 ± 5.6	10 ± 4.3
B/T	1/2.5	1/2.7

*Data adapted from Daniele and co-workers (128).

[†]Determined on purified lymphocyte populations using the sheep erythrocyte rosette technique.

**Determined by the detection of surface immunoglobulin.

[††]Lymphocytes identifiable as neither T nor B cells.

phocytes will stimulate additional and more detailed studies of BAC in a variety of animal species as a function of time, experimental manipulation, and presence of disease activity. The results should help the understanding of how immunity is expressed in the lung and suggest mechanisms of immunopathogenesis of lung diseases. The origin, fate, and relationship of bronchoalveolar lymphocytes to other pulmonary lymphoid tissues are major questions to be answered.

Humoral immune functions of bronchoalveolar cells. Immunoglobulin A is the predominant class of immunoglobulin in secretions of the upper respiratory tract. It is evident that IgG is predominant or increased relative to IgA in the lower respiratory tract (table 5) (42, 64, 67, 129). Canine bronchoalveolar cells synthesize IgG and IgM *in vitro* (43, 78, 82). The synthesis of IgG by rabbit lung slices exceeds that of both IgM and IgA normally and after lower respiratory infection (38). Hamsters infected with *M. pneumoniae* show increased numbers of peribronchial lymphoid cells staining positively for IgM and IgG with immunofluorescent reagents (77). Chronic inflammation of human bronchial mucosa results in an increase in the proportion of IgG-producing cells in the submucosa (70). A study of the distribution of class-specific immunoglobulin markers on human bronchoalveolar lymphocytes revealed IgM and IgG to be the predominant classes, whereas IgA was infrequently observed (128). These studies demonstrate capacity of BAC to synthesize immunoglobulin of 3 major classes (IgG, IgA, and IgM), show that IgG synthesis is quantitatively important in the lower respiratory tract, and suggest that IgG and IgM may be functionally important as well.

In addition to the capacity to synthesize immunoglobulin, specific antibody-forming cells (AFC) have been demonstrated among BAC after local or systemic immunization (reviewed in 130). The appearance of AFC was first demonstrated in alveolar exudates of rabbits immunized via the intratracheal route with sheep erythrocytes (91). The original observations on rabbits have recently been confirmed and extended to include soluble, as well as particulate, antigens (83, 84). The AFC in rabbit alveolar exudates were IgM-secreting during the primary immune response and IgG-secreting during the secondary response (83).

The time courses of appearance and distribution of AFC among various pulmonary and systemic lymphoid tissues as functions of both the immunization route (intrapulmonary versus intravenous) and the dose of sheep erythrocytes administered have been determined in dogs (82). Both immunization routes resulted in a typical IgM-mediated primary immune response (figure 8); however, the tissue distributions of AFC were distinctively different after each route. After intrapulmonary immunization with high doses, AFC appeared in bronchoalveolar cells, the hilar nodes, and blood leukocytes, but not in peripheral nodes or spleen. By contrast, after intravenous immunization, AFC predominated in spleen, bronchoalveolar cells, and blood, whereas few appeared in hilar and peripheral lymph nodes. Both routes resulted in high concentrations of AFC in blood, providing a potential source of these cells for all tissues. The nonrandom tissue distribution of AFC observed may represent either migration into, or generation in, tissues where antigen concentrated after the different immunization routes (131).

As the immunizing dose is decreased (figure

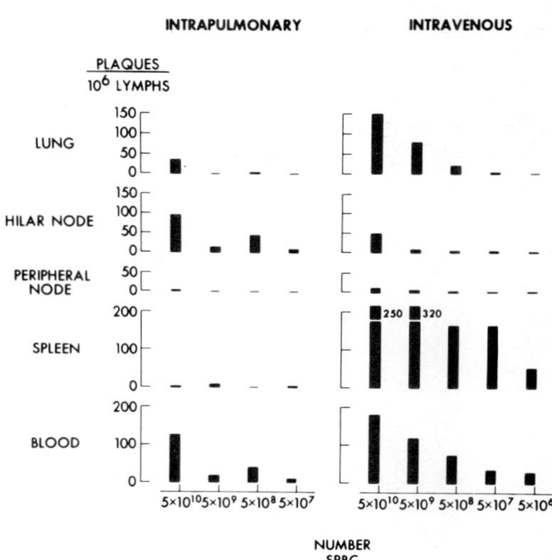

Fig. 9. The effect on the accumulation of antibody-forming cells (plaques) in various canine lymphoid tissues of logfold reductions in the number of sheep red blood cells (SRBC) administered by the intrapulmonary route (*left*) or the intravenous route (*right*). Experiments were performed 4 or 5 days after immunization during the primary immune response. (Modified from Kaltreider and associates [82].)

9), the major tissues concentrating AFC are the hilar nodes after intrapulmonary immunization; the spleen, after intravenous immunization. In addition, the data suggest that at lower doses, the intravenous route is more effective in populating the lung (BAC) with AFC than is the local route (figure 9). Subsequent studies have confirmed this suggestion (132). It appears that a mechanism exists for the translation of intravascular antigen into intra-alveolar cells producing antibody. The physiologic importance of such a mechanism is evident and may be relevant to pulmonary responses to bacteremia or metastasis of neoplasm. The details of the mechanisms involved remain to be elucidated.

These kinds of data show that under appropriate conditions, AFC may be made to appear within the BAC population; however, they do not demonstrate local generation of these cells. In fact, it is not at all clear whether lymphocytes in peripheral lung tissue represent a full complement of precursor cells capable of initiating immune responses, and whether these cells are products of previous antigenic experience. Nor is it clear whether bronchoalveolar lymphocytes are static residents or are the result of the traffic of cells from the blood into bronchoalveolar spaces. The direct confrontation of the

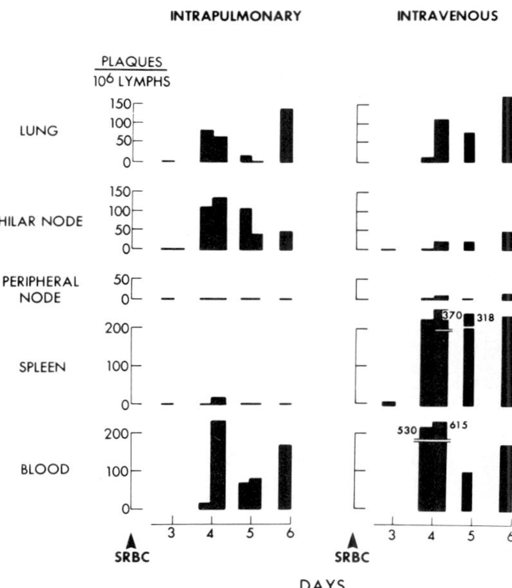

Fig. 8. The appearance, concentration, and distribution of antibody-forming cells (plaques) among various canine lymphoid tissues during the primary immune response to sheep red blood cells (SRBC) administered by the intrapulmonary route (*left*) or the intravenous route (*right*). Each vertical column of bars represents the results of a single experiment on one dog. (Modified from Kaltreider and associates [82].)

issue of full immunocompetence of BAC, namely, the generation of a primary immune response *in vitro,* has not yet been accomplished.

Host-defense function of bronchoalveolar cells. The host-defense system that protects the lower respiratory tract from inhaled organisms is complex, and the role of local humoral antibody in this process is incompletely understood. There is abundant evidence that inhaled bacteria deposited in bronchoalveolar spaces undergo phagocytosis and are killed primarily by alveolar macrophages (45, 54, 58). Humoral antibody, locally synthesized or derived from the circulation, probably functions primarily to enhance phagocytosis through its agglutinative and opsonizing properties. It is clear that specific antibody appears in respiratory secretions during bacterial infections (38, 85, 88), and that these antibodies enhance phagocytosis by alveolar macrophages both *in vivo* and *in vitro* (45, 87, 88). The prominence of IgG antibody in lower respiratory secretions after infection and the presence of receptors for IgG on alveolar macrophages (88) suggest an important role for IgG antibody and the macrophage system interacting to protect against microbial organisms inhaled into the lower respiratory tract. Whether the IgG antibody is locally derived or comes from the serum *in vivo* is an unanswered question. These studies provide a direct demonstration of the cooperation of humoral antibody with mononuclear phagocytes derived from the lower respiratory tract in the defense against bacterial infection.

Hilar Lymph Nodes

The hilar lymph node complex (HLN) includes carinal, tracheobronchial, and paratracheal lymph nodes (29, 30). Anatomically, it is well-organized lymphatic tissue possessing lymphoid follicles, germinal centers, perifollicular regions, a limiting capsule, and afferent and efferent lymphatic channels. The HLN and mesenteric lymph nodes contain greater concentrations of IgA- and IgE-producing cells than do other lymph nodes (62, 71), probably because of their proximity to mucosal surfaces. In other respects, the HLN appear to be identical to lymph nodes elsewhere in the body (43). The HLN receive lymphatic drainage from the entire respiratory tract (29–31). Under normal physiologic conditions, these lymph nodes accumulate some particulate substances (e.g., carbon particles) inhaled into the lower respiratory tract (31, 34). In the presence of inflammation,

the transport of materials to the HLN is greatly enhanced (45, 54). The exact mechanism by which particles transit from bronchoalveolar spaces into interstitial lymphatics and the factors governing this process are not entirely clear. Although controversy exists as to whether particles exit bronchoalveolar spaces within phagocytes or as naked particles, the weight of evidence favors the concept that particulates are engulfed by mononuclear phagocytes after penetration into the interstitium and thereafter traverse lymphatic channels to the HLN (31, 53). The efficiency with which this process occurs under certain circumstances has led some to postulate specialized transport mechanisms located at the bronchoalveolar junction (30, 34, 46).

Hilar lymph node enlargement and involvement is a prominent feature of such common disease conditions as primary tuberculosis or histoplasmosis, sarcoidosis and carcinoma of the lung. Inhaled pathogens, neoplastic cells, or other antigenic materials drain via lymphatic channels. Some material is trapped along the course of lymphatics by small aggregates of lymphatic tissue and give rise to interstitial granulomas. The remainder reaches the HLN, where trapping occurs and immune responses may result. Thus, it appears that the hilar lymph node complex serves as the regional lymph node for the lung in much the same manner as the axillary and inguinal nodes subserve the extremities.

While much information is available regarding the clearance of particles from bronchoalveolar spaces (31, 45–48), little is known about the participation of the HLN in immune responses to antigenic stimulation of the pulmonary parenchyma. In the mouse (44) and the dog (82), immunization of the lower respiratory tract with soluble or particulate antigens results in the evolution of typical primary and secondary antibody-mediated immune responses in the hilar lymph nodes. After instillation of a wide range of inflammation-provoking doses of an organic particulate (radiolabeled sheep red blood cells) into bronchoalveolar spaces of dogs, tissue-bound radioactivity and AFC appear in the hilar lymph nodes within 4 days (55, 56, 131). In addition, serum antibody and antibody-forming cells appear in the circulating blood. These data demonstrate that under appropriate experimental conditions, local deposition of antigen in the lower respiratory tract results in the accumulation of both antigen and antibody-forming cells in the hilar lymph nodes and that both the antibody and the cells appear in the systemic circulation (82). The latter point indicates that the immune response does not, strictly speaking, remain localized to the respiratory tract after local immunization. Thus, inflammatory doses of organic particulates in bronchoalveolar spaces lead consistently to the appearance of antibody-forming cells in the hilar lymph node (figure 9). The same phenomenon may well occur after infection with viable bacteria.

The role of the HLN in the integrated humoral defense of the lung is not entirely clear. If antigenic material bypasses mucosal and bronchoalveolar defenses, it gains access to lymphatics and initiates immune responses in the regional lymph nodes (HLN). The HLN then generate circulating antibody and AFC (figures 8 and 9), either or both of which might re-enter the respiratory tract as secretory antibody or as antibody-producing cells in the submucosa or lamina propria, or among BAC. This formulation provides one possible mechanism for the appearance of AFC in canine bronchoalveolar spaces after either intrapulmonary or intravenous immunization. In fact, the relationship between the AFC in the hilar nodes and those in other lymphoid populations associated with the lung requires clarification.

Cell-mediated Immune Functions of Pulmonary Lymphoid Tissue

In comparison to humoral immunity, relatively little information is available regarding the expression of cell-mediated immunity (CMI) in the lung. Studies of humoral immunity are performed on respiratory secretions that are relatively easily obtained. Exquisitely sensitive assay procedures are available to quantify antibody activity. By contrast, investigation of CMI requires large numbers of lymphoid cells that are technically difficult or impossible to obtain from the respiratory tract. The available *in vitro* assays are cumbersome, insensitive, and only semiquantitative. Hence, whereas cellular immunity in systemic lymphoid tissue (spleen and lymph nodes) is currently the subject of intensive investigation, little of this effort has been successfully directed toward the lung. The available information has been reviewed recently (19, 48, 133).

Cell-mediated Immune Mechanisms

As detailed in a previous section, specifically sensitized T cells are responsible for cell-mediated immunity. Biologically, cell-mediated reactions include delayed-type hypersensitivity (DTH), resistance to intracellular parasites and viruses, rejection of allografts and neoplastic cells (immune surveillance), graft versus host reactions, and the generation of certain granulomas (134). In the lung, CMI is a major defense mechanism against intracellular parasites and viruses.

The degree to which these diverse biologic functions are interdependent is not clear. For example, the question of whether the DTH cutaneous reaction to tuberculoprotein is dissociable from "resistance" to infection with tubercle bacilli is controversial. The opposing arguments have been presented recently (26–28). Perhaps the diverse reactions characteristic of CMI can be understood in light of the recognition that multiple subsets of antigen-reactive T cells exist, each of which probably subserves a distinct cell-mediated function. After antigenic stimulation, any or all of these subsets may be activated simultaneously, resulting in a multiplicity of biologic phenomena (figure 1).

The mechanisms responsible for cell-mediated biologic reactions may be classified into two general categories: lymphokine-mediated reactions, and cell-mediated cytotoxicity. The present state of knowledge suggests that lymphokine-mediated immunity is the major mechanism by which cell-mediated resistance is manifested in the lung (figure 10). The important role of sensitized T cells in the resistance to intracellular parasites (*M. tuberculosis*, *Listeria monocytogenes*) is on firm experimental ground (18). Cytotoxic T cells can destroy neoplastic

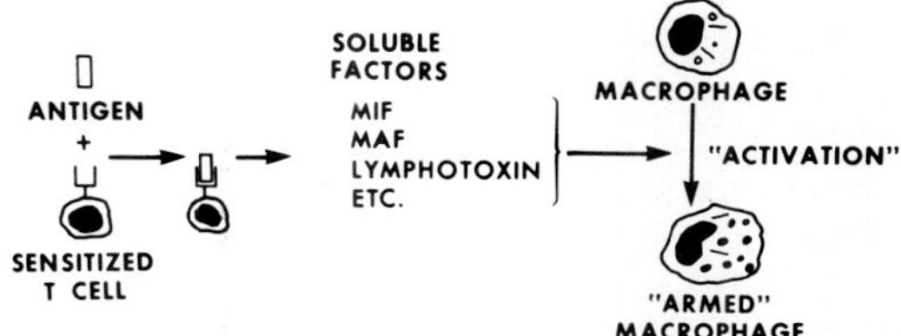

Fig. 10. Diagrammatic representation of the immunologic "activation" of macrophages by various possible soluble factors released by sensitized lymphocytes after interaction with specific antigen (□). The process of activation is immunologically specific. The "armed" macrophage possesses enhanced phagocytic and bactericidal capacity against a wide variety of organisms, and hence functions nonspecifically. MIF = migration inhibition factor; MAF = macrophage activation factor.

cells or cells harboring viruses (20) and in theory, could play an important role in defense against these agents. To date, however, there has been no experimental demonstration of the presence of cytotoxic T cells in any lymphoid tissue associated with the respiratory tract.

Cell-mediated Immunity in the Upper Respiratory Tract

The presence of T cells has been demonstrated directly in nasopharyngeal tonsils (37) and in mucosal lymphoid nodules of large- and medium-sized bronchi (122). The fact that specific secretory IgA antibody is generated locally at mucosal surfaces strongly implies that helper T cells are present or readily available to perform this function (figure 3). There is indirect evidence that sensitized T cells participate in resistance against influenza (135); however, cell-mediated effector mechanisms themselves have not been demonstrated experimentally to occur in the upper respiratory tract. There is no a priori reason to believe that CMI is not occurring in upper airways; however, the technical difficulties of sampling submucosal lymphoid cells render the task of its demonstration difficult.

Cell-mediated Immunity in the Lower Respiratory Tract

In contrast to studies of humoral immunity, most of which have focused on secretory antibody arising from mucosal surfaces of the upper respiratory tract, investigations of the CMI have been performed primarily in the pulmonary parenchyma or have used bronchoalveolar cells obtained by bronchopulmonary lavage.

Production of migration inhibition factor by bronchoalveolar cells. Galindo and Myrvik (136) showed that tubercle bacilli administered to rabbits intravenously in complete Freund's adjuvant resulted in a lymphocytic alveolar exudate that, when cultured *in vitro* in the presence of purified protein derivative, produced MIF. Waldman and Henney (137) demonstrated an apparent dissociation of local and systemic production of MIF. In these experiments, guinea pigs were immunized either locally (intranasal) or systemically (subcutaneous) with a purified protein-hapten antigen. Bronchoalveolar cells obtained by lavage or spleen cells were then assayed for their ability to produce MIF *in vitro* in the presence of the immunizing antigen. The results showed that after intranasal immunization, MIF-producing cells were present among BAC, but not in the spleen. After subcutaneous immunization, MIF-producing cells appeared in the spleen, but not among BAC. The studies supported the notion that CMI responses could be elicited locally in the lower respiratory tract and gave rise to the suggestion that a local system for CMI exists. The observed distribution of MIF-producing cells could equally well have resulted from the organ distribution of the administered antigen; hence, the result might not necessarily indicate an independent CMI system localized to the lung. The demonstration that intravenous administration of tubercle bacilli results in the appearance of MIF-producing cells in rabbit lungs supports the concept that systemic immunization can induce CMI in the respiratory tract if antigen is presented to the lung appropriately (136).

The studies of Waldman and Henney (137) have been extended to include a number of protein (138), viral (139, 140), and bacterial (139, 141–143) antigens in a variety of animal species. Waldman and associates (140) showed that the apparent distinct separation between respiratory and systemic CMI could be minimized or abolished with increasing immunizing doses via either route (140). Bacterial infections or antigenic extracts administered to the lower respiratory tract led to MIF production in both local and splenic lymphocytes (141, 142). Nash and Holle (138) demonstrated that multiple low doses or a single large dose of antigen delivered to the lungs of guinea pigs resulted in MIF-producing cells systemically as well as locally, and that secondary responses appeared in all lymphoid tissues after boosting by either route. Hence, whether a strict separation or compartmentalization of local CMI is manifested clearly depends on the dose and nature of the antigen used.

These studies demonstrate that specifically sensitized cells capable of MIF production do accumulate in bronchoalveolar spaces after the appropriate modes of immunization. Whether these cells arise locally from precursor immunocytes or whether they are recruited into pulmonary parenchyma from the circulating pool of antigen-reactive lymphocytes (7) is an open question. In systemically immunized guinea pigs lacking pulmonary MIF-producing cells, these can be recruited into bronchoalveolar air spaces by local irritation of the lung with an unrelated antigen (138). In the dog, T cells are normally absent from BAC, but may be recruited into the lung by antigenic stimulation (78). Thus, the potential exists for the derivation of MIF-producing cells from the circulation.

The interpretation of the studies described in this section rests partly on the assumption that the production of MIF constitutes a valid measure of T cell function. Until recently, this assumption was generally accepted; however, it is now apparent that both B and T cells may produce soluble mediators, including MIF, under appropriate conditions (144, 145). Hence, MIF production *in vitro* must be cautiously equated with cell-mediated events *in vivo*. Nevertheless, specifically sensitized lymphoid cells clearly do appear in the lower respiratory tract, and the extent to which this occurs is influenced by the immunization route and dose of antigen used.

Resistance to infection by intracellular parasites. With the above studies in mind, the question arises as to how the local presence of the sensitized T cells is translated into a mechanism for defense of the host. Investigations from several laboratories suggest that a major effector of CMI *in vivo* is the accumulation and immunologic activation of alveolar macrophages (figure 10) (18, 19, 146–150).

Alveolar macrophages normally constitute a major phagocytic and bactericidal defense mechanism against microbial organisms inhaled into bronchoalveolar spaces (54, 58). While nonpathogenic organisms are readily engulfed and killed by alveolar macrophages, pathogenic intracellular parasites, such as *L. monocytogenes, M. tuberculosis,* and *Histoplasma capsulatum,* are normally resistant to killing by alveolar macrophages. By contrast, activated macrophages, cells displaying enhanced concentrations of hydrolytic enzymes, phagocytosis, and microbicidal activity, show an augmented ability to engulf and destroy these pathogenic organisms (53, 146, 149, 150).

The proposed mechanism for the immunologic activation of alveolar macrophages as an effector mechanism for CMI is as follows. Sensitization of T cells by antigen (organism) results in an immunologically specific wave of cellular proliferation and differentiation. The enlarged population of sensitized T cells accumulates in the vicinity of the organism, and on their interaction, lymphokines, including MIF and macrophage activating factor, are elaborated and released into the microenvironment. Macrophages accumulate, become enhanced in their bactericidal activity ("activated"), and eradicate

the organism (figure 10). The process of interaction of antigen and T lymphocyte is immunologically specific, that is, only the original sensitizing antigen can stimulate the enlarged T cell population to secrete lymphokines; however, once macrophages are activated by MAF, their action is nonspecific, that is, they display enhanced phagocytosis against a wide variety of microorganisms, not just the original sensitizing organism (149, 150).

Direct experimental evidence in support of this general scheme of a lymphokine-mediated effector mechanism of CMI in defense of the intact host has been presented (18, 19, 149). The lung cells of mice intravenously immunized with the cell walls of BCG produced marked concentrations of MIF. The MIF production showed an excellent correlation with acquired resistance of the immunized animal to a subsequent airborne infection with *M. tuberculosis* strain H37Rv. (151). In a series of elegant studies, Mackaness and North and co-workers (18, 19, 149, 152, 153) showed that in mice, the acquired resistance to *L. monocytogenes,* an intracellular parasite similar to *M. tuberculosis,* was largely mediated by sensitized or immunologically committed T cells and expressed by mononuclear phagocytes that were activated or "armed" by soluble mediator substances released by the lymphocytes. The development of resistance paralelled the acquisition of the delayed type hypersensitivity cutaneous reaction. Both resistance and hypersensitivity to listeria could be adoptively transferred with lymphoid cells.

Truitt and Mackaness (154) extended the general nature of this phenomenon specifically to the respiratory tract. Mice systemically immunized to listeria were given an aerogenic reinfection of this organism. In contrast to the normal control animals, which uniformly succumbed to the infection, the previously sensitized animals demonstrated a high degree of resistance to airborne infection. They observed a massive influx of mononuclear phagocytes and lymphocytes occurring at 24 to 48 hours, consistent with the kinetics of the delayed type hypersensitivity reaction. The organisms in the lung were rapidly phagocytized and killed by the influx of mononuclear phagocytes. The results of their studies suggested that the resident alveolar macrophage population in the lung was considerably less efficient than the influx of mononuclear phagocytes in the effector function of enhanced phagocytosis and killing. It is not clear from these studies whether the apparent lack of efficiency of the alveolar macrophages was due to an intrinsic functional difference between these cells and circulating mononuclear phagocytes, or whether specifically sensitized T cells lacked ready access to the alveolar compartment. Thus, these studies demonstrate the expression of delayed hypersensitivity reactions occurring in the lung, and appear to point to a functional difference between alveolar and systemic macrophages in the efferent limb of the cell-mediated immune response. Further studies to characterize these differences are needed.

A recent study demonstrates that *L. monocytogenes* infection of rabbits produced activation of alveolar macrophages *in vivo*. In addition, lymphoid cells obtained from the lower respiratory tract and regional lymph nodes of such animals produced soluble mediators *in vitro* that activated normal rabbit macrophages (148). Although the soluble mediator was not specifically identified, this evidence obtained *in vitro* supports the *in vivo* studies discussed previously.

Animal Models of Delayed Hypersensitivity Lung Disease

An inflammatory pneumonitis with mononuclear infiltrates histologically resembling those in the delayed hypersensitivity cutaneous reaction have been produced experimentally in a number of animal species (155–157). The models have generally involved an initial systemic sensitization (intramuscular or intravenous) with antigenic materials known to favor the development of CMI. When the sensitized animal is given a local, respiratory challenge with the same antigen, an intense inflammatory reaction consisting of intra-alveolar and interstitial round cell (lymphocytes and macrophages) infiltrate evolves during a period of 1 to 3 days. Miyamoto and associates (158) have performed experiments in which spleen cells from tuberculin-positive guinea pigs were transferred into tuberculin-negative recipients that were then challenged with aerosolized purified protein derivative. A pneumonitis resembling delayed-type hypersensitivity in both kinetics of evolution and morphologic features resulted, suggesting the successful passive transfer of sensitized T cells to the recipient, and that the transferred sensitized cells were responsible for the pulmonary infiltrate after aerosol challenge.

The experimentally produced pulmonary lesions histologically resemble the inflammatory response observed in the delayed-type hypersensitivity cutaneous reaction. The morphologic picture also resembles that seen in hypersensitivity pneumonitis or allergic alveolitis as expressed in humans and has led many investigators to regard CMI as the immunopathogenesis of this group of disorders.

Conclusion

The current state of knowledge with respect to the expression of immune phenomena in the respiratory tract has been reviewed. Existing information is sparse and incomplete. Areas for future investigation have been identified and some general questions have been raised. More detailed information will be required to define the mechanisms of expression of humoral and cell-mediated immunity in the lung. Such information is essential to the understanding of the role of immune reactions in the defense of the host and in the immunopathogenesis of pulmonary disease.

Acknowledgment

The writer wishes to thank Mrs. Veronica Gressani for her excellent and patient secretarial assistance.

References

1. Waksman, B. H.: Presidential Address: Immunology as a basic and applied science, J Immunol, 1971, *107*, 617.
2. Eisen, H. N.: Immunology: An introduction to molecular and cellular principles of the immune responses, in *Microbiology*, B. D. Davis, R. Dulbecco, H. N. Eisen, H. S. Ginsberg, and W. B. Wood, Jr., ed., Harper and Row Publishers, Inc., New York, 1974, pp. 352–624.
3. Roitt, I. M.: Essential Immunology, Blackwell Scientific Publications, Oxford, 1971.
4. Bellanti, J. A.: Immunology, W. B. Saunders Co., Philadelphia, 1971.
5. Bigley, N. J.: Immunologic Fundamentals, Year Book Medical Publishers, Inc., Chicago, 1975.
6. Review of Basic and Clinical Immunology, H. H. Fudenberg, J. L. Caldwell, D. P. Stites, and J. V. Wells, ed., Lange Medical Publications, Los Altos, Calif., in press.
7. Gowans, J. L., and Knight, E. J.: The route of recirculation of lymphocytes in the rat, Proc R Soc Lond [Biol], 1964, *159*, 257.
8. Rowlands, D. T., Jr., and Daniele, R. P.: Surface receptors in the immune response, N Engl J Med, 1975, *293*, 26.
9. Nossal, G. J. V., and Ada, G. L.: Organ distribution of antigens, in *Antigens, Lymphoid Cells, and the Immune Response*, Academic Press, New York, pp. 38–59.
10. Campbell, D. H., and Garvey, J. S.: Nature of

retained antigen and its role in immune mechanisms, Adv Immunol, 1963, *3*, 261.

11. Unanue, E. R.: The regulatory role of macrophages in antigenic stimulation, Adv Immunol, 1972, *15*, 95.

12. Claman, H. N., and Mosier, D. E.: Cell-cell interaction in antibody production, Prog Allergy, 1972, *16*, 40.

13. Miller, J. F. A. P., and Mitchell, G. F.: Thymus and antigen-reactive cells, Transplant Rev, 1969, *1*, 3.

14. Cluff, L. E., and Johnson, J. E., III: Clinical Concepts of Infectious Diseases, The Williams and Wilkins Co., Baltimore, 1972.

15. Jerne, N. K., Nordin, A. A., and Henry, C.: The agar plaque technique for recognizing antibody-producing cells, in *Cell-Bound Antibodies*, B. Amos and H. Koprowski, ed., The Wistar Institute Press, Philadelphia, Pa., 1963, pp. 109–125.

16. Kantor, F. S.: Infection, anergy and cell-mediated immunity, N Engl J Med, 1975, *292*, 629.

17. Bloom, B. R., and Glade, P. R.: In Vitro Methods in Cell-mediated Immunity, Academic Press, New York, 1971.

18. Mackaness, G. B.: Resistance to intra-cellular infection, J Infect Dis, 1971, *123*, 439.

19. Mackaness, G. B.: The J. Burns Amberson lecture. The induction and expression of cell-mediated hypersensitivity in the lung, Am Rev Respir Dis, 1971, *104*, 813.

20. Cerottini, J. C., and Brunner, K. T.: Cell-mediated cytotoxicity, allograft rejection and tumor immunity, Adv Immunol, 1974, *18*, 67.

21. Schwartz, R. S.: Another look at immunologic surveillance, N Engl J Med, 1975, *293*, 181.

22. McCombs, R. P.: Diseases due to immunologic reactions in the lungs (Parts 1 & 2), N Engl J Med, 1972, *286*, 1186 and 1245.

23. Kaltreider, H. B.: Hypersensitivity pneumonitis: Immunologically mediated lung disease resulting from the inhalation of organic antigens, J Occup Med, 1973, *15*, 949.

24. Pepys, J.: Immunologic approaches in pulmonary disease caused by inhaled materials, Ann N Y Acad Sci, 1974, *221*, 27.

25. Gell, P. G. H., and Coombs, R. R. A.: Clinical Aspects of Immunology, Blackwell Scientific Publications, Oxford, 1968.

26. Youmans, G. P.: Relation between delayed hypersensitivity and immunity in tuberculosis, Am Rev Respir Dis, 1975, *111*, 109.

27. Lefford, M. J.: Delayed hypersensitivity and immunity in tuberculosis, Am Rev Respir Dis, 1975, *111*, 243.

28. Salvin, S. B., and Neta, R.: A possible relationship between delayed hypersensitivity and cell-mediated immunity, Am Rev Respir Dis, 1975, *111*, 373.

29. Nagaishi, C.: Functional Anatomy and Histology of the Lung, University Park Press, Baltimore, 1972, pp. 102–180.

30. von Hayek, H.: The Human Lung, Hafner Publishing Co., Inc., New York, 1960, pp. 298–314.

31. Morrow, P. E.: Lymphatic drainage of the lung in dust clearance, Ann N Y Acad Sci, 1971, *200*, 46.

32. Bienenstock, J., Johnston, N., and Perey, D. Y. E.: Bronchial lymphoid tissue. I. Morphologic characteristics, Lab Invest, 1973, *28*, 686.

33. Chamberlain, D. W., Nopajaroonsri, C., and Simon, G. T.: Ultrastructure of the pulmonary lymphoid tissue, Am Rev Respir Dis, 1973, *108*, 621.

34. Macklin, C. C.: Pulmonary sumps, dust accumulations, alveolar fluid and lymph vessels, Acta Anat (Basel), 1954, *23*, 1.

35. Yoffey, J. M., and Courtise, F. C.: Lymphatics, Lymph, and Lymphomyeloid Complex, Academic Press, New York, 1970.

36. Lauweryns, J. M.: The juxta-alveolar lymphatics in the human adult lung, Am Rev Respir Dis, 1970, *102*, 877.

37. Watanabe, T., Yoshizaki, K., Yagura, T., and Yamamura, Y.: In vitro antibody formation by human tonsil lymphocytes, J Immunol, 1974, *113*, 608.

38. Hand, W. C., and Cantey, J. R.: Antibacterial mechanisms of the lower respiratory tract. I. Immunoglobulin synthesis and secretion, J Clin Invest, 1974, *53*, 354.

39. Bienenstock, J., Johnston, N., and Perey, D. Y. E.: Bronchial lymphoid tissue. II. Functional characteristics, Lab Invest, 1973, *28*, 693.

40. Myrvik, Q. N., Leake, E. S., and Fariss, B.: Studies on pulmonary alveolar macrophages from the normal rabbit: A technique to procure them in a high state of purity, J Immunol, 1961, *86*, 128.

41. Finley, T. N., Swenson, E. W., Curran, W. S., Huber, G. L., and Ladman, A. J.: Bronchopulmonary lavage in normal subjects and patients with obstructive lung disease, Ann Intern Med, 1967, *66*, 651.

42. Reynolds, H. Y., and Newball, H. H.: Analysis of proteins and respiratory cells obtained from human lungs by bronchial lavage, J Lab Clin Med, 1974, *84*, 559.

43 Kaltreider, H. B., Turner, F. N., and Salmon, S. E.: A canine model for comparative study of respiratory and systemic immunologic reactions, Am Rev Respir Dis, 1975, *111*, 257.

44. Nash, D. R.: Direct and indirect plaque forming cells in extrapulmonary lymphoid tissue following local vs. systemic injection of soluble antigen, Cell Immunol, 1973, *9*, 234.

45. Green, G. M.: Pulmonary clearance of infectious agents, Annu Rev Med, 1968, *19*, 315.

46. Green, G. M.: Alveolobronchiolar transport mechanisms, Arch Intern Med, 1973, *131*, 109.

47. Lourenco, R. V.: Inhaled aerosol symposium,

Arch Intern Med, 1973, *131*, 21.

48. Cohen, A. B., and Gold, W. M.: Defense mechanisms of the lungs, Annu Rev Physiol, 1975, *37*, 325.

49. Rossen, R. D., and Butler, W. T.: Immunologic responses to infection at mucosal surfaces, in *Viral and Mycoplasmal Infections of the Respiratory Tract*, V. Knight, ed., Lea & Febiger, Philadelphia, Pa., 1973, pp. 23–52.

50. Owen, R. L., and Jones, A. L.: Epithelial cell specialization within Peyer's patches: An ultrastructural study of human intestinal lymphoid follicles, Gastroenterology, 1974, *66*, 189.

51. Owen, R. L., and Jones A. L.: Specialized lymphoid follicle epithelial cells in the human and non-human primate: A possible antigen uptake site, in *Scanning Electron Microscopy*, Part III, Orn Johari, ed., ITT Research Institute, Chicago, Ill., 1974, pp. 697–704.

52. Richardson, J. B., Hogg, J. C., Bouchard, T., and Hall, D. L.: Localization of antigen in experimental bronchoconstriction in guinea pigs, J Allergy Clin Immunol, 1973, *52*, 172.

53. Bowden, D. H.: The alveolar macrophage, Curr Top Pathol, 1971, *55*, 1.

54. Green, G. M.: The J. Burns Amberson Lecture. In defense of the lung, Am Rev Respir Dis, 1970, *102*, 691.

55. Kaltreider, H. B., Adam, E., and Turner, F. N.: Bronchoalveolar clearance of an organic particulate antigen after intrapulmonary immunization (abstract), Clin Res, 1975, *23*, 348A.

56. Kaltreider, H. B., Turner, F. N., Adam, E., and Chan, M. K.: Bronchoalveolar clearance and immunologic reaction to an organic particulate antigen instilled into alveolar spaces of dog lungs, Chest, in press.

57. vanFurth, R.: Mononuclear Phagocytes, F. A. Davis Co., Philadelphia, Pa., 1970.

58. Green, G. M., and Kass, E. H.: The role of the alveolar macrophage in the clearance of bacteria from the lung, J Exp Med, 1964, *119*, 167.

59. Cohn, Z. A.: The structure and function of monocytes and macrophages, Adv Immunol, 1968, *9*, 163.

60. Tomasi, T. B., Jr.: Secretory immunoglobulins, N Engl J Med, 1972, *287*, 500.

61. Hauptman, S. P., and Tomasi, T. B., Jr.: The secretory immune system, in *Review of Basic and Clinical Immunology*, H. H. Fudenberg, J. L. Caldwell, D. P. Stites, and J. V. Wells, ed., Lang Medical Publications, Los Altos, Calif., in press.

62. Tomasi, T. B., Jr., and Grey, H. M.: Structure and function of immunoglobulin A, Prog Allergy, 1972, *16*, 81.

63. Tomasi, T. B., Jr., and Bienenstock, J.: Secretory immunoglobulins, Adv Immunol, 1969, *9*, 1.

64. Masson, P. L., and Heremans, J. F.: Sputum proteins, in *Sputum: Fundamentals and Clinical Pathology*, J. J. Dulfano, ed., Charles C Thomas, Springfield, Ill., 1973, pp. 412–475.

65. Mastecky, J., and Lawton, A. R.: The immunoglobulin A system, in *Advances in Experimental Medicine and Biology*, Plenum Press, New York, 1974.

66. Chanock, R. M.: The respiratory system, in *The Secretory Immunologic System*, D. H. Dayton, Jr., P. A. Small, Jr., R. M. Chanock, H. E. Kaufman, and T. B. Tomasi, Jr., ed., U. S. Government Printing Office, Washington, D. C., 1970, pp. 83–244.

67. Kaltreider, H. B., and Chan, M. K. L.: The class-specific immunoglobulin composition of fluids obtained from various levels of the canine respiratory tract, J Immunol, in press.

68. Halpern, M. S., and Koshland, M. E.: Novel subunit in secretory IgA, Nature, 1970, *228*, 1276.

69. Newcomb, R. W., and Ishizaka, K.: Physicochemical and antigenic studies on human γE in respiratory fluid, J Immunol, 1970, *105*, 85.

70. Martinez-Tello, F. J., Braun, D. G., and Blanc, W. A.: Immunoglobulin production in bronchial mucosa and bronchial lymph nodes, particularly in cystic fibrosis of the pancreas, J Immunol, 1968, *101*, 989.

71. Tada, T., and Ishizaka, K.: Distribution of IgE-forming cells in lymphoid tissues of the human and monkey, J Immunol, 1970, *104*, 377.

72. Tourville, D. R., Adler, R. H., Bienenstock, J., and Tomasi, T. B.: The human secretory immunoglobulin system: Immunohistological localization of γA, secretory "piece" and lactoferrin in normal human tissues, J Exp Med, 1969, *129*, 411.

73. Rossen, R. D., Morgan, C., Hsu, K. C., Butler, W. T., and Rose, H. M.: Localization of 11S external secretory IgA by immunofluorescence in tissues lining the oral and respiratory passages in man, J Immunol, 1968, *100*, 706.

74. Vaerman, J. P., and Heremans, J. F.: Origin and molecular size of immunoglobulin-A in the mesenteric lymph of the dog, Immunology, 1970, *18*, 27.

75. Bonomo, L., and D'Addabbo, A.: ^{131}I-albumin turnover and loss of protein into the sputum in chronic bronchitis, Clin Chim Acta, 1964, *10*, 214.

76. Butler, W. T., Rossen, R. D., and Waldmann, T. A.: The mechanism of appearance of immunoglobulin A in nasal secretions in man, J Clin Invest, 1967, *46*, 1883.

77. Fernald, G. W., Clyde, W. A., Jr., and Bienenstock, J.: Immunoglobulin-containing cells in lungs of hamsters infected with *Mycoplasma pneumoniae*, J Immunol, 1972, *108*, 1400.

78. Kaltreider, H. B., and Salmon, S. E.: Immunology of the lower respiratory tract: Functional

properties of bronchoalveolar lymphocytes obtained from the normal canine lung, J Clin Invest, 1973, *52*, 2211.

79. Platts-Mills, T. A. E., and Ishizaka, K.: IgG and IgA diphtheria antitoxin responses from human tonsil lymphocytes, J Immunol, 1975, *114*, 1058.

80. Falk, G. H., Okinaka, A. J., and Siskind, G. W.: Immunoglobulins in the bronchial washings of patients with chronic obstructive pulmonary disease, Am Rev Respir Dis, 1972, *105*, 14.

81. Ishizaka, K., and Newcomb, R. W.: Presence of γE in nasal washings and sputum from asthmatic patients, J Allergy, 1970, *46*, 197.

82. Kaltreider, H. B., Kyselka, L., and Salmon, S. E.: Immunology of the lower respiratory tract. II. The plaque-forming response of canine lymphoid tissues to sheep erythrocytes after intrapulmonary or intravenous immunization, J Clin Invest, 1974, *54*, 263.

83. Ford, R. J., Jr., and Kuhn, C.: Immunologic competence of alveolar cells. I. The plaque-forming response to particulate and soluble antigens, Am Rev Respir Dis, 1973, *107*, 763.

84. Ford, R. J., Jr., and Kuhn, C.: Immunologic competence of alveolar cells. II. Modification of the plaque-forming response by inhibitors, tolerance, and chronic stimulation, Am Rev Respir Dis, 1973, *107*, 772.

85. Reynolds, H. Y., Kazmierowski, J. A., and Newball, H. H.: Specificity of opsonic antibodies to enhance phagocytosis of *Pseudomonas aeruginosa* by human alveolar macrophages, J Clin Invest, 1975, *56*, 376.

86. Reynolds, H. Y., and Thompson, R. E.: Pulmonary host defenses. I. Analysis of protein and lipids in bronchial secretions and antibody responses after vaccination with *Pseudomonas aeruginosa*, J Immunol, 1973, *111*, 358.

87. Reynolds, H. Y., and Thompson, R. E.: Pulmonary host defenses. II. Interaction of respiratory antibodies with *Pseudomonas aeruginosa* and alveolar macrophages, J Immunol, 1973, *111*, 369.

88. Reynolds, H. Y., Atkinson, J. P., Newball, H. H., and Frank, M. M.: Receptors for immunoglobulin and complement on human alveolar macrophages, J Immunol, 1975, *114*, 1813.

89. Brandtzaeg, P., Fjellanger, I., and Gjeruldsen, S. T.: Human secretory immunoglobulins. I. Salivary secretions from individuals with normal or low levels of serum immunoglobulins, Scand J Haematol, 1970, *12* (Supplement, p. 4).

90. Stobo, J. D., and Tomasi, T. B.: A low molecular weight immunoglobulin antigenically related to 19S IgM, J Clin Invest, 1967, *46*, 1329.

91. Holub, M., and Hauser, R. E.: Lung alveolar histiocytes engaged in antibody production, Immunology, 1969, *17*, 207.

92. Brandtzaeg, P.: Human secretory immunoglobulins. II. Salivary secretions from individuals with selectively excessive or defective synthesis of serum immunoglobulins, Clin Exp Immunol, 1970, *8*, 901.

93. Tomasi, T. B., Tan, E. M., Solomon, A., and Prendergast, R. A.: Characteristics of an immune system common to certain external secretions, J Exp Med, 1965, *121*, 101.

94. Johansson, S. G. O., Bennich, H. H., and Berg, T.: The clinical significance of IgE, in *Progress in Clinical Immunology*, vol. 1, R. S. Schwartz, ed., Grune and Stratton, Inc., New York, 1972, pp. 157–181.

95. Ishizaka, K.: Chemistry and biology of immunoglobulin E, in *Antigens*, vol. 1, M. Sela, ed., Academic Press Inc., New York, 1973, pp. 479–528.

96. Bennich, H., and Johansson, S. G. O.: Structure and function of human immunoglobulin E, Adv Immunol, 1971, *13*, 1.

97. Ishizaka, K.: Function of IgE antibody and regulation of IgE antibody response, in *New Directions in Asthma*, M. Stein, ed., American College of Chest Physicians, Park Ridge, Ill., 1975, pp. 133–148.

98. Austen, K. F., and Orange, R. P.: Bronchial asthma: The possible role of the chemical mediators of immediate hypersensitivity in the pathogenesis of subacute chronic disease, Am Rev Respir Dis, 1975, *112*, 423.

99. Austen, K. F., and Lichtenstein, L. M.: Asthma: Physiology, Immunopharmacology and Treatment, Academic Press, Inc., New York, 1973.

100. Levine, B. B., Stember, R. H., and Fotimo, M.: Ragweed hay fever: Genetic control and linkage to HL-A haplotypes, Science, 1972, *178*, 1201.

101. Donovan, R., Johansson, S. G. O., Bennich, H., and Soothill, J. F.: Immunoglobulins in nasal polyp fluid, Int Arch Allergy, 1970, *37*, 154.

102. Brown, W. R., Newcomb, R. W., and Ishizaka, K.: Proteolytic degradation of exocrine and serum immunoglobulins, J Clin Invest, 1970, *49*, 1374.

103. Medici, T. C., and Bürgi, H.: The role of immunoglobulin A in endogenous bronchial defense mechanisms in chronic bronchitis, Am Rev Respir Dis, 1974, *103*, 784.

104. Walker, W. A., Isslebacker, K. J., and Block, K. J.: Intestinal uptake of macromolecules: Effect of oral immunization, Science, 1972, *177*, 608.

105. Tomasi, T. B., Jr., and Katz, L.: Human antibodies against bovine immunoglobulin M and IgA deficient sera, Clin Exp Immunol, 1971, *9*, 3.

106. Huntley, C. C., Robbins, J. B., Leverly, A. D., and Buckley, R. H.: Characterization of precipitating antibodies to ruminant serum and milk proteins in humans with selective IgA deficiency, N Engl J Med, 1971, *284*, 7.

107. Dolovich, J., Tomasi, T. B., and Abesman, C. E.: Antibodies of nasal and parotid secretions of ragweed-allergic subjects, J Allergy, 1970, *45*, 286.

108. Turk, A., Lichtenstein, L. M., and Norman, P. S.: Nasal secretory antibody to inhalant allergens in allergic and non-allergic patients, Immunology, 1970, *19*, 85.

109. Freter, R.: Parameters affecting the association of vibrios with the intestinal surface in experimental cholera, Infect Immunol, 1972, *6*, 134.

110. Williams, R. C., and Gibbons, R. J.: Inhibition of bacterial adherence by secretory immunoglobulin A: Mechanism of antigen disposal, Science, 1972, *177*, 697.

111. Schwartz, D. P., and Buckley, R. H.: Serum IgE concentrations and skin reactivity to anti-IgE antibody in IgA deficient patients, N Engl J Med, 1971, *284*, 513.

112. Ammann, A. J., and Hong, R.: Selective IgA deficiency: Presentation of 30 cases and a review of the literature, Medicine (Baltimore), 1971, *50*, 223.

113. Rockey, J. H., Hanson, L. A., Heremans, J. F., and Kunkel, H. G.: Beta-2A-aglobulinemia in 2 healthy men, J Lab Clin Med, 1964, *63*, 205.

114. Ogra, P. L., and Karzon, D. T.: Formation and function of poliovirus antibody in different tissues, in *Progress in Medical Virology*, vol. 13, J. L. Melnick, ed., S. Karger, New York, 1971, pp. 156–193.

115. Panusarn, C., Stanley, E. D., Dirda, V., Rubenis, M., and Jackson, G. G.: Prevention of illness from rhinovirus infection by a topical interferon inducer, N Engl J Med, 1974, *291*, 57.

116. Merigan, T. C.: Host defenses against viral disease, N Engl J Med, 1974, *290*, 323.

117. Mostow, S. R.: The control of influenza, Am Rev Respir Dis, 1974, *110*, 542.

118. Craig, S. W., and Cebra, J. J.: Peyer's patches: An enriched source of precursors for IgA-producing immunocytes in the rabbit, J Exp Med, 1971, *134*, 188.

119. Ogra, P. L.: Effect of tonsillectomy and adenoidectomy on nasopharyngeal antibody response to poliovirus, N Engl J Med, 1971, *284*, 59.

120. Ogra, P. L., Kerr-Grant, D., Umana, G., Dzierba, J., and Weintraub, D.: Antibody response in serum and nasopharynx after naturally acquired and vaccine-induced infection with rubella virus, N Engl J Med, 1971, *285*, 1333.

121. Clancy, R., and Bienenstock, J.: The proliferative response of bronchus-associated lymphoid tissue after local and systemic immunization, J Immunol, 1974, *112*, 1997.

122. Rudzik, O., Clancy, R. L., Perey, D. Y. E., Bienenstock, J., and Singal, D. P.: The distribution of a rabbit thymic antigen and membrane immunoglobulins in lymphoid tissue, with special reference to mucosal lymphocytes, J Immunol, 1975, *114*, 1.

123. Rudzik, R., Clancy, R. L., Perey, D. Y. E., Day, R. P., and Bienenstock, J.: Repopulation with IgA-containing cells of bronchial and intestinal lamina propria after transfer of homologous Peyer's patch and bronchial lymphocytes, J Immunol, 1975, *114*, 1599.

124. Bienenstock, J., Clancy, R. L., and Perey, D. Y. E.: Bronchial associated lymphoid tissue: Its relationship to mucosal immunity, in *The Immunologic and Infectious Reactions in the Lung*, C. Kirkpatrick and H. Y. Reynolds. ed., Marcel Dekker, Inc., New York, 1976.

125. Brain, J. D.: Free cells in the lungs: Some aspects of their role, quantitation and regulation, Arch Intern Med, 1970, *126*, 477.

126. Harris, J. O., Swenson, E. W., and Johnson, J. E., III: Human alveolar macrophages: Comparison of phagocytic ability, glucose utilization, and ultrastructure in smokers and nonsmokers, J Clin Invest, 1970, *49*, 2086.

127. Davis, G. S., Landis, J. N., Brody, A. R., Graham, W. G. B., Craighead, J. E., and Green, G. M.: Characteristics of diffuse lung disease reflected by pulmonary lavage (abstract), Am Rev Respir Dis, 1975, *111*, 933.

128. Daniele, R. P., Altose, M. D., and Rowlands, D. T., Jr.: Immunocompetent cells from the lower respiratory tract of normal human lungs, J Clin Invest, 1975, *56*, 986.

129. Waldman, R. H., Jurgensen, P. F., Olsen, G. N., Ganguly, R., and Johnson, J. E., III: Immune responses of the human respiratory tract. I. Immunoglobulin levels and influenza virus vaccine antibody response, J Immunol, 1973, *111*, 38.

130. Kaltreider, H. B.: Initiation of immune responses in the lower respiratory tract with red cell antigen, in *Immunologic and Infectious Reactions in the Lung*, C. H. Kirkpatrick and H. Y. Reynolds, ed., Marcel Dekker, Inc., New York, 1976, pp. 73–100.

131. Kaltreider, H. B., Turner, F., and Chan, M.: Concentrations of antigen and antibody-forming cells in two pulmonary lymphoid tissues after intrapulmonary or i.v. immunization (abstract), Clin Res, 1975, *23*, 348A.

132. Kaltreider, H. B., and Turner, F. N.: The appearance of antibody-forming cells in two populations of lymphocytes associated with the lower respiratory tract of the dog after intrapulmonary or intravenous immunization with sheep erythrocytes, Am Rev Respir Dis, in press.

133. Henney, C. S.: Cell-mediated immune reaction in the lung, in *Immunologic and Infectious Reactions in the Lung*, C. H. Kirkpatrick and H. Y. Reynolds, ed., Marcel Dekker, Inc., New York, 1976, pp. 59–71.

134. Boros, D. L., Pelley, R. P., and Warren, K. S.:

Spontaneous modulation of granulomatous hypersensitivity in schistosomiasis mansoni, J Immunol, 1975, *114*, 1437.

135. Cate, T. R.: Interferons, in *Viral and Mycoplasmal Infections of the Respiratory Tract*, V. Knight, ed., Lea and Febiger, Philadelphia, 1973, pp. 53–64.

136. Galindo, B., and Myrvik, Q. N.: Migratory response of granulomatous alveolar cells from BCG-sensitized rabbits, J Immunol, 1970, *105*, 227.

137. Waldman, R. H., and Henney, C. S.: Cell-mediated immunity and antibody response in the respiratory tract after local and systemic immunization, J Exp Med, 1971, *134*, 482.

138. Nash, D. R., and Holle, B.: Local and systemic cellular immune responses in guinea pigs given antigen parenterally or directly into the lower respiratory tract, Clin Exp Immunol, 1973, *13*, 573.

139. Jurgensen, P. F., Olsen, G. N., Johnson, J. E., III, Swenson, E. W., Ayoub, E. M., Henney, C. S., and Waldman, R. H.: Immune response of the human respiratory tract. II. Cell-mediated immunity in the lower respiratory tract to tuberculin, mumps, and influenza viruses, J Infect Dis, 1973, *128*, 730.

140. Waldman, R. H., Spencer, C. S., and Johnson, J. E., III: Respiratory and systemic cellular and humoral immune responses to influenza virus vaccine administered parenterally or by nose drops, Cell Immunol, 1972, *3*, 294.

141. Reynolds, H. Y., Thompson, R. E., and Devlin, H. B.: Development of cellular and humoral immunity in the respiratory tract of rabbits to *Pseudomonas* lipopolysaccharide, J Clin Invest, 1974, *53*, 1351.

142. Cantey, J. R., and Hand, W. L.: Cell-mediated immunity after bacterial infection of the lower respiratory tract, J Clin Invest, 1974, *54*, 1125.

143. Spencer, J. C., Waldman, R. H., and Johnson, J. E., III: Local and systemic cell-mediated immunity after immunization of guinea pigs with live or killed M. tuberculosis by various routes, J Immunol, 1974, *112*, 1322.

144. Rocklin, R. E., MacDermott, R. P., Chess, L., Schlossman, S. F., and David, J. R.: Studies on mediator production by highly purified human T and B lymphocytes, J Exp Med, 1974, *140*, 1303.

145. Wahl, S. M., Iverson, G. M., and Oppenheim, J. J.: Induction of guinea pig B-cell lymphokine synthesis by mitogenic and non-mitogenic signals to Fc, Ig, and C3 receptors, J Exp Med, 1974, *140*, 1631.

146. Myrvik, Q. N.: Function of the alveolar macrophage in immunity, J Reticuloendothel Soc, 1972, *11*, 459.

147. Myrvik, Q. N.: The role of the alveolar macrophage, J Occup Med, 1973, *15*, 190.

148. Johnson, J. D., Hand, W. L., King, N. L., and Hughes, C. G.: Activation of alveolar macrophages after lower respiratory tract infection, J Immunol, 1975, *115*, 80.

149. North, R. J.: Cell-mediated immunity and the response to infection, in *Mechanisms of Cell-Mediated Immunity*, R. T. McCluskey and S. Cohen, ed., John Wiley and Sons, Inc., New York, 1974, pp. 185–219.

150. Dannenberg, A. M., Jr.: Macrophages in inflammation and infection, N Engl J Med, 1975, *293*, 489.

151. Yamamoto, K., Anacker, R. L., and Ribi, E.: Macrophage migration inhibition studies with cells from mice vaccinated with cell walls of *Mycobacterium bovis* BCG: Relationship between inhibitory activity of lung cells and resistance to airborne challenge with *Mycobacterium tuberculosis* H37Rv, Infect Immun, 1970, *1*, 595.

152. Mackaness, G. B.: The influence of immunologically committed lymphoid cells on macrophage activation in vivo, J Exp Med, 1969, *129*, 973.

153. North, R. J.: The relative importance of blood monocytes and fixed macrophages to the expression of cell-mediated immunity to infection, J Exp Med, 1970, *132*, 521.

154. Truitt, G. L., and Mackaness, G. B.: Cell-mediated resistance to aerogenic infection of the lung, Am Rev Respir Dis, 1971, *104*, 829.

155. Richerson, H. B.: Varieties of acute immunologic damage to the rabbit lung, Ann N Y Acad Sci, 1974, *221*, 340.

156. Moore, V. L., Hensley, G. T., and Fink, J. N.: An animal model of hypersensitivity pneumonitis in the rabbit, J Clin Invest, 1975, *56*, 937.

157. Johnson, K. J., and Ward, P. A.: Acute immunologic pulmonary alveolitis, J Clin Invest, 1974, *54*, 349.

158. Miyamoto, T., Junzaburo, K., Noda, M., Kobayashi, N., and Miura, K.: Physiologic and pathologic respiratory changes in delayed-type hypersensitivity reaction in guinea pigs, Am Rev Respir Dis, 1971, *103*, 509.

State of the Art

Pulmonary Infection in the Compromised Host

Part I

D. M. WILLIAMS, J. A. KRICK, and J. S. REMINGTON

Contents

[1] From the Department of Medicine, Division of Infectious Diseases, Stanford University School of Medicine, Stanford, Calif.; the Division of Allergy, Immunology and Infectious Diseases, Palo Alto Medical Research Foundation, Palo Alto, Calif.; and the Alamo Medical Clinic, Alamo, Calif.

[2] This work was supported by grant no. AI04717 from the National Institutes of Health.

[3] Requests for reprints should be addressed to Jack S. Remington, M.D., Palo Alto Medical Research Foundation, 860 Bryant St., Palo Alto, Calif. 94301.

Introduction

A wide variety of opportunistic pathogens cause pulmonary infection in the compromised host. For purposes of the present discussion, the compromised host is defined as a patient who has a primary underlying condition or is receiving therapy that impairs resistance to infection. Unfortunately, for many of these opportunistic pathogens, little is known about (1) host mechanisms of resistance (particularly, the specific immune defect leading to infection); (2) safe and accurate methods of premortem diagnosis and the proper time to use these methods; (3) the epidemiology and effective means of prevention; and (4) the optimal type and duration of therapy. This review will be addressed to what is known about these questions as they relate to the compromised host and includes a summary of the available literature on the pathologic and clinical aspects of these infections. No new clinical data are provided, but an effort has been made to gather a variety of existing material together in a single source. Because of the huge volume of material available, no attempt has been made to be exhaustively complete; however, representative data have been selected to provide an overview of a vast and complex field. Opinions are offered on controversial points, but the distinction between fact and opinion is maintained. The length of each section does not necessarily relate to the clinical incidence or importance of the infection or pathogen discussed. A discussion of the common bacterial pathogens causing pulmonary infections is beyond the scope of this article. Aerobic gram-negative bacillary pneumonia, a significant problem in the compromised host, has recently been extensively discussed in this journal by Pierce and Sanford (1).

The subject of pulmonary defense mechanisms has recently been discussed by Green (2) and Kaltreider (3) and will be dealt with only briefly here. Pulmonary defense begins with aerodynamics; the considerable turbulence experienced by the incoming airstream causes the removal (by inertial impaction) of most particles larger than 2 to 3 μm, which include large fungal spores. These particles are transported (either alone, or intracellularly after phagocytosis) by complex systems to the outside, to the reticuloendothelial system, or to retained deposits in the lung. Alveolar macrophages appear to be the major initial line of defense against particles deposited on the respiratory membrane. Presumably, specific immune responses are required if the alveolar macrophage mechanism fails. There is evidence that local, specific immune responses do occur in the lung. For example, in the guinea pig, inhaled antigen was shown to lead to the presence of sensitized lymphocytes in the lower respiratory tract, whereas antigen injected into the footpad resulted in sensitized lymphocytes in the spleen, but not in the lower respiratory tract (4, 5). In extending these studies to man, Jurgensen and associates (6) obtained lymphocytes by bronchoalveolar lavage and circulating lymphocytes from volunteers who had positive reactions to skin tests with mumps antigen tuberculin; they demonstrated that lymphocytes from both sources were sensitized to these antigens. Immunization of volunteers with influenza vaccine by the aerosol route was more effective at sensitizing lower respiratory tract lymphocytes than was immunization by the subcutaneous route (6). Unfortunately, the actual roles of alveolar macrophages and local specific, humoral, and cell-mediated immunity in protecting against most opportunistic pathogens discussed below is not clearly defined.

It is evident that the therapy being given to many of these compromised patients to treat their underlying diseases (e.g., corticosteroids, cytotoxic drugs, and antimicrobial agents) contributes to their susceptibility to opportunistic infection. A complete discussion of the immunologic alterations produced by corticosteroids and cytotoxic agents is beyond the scope of this paper, and the reader is referred to other sources (7–18). Specific defects produced by these agents that render the host susceptible to individual infections, in cases in which they are known, will be discussed under *Immunopathologic Aspects* in each section.

The approach to recognition and diagnosis of pulmonary infection in the compromised host is different from that in the normal host. It should be emphasized that no symptoms, signs, or roentgenographic features are specific for a given opportunistic infection in the compromised host, although, as will be discussed, certain patterns are suggestive. Concurrent and sequential infections of the lung are notoriously common in this population, making the relationship of disease manifestations to any single pathogen difficult to define.

The suspicion of infection in the compromised host should be pursued far beyond the routine "fever work-up" (19). Routine evaluation primarily includes obtaining material for appropriate stain and culture from multiple, easily accessible sites, such as sputum (when it is produced), blood, throat, nares, stool, urine, and skin. In cases of pneumonia, skin testing for tuberculosis, measurement of cold agglutinins, and serologic tests for *Toxoplasma gondii*, candida, cryptococcus (and, depending on exposure, *Coccidioides immitis* and *Histoplasma capsulatum*) and stool examination for strongyloides should be considered. In some cases, serial serologic studies for the deoxyribonucleic acid viruses (herpes simplex, varicella-zoster, and cytomegalovirus) or indirect fluorescent antibody studies of material from viral skin lesions may be helpful. After "routine work-up," the severely compromised patient with apparent infection is started on antibacterial chemotherapy. However, if an etiology has not been established quickly by "routine work-up," the need for repeated physical examinations, chest radiographs, and further cultures during empiric therapy must be emphasized (20). The etiologic agent may be recovered for the first time after antimicrobial drugs have been started, and repeated cultures may be successful in detecting multiple infections or superinfection. When the infection is pulmonary, and when a diagnosis has not been obtained in the "routine work-up," then there should be a graduated pursuit of invasive methods. This is particularly true if a course of empiric antibacterial agents has been administered without adequate response. Others have also stressed this approach, and platelet transfusion should be used in the thrombocytopenic patient to protect against hemorrhagic complications of these invasive procedures (21–23).

With regard to invasive procedures, there are few available data concerning the frequency of success or failure in the antemortem diagnosis of opportunistic pulmonary infection in the compromised host. Transtracheal aspiration appears to be the next logical step when sputum examination is unrewarding or when there is no sputum production; the latter occurs often in many patients, perhaps because of the inadequacy of the inflammatory response (23).

Needle aspiration should be considered next. Bandt and co-workers (24) reported the results of needle aspiration in 25 episodes of pneumonitis (with localized lung lesions) in 21 compromised hosts . In 16 of 22 aspiration specimens and each of 3 core biopsies, an infectious agent was identified (72 per cent). In the 22 aspirations using a thin-walled, 18-gauge, noncutting needle, there was only one major complication, a 30 per cent pneumothorax in one patient. Two of the 3 biopsies with the modified Vim-Silverman cutting needle led to serious complications (hemoptysis requiring transfusions and significant pneumothorax). Isolates in the 22 aspirations included fungi and nocardia, as well as gram-negative and gram-positive bacteria. Both isolates of *Pneumocystis carinii* were obtained by core biopsy.

Greenman and associates (21) and Greenman (Personal communication, 1975) reviewed the records of 78 compromised hosts undergoing 95 invasive diagnostic lung procedures at Stanford Medical Center. There were 34 needle aspirates, 13 cutting needle biopsies, and 48 open biopsies. Specific infection was diagnosed by 60 per cent of the aspirates, 75 per cent of the needle

biopsies, and 79 per cent of the open biopsies. Needle aspiration led to the diagnosis of 2 of 2 *P. carinii* infections and 3 of 4 fungal infections; needle biopsy diagnosed 3 of 3 *P. carinii* infections and missed one fungal infection; open biopsy diagnosed 4 of 4 *P. carinii* infections and 5 of 6 fungal infections. Open biopsy, performed 6 times, was successful in diagnosing 2 candida infections missed by needle aspiration and cutting needle, one case of aspergillosis, and 2 cases of coccidioidomycosis. One patient with coccidioidomycosis, in whom the needle aspirate was negative on stain, but positive on culture 10 days after the procedure, underwent open biopsy that revealed the organism in the interim. A diagnosis of disseminated phycomycosis, made at autopsy, was missed on open biopsy. Bleeding complications occurred with 3 of 34 aspirates, 2 of 13 needle biopsies, and 2 of 48 open biopsies. Pneumothorax occurred in 3 of 34 aspirates and 4 of 13 needle biopsies. One fatality occurred (a hemothorax due to needle biopsy). The risk of complications with needle biopsy, therefore, seems somewhat greater than with the other 2 procedures, both of which had acceptable complication rates and provided useful information.

Other procedures for diagnosis of pulmonary infections in the compromised host have advantages and disadvantages, proponents and opponents, and their use and effectiveness depend, in part, on the skill of the operator, the distribution of lung lesions, and appropriate caution in interpretation of results. Bronchoscopy has been opposed because organisms from the mouth are carried with the instrument, and because the topical anesthetics used are inhibitory to pathogens (25–27). Experience with 57 bronchial brushings in 55 compromised hosts with pulmonary lesions has recently been published (28). The diagnosis was made in 8 of 10 patients with *P. carinii* infection. Nocardia was isolated in 2 of 3 patients with nocardiosis; aspergillus, in 1 of 2 patients with aspergillosis. Viral isolations were always associated with pulmonary disease but were more difficult to evaluate. Of 750 patients, one required a chest tube, one had a respiratory arrest, and 2 had major hemorrhage. The procedure thus seemed relatively safe and effective in the diagnosis of pneumocytosis, nocardiosis, and fungal disease, but contamination by oral flora remained a problem shared by bronchial lavage.

Contamination by mouth flora is avoided by the technique of transtracheal selective bronchial brushing described by Aisner and associates (29). Twenty-seven patients believed to have pulmonary infection underwent this procedure. In 10 (8 of whom were receiving broad-spectrum antimicrobial drugs before or during the procedure), no infection was ever documented. In the remaining 17 patients, transtracheal selective bronchial brushing led to a correct diagnosis in 14. The 3 false-negative results occurred in patients with fungal pneumonias (2 with aspergillosis, and one with phycomycosis). These 3 represented a 30 per cent false-negative rate among patients with proved fungal infections, excluding 2 patients with torulopsis isolated by the procedure. Correct diagnoses were made in 5 cases of aspergillosis, 2 of phycomycosis, 2 of tuberculosis, 2 of *Torulopsis glabrata* infection, and one of pneumocystosis. The patients from whom torulopsis was isolated recovered from their apparent infection without antifungal treatment, thus raising doubt about the etiologic role of these yeasts in the infection. Seven patients had significant but nonfatal complications, including hemoptysis, pneumothorax, and cervical cellulitis (29). Blood transfusion was required in one patient; chest tube placement, in 2.

Transbronchoscopic lung biopsy has been reported to be successful in the diagnosis of various lung diseases, but suppurative pulmonary disease has been considered a contraindication (30).

Open lung biopsy is the ultimate antemortem procedure, and its effectiveness in diagnosing a large number of different lung diseases has been recently stressed (30–32). If the infected area of lung is biopsied, and if the tissue obtained is distributed to the appropriate laboratories for the necessary stains and culture, there should, theoretically, be no false-negative results, although practice has fallen short of theory.

The relative merits and risks of these various procedures are difficult to assess. Because of relative safety of the procedure and the need to avoid oral contamination, when transtracheal aspiration was unrewarding, we have favored percutaneous pulmonary aspiration before proceeding to open lung biopsy. Transtracheal selective bronchial brushing may well be a useful addition (in experienced hands), although its safety requires further evaluation. Also, the false-negative rate in fungal infections appears, at least in the one study cited (29), to be significant.

The optimal method of diagnosis must be individualized for each patient and will depend, in part, on the urgency of the clinical situation. In all cases, this decision requires an awareness by all physicians caring for such patients of the variety of pathogens that may cause such infections and the methods necessary for diagnosing each of them. It is usually necessary to use a "team approach," in which the patient's attending physician, in consultation with a surgeon, a pathologist, and the personnel of the microbiology laboratory, work together to establish an early definitive diagnosis. The lack of such team effort and cooperation may result in delay in establishing a specific infectious etiology in patients for whom appropriate therapy may be available. Unfortunately, it is not uncommon in hospitals where such patients are treated for the primary physician to be unable to obtain the appropriate biopsy material at the optimal time. Even if a procedure such as an emergency open lung biopsy is done, the preparation of special stains (e.g., of frozen sections on tissue imprints) by the pathology laboratory may be delayed until regular working hours. This is to be deplored. An aggressive team approach toward establishing an early diagnosis and instituting appropriate treatment of infectious episodes is crucial for improving the patient's chance of survival.

In the following sections, the immunologic, pathologic, clinical, diagnostic, and preventive and therapeutic aspects of selected pulmonary pathogens and infections of importance in the compromised host will be discussed. The emphasis will be primarily on infections as they occur in adult patients.

Fungi

Cryptococcus neoformans

Cryptococcosis is defined as invasion of otherwise viable tissue by *C. neoformans*. Rarely, however, other species of cryptococcus have been implicated in human pulmonary disease (33). Cryptococcosis is considered to occur most frequently by inhalation of the organism. It is frequently found in soil contaminated by pigeon and chicken excreta (34–37). The organism has also been isolated from fruit juice, milk, and ordinary soil. Therefore, it has not been established that most persons become infected through exposure to pigeons (38). Human-to-human transmission has not been reported (37). It has been stated that pathogenic *C. neoformans* has been recovered from normal skin, vagina, gastrointestinal tract, and oropharynx (37); however, this occurrence must be rare. Kahanpää (39), for example, isolated *C. neoformans* from only 1 of 3,729 sputum specimens and only once from 62 cultures of material from the maxillary sinus and nasal cavities in a group of patients with a variety of chronic pulmonary diseases. It has been postulated that *C. neoformans* may remain dormant in lung tissue for prolonged periods and become activated with changes in host defenses. In such cases the infection would be from an endogenous site (40, 41).

Immunopathologic aspects. A clinical association has been found between Hodgkin's disease and disseminated cryptococcosis. For example, in 51 patients with Hodgkin's disease seen at the National Cancer Institute, disseminated mycotic infection occurred in 5 patients, and cryptococcus was responsible for 4 of these (42). Feld and associates (43) identified cryptococcus as the cause of 2 of 4 fatal fungal infections in patients with Hodgkin's disease, and Hart and coworkers (44) found cryptococcus in 2 of 10 patients with underlying Hodgkin's disease who had acquired deep fungal infections. Because of the known defects in specific cellular immunity in patients with untreated Hodgkin's disease (45), this clinical association has led to speculation that cell-mediated immunity is important in resistance to cryptococcosis. In support of this theory, patients without known underlying disease who had been successfully treated for disseminated cryptococcosis have been found to have reduced antigen-specific lymphocyte transformation when compared to normal subjects with positive skin tests (46). Also, patients who recovered from disseminated cryptococcosis have exhibited decreased lymphocyte counts, decreased rosetting lymphocytes, and reduced skin test responsiveness to candida and histoplasma antigens (in an area in which histoplasma was endemic), thus suggesting a generalized decrease in responsiveness of the cellular immune system (47). The antigen-specific lymphocyte transformation, however, was not different from that of control subjects.

In addition to Hodgkin's disease, other factors that seem to predispose to cryptococcal infection have been identified. Goldstein and Rambo (48) reported that from 1950 to 1960, 5 per cent of 147 patients with cryptococcosis without known underlying malignancy had received corticosteroids (48). Controlled studies designed to prove definitively the association between pharma-

cologic corticosteroid therapy and cryptococcosis are lacking, and conflicting data have been reported. For example, Bodey (49) found that 5 patients with cryptococcosis had received corticosteroids only briefly (for an average of less than 1 per cent of the days of the month before infection); in contrast, a control group, which had received corticosteroids for 22 per cent of days of the month before death, did not develop fungal infection (49). In an animal model, Gadebusch and Gikas (50) demonstrated that animals treated with corticosteroids had an increased mortality when cryptococcosis was induced by inhalation.

In a murine model, protection against cryptococcosis has been demonstrated by prior immunization (51–54, 55); however, sufficient data are not available to define precisely the mechanisms of resistance to cryptococcosis in these models, although cell-mediated immunity has been believed to be of prime importance (55). Gentry and Remington (55) demonstrated that in mice, heterologous infection with listeria, besnoitia (known to activate the macrophages of the host) or the protozoa, toxoplasma, conferred protection against challenge with cryptococcus (55). Furthermore, mouse peritoneal macrophages activated *in vivo* by infection with listeria, toxoplasma, or besnoitia were resistant *in vitro* to destruction by cryptococcus. These data suggest a role for the macrophage in resistance to cryptococcal infection (55). On the other hand, Diamond and Bennett (56) and Diamond and associates (57) found that human macrophages derived from peripheral blood monocytes and activated *in vitro* by cryptococcal antigen could not kill ingested cryptococcus, even though the blood monocytes from which they had been derived could kill this yeast. The definitive role of the macrophage in resistance to infection therefore remains to be clarified.

Studies have been performed to determine the role of human blood phagocytes in resistance to this infection. Cline and Lehrer (58) demonstrated that monocytes, but not polymorphonuclear leukocytes, were able to phagocytose cryptococcus in the presence of serum (58). Bulmer and Sans (59) and Diamond and associates (57) showed phagocytosis by both cell types. Ingestion did not appear to be affected by specific anticryptococcal antibody (57), but was dependent on the size of the yeast capsule. In a later study, however, opsonization was shown to be required for optimal phagocytosis (60). Diamond and co-workers (57) and Tacker and associates (61) demonstrated that monocytes and polymorphonuclear cells were able to kill intracellular, encapsulated cryptococcus. Killing appeared to be dependent on generation of hydrogen peroxide, and the rate of killing, on myeloperoxidase function (57), although a defect in this mechanism could not be demonstrated in patients with cryptococcosis and no detectable predisposing condition (57). Diamond (62) has recently shown that mononuclear cells and specific antibody can kill cryptococcus without phagocytosis. The exact cell type (monocyte or lymphocyte) was not determined, and the mechanism of killing was not identified; however, this may be a possible mechanism by which the host deals with large-capsule cryptococcus. Also, Kalina and associates (63) demonstrated that rabbit peritoneal polymorphonuclear leukocytes and mononuclear phagocytes, both *in vivo* after intraperitoneal challenge with cryptococcus and *in vitro*, formed tight rings around large-capsule cryptococcus, with penetration of the capsule by pseudopodia from the phagocytes (63). There was subsequent degeneration of the capsule and yeast cytoplasm, without phagocytosis of whole yeasts. Capsular-like material was seen in phagocytic vacuoles.

A pathogenesis of cryptococcal infection has been suggested that includes a major role for circulating phagocytes in resistance. Cryptococcus in the soil is normally not encapsulated. This form is inhaled into the lungs, whereupon a capsule may be produced. Alveolar macrophages, normal and activated, are unable to kill ingested unencapsulated cryptococci, but by virtue of phagocytosis alone, may wall off the infection. Circulating phagocytes, by contrast, are able to kill unencapsulated cryptococci, but capsular material inhibits phagocytosis. Therefore, an early inflammatory response in the lung may be instrumental in protecting the normal host against inhaled organisms. Finally, cryptococci walled off by alveolar macrophages may persist in the lung in an inactive state for a prolonged period and may become active and invasive owing to some change in the host-parasite relationship (64, 65).

No clinical data are available relating cryptococcosis to neutropenia (43, 49).

Data on serum factors in resistance to cryptococcal infection are not clear. A factor in normal serum that inhibits cryptococcal growth has been described (66). Tacker and co-workers (61) demonstrated that normal human serum had a fungicidal effect that was abolished by heating. On the other hand, Diamond and co-workers (57) were unable to demonstrate a cryptococcocidal effect of human serum, even though 90 per cent of the serum was from cryptococcal antibody–positive healthy subjects (57).

Pathologic features. In studies primarily involving the normal host with cryptococcosis, a wide variety of pulmonary pathologic findings have been described (67, 68). In some cases, little or no inflammatory reaction has been seen, particularly when the organisms are encapsulated (69), whereas in others, macrophages, lymphocytes, plasma cells, and infiltrates of polymorphonuclear leukocytes have been noted. The histologic appearance may depend on the duration of the lesion. Necrosis has varied from none to extensive caseation and cavitation, although the latter characteristics have been seen only occasionally. Granuloma formation without calcification has been common (68) and is perhaps most typical of older lesions (70). Giant cells have been found frequently, but epithelioid cells have not. The fungus may be intracellular or extracellular in masses. A case has been described in which the pathologic features were indistinguishable from those seen in histoplasmosis (67).

Similar pathologic findings have been seen in the compromised host. MacGillivray (71) and Mills and co-workers (72), for example, noted granulomas containing cryptococci in the lungs of renal transplant patients receiving immunosuppressive therapy. Kent and Layton (73) described 2 cases of "massive" pulmonary cryptococcosis in immunosuppressed patients. Bronchioles and alveoli were filled with edema fluid and red blood cells. Polymorphonuclear leukocytes and mononuclear phagocytes were present, with large numbers of budding yeasts found throughout bronchioles, alveoli, and blood vessels (73). Clumps of organisms were seen in small arteries, capillaries, and veins. *C. neoformans* was cultured from the lung. In contrast, Lomvardias and Lurie (74) reported a case of epipleural cryptococcosis in a patient with Hodgkin's disease in whom epipleural connective tissue and numerous encapsulated yeast cells were noted without significant penetration into the lung parenchyma. Occasional yeast cells were seen in the alveoli beneath the pleural nodules, but no associated tissue reaction was found.

With Mayer's mucicarmine stain, considered to be diagnostic for *C. neoformans*, the fungus cell wall and a small amount of the capsule stain red (68).

Clinical manifestations. Cryptococcosis, as stated, has been found in a variety of types of compromised hosts, including patients with acute leukemia (49, 75), Hodgkin's disease (74), and lymphosarcoma (70). Although chronic lymphocytic leukemia and multiple myeloma are only rarely complicated by fungal infections, cryptococcosis has been reported in these patients during therapy with corticosteroids (44, 76, 77). Mills and associates (72), in examining 16 cases of pulmonary mycosis in renal allograft patients, found infection with *C. neoformans* in 4.

The range of symptoms in pulmonary cryptococcosis in a basically nonimmunosuppressed population has been well described in a review of 101 cases of cryptococcosis limited to the lungs (78). Symptoms included cough in 54 per cent, chest pain in 46 per cent, sputum production in 32 per cent, and weight loss and fever in 26 per cent each. Hemoptysis was noted in 18 per cent, dyspnea in 16 per cent, and night sweats in 9 per cent. It is of note that 32 per cent of patients had no symptoms. Disease was limited to one lobe in 68 patients and was localized in the right lower lobe in one third of these. Among the patients in whom this could be determined, disease had been present for at least 3 months in 47 per cent and for more than 18 months in 17 per cent. One patient had documented disease for 6 years, demonstrating the chronicity of disease in some normal hosts. Sixty-three per cent of patients were 30 to 50 years of age, 87 per cent were white, and 82 per cent were male. Campbell (78) reported physical findings in his cases that ranged from a normal physical examination to crepitant rales and a pleural friction rub. Gordonson and co-workers (79) described the radiographic findings in a series of 26 patients, 14 of whom had no underlying systemic disease. Thirty-five per cent had single mass lesions that occasionally cavitated. Eight per cent had multiple unilateral or bilateral small, discrete masses. Lobar or segmental consolidation was found in 35 per cent, with cavitation in 8 per cent. Extensive pulmonary lymphadenopathy was found in 12 per cent; pleural effusions, in 4 per cent of patients. Diffuse, nonlocalized disease was noted in 23 per cent and could not be differentiated from a variety of other pneumonias with a similar pattern. Seventy-seven per cent had no coexisting pulmonary disease. Cryptococcosis may also be found in asymptomatic patients with only a subpleural nodule or focus in a hilar lymph node that are beyond the resolving power of the routine chest radiograph. Clinically apparent infection often follows a subacute course (68); but on rare occasions, progressive pulmonary cryptococcosis has resulted in death (37, 78). Hematologic values were frequently normal and nondiagnostic.

The spectrum of cryptococcal pulmonary infection in compromised patients has been similar, although it must be emphasized that pulmonary involvement alone is uncommon in this setting, most cases being associated with dissemination. Mills and associates (72) reported 4 cases of pulmonary involvement with cryptococcus in renal allograft patients, 3 of whom also had meningeal infection. In one patient, nocardia was also present in sputum. Symptoms varied from none to fever and cough. Chest radiographs revealed pulmonary infiltrates in 3, nodules in 2, and cavitation in one. The histologic features in one patient with a solitary mass lesion consisted of granulomas containing cryptococcus (72). Hematologic values were unremarkable, although anemia and increased sedimentation rate may be observed (68). Two patients died, both of whom had cryptococcal meningitis. Lomvardias and Lurie (74) described a case of epipleural cryptococcosis in a patient with Hodgkin's disease. An example of much more virulent disease in the compromised host is given by Kent and Layton (73), who describe a 21-year-old white man with acute lymphatic leukemia who was admitted to the hospital with a 4-day history of malaise and cough. The night before admission, he developed fever and was brought to the hospital obtunded and with a temperature of 106° F. The lungs were clear on physical examination. The patient died within 12 hours. *C. neoformans* was grown from 4 blood cultures. At autopsy, the lungs were found to contain huge amounts of proteinaceous material, as well as hemorrhage in bronchioles and alveoli. Large numbers of budding yeasts were seen, and cultures from multiple organs were positive for *C. neoformans*.

The most feared complication of pulmonary cryptococcosis is the dissemination of the organism, particularly to the meninges. This may occur from minute pulmonary foci (41). In a review of 101 cases of cryptococcosis initially limited to the lung, Campbell (78) noted that 7 of 62 patients treated surgically developed meningitis. Two of 31 (6 per cent) developed meningitis in the absence of surgical excision or amphotericin B therapy. It is not stated whether any of those who went on to develop meningitis were compromised hosts. None of 10 treated with amphotericin B developed meningitis, and Campbell (78) states that no patients reported in the literature to that time (1966) developed meningitis if they had received amphotericin B for pulmonary cryptococcosis. Hammerman and associates (80) described 28 patients with definite or probable pulmonary cryptococcosis of whom 5 received no treatment; 8, pulmonary resection; the remainder, amphotericin B with or without surgery. None developed meningitis; however, in their review of the literature, a few patients were found in whom meningitis appeared to develop after surgical resection of pulmonary lesions.

Diagnosis. Definitive diagnosis of invasive pulmonary cryptococcosis requires the demonstration of the organism in pulmonary tissue. Because *C. neoformans* is found in the sputum of some patients with chronic lung disease but with no evidence of cryptococcosis (39, 80–82), the recovery of the organism from sputum in such patients is unreliable in establishing the diagnosis. Open lung biopsy and transbronchial brush biopsy have been successful techniques (40, 78, 79, 83–85). Pulmonary cryptococcosis may appear as a mass lesion, in which case cancer must be excluded, particularly when predisposing factors to opportunistic infection do not exist. When such patients are otherwise apparently normal, demonstration of the yeast in material obtained by percutaneous needle aspiration of the pulmonary lesion is probably a sufficient reason for following the patient with periodic radiographs, rather than proceeding with immediate thoracotomy. In the immunocompromised host, a positive result after needle aspiration is probably sufficient indication for beginning antifungal therapy. In the compromised host, aspiration of pleural fluid has disclosed budding yeast cells surrounded by capsules (86).

Other diagnostic methods are clearly less direct and less definitive in terms of determining the exact cause of the pulmonary component of the infection. In patients with disseminated disease, *C. neoformans* has been isolated from sputum (in the absence of infiltrate on radiographs), stool, blood, urine, skin lesions, and prostatic fluid (44, 49, 87–90). It is of interest that a patient has been reported with cancer and clinical illness from whose blood *C. neoformans* was isolated on one occasion, but who at autopsy had no evidence of cryptococcal infection (90). He had not been treated with antifungal agents. At least in this patient, cryptococcemia did not establish a diagnosis of deep-seated cryptococcosis.

It is now generally agreed that an unequivocally positive test for cryptococcal antigen in the serum or cerebrospinal fluid is diagnostic of cryptococcosis (91). Bindschadler and Bennett (77) reported that 92 per cent of 75 patients with proved cryptococcosis had cryptococcal capsular antigen or antibody to capsular antigen in serum or cerebrospinal fluid or both. No correlation was found between the results of tests for antigen and antibody and the presence or absence of underlying disease. They found that the complement fixation test for antigen lacked sensitivity and was positive in only 63 per cent. Previously, no false-positive results had been found in 62 patients with systemic mycoses not due to cryptococcus or in 48 patients with miscellaneous diseases (92). A latex agglutination test is available to test for antigen. A 50 per cent false-positive rate has been noted in patients with rheumatoid factor, and control tests for this must be run. In a series of 30 patients with active cryptococcosis, the complement fixation test for antigen alone was positive in 26; the latex agglutination test alone, in 27; and both complement fixation and latex agglutination tests, in 28. This led to a combined sensitivity of 93 per cent (93). An occasional low titer (less than 1:4) false-positive latex agglutination test was found not associated with rheumatoid factor; however, the complement fixation test was negative in these patients. For optimal sensitivity, therefore, it was suggested that both of these tests were needed; however, if proper controls for the latex agglutination test were run, it, by itself, would probably be adequate for the average clinical laboratory. Gordon and Lapa (94) suggested further refinements in the latex agglutination test to eliminate false-positive results associated with rheumatoid factor.

In contrast to the data presented for antigens, serologic tests for antibody to capsular antigen have a significant false-positive rate. For example, the test has been positive in 12 per cent of patients with histoplasmosis and 6 per cent of patients with blastomycosis (77). A positive test, therefore, can be considered only suggestive evidence of cryptococcal infection.

Because of the difficulty encountered at times in interpretation of serologic test results of immunosuppressed patients, it is suggested that banks of serum be established as early as possible in the disease course, before immunosuppressive therapy has begun, so that serum specimens can later be run in parallel with those obtained after infectious complications have arisen.

Prevention and treatment. Patients known to be compromised hosts should be instructed to avoid contact with pigeons and chickens and their excreta, and hospital air inlets should be kept as free as possible of these substances as well. Many other potential sources of infection exist, however, and activation of latent infection has not been excluded as a pathogenic mechanism.

Amphotericin B Susceptibility

To our knowledge, all clinical isolates of *C. neoformans* tested to date have been susceptible to amphotericin B. A minimal inhibitory concentration (MIC) of 0.64 μg per ml was reported by Bennett (95) against 33 clinical isolates. The mean concentration of amphotericin B that produced 50 per cent inhibition was 0.04 μg per ml (range, 0.0064 to 0.094 μg per ml), less than one tenth of the MIC. No significant change in MIC occurred in patients during therapy with amphotericin B, although a modest increase in the concentration needed for 50 per cent inhibition occurred, the highest being 0.36 μg per ml. Rhoades and co-workers (96) found MICs from 0.024 to 0.39 μg per ml in 89 isolates of *C. neoformans.* Shadomy and associates (97) determined the mean MIC against 77 strains to be 0.19 μg per ml. The mean minimal fungicidal concentration was 0.40 μg per ml. Hoeprich and Huston (98), looking at 21 strains of *C. neoformans,* found a mean MIC of 0.86 μg per ml (range, 0.24 to 0.96 μg per ml).

We agree with the often-expressed opinion that patients with pulmonary cryptococcosis and impaired host defenses should be treated with amphotericin B to prevent possible dissemination (78, 99) and to treat already present, but clinically silent, metastatic foci. Definitive data supporting this opinion do not appear to be readily available. In contrast, in the apparently normal host, spontaneous resolution of proved invasive pulmonary cryptococcosis is well documented (40). This fact should lead to caution in claims of treatment success (100). The optimal dosage of amphotericin B and the duration of therapy for treatment of pulmonary disease have not been determined and must be dictated by the response of the patient and the toxicity of the drug. More extensive data have been accumulated from studies in patients with cryptococcal meningitis regarding amount and duration of therapy. Discussion of these data is beyond the scope of this review; the reader is referred to references 88 and 101.

5-Fluorocytosine

Cryptococcus not previously exposed to 5-fluorocytosine is rarely resistant to this drug; however, development of resistance during therapy is common and may result in treatment failure. For patients with hematologic and lymphoproliferative malignancies, which are important prognostic indicators (88, 101), only anecdotal experience is available (102, 103). With regard to cryptococcosis confined to the lung, Utz and co-workers (104) reported improvement without relapse in 3 patients, and Harder and Hermans (105) noted cure or improvement in 4, 2 of whom had received prednisone therapy for nonmalignant disease. In the absence of data for a large number of patients with pulmonary cryptococcosis treated with a dose of 150 mg per kg per day, however, we believe that this drug should not be used alone to treat this infection in the compromised host.

The combination of 5-fluorocytosine (150 mg per kg per day) and low doses of amphotericin B (20 mg per day) has been used against cryptococcosis in a preliminary study with encouraging results. Eleven of 15 patients were free of infection clinically or at autopsy after death from underlying diseases (106). In a murine model, the 2 drugs in combination were additive and possibly synergistic (107); however, caution is suggested by recent reports that the 2 drugs may be antagonistic both *in vitro* and in an animal model (108, 109).

Aspergillus

Aspergillosis is the invasion of otherwise viable tissue by any species of the aspergillus organism, most commonly *Aspergillus fumigatus,* in the compromised host with pulmonary infection (49, 110, 111). *A. flavus* and *A. glaucus* are the next most common causes of this disease entity. Occasional cases due to other species have been noted, however, and it is probable that any aspergillus species may be pathogenic in the compromised host (112). The respiratory tract (inhalation of spores) is believed to be the significant portal of entry in man (35). Because of this, a variety of studies have been done to determine the frequency with which aspergillus species, including *A. fumigatus*, could be isolated from hospital air (39, 113–115). Four studies have attempted to correlate environmental contamination with spores and the development of disease in the compromised host. Gage and co-workers (116) described 3 cases of aspergillus endocarditis after open heart surgery (116). They were able to isolate *A. fumigatus* from pigeon excreta near the intake of the ventilating system in the operating room. Rose (117) studied the incidence of *A. fumigatus* infection in a new hospital in which no cases were found and an old hospital in which 11 cases were found during a similar period of time. Spores of *A. fumigatus* were present in the air of the old hospital but could not be found in the new one, suggesting a direct relationship to the relative incidence of the disease in the 2 hospitals. Burton and co-workers (118) found *A. fumigatus* spore contamination of air ducts leading to an isolation room in which renal transplant patients apparently had developed aspergillosis. After changes were made to eliminate this contamination, no further cases of aspergillosis were found. Aisner and co-workers (83) in a population with acute luekemia, found a 3- to 4-fold increase in the incidence of aspergillosis on moving to a new hospital facility, which was found to be heavily contaminated with *A. fumigatus* and *A. flavus.*

It is also possible in some cases that infection results from an endogenous or gastrointestinal source. Aspergillus species were found in the sputum of 16 per cent of 103 normal men (119), and Kahanpää (39) isolated aspergillus from 0.7 to 6.1 per cent of patients with chronic lung disease and normal control subjects, depending on where in the respiratory tree the specimen was obtained. Aspergillus has also been isolated occasionally from normal human gastrointestinal tracts (120) and has been found in a high percentage of commercial packages of spaghetti, macaroni, noodles, and similar products (121). The sinuses have also been implicated as a possible primary site (39), and cases of rhinocerebral aspergillosis have been reported in patients with leukemia in whom the sinuses appeared to be the primary site of infection (49).

Immunopathologic aspects. Immune defenses against aspergillosis have not been well defined. Epstein and co-workers (122) obtained alveolar macrophages from mice given an inhalation challenge of aspergillus and determined that virtually all spores were ingested by the macrophages. Intracellular germination was occasionally seen. Aspergillus spores were also readily phagocytosed *in vitro;* however, after 75 min of incubation, no apparent killing was seen. Normal mouse alveolar macrophages, therefore, seemed able to ingest the organism and to inhibit germination, but were not sporicidal.

After intravenously injecting *A. flavus* spores into mice, Ford and co-workers (123) found that colony counts in the liver and spleen sequentially decreased, suggesting killing of the organism. Four hours after inoculation, neutrophils were observed in the liver, before fungal hyphae were seen. In the brain and kidney, however, where fungus multiplication was noted, no polymorphonuclear cells were seen before the appearance of hyphae. This was interpreted to indicate that a delay in polymorphonuclear response, such as occurred in the brain and kidney, might have permitted hyphal growth until it was beyond the control of polymorphonuclear leukocytes, whereas a prompt polymorphonuclear response in liver and spleen may have permitted sporicidal activity. A possible clinical correlation exists in chronic granulomatous disease (124). An important cellular defect in this disease is the inability to generate hydrogen peroxide after phagocytosis by polymorphonuclear leukocytes. The not infrequent occurrence of aspergillosis in this group of patients may suggest that the polymorphonuclear leukocyte is important as a defense mechanism in the human population as well. It must also be noted, however, that these patients commonly take prophylactic antimicrobial drugs, and other reasons for their susceptibility to aspergillosis can certainly be suggested.

Data from other experiments performed *in vitro* have not supported the importance of the polymorphonuclear leukocyte in normal host defense against aspergillosis. Lehrer and Jan (125) were unable to detect killing of spores of *A. fumigatus in vitro* by human blood phagocytes (both polymorphonuclear leukocytes and monocytes). A combination of hydrogen peroxide, potassium iodide, and human myeloperoxidase was rapidly sporicidal in a cell-free system, but chloride, which may be the naturally occurring intracellular halide, was unable to substitute for the iodide (126).

Smith (127) has suggested that specific immunity against aspergillosis may exist. An intravenous sublethal dose of spores of *A. fumigatus* in a murine model protected against subsequent lethal intravenous challenge. The mechanism of this resistance, however, was not investigated. Normal immunoglobulin concentrations have been found in most patients with aspergillosis (110, 128); however, in severely compromised patients with advanced disease in the last weeks of life, significant titers of antibody often cannot be detected (129). The clinical implications of this are unclear. To our knowledge, there are no further data that might implicate specific humoral or cellular immunity in resistance to *Aspergillus.*

Attempts have been made to look at predisposing factors to invasive aspergillosis. Immunosuppressive drugs, cytotoxic chemotherapy, corticosteroids, concurrent antimicrobial drug treatment, and recent bacterial infections have all been implicated (72, 110, 118, 128, 130–132). It is impossible to identify any one factor in this complex group of patients as being most important in leading to invasive disease (44, 128). It has been suggested that in heart transplant patients with aspergillosis, local pulmonary factors, such as pulmonary edema, effects of thoracotomy, and prolonged mechanical ventilation may be important in predisposing to disease (131). Radiation fibrosis, intrapulmonary hemorrhage, pulmonary drug toxicity, tumor infiltration of pulmonary tissue, and prior and concurrent infections might also be important local predisposing factors. Corticosteroids have been shown to be an important predisposing factor to aspergillosis in animal models (133–135). In the murine model, it has been shown that prior treatment with corticosteroids leads to defective fusion of lysosomes with phagosomes containing spores (136). Phagocytosed spores in normal macrophages remain dormant or degenerated, whereas those in macrophages from animals treated with steroids showed evidence of germination. Hart and associates (44), for example, found that 7 of 8 patients were receiving corticosteroids at the onset of aspergillus infection. Many other factors, however, are operative, as indicated by the series of Young and associates (110), in which 2 patients with disseminated aspergillus infection were not receiving corticosteroids.

Pathologic features. The lung is the most common site of infection with aspergillus in patients with leukemia and lymphoma, being involved in more than 90 per cent of cases (49, 110, 128). It is also an important site of infection in cardiac and renal transplant patients (72, 118, 131, 137). At autopsy, necrotizing bronchopneumonia, including necrotizing bronchitis and invasion of small blood vessels, and pulmonary infarction due to invasion and occlusion of large- or medium-sized blood vessels, are the 2 most common lesions. Each has been observed in approximately one third of patients (110, 128). Other lesions have included miliary microabscesses, bronchitis, lobular and lobar pneumonia, aspergillomas, solitary granulomas, and lung abscesses (110, 128). Rarely, multiple cavitating aspergillomas (fungus balls) have been described in the immunosuppressed population, but it is frequently difficult to determine whether the fungus has invaded normal or diseased tissue (138, 139).

The microscopic appearance has been characterized by areas of tissue necrosis containing hyphae, neutrophils, and evidence of hemorrhage; hyphal invasion of tracheobronchial mucosa and cartilage; and thrombi in all sizes of pulmonary vessels containing hyphae that grow through vessel walls into lung parenchyma (128). Mycelial growth in pulmonary tissue usually does not produce fructification (68).

Clinical manifestations. Because multiple infections occur frequently in the immunosuppressed population, the clinical situation is quite complex with regard to aspergillosis. Bodey (49) stated that in 74 per cent of leukemic patients reviewed at autopsy, pulmonary aspergillosis had occurred in proximity of time or place with other pulmonary infections. As noted previously, necrotizing bronchopneumonia and hemorrhagic pulmonary infarction have been the most frequent clinical presentations (110, 128). Symptoms have commonly included dyspnea, tachypnea, fever, and nonproductive cough (72, 110, 118, 128, 130, 139, 140). Pleuritic chest pain and hemoptysis have also been described (110, 118, 128, 130, 139). For example, Young and associates (110), in a survey of 92 patients who had pulmonary aspergillosis at autopsy, noted a pattern of hemorrhagic pulmonary infarction in 29, 61 per cent of whom had experienced pleuritic chest pain. Three of this group had had hemoptysis. Meyer and associates (128) noted among 93 cases of aspergillosis the onset of sudden pleuritic chest pain in 6 and hemoptysis in 2; of these patients, 3 had hemorrhagic infarction, 2 had necrotizing bronchopneumonia, and one had lobar consolidation. When the pleuritic chest pain and hemoptysis occur, the chest radiograph may be normal, lung scan may show perfusion defects, and differentiation from bland pulmonary embolus and infarction may be impossible (110, 139). Aslam and associates (138) noted that hemoptysis was common in patients with aspergillosis, except those with lymphoma or leukemia, and Carbone and co-workers (130) found hemoptysis in only one of 22 such patients. Physical findings have, at times, been correlated with pulmonary symptoms. Carbone and associates (130) observed rales, chest pain, wheezes, or cough in 14 of 22 patients at a time when the chest film indicated disease. They noted a pleural friction rub in 6 of 21 patients. Meyer and co-workers (128) heard a pleural rub in 3 of 90 patients. Physical findings, however, may be minimal, as exemplified by 2 cases of cavitary disease, but normal physical examination (118). Fever greater than 100.4° F was noted in 12 of 22 patients (130). Hematologic values have been nonspecific. The roentgenographic picture has been variable. Carbone and associates (130) noted that pulmonary infiltrates were seen only in the last 2 weeks of life in 11 patients and were nonspecific, including patchy or nodular infiltrates, consolidation, atelectasis, and solitary or multiple nodules. Young and co-workers (110) stated that in 17 per cent of patients with bronchopneumonia, radiographic changes were absent, although pulmonary symptoms were present; again, they noted that changes tended to be seen very late in the disease, when the patient was critically ill. Seven of their patients, however, had persistent bronchopneumonia (later verified by autopsy in 6), which lasted 19 to 43 days. Meyer and co-workers (128), investigating this point, looked at 63 radiographs taken in 90 patients with aspergillosis and pulmonary involvement within 3 days of death. New infiltrates were seen in 47 of the 63. In 41 of these 47, the infiltrates were correlated with aspergillosis and included bronchopneumonia (12 cases), patchy infiltrates (11 cases), nodular densities (7 cases), consolidation (6 cases), aspergilloma with cavitation (4 cases), and reticular interstitial pneumonitis (1 case). Burke and Coltman (139) reported a case in which the radiograph was normal when the pleuritic pain first appeared; however, multiple aspergillomas later developed. Young and co-workers (110) stated that in the patients with the hemorrhagic infarction pattern of infection, almost one-third had no radiographic changes acutely, although pleuritic chest pain was present in 61 per cent. Zimmerman and Miller (140) re-emphasized that the disease may

be diffuse, lobar, nodular, or central, and that it cannot be distinguished from other types of pneumonia radiographically. Crescent-shaped areas of air may occasionally be seen in primary aspergillosis (68). The clinical and radiographic presentation is therefore variable and may be either acute or chronic (141). As previously noted, mixed infections often occur (44, 72, 131), making the separation of individual clinical or radiographic presentations even more difficult. Descriptions of "characteristic" pictures have varied from multiple nodular infiltrates, rapidly progressive and crossing fissures (112), to an ill-defined mass lesion proceeding to cavitation (142). It seems clear that there is no one typical clinical presentation.

Dissemination has been reported to occur in 20 to 50 per cent of patients (22, 44, 49, 110, 128). The lung is the site of origin of most disseminated cases.

The reported death rate among patients with aspergillosis has varied widely, according to the study. Carbone and co-workers (130) noted a 32 per cent mortality rate, whereas Meyer and associates (128) found a rate of 89 per cent. Part of the reason for the discrepancy in the literature is that the precise mode of death has been difficult to determine in many cases. Young and associates (110) stated that 30 per cent of patients with pulmonary aspergillosis died from consequent respiratory insufficiency.

Diagnosis. Requirements for definitive diagnosis involve both demonstration of characteristic hyphae in otherwise viable tissue and identification of the fungus as aspergillus by culture. The first is necessary because positive culture alone may reflect laboratory contamination or colonization of the respiratory tract; the second, because conidiophores are only rarely seen in tissue, and characteristic hyphae permit only a presumptive identification (143). These rigid criteria, of course, may have to be modified in individual clinical cases, particularly in the compromised patient with progressive pulmonary infiltration. Cases such as those noted by Gurwith and associates (131), in which needle aspiration of the lung produced material with positive histologic features, and cultures were positive for aspergillus, are sufficient for a diagnosis of invasive infection. Tissue has been obtained by open lung biopsy even in severely ill patients (118). Much greater modification of the criteria for diagnosis (unacceptable for definitive diagnosis, but probably adequate as an indication for starting therapy immediately) is exemplified by a patient with contraindications to an invasive procedure whose sputum contains characteristic hyphae or yields aspergillus on culture. In patients capable of withstanding this procedure, transtracheal aspiration has been useful in suggesting the diagnosis (131). We believe that there is a need, however, to state clearly the criteria for diagnosis and indications for starting therapy in cases reported in the literature.

Unfortunately, negative antemortem cultures are the rule in invasive pulmonary aspergillosis. For this reason, the diagnosis has often not been suspected before death. For example, Bodey (49) reported 38 leukemia patients in whom the diagnosis was established in only one before death. This patient had rhinocerebral aspergillosis. Six other patients with documented disease had positive antemortem cultures, but the fungus was not believed to be of clinical significance. Young and co-workers (110) stated that 34 per cent of their patients had one positive culture ante mortem; however, only 9 per cent had more than one positive culture. Meyer and associates (128) reported 59 patients with documented aspergillosis in whom antemortem fungal cultures of throat, sputum, or tracheal secretions were performed. Of these, 12 per cent were positive. In cases of disseminated disease, culture of other fluids may, at times, be useful. For example, in patients with renal involvement from dissemination, urine cultures were positive in 2 of 8 patients. In one series, hyphae were demonstrated by biopsy of skin lesions in 2 of 98 patients (110), and aspiration of vitreous humor yielded aspergillus in 2 patients with endophthalmitis due to dissemination (118, 144).

With regard to interpretation of positive cultures for aspergillus, Bodey (49) reported that invasive aspergillosis was found at autopsy in every patient with a positive antemortem culture from sputum, urine, or feces. On the other hand, Meyer and associates (128) reported 3 patients receiving no antifungal therapy in whom aspergillus was isolated from the sputum, but in whom aspergillosis was not present at autopsy. In this latter series, therefore, among 9 patients in whom aspergillus was isolated from pulmonary secretions, there were 3 false-positive results. We have described a heart transplant patient with a pulmonary infiltrate in whom percutaneous needle aspirate yielded a rare colony of aspergillus (145). Amphotericin B therapy, however, was ineffective, and the infiltrate progressed. When a repeat aspiration was done, *No-*

cardia asteroides was found. The positive isolates for aspergillus proved to be due to laboratory contamination.

The records of blood cultures for fungus at the National Institutes of Health from 1962 to 1972 were reviewed by Young and associates (90). All of 6 positive antemortem blood cultures were proved to be contaminants when aspergillosis was not found in any of the patients at autopsy.

We believe that a positive culture from any body fluid, even from a space not normally connected to the outside, strongly suggests evidence of invasive infection in the compromised host; however, culture alone does not constitute definitive evidence.

Serologic tests have not been useful in the diagnosis of invasive aspergillosis (91, 146). When Young and Bennett (129) obtained serum late in the course of disease from 16 patients, 12 of whom had acute leukemia and all of whom had proved invasive aspergillosis, no differences were found between infected and control groups by a variety of tests for antibody. Negative tests or low antibody titers were commonly found. Gurwith and co-workers (131) reported 5 cardiac transplant patients with proved invasive disease in whom precipitins were found in only one. Coleman and Kaufman (147) reported that 14 of 16 patients with invasive aspergillosis had positive precipitins; however, it is not clear that the diagnosis of invasive disease was proved in most of the patients.

In another report of pulmonary infection in cancer patients, Bardana and co-workers (148) surveyed a variety of immunologic techniques for demonstrating antibody in the serum of 79 patients with pulmonary aspergillosis. In their hands, immunodiffusion to demonstrate precipitins was the most valuable test in the invasive or disseminated form of the disease, with positive tests in 4 of 7 sera. Only one of 5 serum samples from patients with invasive aspergillosis had antibodies detectable by specific complement fixing techniques. An increased concentration of complement component C3 was also noted in patients with locally invasive or disseminated disease (148). Recently, Schaefer and co-workers (149) published the results of an *A. fumigatus* immunodiffusion test performed every 2 weeks for 1 year in 80 patients with acute leukemia. In 10 patients proved to have invasive aspergillosis, 6 converted from negative to positive by this test, and a seventh patient had a change from weakly positive to strongly positive.

The test appeared to be specific in cases in which this could be evaluated, but further study is required.

Aspergillus has also been reported to take up strontium during lung scans with this material (150, 151). The clinical usefulness of this procedure has not been determined.

Prevention and treatment. A primary concern with regard to this infection should be prevention. In accordance with data previously mentioned in this paper, hospital epidemics of aspergillosis should be investigated, and contamination of air, possibly due to contamination of air ducts, should be considered. Patients should also be warned against contact with pigeons. The efficacy of these procedures, however, is unclear.

Determinations of the MIC of amphotericin B for aspergillus species have varied in different reports, probably due to different methodology. Brandsberg and French (152) found an MIC range of 0.14 to 0.60 μg per ml against 21 clinical isolates of *A. fumigatus*. Howarth and associates (153) reported an MIC of 0.5 μg per ml against one strain of *A. niger* and one of *A. fumigatus* in the mycelial phase; however, the minimal fungicidal concentrations were 10 μg per ml and 5 μg per ml, respectively. Fields and co-workers (154) tested 7 patient-isolates of aspergillus species from clinical material and reported MICs of 1 μg per ml for 2 isolates and 2 μg per ml for 5 isolates. Carrizosa and associates (155) reported an isolate of *A. ustus* from a case of aspergillus endocarditis with an MIC of 12.5 μg per ml. Abernathy (99) has reported an MIC of amphotericin against aspergillus species of 6.25 μg per ml.

The susceptiblity to 5-fluorocytosine in different reports has ranged from zero to 100 per cent (43, 156–158). These differences probably also represent differences in technique and method.

Results of therapy. Although rare spontaneous resolution of invasive aspergillosis has been reported in the normal host (159, 160), to our knowledge this has not occurred in the compromised host. Results of treatment of patients with lymphoma and leukemia have not been encouraging, but data are meager. Seven patients treated with amphotericin B in one study did not survive longer than control untreated patients (49). Young and co-workers (110) reported a study of 14 patients, of whom 11 received the drug in the last 6 days of life. No therapeutic benefit was evident in this group. One patient received a dose of 486 mg during 2 weeks. Slight improvement was noted, but death resulted eventually from progressive, disseminated infection. Another patient received 2 g during 6 weeks. Four months later, after death from bacterial infection, hyphae were still demonstrable in the lung. In a study of 14 patients, Meyer and associates (128) concluded that administration of amphotericin B had no discernible effect on the outcome of the disease. Burke and Coltman (139) described a patient who developed multiple aspergillomas during remission induction for acute myelogenous leukemia; this patient received 435 mg of amphotericin B in addition to nystatin by aerosol, with improvement and survival. The original lung damage, however, might not have been due to aspergillosis, and the patient achieved concurrent remission of the leukemia. In uncompromised hosts, spontaneous lysis of fungus balls has been reported in 10 per cent of patients (161). Finally, Gercovich and co-workers (162) described a man with acute progranulocytic leukemia who developed bilateral patchy pulmonary densities in both upper lobes with biopsy-proved *A. niger* in a necrotic leg lesion and culture-proved hepatic involvement, all of which cleared after 3 weeks of granulocyte transfusions, achievement of complete remission, and administration of 1.6 g of amphotericin B. Schaefer and co-workers (149) recently described 4 patients with documented aspergillosis who responded to early therapy with amphotericin B. Three achieved a complete remission of their leukemia; the other, partial remission. Further details are not given with regard to clinical course, amount of therapy, or follow-up.

The use of 5-fluorocytosine has not been well investigated in the compromised host. Atkinson and Israel (163) reported favorable results, whereas Fields and co-workers (164) reported lack of success using this drug. In these patients, however, the diagnosis of invasive disease is not beyond question, and the patients were not compromised hosts. We believe that there is currently no defined role for the use of 5-fluorocytosine in the treatment of invasive aspergillosis.

In contrast to the poor results in patients with lymphoma and leukemia, the results of treatment of invasive pulmonary infection in heart and kidney transplant patients receiving immunosuppressive therapy have been more encouraging. Control of disease and even clinical cures have been reported in this population, and administration of amphotericin B for 1 year or more may play a significant role (118, 131). Further study of aspergillosis, especially when definitively diagnosed by aggressive procedures early in the clinical course, is needed to evaluate further the role of amphotericin B therapy, particularly in patients with lymphoma and leukemia.

Phycomycetes

Phycomycosis is defined as the invasion of tissue by any genus of the class, *Phycomycetes*. In culture-positive cases, the genera, *Rhizopus* and *Mucor,* have almost always been the causal agents in patients with leukemia and lymphoma. Occasionally, infection has been produced by the genera, *Absidia, Mortierella,* and *Basidiobolus* (164). In the compromised patient, it is assumed that phycomycosis is an exogenous infection acquired primarily by inhalation, with the lungs being the initial site of invasion. The only clearly defined exception to this is the occasional rhinocerebral infection in this group of patients. Spores of phycomycetes are small enough to be deposited in the lower respiratory tract (115). Occasional rhizopus and mucor have been isolated from outside air or ward air in hospitals (114, 115, 165). This suggests the possibility of nosocomial infection in some cases. From 3,729 patients, most of whom had chronic lung diseases, Kahanpää (39) isolated rhizopus only 5 times and mucor only twice from sputum. Rhizopus was found in 3 per cent of sputum specimens from normal men (119). Therefore, the organism does not appear to be a saprophyte.

Immunopathologic aspects. The lack of information in the literature concerning mechanisms of resistance to this infection makes a meaningful discussion of individual factors predisposing to infection impossible. In a review of experimental fungal infections, acidosis was reported to be a significant predisposing factor in the experimental animal (166). A high concentration of glucose did not affect the growth of phycomycetes *in vitro* or *in vivo* in the rabbit. Corticosteroid administration did not significantly worsen rhizopus infection in mice, rats, or guinea pigs. By contrast, in a recent report, cortisone did increase the mortality rate in mice infected with absidia (167). These discrepant results may be partly due to differences in experimental design. Reticuloendothelial blockade also increased mortality. Treatment with azathioprine, cyclophosphamide, and antithymocyte serum did not increase susceptibility to infec-

tion, suggesting that cell-mediated immunity may not play a significant role in resistance to the experimental infection. Phagocytic cells were considered to be the most significant defense mechanism.

Bartrum and co-workers (168) found 69 cases of phycomycosis with pulmonary involvement in the literature to 1973. In 62 cases, an underlying disease was present, and only one case occurred in a patient who was known to be definitely healthy. Underlying diseases included leukemia in 36 cases, diabetes mellitus in 14 cases, Hodgkin's disease in 2, and severe uremia in 2. Meyer and associates (169) reported 26 cases of phycomycosis in patients with leukemia or lymphoma, some of whom also had diabetes. Seventeen of the 26 patients had acute leukemia that was in relapse with leukopenia. Fourteen of the 26 had diabetes, although in general, it was well controlled. No case of diabetic acidosis was described. Two of 26 had acidosis due to renal failure. All of the 26 patients had received antimicrobial drugs, and 25 had received corticosteroids. Beathard and associates (170) described a patient in renal failure treated with antilymphocyte globulin and lymphocyte depletion by chronic thoracic duct lymph drainage who also had decreased IgM concentrations and who developed extensive pulmonary phycomycosis. These data emphasize that only a generalization can be made with regard to predisposing factors, namely, that pulmonary and disseminated phycomycosis occur only in the seriously compromised host.

Pathologic features. The pathologic features of this infection were summarized by Meyer and associates (169). They noted that infarction secondary to invasion of blood vessels in the lung is the hallmark of pulmonary phycomycosis. On gross examination, the involved areas were often dark red and usually firm, with occasional areas of yellow discoloration. If the lesion extended to the pleural surface, a fibrinous exudate was present. Of 16 lesions believed to be predominantly infarcts, 6 were solitary. Microscopically, the zones of infarction often had diffuse hemorrhage, and hyphae of phycomyces were seen growing in and through blood vessels and extending into the lung parenchyma. The hyphae are characteristically broad and nonseptate. Occlusion of these vessels was due either to massive growth of fungi or to thrombus formation superimposed on the mass of hyphae. In this series of compromised patients, areas of infarction generally did not have an inflammatory reaction or "elements of bronchopneumonia and abscess formation." Bronchopneumonia, however, was seen, and in one case was bilateral. Phycomycotic lesions did not occur in areas of pulmonary involvement by leukemia or lymphoma. In only one of their cases was pulmonary infection caused by more than one organism (in combination with aspergillus). Bartrum and co-workers (168) described pathologic findings in 21 cases of pulmonary phycomycosis gathered from the literature to 1973 (168). In all of their cases, pulmonary vascular thrombosis and infarction were found. Extensive pulmonary infection with consolidation and cavitation were also seen (168). A solitary pulmonary nodule due to phycomycosis has also been described (171). In that case, histologic study showed an ischemic pulmonary infarct due to arterial invasion and occlusion by the fungus. Giant cells, eosinophils, and lymphocytes have been seen occasionally in lesions that are a mixture of mild inflammation and infarction (170).

Clinical manifestations. In contrast to the frequent nasopharyngeal involvement in diabetics, patients with leukemia and lymphoma with phycomycosis most commonly have involvement of the lungs. The reason for these characteristic locations is unknown (27, 44, 49, 169, 172, 173).

Meyer and co-workers (169) reported 21 cases of pulmonary phycomycosis in patients with leukemia and lymphoma. Findings were often nonspecific. Three patients had symptoms suggestive of pulmonary infarction and complained of pleural pain. Hemoptysis was observed in one patient with pleural involvement, as well as in another with bronchopneumonia. Pleural rubs were heard in several patients. The clinical picture was otherwise unremarkable, most commonly consisting of persistent fever and pulmonary infiltration that was unresponsive to antimicrobial drug therapy. In 2 patients, fungus balls developed. The clinical picture, therefore, is similar to that seen with pulmonary aspergillosis, and histologic or cultural data must be used to separate the 2 entities. Unfortunately, sputum cultures are rarely positive (169).

In patients without leukemia, leukocytosis, with a shift to the left, is frequently seen; however, in general, laboratory values are not helpful.

Bartrum and associates (168) described the radiologic features of 13 cases of pulmonary phycomycosis and emphasized that the radiographic picture is nonspecific. The radiographic picture was an "infiltrate" in 5 cases, a "patchy" or nonhomogeneous infiltrate in 4 cases, and consolidation in 3 cases. In 4 patients, a cavity was seen. One pleural effusion was noted. Among their own 6 cases, they found consolidation in 5. Meyer and co-workers (169) described chest radiographic abnormalities associated with progressive phycomycosis in 10 patients. Patchy infiltrates were seen in 4, bronchopneumonia in 2, consolidation in one, and consolidation with pleural effusion in another. Cavitation was seen in 2 patients, with fungus ball formation in one. Bartrum and associates (168) noted that the distribution of infection in the lung was random; for example, the right and left lower lobes were involved in 4 cases each; the right upper lobe in 3; and the left lower lobe in 2. In at least 5 of 12 cases, more than one lobe was involved. It has been stated that individual lesions tend to be larger, and roentgenologic progression faster, in pulmonary phycomycosis than in aspergillosis or nocardiosis (142). It must also be remembered that a negative chest radiograph does not exclude pulmonary phycomycosis (49).

Fever was present in 17 of 21 patients with pulmonary phycomycosis reviewed by Meyer and associates (169). Five of these had severe concurrent bacterial infections. Concurrent infections have been frequently observed by others (22, 44, 174). Dissemination of infection from a pulmonary focus occurred in 11 of 21 patients with pulmonary phycomycosis (169). Spleen, kidney, brain, and heart were the organs most frequently involved.

Diagnosis. The definitive diagnosis of pulmonary phycomycosis requires the demonstration of characteristic broad, nonseptate hyphae in lung tissue. With regard to cultures, phycomyces have been isolated ante mortem only rarely in other than rhino-orbital infection. In fact, it should be stressed that negative cultures are the overwhelming rule in this infection. Bodey (49) reported one leukemic patient with a positive blood culture for rhizopus, but the organism was considered to be a contaminant. At autopsy, a phycomycotic infarction of the appendix was found. Medoff and Kobayashi (175) describe a patient with acute lymphocytic leukemia and pulmonary phycomycosis in whom cultures of sputum and lung biopsy material yielded the organism. In contrast, Meyer and co-workers (169) not only did not isolate the fungus during life from 26 patients with phycomycosis, even by examining multiple cultures of sputum, blood, urine, and cerebrospinal fluid, but also did not culture it from tissue from 13 autopsy patients. As stated above previously, the diagnosis is established by demonstration of the hyphae in tissue. Invasive techniques must be used to obtain pulmonary tissue if an antemortem diagnosis is to be made (68, 112, 169, 176). Demonstration of the fungus by stain of material obtained by needle aspirate probably suffices to make the diagnosis, even though intact lung tissue is not seen.

In a case with pleural effusion, the organism was cultured from pleural fluid (177). Thoracentesis and culture should therefore be attempted when pleural fluid is present. Skin lesions resulting from hematogenous dissemination have also been described in a patient (at autopsy), suggesting that the antemortem diagnosis might be made by biopsy of skin lesions (178).

Prevention and treatment. With the possible exception of the control of diabetes mellitus or acidosis in cases in which they coexist with phycomycosis, to our knowledge no suggestions have been made with regard to prevention of this infection.

Because antemortem diagnosis of pulmonary phycomycosis has been uncommon, few data exist with regard to therapy. Amphotericin B should be used. Howarth and co-workers (155) found that the MIC of amphotericin B against 5 strains of rhizopus was 0.5 μg per ml; against a strain of mucor, 0.1 μg per ml. Similarly, Medoff and Kobayashi (175) found an MIC of 0.1 μg per ml against an isolate of mucor. Medoff and Kobayashi (175) also described the successful treatment of a patient with acute lymphocytic leukemia and pulmonary mucormycosis treated with approximately 1.2 g of amphotericin B. Bogard (179) reported the cure of a patient with hypogammaglobulinemia and pulmonary mucormycosis by the administration of 570 mg of amphotericin B. The diagnosis in this case was made by positive sputum culture alone. Lombardi and associates (177) described a patient with absidiosis involving the right lung base and right pleural cavity who died despite antemortem diagnosis and treatment with amphotericin B (total dose unknown). The MIC of amphotericin B against the organism was greater than 50 μg per ml, suggesting to Lombardi and associates (177) that adequate doses of amphotericin B could not be delivered to the patient. Surgical removal of involved tissue in cases in which this is possible may be helpful (168). Surgical resection of isolated lung tissue has been performed in diabetic patients, with

survival (180). Surgical treatment of other localized infections has also been stressed (181). Except, perhaps, in the rhinocerebral form, and in cases in which traditional surgical therapy of accessible abscesses is indicated, the precise role of surgery in dealing with the infection in the compromised host is not well defined.

It should be stressed that an adequate study of amphotericin B (with or without other ancillary measures) in the treatment of early and definitively diagnosed pulmonary phycomycosis in the compromised host has not yet been published.

No clinical data exist with regard to the use of 5-fluorocytosine alone in the treatment of pulmonary phycomycosis. The agent was not useful in a murine model (182). Hammer and associates (183) tested an isolate of *Rhizopus arrhizus* isolated from a case of phycomycosis in a transplant recipient, as well as 2 other isolates of *R. arrhizus* that had been recovered from infections in patients with diabetes; all were "highly resistant" to 5-fluorocytosine. No synergy could be demonstrated on addition of amphotericin B. At this time, therefore, 5-fluorocytosine does not appear to be useful in the treatment of phycomycosis.

Candida albicans

Candidiasis is defined as the invasion of viable tissue by any species of the genus *Candida*. *C. albicans* is the most common species responsible for invasive infection in the compromised host.

C. albicans is found in the mouth and gastrointestinal tract of most normal humans (120). It is also found on the skin in hospitalized patients, particularly those with skin disease (184, 185). In patients with chronic bronchopulmonary disorders (39) and in markedly debilitated patients (186), it may be found in the tracheobronchial tree. Candidiasis, therefore, has generally been assumed to be an endogenous infection. In contrast, other species of candida, such as *C. tropicalis* and *C. parapsilosis,* are found in soil and water, as well as in human hosts (187).

The finding of *C. albicans* and other yeasts at sites in the patient during hospitalization where none had been found on hospital admission suggests that they may occasionally be acquired during hospitalization, from person-to-person spread or by means of fomites (185, 188, 189). In this regard, it is of interest that *C. albicans* was cultured from the fingers of 17 per cent of healthy medical students (190). *C. albicans* has been cultured from 3 per cent of samples of hospital air (115), a finding of uncertain epidemiologic significance. Further epidemiologic study awaits a method of subgrouping these yeasts, so that organisms acquired from the external environment can be differentiated from those compromising the patient's initial flora.

Immunopathologic aspects. Initial studies by Louria and Brayton (191) in 1964 indicated that polymorphonuclear leukocytes in whole blood were able to phagocytose *C. albicans;* but in 40 to 70 per cent of the cells, pseudohyphae were growing after incubation for 4 hours. This led Louria and Brayton (191) to question the effectiveness of the polymorphonuclear leukocyte as a defense mechanism against candida. Subsequent studies, however, have established that circulating human polymorphonuclear leukocytes, monocytes, and eosinophils can kill candida *in vitro* under carefully defined conditions (192–196). Killing of candida by neutrophils and monocytes apparently can occur by at least 2 mechanisms. The first is dependent on the myeloperoxidase-halide-hydrogen peroxide system and the other, which seems important primarily against species of candida other than *C. albicans,* is independent of that system (194, 197).

Suggestive *in vivo* evidence of the importance of the polymorphonuclear leukocyte in defense against *C. albicans* is the common occurrence of deep-seated candidiasis in patients with severe neutropenia and the occasional occurrence in patients whose polymorphonuclear leukocytes have been shown to have impaired candidacidal activity, e.g., the neutrophil defects of chronic granulomatous disease and myeloperoxidase deficiency (196, 198). Defective candidacidal activity has also been demonstrated in patients with advanced Hodgkin's disease, acute leukemia, and metastatic cancer who were undergoing chemotherapy, suggesting that defects in cellular function, as well as neutropenia, may be important in acquisition of candidal infection in these severely compromised hosts (199). The published evidence that granulocyte transfusions do not appear to be beneficial in treating established deep-seated candidiasis in patients with severe neutropenia does not exclude the granulocyte as an important defense mechanism in this infection.

The role of serum factors in resistance to invasive candida infection is not well established. Factors necessary for optimal phagocytosis of candida *in vitro* are found in normal human serum and are both specific (absorbable) and nonspecific (heat labile) (58, 196). Dobias (200) used a candida cell wall extract to produce specific immunity to candida infection. The resistance produced by this immunizing procedure was assumed to be due to specific antibody, but this was not demonstrated. He also reviewed prior reports claiming passive transfer of specific immunity with serum. In this regard, it is of interest that Laforce and co-workers (201) found suppression of killing of candida by normal polymorphonuclear leukocytes, as tested *in vitro* in the presence of serum specimens from 7 patients with disseminated candidiasis. An anti-candida IgG antibody was considered by Laforce and associates (201) to be a possible cause of this defect. Abnormal phagolysosomes containing yeast forms were noted in polymorphonuclear leukocytes in these experiments and were believed possibly to be related to the candidacidal defect. Thus, proposals have been made that specific antibody may be contributory or detrimental to host resistance.

Studies have been performed in an attempt to define the importance of specific cell-mediated immunity in defense against candida infection (excluding the syndrome of mucocutaneous candidiasis). Pearsall and Lagunoff (202), in a murine model, found that transfer of immune lymphoid cells did not protect against *C. albicans* infection; however, it has also recently been shown in the mouse, that nonspecific stimulation of the cellular immune system with bacille Calmette-Guérin and *C. parvum* appears to prolong survival after intravenous candidal challenge (203). These agents induce a population of activated macrophages (the effector arm of cellular resistance to microorganisms), and it is therefore possible that such macrophages have a role in defense of the host against candida. In this regard, it is of interest that lymphokines from stimulated lymphocytes were shown to be able to kill *C. albicans in vitro* (204). The clinical significance of these data is unclear.

Studies have also been undertaken to investigate the function of the reticuloendothelial system in defense against *C. albicans* infection. Increased reticuloendothelial phagocytic activity in response to *C. albicans* was demonstrated in a murine model by Bird and Sheagren (205). Baine and associates (206) showed that candida injected intravenously into rabbits was rapidly removed from the bloodstream by the lung when the yeast was injected into a peripheral vein, and by the liver when the injection was into a mesenteric vein. When candida was inoculated into the isolated perfused liver, organisms were found in polymorphonuclear leukocytes, as well as in Kupffer cells, suggesting that both cell types might be responsible for clearance of this organism. Furthermore, a rapid decrease in the polymorphonuclear leukocyte count was seen within minutes after challenge with *C. albicans in vivo*, suggesting to Baine and co-workers (206) that phagocytosis of candida by these cells and subsequent sequestration might have occurred. Stanley and Hurley (207) showed that mouse peritoneal macrophages readily phagocytosed *C. albicans in vitro*. Within 2 hours, however, 95 percent of the ingested yeast formed had pseudohyphae, with subsequent destruction of the macrophages. Destruction of macrophages after phagocytosis was also noted with other species of candida. Ozato and Vesaka (208) confirmed the ability of *C. albicans* to multiply within mouse peritoneal macrophages, leading to the destruction of the macrophages. The ability of macrophages activated nonspecifically *in vivo* to enhance resistance to candida infection has been studied, but the results are not clear cut. In one study, nonspecific activation of macrophages in mice was shown to provide some protection against subsequent challenge with *C. albicans* (209).

Morelli and Rosenberg (210) noted that mice deficient in complement were more susceptible to candida infection. *In vitro,* antibody and complement together were not fungicidal.

A variety of factors appear to increase the host's susceptibility to infection with candida or to increase the severity of disease. Using a guinea pig model to compare the effects of short- and long-acting corticosteroids, Hurley and co-workers (211) found that whereas short-acting glucocorticoids did not lead to an increased death rate due to candidiasis or increased renal colony counts of candida and did not affect the development or expression of immunity, long-acting corticosteroids led to an increased mortality rate and increased colony counts in renal and other tissues, as well as suppression of existing cellular immunity. The development of cellular immunity to candida, however, was not impaired. These studies in the guinea pig, which perhaps more closely relate to man in terms of response to steroids than does the murine model, provide some experimental evidence concerning the role of immunosuppression in increased susceptibility to this infection. This association is underscored in the clinical literature.

Intravenous catheters also predispose to candida infection (44, 212–215). The precise mechanism by which catheters lead to candidemia is unclear. They may act as conduits from skin to bloodstream or a site of colonization during transient candidemia. Mucosal lesions in the gastrointestinal tract increase the risk of infection with candida. Such lesions might be due to an underlying malignancy or to chemotherapeutic drugs. Steinberg and co-workers (216) demonstrated invasion of the blood vessels in the wall of the ileum by candida in a patient with leukemia with necrotizing enterocolitis. Myerowitz and associates (217), examining 24 patients with disseminated infection (18 of whom had acute leukemia), found that all had invasive gastrointestinal tract candidiasis. This suggested that the initial portal of entry might have been the gastrointestinal tract. It has also been shown that antimicrobial drugs lead to the overgrowth of *C. albicans* in the gastrointestinal tract and on the skin (185, 218, 219). The mechanism by which overgrowth relates to or predisposes to deep-seated infection with *C. albicans* has not been established.

Although some cases of pulmonary candidiasis may be secondary to aspiration (214), it may be impossible to exclude hematogenous dissemination as the mechanism of delivery of the organism to the lung in the compromised host.

Pathologic features. Ramirez and co-workers (220) described apparent *C. albicans* bronchopneumonia in a patient not known to be immunosuppressed. At autopsy, many "nodular and whitish infiltrates" were found in both lungs. Typical budding yeast-like cells and pseudohyphae were seen within the nodules. Fungal elements were mixed with an acute inflammatory exudate (220). *C. albicans* was recovered in pure culture. In a patient with probable candida pneumonia, Lau and associates (221) noted diffuse pulmonary inflammation consisting of neutrophils and some histiocytes. Pseudohyphae, as well as yeast forms, were seen in bronchioles, alveolar ducts, and, occasionally, in alveoli. Law and co-workers (222) noted large colonies of pseudohyphae and yeast forms in pulmonary candida abscesses in burn patients. Louria and associates (214) found lung involvement in 9 of 19 patients dying with disseminated candidiasis in whom autopsies were performed. Bronchopneumonia was noted in some lungs, with neutrophils, edema fluid, and the yeast form and pseudohyphae in bronchioles and alveoli. In other cases, the pulmonary parenchyma appeared to be invaded from thrombosed blood vessels containing candida, suggesting that the infection was due to a hematogenous dissemination, although thrombosis occurring in an already infected areas, with subsequent invasion of the thrombosed vessel by candida, cannot be excluded. Similar thrombotic disease has been described by others (223).

Clinical manifestations. Pulmonary infection with candida in the normal host has been reported in 2 cases (220, 224). Both patients were predisposed to aspiration pneumonia. Symptoms included tachypnea, chills, and fever, and physical findings included rhonchi, crepitant rales, and cyanosis.

Within the compromised population, candida pulmonary infection has been described complicating acute leukemia (23, 49, 214), after renal allografts (72, 132), and in patients with extensive burns, lupus erythematosus, and diabetes mellitus (214, 222). The lung is among the organs most frequently involved in disseminated infection (44, 49) and is probably most frequently infected in this manner in the compromised host. Severe tracheobronchitis, bronchopneumonia, and pulmonary abscess formation have been reported. Hart and co-workers (44), in a survey of fungal infection in the compromised host, found 5 cases of candidiasis involving only the lung, all confirmed at autopsy. Sickles and associates (23) observed that extremely extensive pneumonia was caused by this agent in acute leukemia. An average of 3.6 lobes were involved per case, but few symptoms or signs were noted, although rales have been described (221). The chest radiograph showed an abnormality suggesting pneumonia in 96 per cent of 52 cases of pneumonia in acute leukemia, of which 12 were believed to be due to candida (23). Bodey (49), on the other hand, initially found no evidence of pulmonary disease in 46 per cent of radiographs at the onset of candida infection involving the lungs in leukemic patients. Approximately one half of the patients, however, subsequently developed abnormal radiographs. He also noted that the candida pulmonary infections in his series frequently (28 per cent) occurred after resolution of a previous bacterial pneumonia. Mills and co-workers (72) described the onset of an extensive cavitary candida bronchopneumonia in a renal transplant patient who was undergoing therapy for threatened rejection with prednisone and azathioprine. Law and associates (222) found candidal abscesses in the lungs of 53 per cent of burn patients dying with disseminated candidiasis (222). Gaines and Remington (225) found involvement of the lung in 12 of 33 surgical patients with systemic candidiasis. Most were immunosuppressed.

Because of the lack of a characteristic clinical picture, because early miliary abscesses may be minute and difficult to appreciate on chest radiographs, and because of other difficulties in diagnosis (to be discussed), candida is often discovered only at autopsy (72). Clearly, if an antemortem diagnosis is to be definitively established, more than a chest roentgenogram is required.

Diagnosis. The most reliable criterion for the definitive diagnosis of pulmonary candidiasis is histologic demonstration of the fungus in otherwise viable lung tissue. Diagnosis on the basis of positive culture from material taken anywhere in the respiratory tree is unreliable. The isolation of candida from 20 per cent of specimens of lung tissue obtained at biopsy or surgery in patients with chronic lung disease not due to candida emphasizes this fact (39). Candida has also been cultured from lung at autopsy without antecedent clinically consistent disease or histiologic evidence of invasion of tissue (226). The value of the demonstration of candida pseudohyphae in sputum, as distinct from the presence only of yeast forms, as evidence of tissue invasion has also been questioned (227, 228). Even the results of transtracheal aspiration can be questioned in the patient with oral thrush, in whom a positive result may represent colonization from the upper airway (224). In this situation, a specific diagnosis of invasive pulmonary candidiasis may require collection of pulmonary tissue by aspiration (224) or open lung biopsy. Even so, only the latter may fulfill the criterion for definitive diagnosis set forth in the beginning of this section, because the former does not provide intact lung tissue for histologic preparation. A positive culture of lung aspirate when skin contamination is excluded may be an indication for starting therapy.

Cultures of candida from abscess material, pleural fluid, or peritoneal fluid when inflammation is present and contamination by skin or surgical drains is absolutely excluded establishes the diagnosis of candidal infection (44).

The presence of candida in the urine is abnormal. Because the kidney is a very common site for metastatic infection during candidemia, the finding of candida in a clean-catch, midstream urine specimen in the absence of an indwelling bladder catheter may suggest the presence of renal candidiasis. In contrast, candiduria in the presence of an indwelling bladder catheter is common and may represent harmless colonization promulgated by the foreign body. If a catheter is in place, however, candiduria is of value in the diagnosis of renal candidiasis if the same species of candida is found in the blood sampled before (or at the same time as) the candiduria. In general, a positive culture of candida from any site in an immunocompromised patient should never be ignored and should be a signal for the consideration of further diagnostic studies.

Because, as stated previously, the lung is a common site of metastatic infection, it is important to discuss the significance of candidemia. Candidemia may be benign, may lead to invasive candidiasis, or may result from established, deep-seated infection. In the presence of an indwelling venous catheter, candidemia, even when associated with fever, may be transient and benign (44, 90, 229–31).

Although benign candidemia occurs in compromised patients, candidemia frequently indicates significant, frequently rapidly fatal infection in this population (44). Young and co-workers (90), studying 48 patients with cancer in whom candidemia was noted, found that only 23 per cent had transient, benign candidemia (90). Clearly, in this setting, candidemia often is evidence of or will lead to invasive disease. Therefore, it should be emphasized that a positive blood culture for candida (although not a reliable diagnostic criterion for deep-seated infection) may be an indication for starting antifungal therapy in a compromised patient who is seriously ill.

It should be clearly understood that negative blood cultures do not exclude the diagnosis of deep-seated candidiasis. In 3 separate autopsy series of patients with acute leukemia and deep-seated candidiasis, blood cultures were negative in 100 per cent (22), 75 per cent (49), and 62 per cent (217). In contrast, in a study of burn patients with disseminated disease documented at autopsy, only 21 per cent had negative antemortem blood cultures. Recently, suggestions have been made to improve the yield of positive cultures (232, 233). Other diagnostic studies that, if positive for candida, provide definitive evidence of the presence of disseminated infection, are biopsy of characteristic skin lesions (20, 234), liver biopsy (217), and ophthalmologic examination, showing eye lesions typified by white, fluffy exudative lesions in the chorioretina, often accompanied by an overlying vitreous haze (235, 236). Involvement of the anterior chamber of the eye is frequent (236), and the organism has been grown from aspirates of aqueous humor (105, 237).

With regard to serologic tests, interpretation of serologic data in patients stated in the literature to have invasive candidasis is difficult. Different antigenic preparations have been used, and the criteria for the diagnosis of invasive infection have often not been rigorous. As elaborated subsequently, none of the serologic methods used at present provides diagnostic information in the absence of other evidence of infection.

Agglutinating antibodies do not appear to be specific (227–240). The precipitin test for antibody appears to be the procedure of choice.

False-negative precipitin tests have been found in zero to 20 per cent of patients with candidiasis (227, 238, 239, 241–243). Increasing sensitivity in these tests may decrease specificity (241). The reason for the false-negative results is unknown, but reflects very early disease or the inability of the compromised host to produce antibodies against candidal challenge. False-positive precipitin tests determined by the immunodiffusion method have ranged from zero to 20 per cent in a wide variety of patient and subject types (238–244). Using counterimmunoelectrophoresis, Remington and associates (245) found no false-positive results in patients undergoing general surgery; however, Dee and Rytel (241) found 63 per cent false-positive results in patients with candida colonization or transient candidemia and 14 per cent in normal subjects using this method (241). Titering the sera proved useful in dealing with this problem; they concluded that a counterimmunoelectrophoresis titer $\geq$1:8 provided satisfactory presumptive evidence for significant candida. We have drawn similar conclusions from our experience. Recently, Marier and Andriole (246) found antibody by counterimmunoelectrophoresis in 20 per cent of control patients, 48 per cent of patients colonized with candida, and 52 per cent of patients infected with yeast; however, significant increase in antibody by counterimmunoelectrophoresis occurred in 0.03 per cent of control patients, none of the patients colonized with C. albicans, and 62 per cent of patients infected with candida, including all with disseminated infection. Weiner and co-workers (247) recently described a hemagglutination inhibition assay for mannan, a surface polysaccharide of candida. Mannan antigenemia was detected in 4 of 14 patients early in the course of systemic candidiasis and in 2 of 5 patients with invasive gastrointestinal candidiasis, but in only 3 of 234 control sera and in none of 49 patients with noninvasive candida infections or other systemic mycotic infections, indicating good specificity but only fair sensitivity. Gas-liquid chromatography of serum from patients with candidemia has recently been reported to give a characteristic pattern (248). Sera from 2 of 4 patients with invasive, but not widely disseminated, candidiasis were positive, whereas blood cultures were negative. The test reportedly detected circulating components of the yeast cell. These preliminary results are promising, and more data are needed. Sensitive and specific serologic tests for candida antigen and antibody are essential if blood culture–negative invasive candidiasis is to be diagnosed antemortem.

Clearly, at this time, a positive serologic test should increase the index of suspicion of the disease, but is not, by itself, an indication for treatment. That decision must be based on the total clinical picture. As previously discussed, further diagnostic studies are needed to establish the specific etiology of pulmonary involvement in these patients.

Treatment. Pulmonary candidiasis in the compromised host should be considered a metastatic focus of infection from hematogenous dissemination and should be treated as a life-threatening infection. Amphotericin B should be administered immediately, and time should not be wasted building up from small initial doses (182).

Candidemia, on the other hand, does not necessarily reflect deep-seated infection. Immediate therapy in patients with candidemia may be withheld (*1*) if the patient's condition is not deteriorating rapidly clinically; (*2*) if there is no evidence of deep-seated invasion, such as endophthalmitis, biopsy-positive skin lesions, candiduria in the absence of bladder catheter, or, possibly, positive candida precipitins; (*3*) if there is an indwelling venous catheter in place; and (*4*) if candidemia resolves within 2 or 3 days after removal of the catheter. Even if all 4 criteria for the diagnosis of benign, catheter-related candidemia are met, however, there is no assurance that the transient episode of candidemia did not produce a deep-seated focus (44, 249). Thus, prolonged follow-up is required to exclude the latter event.

Amphotericin B

The MIC of amphotericin B of most strains of candida has ranged from 0.5 μg per ml to as low as 0.02 μg per ml (99, 153, 215, 231). Higher values have also been reported, ranging from 0.4 to 3 μg per ml (98, 250). The significance of the higher values is unclear. To our knowledge, there is only one report in the literature of amphotericin B resistance developing during therapy of candidiasis (251).

The total dose of amphotericin B that should be used to treat candidiasis in the compromised host is not known. It is of note that Taschdjian and associates (227) reported that, at autopsy, intracellular candida organisms were seen in 2 patients with acute leukemia (of 2 years' duration in one, 3 months in the other) after apparent recovery from systemic infection (227). The question of lifelong therapy with amphotericin B in patients with invasive candidasis receiving immunosuppressive therapy must be raised. On the other hand, using clinical criteria for diagnosis (in conjunction with candidemia), rather than demonstration of the organism in tissue, Young and co-workers (90) treated 8 cancer patients who had cadidemia with amphotericin B. Duration of therapy ranged from 5 to 60 days, and contaminated intravenous catheters were removed from several patients. No patient had subsequent evidence of persistent candida infection. Hart and co-workers (44) also described a patient with multiple abdominal operations and candidemia who had no evidence of candidiasis at autopsy, although she had been given only 65 mg of amphotericin B. It is unclear whether these patients were "cured" with these low doses, or whether, in fact, they had invasive candidiasis.

5-Fluorocytosine

The role of 5-fluorocytosine in treatment of the compromised host with invasive candidiasis has not yet been determined (100). Resistance both de novo and emerging during treatment has been described and has been associated with therapeutic failures (252–254). Few data are available on treatment of candidiasis in the compromised host with this agent alone. Vandevelde and associates (255) described a patient with acute lymphocytic leukemia and candida meningitis considered cured after administration of 6 g of 5-fluorocytosine daily for 25 days. Failures have occurred (256). The combination of amphotericin B with 5-fluorocytosine has been used to treat deep mycoses. Synergism of amphotericin B and 5-fluorocytosine has been demonstrated (250, 257) for candida species, even with resistance to 5-fluorocytosine alone; however, the possibility of antagonism between the 2 drugs must also be considered (258). The ability of 5-fluorocytosine combined with amphotericin B, as opposed to amphotericin B alone to enhance survival in man with deep-seated candidiasis remains to be proved.

Miscellaneous Fungi

Histoplasma capsulatum

Chronic disseminated histoplasmosis is an infrequent pulmonary and systemic fungal infection in immunocompromised patients (49, 259, 260), even in endemic areas (75, 261). It has been reported in association with renal transplantation and lupus erythematosus as well as malignancy (49, 261). Signs and symptoms, if present, consist of nonproductive cough, respiratory distress, and in a patient with concurrent *P. carinii* infection, rales and pleuritic chest pain; but signs and symptoms are frequently minimal or absent (261). Chest radiographs have shown diffuse alveolar disease bilaterally in a miliary, granular, or confluent pattern (261), or "patchy" or reticulonodular infiltrates (49). Granulocytopenia, lymphocytopenia, corticosteroid therapy, and administration of antimicrobial drugs have not been shown to be correlated with the development of histoplasmosis in patients with acute leukemia (49). The diagnosis of histoplasmosis is based on microscopic or cultural demonstration of the organism (176), which may be present in sputum (49). Unfortunately, diagnostic pulmonary aspiration in children has been unsuccessful in many cases (261). Bone marrow culture has been more helpful (49, 261), and blood cultures have been positive (49). A positive complement fixation test to either yeast or mycelial phase antigen greater than 1:16 or an increasing titer is considered strong presumptive evidence of infection but is not definitive because of the occasional occurrence of false-positive results (91). With regard to therapy, the susceptibility of the organism to amphotericin B is well documented, the MIC being 0.5 μg per ml or less for 40 of 41 strains tested in 3 studies (66, 153, 262). Results of therapy in disseminated histoplasmosis were recently reviewed, although underlying diseases were not specified (99). Of 63 treated patients in 3 studies, 30 patients died; in 10 of

these (16 per cent of treated patients), the infection was considered to be the cause of death. Nine of the 10 had received less than 900 mg of amphotericin B. In another study, 2 patients with disseminated histoplasmosis and acute leukemia survived their infection. One was treated with amphotericin B and achieved remission of leukemia. The other was treated with a sulfonamide, and his leukemia was in remission throughout the infection (49). A recent study of disseminated histoplasmosis in 6 children with acute lymphocytic leukemia emphasized that the infection most commonly occurred during remission of leukemia. All children were treated with amphotericin B and recovered (261).

Coccidioides immitis

Pulmonary coccidioidomycosis may occasionally be seen in immunocompromised patients. Experience with this association at Stanford University Hospital and the pertinent literature have recently been reviewed and extensively discussed in a series of 13 cases, of which 6 had disseminated coccidioidomycosis (263). Three of these had Hodgkin's disease, one was post-renal transplantation, one had acute renal failure, and one had pemphigus vulgaris under treatment. Five of these 6 patients had radiographic evidence of fungal infection at some time during their illness, but 4 had this evidence only within 12 days of their death. Changes included localized or diffuse alveolar infiltrates, nodules, and pleural effusions, and progression was often very rapid. A patient with a stable pulmonary nodule, presumably due to the primary coccidioidomycosis, which was not exacerbated, despite irradiation and chemotherapy, was also presented. The data discussed make it clear that patients with prior infection with *C. immitis* are at risk of reactivation of a latent focus, although quantification of the risk, apparently small, is not currently possible. Dissemination may take place. The occurrence of complement fixing antibody in disseminated infection did not appear to be affected by immunosuppression, although the possibility of a blunted response occurred in one patient. The importance of the fact that the humoral immune response was preserved in disseminated infection in the compromised host was 2-fold. (1) The chest radiograph frequently revealed no evidence of active progressive infection until shortly before death, indicating that serologic tests may be the only way to establish the diagnosis and therefore should be performed in any person with a history of exposure who is a compromised host with a febrile illness. (2) It was suggested that in a compromised host known to have been previously exposed to or infected by *C. immitis* who develops a pulmonary infiltrate, an emergency serologic test, if positive, may avert the need for an invasive lung procedure, during which *C. immitis* may disseminate.

The need to consider coccidioidomycosis as a possible cause of severe infection in the compromised host who has been to an endemic area, and the need to use serologic tests for *C. immitis* freely in the evaluation of apparent infection in such a patient, have also been strongly emphasized by Pappagianis (264).

Blastomyces dermatitidis

Disseminated pulmonary blastomycosis has been reported in the compromised host (265). In one example (265) a 73-year-old man with lymphocytic lymphoma undergoing immunosuppressive therapy developed cough and sputum production. Rales were heard at both lung bases, and chest radiographs disclosed diffuse reticulonodular infiltrates. Sputum cultures yielded only normal respiratory flora. The diagnosis was made by demonstrating *B. dermatitidis* in bronchial brush and transbronchial lung biopsy specimens and was confirmed by culture. The infection was fulminant, and the patient died of acute respiratory failure before specific therapy could be instituted (265).

Torulopsis glabrata

T. glabrata is an opportunistic yeast that has been implicated in an increasing number of cases of pulmonary infection in immunocompromised patients (266–269). Because the organism is found in the normal human flora (188, 270), the problems involved in establishing the diagnosis of invasive infection are similar to those encountered with candida.

Penicillium

Reports of pulmonary infection caused by the opportunistic fungus, penicillium (271), in immunocompromised patients have appeared in the literature. Penicillium species caused pulmonary lesions in one heart transplant patient at Stanford University Hospital. These infections are extremely rare.

Bacteria

Nocardia

Nocardia asteroides is a gram-positive, nonmotile, frequently acid-fast bacterium that is an increasingly recognized cause of infection in the compromised host (272–277). Although more than 30 species of nocardia exist, the great majority of reported cases in compromised patients have been caused by *N. asteroides*. Nevertheless, some compromised hosts have been infected with *N. brasiliensis* (278). *N. farcinica* (279), and *N. caviae* (280). It is interest that *N. asteroides*, *N. caviae*, and *N. brasiliensis* have been reported to exhibit similar, although not identical, virulence during intraperitoneal infection in mice (281).

The respiratory tract is believed to be the usual site of entry of *N. asteroides*. This organism is present in the soil worldwide and may be inhaled. Other suggested mechanisms of entry to the body may be contaminated food or traumatic inoculation (282). Cox and Hughes (282) reported a cluster of 3 cases in a group of compromised hosts, including a patient with a laryngeal lesion (282). This raised the possibility of human-to-human transmission.

N. brasiliensis involves lymphocutaneous sites. Pulmonary disease with this species is often produced by penetration through the chest wall (283).

Immunopathologic aspects. Infection with nocardia has occurred in many settings, including chronic granulomatous disease of childhood (284), dysgammaglobulinemia (272, 275, 285), pulmonary alveolar proteinosis (286), in patients with neoplasia or connective tissue disease who are receiving immunosuppressive therapy (275, 283, 286–288), or after organ transplantation (132, 273, 276, 277, 289–291).

Disease in humans in association with the use of immunosuppressive therapy has been observed in renal transplant recipients. In some studies, a correlation has been noted between frequency of rejection requiring increased immunosuppression and development of nocardia infection (276). In a review of 243 cases of nocardiosis in the literature, 23 per cent had a history of prior corticosteroid therapy (286). An additional 17 per cent had immunologic impairment on the basis of their underlying disease (286). Forty-nine per cent had no recognizable underlying conditions, indicating that nocardiosis is not only an opportunistic infection. In fact, fulminant disease has occurred in patients with no known underlying disease (292).

The mechanisms of normal host defense against *N. asteroides* are not known. Circulating antibodies and delayed hypersensitivity have both been demonstrated in animals (293) and in humans (294, 295), but the roles of humoral and cellular immunity have not been established. In 1922, Nelson and Henrici (296) reported that serum from previously specifically vaccinated rabbits could transfer immunity to recipient animals, but these results remain to be confirmed. In 1974, Bourgeouis and Beaman (297) demonstrated that *N. asteroides* could remain viable within normal mouse peritoneal macrophages. Krick and Remington (298) showed that mice immunized with *N. asteroides* were resistant to homologous challenge (298). Although Krick and Remington (298) were unable to demonstrate the transfer of resistance by either serum or spleen cells, a population of activated macrophages was generated by nocardial infection, as evidenced by resistance of mice infected with nocardia to heterologous challenge with intracellular bacteria. The direct application of these animal data to human disease is not possible, but an important role for cell-mediated immunity in resistance to infection with nocardia is suggested.

Recent data from our laboratory suggest that neutrophils may be better able to phagocytose *N. asteroides in vitro* than are monocytes. Human neutrophils *in vitro* did not exert a significant killing effect against the strains of this organism used in these studies. Monocytes, on occasion, but not usually, did appear to be capable of killing these strains of nocardia (299).

Pathologic features. Although the pathologic features may vary somewhat with the form of disease produced (see *Clinical Manifestations*) nocardial infection generally calls forth a purulent inflammatory response. The organisms are seen in tissue as coccobacillary forms or branching filaments and are gram positive. Hyphae often appear to be beaded. Regions of chronic pneumonitis may be adjacent to areas with abscess formation and show lymphocytes, occasional giant cells, and scar tissue. Multiple abscesses of varying size may be present and may consist of centrally located polymorphonuclear leukocytes surrounded by histiocytes, epithelioid cells, lymphocytes, and fibroblasts (292). Many coccobacillary forms and filaments may be seen around the abscess (292). Neu and co-workers (285) describe "slight inflammatory exudates surrounding extensive necrotizing abscesses" in the compromised patient.

Clinical manifestations. The lung has been the most commonly affected initial site of involvement, being involved in more than 70 per cent of human cases reported in the literature (286). Symptomatology has varied widely. In some patients, there have been no symptoms, and infection was detected only after a chest radiograph was taken or at autopsy (277). In others, malaise, dry or productive cough, fever, and, rarely, pleuritic chest pain have been prominent (277, 285, 287, 288, 290). Rales or evidence of consolidation or both have been found on physical examination (285, 287). Almost all symptomatic cases have shown abnormalities on chest radiographs. Localized infections, such as segmental or lobar infiltrates or thick walled cavities, are common (283, 288, 290, 291). Necrotizing bronchopneumonia, lobar pneumonia, abscess formation, single nodules, multiple nodules, consolidation, masses with central cavities, pleural effusions, empyema, and consolidation have all been reported (68, 273, 275, 277, 283, 285, 288, 291, 292, 300). It should be stressed that the chest radiographic abnormalities in pulmonary nocardiosis are nonspecific; furthermore, in the compromised host, they may reflect nocardial infection alone or a combination of this organism with any opportunistic pathogen. Bowing of the major fissure, mimicking klebsiella pneumonia, may be seen (288). Pleural involvement may be detected (285, 295), but hilar involvement and calcification are rare (288).

Hematologic data are variable and nondiagnostic (275). Mild anemia is common. The white blood cell count has been variable, showing leukocytosis in some cases (300); the sedimentation rate may be increased (68).

Diagnosis. Isolation of nocardia from sputum may be difficult, in part because the culture plate may be overgrown by more rapidly growing mouth flora. Repeated attempts should be made (286, 287), using ultrasonic nebulization to induce sputum if necessary (276). Cultural confirmation is necessary, because actinomyces and nocardia cannot be definitively separated by staining and morphologic criteria alone (301). Nocardia may be difficult to identify on examination of Gram-stained sputum, even when the sputum is copious and is filled with polymorphonuclear leukocytes. Culture of sputum may also be falsely negative (275, 277, 287). If these procedures are unrewarding, invasive procedures, such as thoracocentesis, transtracheal aspiration (287), and lung aspiration or biopsy should be pursued (273, 277). In a Stanford University Medical Center series, transtracheal aspiration was performed in 5 patients with pulmonary nocardiosis (277). The Gram stain was positive in 1 patient; culture of aspirated material was positive in 2 patients. Stains and cultures were both falsely negative in 3 patients. Formation of paratracheal nocardial abscess has been described as a complication of transtracheal aspiration (302). As is true of other opportunistic pathogens, lung aspiration may occasionally yield false-negative results (2 of 6 cases) (277). Material should be stained with Gomori silver methenamine stain in order to search for fungi and *P. carinii,* as well as Gram and acid-fast stains (decolorizing with 1 per cent sulfuric acid) (283). Cultures should be kept for at least 2 weeks, and care should be taken not to confuse nocardia with rapidly growing atypical mycobacteria or streptococci, filaments of which do not branch (273, 275, 285–287, 292).

Patients with sputum positive for *N. asteroides* or *N. brasiliensis,* but with a negative chest film, have been reported. In most cases, such patients remained asymptomatic without treatment, and the relationship of the positive culture to possible infection is unclear (283). Hosty and co-workers (303) reported isolation of *N. asteroides* from 134 patients, none of whom was said to have disease due to that organism. In contrast, Raich and co-workers (304) did not find nocardia to be a common contaminant; this has also been our experience and that of others as well (285, 286). It is our opinion that isolation of *N. asteroides* from the sputum in a compromised host must be interpreted, at least initially, as indicating infection. A vigorous attempt should then be made to identify an infected site, both with repeated chest radiographs and thorough evaluation of the skin and central nervous system (looking for metastatic foci). A negative chest film does not exclude disseminated nocardiosis (305).

The combination of pulmonary and central nervous system disease or skin infection in the compromised host should prompt a vigorous diagnostic search for this infection (277). Blood cultures are usually not helpful (286), but 6 cases of *N. asteroides* bacteremia have been reported (290), and special culture techniques have been suggested to increase the chances of isolation from blood (291).

Precipitating antibodies can be demonstrated in sera from patients with active nocardiosis, but the sensitivity is poor in the immunologically compromised population (22 per cent positive), and false-positive results occur in patients with leprosy and tuberculosis (306). Therefore, serologic tests, and also skin tests, are not currently of value in the diagnosis of acute nocardial infection.

Treatment. Little question exists with regard to the efficacy of sulfonamide therapy for most cases of nocardiosis (307), but the duration of therapy required for cure has not been clearly defined (277, 307). It has been considered that most sulfonamides inhibit the growth of 95 to 100 per cent of nocardia strains at a concentration of 10 mg per 100 ml (286). Lerner and Baum (308), examining 30 isolates of *N. asteroides* (21 from human sources) and 6 isolates of *N. brasiliensis* found that 46 per cent were inhibited by sulfadiazine concentrations of 3.12 μg per ml and 6 per cent by sulfadiazine concentrations of 12.5 μg per ml (308). Although the possibility of sulfonamide resistance has been raised (309), the test for susceptibility is not well standardized, and results vary with inoculum size (308). Results with low inoculum size (308) (100 per cent susceptibility) correlate well with clinical results. Patients should receive a dose of sulfonamide that produces peak serum concentrations in the range of 12 to 15 mg per 100 ml. In general, this requires 6 to 10 g of sulfonamide per day, but laboratory determinations of concentrations should be made. In 5 Stanford heart transplant patients treated for 5 to 15 months, no relapses were noted (277).

Drugs other than sulfonamides, the combination of a sulfonamide with trimethoprim, and the addition of antimicrobial drugs to a sulfonamide regimen have been used in the treatment of nocardiosis. Nevertheless, we agree with others (272, 274) who have concluded that there is no evidence that any of these regimens improve survival rates in this infection when compared to those with sulfonamide alone. There is one case report, to our knowledge, in which minocycline alone may have cured disseminated nocardiosis (a 13-month follow-up) in a compromised host (310, 311). In other reports, the effectiveness of minocycline is moot, except perhaps in the short-term suppression of this infection (305). In cases in which the trimethoprim-sulfamethoxazole combination has been used, there is usually no reason to believe that sulfonamides alone used in maximal doses would have been ineffective. In cases in which brain abscess was proved, it was also managed surgically (312). An aminoglycoside has occasionally been added to a sulfonamide in the therapy of nocardiosis (277). These substitute, or allegedly adjunctive, drugs have potentially untoward side effects, and their use in a patient already ill with infection and underlying disease should not be instituted uncritically, without *in vivo* evidence of greater benefit than can be achieved with sulfonamide alone. In any case, when drugs are used in combination with sulfonamides, claims for success due to the added agents should be made with caution.

Goodman and Koenig (274) reported that patients with minor infections were treated for 3 weeks, whereas those with serious infections were treated for 1 year. The determination of degree of severity (in fact, to be certain that minute foci of dissemination are not present) is difficult, and it is our opinion that all immunosuppressed patients with nocardiosis should receive treatment for perhaps as long as 1 year to prevent relapse of latent infection, in view of the possible fulminant course of the disease in this population. It is important to recognize that prompt diagnosis and appropriate therapy often lead to successful treatment, even in the compromised host (275, 277, 285) and even with significant disease involving cavitation and empyema (285).

References

1. Pierce, A. K., and Sanford, J. P.: Aerobic gramnegative bacillary pneumonias, Am Rev Respir Dis, 1974, *110*, 647.
2. Green, G. M.: Lung defense mechanism, Med Clin North Am, 1973, *57*, 547.
3. Kaltreider, H. B.: Expression of immune mechanism in the lung, Am Rev Respir Dis, 1976, *113*, 347.
4. Henney, C. S., and Waldman, R. H.: Cell-mediated immunity shown by lymphocytes from the respiratory tract, Science, 1970, *169*, 696.
5. Waldman, R. H., and Henney, C. S.: Cell-mediated immunity and antibody responses in the respiratory tract after local and systemic immunization, J Exp Med, 1971, *134*, 482.
6. Jurgensen, P. F., Olsen, G. N., Johnson, J. E., III, Swenson, E. W., Ayoub, E. M., Henney, C. S., and Waldman, R. H.: Immune response of the human respiratory tract. II. Cell-mediated immunity in the lower respiratory tract to tuberculin and mumps and influenza viruses, J Infect Dis, 1973, *128*, 730.
7. Armstrong, D.: Infectious complications in cancer patients treated with chemical immunosuppressive agents, Transplant Proc, 1973, *5*, 1245.
8. Dale, D. C., and Petersdorf, R. G.: Corticosteroids and infectious diseases, Med Clin North Am, 1973, *57*, 1277.
9. Zurier, R. B., and Weissman, G.: Anti-immunologic and anti-inflammatory effects of steroid therapy, Med Clin North Am, 1973, *57*, 1295.
10. Atkinson, J. P, and Frank, M. M.: Effect of cortisone therapy on serum complement components, J Immunol, 1973, *111*, 1061.
11. Thompson, J., and Van Furth, R.: The effect of glucocorticosteroids on the kinetics of mononuclear phagocytes, J Exp Med, 1970, *131*, 429.
12. MacGregor, R. R., Spagnuolo, P. J., and Lentnek, A. L.: Inhibition of granulocyte adherence by ethanol, prednisone and aspirin, measured with an assay system, N Engl J Med, 1974, *291*, 642.
13. Balow, J. E., and Rosenthal, A. S.: Mechanisms of steroid suppression of cellular immunity, Clin Res, 1972, *20*, 506.
14. Boggs, D. R., Athens, J. W., Cartwright, G. E., and Wintrobe, M. M.: Leukokinetic studies. IX. Experimental evaluation of a model of granulopoiesis, J Clin Invest, 1965, *44*, 643.
15. Casey, W. J., and McCall, C. E.: Suppression of cellular interactions of delayed hypersensitivity by corticosteroids, Immunology, 1971, *21*, 225.
16. Hersh, E. M., Wong, V. G., and Freireich, E. J.: Inhibition of the local inflammatory response in man by antimetabolites, Blood, 1966, *27*, 38.
17. Gershwin, M. E., Goetzl, E. J., and Steinberg, A. D.: Cyclophosphamide: Use in practice, Ann Intern Med, 1974, *80*, 531.
18. Hersh, E. M., and Oppenheim, J. J.: Inhibition of *in vitro* lymphocyte transformation during chemotherapy in man, Cancer Res, 1967, *27*, 98.
19. Remington, J. S.: The compromised host, Hosp Pract, 1972, *7*, 59.
20. Bodey, G. P.: Microbiologic aspects in patients with leukemia, Hum Pathol, 1974, *5*, 687.
21. Greenman, R. L., Goodall, P. T., and King, D.: Lung biopsy in immunocompromised hosts, Am J Med, 1975, *59*, 488.
22. Mirsky, H. S., and Cuttner, J.: Fungal infection in acute leukemia, Cancer, 1972, *30*, 348.
23. Sickles, E. A., Young, V. M., Greene, W. H., and Wiernik, P. H.: Pneumonia in acute leukemia, Ann Intern Med, 1973, *79*, 528.
24. Bandt, P. D., Blank, N., and Castellino, R. A.: Needle diagnosis of pneumonitis. Value in high-risk patients, JAMA, 1972, *220*, 1578.
25. Baum, G. L.: The significance of *Candida albicans* in human sputum, N Engl J Med, 1960, *263*, 70.
26. Hoeprich, P. D.: Etiologic diagnosis of lower

respiratory tract infections, Calif Med, 1970, *112*, 1.

27. Murray, J. F., Haegelin, H. F., Hewitt, W. L., Latta, H., McVickar, D., Rasmussen, A. F. Jr., and Rigler, L. G.: Opportunistic pulmonary infections, Ann Intern Med, 1966, *65*, 566.

28. Finley, R., Kieff, E., Thomsen, S., Fennessy, J., Beem, M., Lerner, S., and Morello, J.: Bronchial brushing in the diagnosis of pulmonary disease in patients at risk for opportunistic infection, Am Rev Respir Dis, 1974, *109*, 379.

29. Aisner, J., Kvols, L. K., Sickles, E. A., Schimpff, S. C., and Wiernik, P. H.: Transtracheal selective bronchial brushing for pulmonary infiltrates in patients with cancer, Chest, in press.

30. Andersen, H. A., Miller, W. E., and Bernatz, P. E.: Lung biopsy: Transbronchoscopic, percutaneous, open, Surg Clin North Am, 1973, *53*, 785.

31. Aaron, B. L., Bellinger, S. B., Shepard, B. M., and Doohen, D. J.: Open lung biopsy: A strong stand, Chest, 1971, *59*, 18.

32. Baker, R. R., Lee, J. M., and Carter, D.: An evaluation of open lung biopsy, Johns Hopkins Med J, 1973, *132*, 103.

33. Krumholz, R. A.: Pulmonary cryptococcosis: A case due to *Cryptococcus albidus*, Am Rev Respir Dis, 1972, *105*, 421.

34. Ajello, L.: Soil as a natural reservoir for human pathogenic fungi, Science, 1956, *123*, 876.

35. Ajello, L.: A comparative study of the pulmonary mycoses of Canada and the United States, Public Health Rep, 1969, *84*, 869.

36. Littman, M. L., and Walter, J. E.: Cryptococcosis: Current status, Am J Med, 1968, *45*, 992.

37. Littman, M. L., and Zimmerman, L. E.: Cryptococcosis: Torulosis or European Blastomycosis, Grune and Stratton, New York, 1956.

38. Buechner, H. A., Furcolow, M. L., Farness, O. J., Reagan, W. P., Saliba, N. A., and Abernathy, R.: Epidemiology of the pulmonary mycoses, Chest, 1970, *58*, 68.

39. Kahanpää, A.: Bronchopulmonary occurrence of fungi in adults especially according to cultivation material, Acta Pathol Microbiol Scand [B], 1972 (Supplement 227, p. 1).

40. Houk, V. N., and Moser, K. M.: Pulmonary cryptococcosis: Must all receive amphotericin B? Ann Intern Med, 1965, *63*, 583.

41. Salyer, W. R., Salyer, D. C., and Baker, R. D.: Primary complex of Cryptococcus and pulmonary lymph nodes, J Infect Dis, 1974, *130*, 74.

42. Casazza, A. R., Duvall, C. P., and Carbone, P. P.: Infection in lymphoma: Histology, treatment and duration in relation to incidence and survival, JAMA, 1966, *197*, 710.

43. Feld, R., Bodey, G. P., Rodriguez, V., and Luna, M.: Causes of death in patients with malignant lymphoma, Am J Med Sci, 1974, *268*, 97.

44. Hart, P. D., Russell, E., Jr., and Remington, J. S.: The compromised host and infection. II. Deep fungal infection, J Infect Dis, 1969, *120*, 169.

45. Gaines, J. D., Gilmer, M. A., and Remington, J. S.: Deficiency of lymphocyte antigen recognition in Hodgkin's disease, Natl Cancer Inst Monogr, 1973, *36*, 117.

46. Diamond, R. D., and Bennett, J. E.: Disseminated cryptococcosis in man: Decreased lymphocyte transformation in response to *Cryptococcus neoformans*, J Infect Dis, 1973, *127*, 694.

47. Graybill, J. R., and Alford, R. H.: Cell-mediated immunity in cryptococcosis, Cell Immunol, 1974, *14*, 12.

48. Goldstein, E., and Rambo, O. N.: Cryptococcal infection following steroid therapy, Ann Intern Med, 1962, *56*, 114.

49. Bodey, G. P.: Fungal infections complicating acute leukemia, J Chronic Dis, 1966, *19*, 667.

50. Gadebusch, H. H., and Gikas, P. W.: The effect of cortisone upon experimental pulmonary cryptococcosis, Am Rev Respir Dis, 1965, *92*, 64.

51. Abrahams, I., and Gilleran, T. G.: Studies on actively acquired resistance to experimental cryptococcosis in mice, J Immunol, 1960, *85*, 629.

52. Louria, D. B.: Specific and non-specific immunity in experimental cryptococcosis in mice, J Exp Med, 1960, *111*, 643.

53. Louria, D. B., Kaminski, T., and Finkel, G.: Further studies on immunity in experimental cryptococcosis, J Exp Med, 1963, *117*, 509.

54. Perceval, A. K.: Experimental cryptococcosis: Hypersensitivity and immunity, J Pathol, 1965, *89*, 645.

55. Gentry, L. O., and Remington, J. S.: Resistance against cryptococcus conferred by intracellular bacteria and protozoa, J Infect Dis, 1971, *123*, 22.

56. Diamond, R. D., and Bennett, J. E.: Growth of *Cryptococcus neoformans* within human macrophages in vitro, Infect Immun, 1973, *7*, 231.

57. Diamond, R. D., Root, R. K., and Bennett, J. E.: Factors influencing killing of *Cryptococcus neoformans* by human leukocytes *in vitro*, J Infect Dis, 1972, *125*, 367.

58. Cline, M. J., and Lehrer, R. I.: Phagocytosis by human monocytes, Blood, 1968, *32*, 423.

59. Bulmer, G. S., and Sans, M. D.: *Cryptococcus neoformans*. II. Phagocytosis by human leukocytes, J Bacteriol, 1967, *94*, 1480.

60. Diamond, R. D., May, J. E., Kane, M., Frank, M. M., and Bennett, J. E.: The role of late complement components and the alternate complement pathway in experimental cryptococcosis, Proc Soc Exp Biol Med, 1973, *144*, 312.

61. Tacker, J. R., Farhi, F., and Bulmer, G. S.: Intracellular fate of *Cryptococcus neoformans*, Infect Immun, 1972, *6*, 162.

62. Diamond, R. D.: Antibody-dependent killing

of *Cryptococcus neoformans* by human peripheral blood mononuclear cells, Nature, 1974, *247*, 148.

63. Kalina, M., Kletter, Y., and Aronson, M.: The interaction of phagocytes and large-sized parasite *Cryptococcus neoformans*: Cytochemical and ultrastructural study, Cell Tissue Res, 1974, *152*, 165.

64. Bulmer, G. S., and Sans, M. D.: *Cryptococcus neoformans*. III. Inhibition of phagocytosis, J Bacteriol, 1968, *95*, 5.

65. Bulmer, G. S., and Tacker, J. R.: Phagocytosis of *Cryptococcus neoformans* by alveolar macrophages, Infect Immun, 1975, *11*, 73.

66. Baum, G. L., and Arits, D.: Characterization of the growth inhibition factor for *Cryptococcus neoformans* (GIF) in human serum, Am J Sci, 1963, *246*, 87.

67. Gutierrez, F., Fu, Y. S., and Lurie, H. I.: Cryptococcosis histologically resembling Histoplasmosis, Arch Pathol, 1975, *99*, 347.

68. Conant, N. F., Smith, D. T., Baker, R. D., and Callaway, J. L.: Manual of Clinical Mycology, ed. 3, W. B. Saunders Co., Philadelphia, 1971.

69. Farmer, S. G., and Komorowski, R. A.: Histologic response to capsule-deficient *Cryptococcus neoformans*, Arch Pathol, 1973, *96*, 383.

70. Baker, R. D., and Haugen, R. K.: Tissue change and tissue diagnosis in cryptococcosis: A study of 26 cases, Am J Clin Pathol, 1955, *25*, 14.

71. MacGillivray, J. B.: Two cases of cryptococcosis, J Clin Pathol, 1966, *19*, 424.

72. Mills, S. A., Seigler, H. F., and Wolfe, W. G.: The incidence and management of pulmonary mycosis in renal allograft patients, Ann Surg, 1975, *182*, 617.

73. Kent, T. H., and Layton, J. M.: Massive pulmonary cryptococcosis, Am J Clin Pathol, 1962, *38*, 596.

74. Lomvardias, S., and Lurie, H. I.: Epipleural cryptococcosis in a patient with Hodgkin's disease: A case report, Sabouraudia, 1972, *10*, 256.

75. Hughes, W. T.: Fatal infections in childhood leukemia, Am J Dis Child, 1971, *122*, 283.

76. Bennington, J. L., Haber, S. L., and Morgenstern, N. L.: Increased susceptibility to cryptococcosis following steroid therapy, Dis Chest, 1964, *45*, 262.

77. Bindschadler, D. D., and Benett, J. E.: Serology of human cryptococcosis, Ann Intern Med, 1968, *69*, 45.

78. Campbell, G. D.: Primary pulmonary cryptococcosis, Am Rev Respir Dis, 1966, *94*, 236.

79. Gordonson, J., Birnbaum, W., Jacobson, G., and Sargent, E. N.: Pulmonary cryptococcosis, Radiology, 1974, *112*, 557.

80. Hammerman, K. J., Powell, K. E., Christianson, C. S., Huggin, P. M., Larsh, H. W., Vivas, J. R., and Tosh, F. E.: Pulmonary cryptococcosis: Clinical forms and treatment. A Center for Disease Control cooperative mycoses study, Am Rev Respir Dis, 1973, *108*, 1116.

81. Tynes, B., Mason, K. N., Jennings, A. E., and Bennett, J. E.: Variant forms of pulmonary cryptococcosis, Ann Intern Med, 1968, *69*, 1117.

82. Warr, W., Bates, J. H., and Stone, A.: The spectrum of pulmonary cryptococcosis, Ann Intern Med, 1968, *69*, 1109.

83. Aisner, J., Schimpff, S. C., Bennett, J. E., Sutherland, J. C., Young, V. M., and Wiernik, P. H.: Increased incidence of aspergillus infections in cancer patients: An association with fireproofing material, JAMA, in press.

84. Bahr, R. D., Satz, H., and Purlia, V. L.: Primary pulmonary cryptococcosis, Am J Roentgenol Radium Ther Nucl Med, 1962, *5*, 859.

85. Soll, E. L., and Bergeron, R. B.: Pulmonary cryptococcosis: A case diagnostically confirmed by transbronchial brush biopsy, Chest, 1971, *59*, 454.

86. Smilack, J. D., Bellet, R. E., and Talman, W. T., Jr.: Cryptococcal pleural effusion, JAMA, 1975, *232*, 639.

87. Brooks, M. H., Scheerer, P. P., and Linman, J. W.: Cryptococcal prostatitis, JAMA, 1965, *192*, 639.

88. Diamond, R. D., and Bennett, J. E.: Prognostic factors in cryptococcal meningitis: A study of 111 cases, Ann Intern Med, 1974, *80*, 176.

89. Sarosi, G. A., Silberfarb, P. M., and Tosh, F. E.: Cutaneous cryptococcosis: A sentinel of disseminated disease, Arch Dermatol, 1971, *104*, 1.

90. Young, R. C., Bennett, J. E., Geelhoed, G. W., and Levine, A. S.: Fungemia with compromised host resistance: A study of 70 cases, Ann Intern Med, 1974, *80*, 605.

91. Buechner, H. A., Seabury, J. H., Campbell, C. C., Georger, L. K., Kaufman, L., and Kaplan, W.: The current status of serologic, immunologic, and skin tests in the diagnosis of pulmonary mycoses: Report of the Committee of Fungus Diseases and Subcommittee on Criteria for Clinical Diagnosis, American College of Chest Physicians, Chest, 1973, *63*, 259.

92. Bennett, J. E., Hasenclever, H. F., and Tynes, B. S.: Detection of cryptococcal polysaccharide in serum and spinal fluid: Value in diagnosis and prognosis, Trans Assoc Am Physicians, 1964, *77*, 145.

93. Bennett, J. E., and Bailey, J. W.: Control for rheumatoid factor in the latex test for cryptococcosis, Am J Clin Pathol, 1971, *56*, 360.

94. Gordon, M. A., and Lapa, E. W.: Elimination of rheumatoid factor in the latex test for cryptococcosis, Am J Clin Pathol, 1974, *61*, 488.

95. Bennett, J. E.: Susceptibility of *Cryptococcus neoformans* to amphotericin B, Antimicrob Agents Chemother, 1966, 405.

96. Rhoades, E. R., Felton, F. G., Wilkus, J., and

Muchmore, H. G.: Susceptibility of human and environmental isolates of *Cryptococcus neoformans* to amphotericin B, Antimicrob Agents Chemother, 1967–1968, 736.

97. Shadomy, S., Shadomy, H. H., McCay, J. A., and Utz, J. P.: *In vitro* susceptibility of *Cryptococcus neoformans* to amphotericin B, hamycin, and 5-fluorocytosine, Antimicrob Agents Chemother, 1968–1969, 452.

98. Hoeprich, P. D., and Huston, A. C.: Susceptibility of *Coccidioides immitis, Candida albicans,* and *Cryptococcus neoformans* to amphotericin B, flucytosine, and clotrimazole, J Infect Dis, 1975, *132,* 133.

99. Abernathy, R. S.: Treatment of systemic mycoses, Medicine (Baltimore), 1973, *52,* 385.

100. Krick, J. A., and Remington, J. S.: Treatment of fungal infections, Arch Intern Med, 1975, *135,* 344.

101. Sarosi, G. A., Parker, J. D., Doto, I. L., and Tosh, F. E.: Amphotericin B in cryptococcal meningitis: Long-term results of therapy, Ann Intern Med, 1969, *71,* 1079.

102. Tassel, D., and Madoff, M. A.: Treatment of candida sepsis and cryptococcus meningitis with 5-fluorocytosine, JAMA, 1968, *206,* 830.

103. Halkin, J., Ravid, M., Zulman, J., and Reichert, N.: Cryptococcal meningitis treated with 5-fluorocytosine and amphotericin B, Isr J Med Sci, 1974, *10,* 1148.

104. Utz, J. P., Tynes, B. S., Shadomy, H. J., Duma, R. J., Kannan, M. M., and Mason, K. N.: 5-Fluorocytosine in human cryptococcosis, Antimicrob Agents Chemother, 1968, 344.

105. Harder, E. J., and Hermans, P. E.: Treatment of fungal infections with flucytosine, Arch Intern Med, 1975, *135,* 231.

106. Garriques, I. L., Sande, M. A., Utz, J. P., Mandell, G. L., Warner, J. F., McGehee, R. F., and Shadomy, S.: Combined amphotericin B-flucytosine chemotherapy in human cryptococcosis, Thirteenth Interscience Conference on Antimicrobial Agents and Chemotherapy, 1973, Abstract No. 239.

107. Block, E. R., and Bennett, J. E.: The combined effect of 5-fluorocytosine and amphotericin B in the therapy of murine cryptococcosis, Proc Soc Exp Biol Med, 1973, *142,* 476.

108. Hamilton, J. D., and Elliott, D. M.: Combined activity of amphotericin B and 5-fluorocytosine against *Cryptococcus neoformans in vitro* and in mice, J Infect Dis, 1975, *131,* 129.

109. Shadomy, S., Wagner, G., Espinel-Ingroff, A., and Davis, B. A.: *In vitro* studies with combinations of 5-fluorocytosine and amphotericin B, Antimicrob Agents Chemother, 1975, *8,* 117.

110. Young, R. C., Bennett, J. E., Vogel, C. L., Carbone, P. P., and DeVita, V. T.: Aspergillosis: The spectrum of the disease in 98 patients, Medicine (Baltimore), 1970, *49,* 147.

111. Young, R. C., Jennings, A., and Bennett, J. E.: Species identification of invasive aspergillosis in man, Am J Clin Pathol, 1972, *58,* 554.

112. Levine, A. S., Schimpff, S. C., Graw, R. G., Jr., and Young, R. C.: Hematologic malignancies and other marrow failure states: Progress in management of complicating infections, Semin Hematol, 1974, *11,* 141.

113. Hughes, W. T., and Crosier, J. W.: Thermophilic fungi in the mycoflora of man and environmental air, Mycopathol Mycol Appl, 1973, *49,* 147.

114. Noble, W. C., and Clayton, Y. M.: Fungi in the air of hospital wards, J Gen Microbiol, 1963, *32,* 397.

115. Sayer, W. J., Shean, D. B., and Ghosseiri, J.: Estimation of airborne fungal flora by the Andersen sampler versus the gravity settling culture plate, J Allergy, 1969, *44,* 214.

116. Gage, A. A., Dean, D. C., Schimert, G., and Minsley, N.: Aspergillus infection after cardiac surgery, Arch Surg, 1970, *101,* 384.

117. Rose, H. D.: Mechanical control of hospital ventilation and aspergillus infections, Am Rev Respir Dis, 1972, *105,* 306.

118. Burton, J. R., Zacher, J. B., Bessin, R., Rathbun, H. K., Greenough, W. B., III, Sterioff, S., Wright, J. R., Slavin, R. E., and Williams, G. M.: Aspergillosis in four renal transplant recipients: Diagnosis and effective treatment with amphotericin B, Ann Intern Med, 1972, *77,* 383.

119. Comstock, G. W., Palmer, C. E., Stone, R. W., and Goodman, N. L.: Fungi in the sputum of normal men, Mycopathol Mycol Appl, 1974, *54,* 55.

120. Cohen, R., Roth, F. J., Delgado, E., Ahearn, D. G., and Kalser, M. H.: Fungal flora of the normal human small and large intestine, N Engl J Med, 1969, *280,* 638.

121. Christensen, C. M., and Kennedy, B. W.: Filamentous fungi and bacteria in macaroni and spaghetti products, Appl Microbiol, 1971, *21,* 144.

122. Epstein, S. M., Verney, E., Miale, T. D., and Sidransky, H.: Studies on the pathogenesis of experimental pulmonary aspergillosis, Am J Pathol, 1967, *51,* 769.

123. Ford, S., Baker, R. D., and Friedman, L.: Cellular reactions and pathology in experimental disseminated aspergillosis, J Infect Dis, 1968, *118,* 370.

124. Bujak, J. S., Kwon-Chung, K. J., and Chusid, M. J.: Osteomyelitis and pneumonia in a boy with chronic granulomatous disease of childhood caused by a mutant strain of *Aspergillus nidulans,* Am J Clin Pathol, 1974, *61,* 361.

125. Lehrer, R. I., and Jan, R. G.: Interaction of *Aspergillus fumigatus* spores with human leukocytes and serum, Infect Immun, 1970, *1,* 345.

126. Lehrer, R. I.: Antifungal effects of peroxidase systems, Bacteriol Rev, 1969, *99*, 361.

127. Smith, G. R.: Experimental aspergillosis in mice: Aspects of resistance, J Hyg (Camb), 1972, *70*, 741.

128. Meyer, R. D., Young, L. S., Armstrong, D., and Yu, B.: Aspergillosis complicating neoplastic disease, Am J Med, 1973, *54*, 6.

129. Young, R. C., and Bennett, J. E.: Invasive aspergillosis: Absence of detectable antibody response, Am Rev Respir Dis, 1971, *104*, 710.

130. Carbone, P. P., Sabesin, S. M., Sidransky, H., and Frei, E., III: Secondary aspergillosis, Ann Intern Med, 1964, *60*, 556.

131. Gurwith, M. H., Stinson, E. B., and Remington, J. S.: Aspergillus infection complicating cardiac transplantation: Report of five cases, Arch Intern Med, 1971, *128*, 541.

132. Gallis, H. A., Berman, R. A., Cate, T. R., Hamilton, J. D., Gunnells, J. C., and Stickels, D. L.: Fungal infection following renal transplantation, Arch Intern Med, 1975, *135*, 1163.

133. Sidransky, H., Verney, E., and Beede, H.: Experimental pulmonary aspergillosis, Arch Pathol, 1965, *79*, 299.

134. Merkow, L., Pardo, M., Epstein, S. M., Verney, E., and Sidransky, H.: Lysosomal stability during phagocytosis of *Aspergillus flavus* spores by alveolar macrophages of cortisone-treated mice, Science, 1968, *160*, 79.

135. Sidransky, H., Epstein, S. M., Verney, M. S., and Horowitz, C.: Experimental visceral aspergillosis, Am J Pathol, 1972, *69*, 55.

136. Merkow, L. P., Epstein, S. M., Sidransky, H., Verney, E., and Pardo, M.: The pathogenesis of experimental pulmonary aspergillosis, Am J Pathol, 1971, *62*, 57.

137. Castellino, R. A., Goldstein, H. M., Stinson, E. B., and Griepp, R. A.: Needle aspiration biopsy technique in pulmonary disease, JAMA, *213*, 463.

138. Aslam, P. A., Eastridge, C. E., and Hughes, F. A., Jr.: Aspergillosis of the lung: An eighteen-year experience, Chest, 1971, *59*, 28.

139. Burke, P. S., and Coltman, C. A., Jr.: Multiple pulmonary aspergillomas in acute leukemia, Cancer, 1971, *28*, 1289.

140. Zimmerman, R. A., and Miller, W. T.: Pulmonary aspergillosis, Am J Roentgenol Radium Ther Nucl Med, 1970, *109*, 505.

141. Khoo, T. K., Sugai, K., and Leong, T. K.: Disseminated aspergillosis, Am J Clin Pathol, 1966, *45*, 697.

142. Bragg, D. G., and Janis, B.: The radiographic presentation of pulmonary opportunistic inflammatory disease, Radiol Clin North Am, 1973, *11*, 357.

143. Emmons, C. W., Binford, C. H., and Utz, J. P.: Medical Mycology, Lea and Febiger, Philadelphia, 1970.

144. Naidoff, M. A., and Green, W. R.: Endogenous aspergillus endophthalmitis occurring after kidney transplant, Am J Ophthalmol, 1975, *79*, 502.

145. Krick, J. A., and Remington, J. S.: Nocardia infection in heart transplant patients, Ann Intern Med, 1975, *82*, 18.

146. Bardana, E. J., Jr.: Measurement of humoral antibodies to aspergilli, Ann NY Acad Sci 1974, *221*, 64.

147. Coleman, R. M., and Kaufman, L.: Use of the immunodiffusion test in the serodiagnosis of aspergillosis, Appl Microbiol, 1972, *23*, 301.

148. Bardana, E. J., Jr., Gerber, J. D., Craig, S., and Cianciulli, F. D.: The genera and specific humoral immune response to pulmonary aspergillosis, Am Rev Respir Dis, 1975, *112*, 799.

149. Schaefer, J. C., Yu, B., and Armstrong, D.: An aspergillus immunodiffusion test in the early diagnosis of aspergillosis in adult leukemic patients, Am Rev Respir Dis, 1976, *113*, 325.

150. Adiseshan, N., and Oliver, W. A.: Strontium lung scans in the diagnosis of pulmonary aspergillosis, Am Rev Respir Dis, 1973, *108*, 441.

151. Ray, G. R., DeNardo, G. L., and King, G. H.: Localization of strontium 85 in soft tissue infected by *Aspergillus niger*, Radiology, 1971, *101*, 119.

152. Brandsberg, J. W., and French, M. E.: *In vitro* susceptibility of isolates of *Aspergillus fumigatus* and *Sporothrix schenkii* to amphotericin B, Antimicrob Agents Chemother, 1972, *2*, 402.

153. Howarth, W. R., Tewari, R. P., and Solotrovsky, M.: Comparative *in vitro* antifungal activity of amphotericin B and amphotericin B methyl ester, Antimicrob Agents Chemother, 1975, *7*, 58.

154. Fields, B. T., Jr., Meredith, W. R., Galbraith, J. E., and Hardin, H. F.: Studies with amphotericin B and 5-fluorocytosine in aspergillosis, Clin Res, 1974, *22*, 32A.

155. Carrizosa, J., Levinson, M. E., Lawrence, T., and Kaye, D.: Cure of *Aspergillus ustus* endocarditis on a prosthetic valve, Arch Intern Med, 1974, *133*, 486.

156. Jones, B. R.: Principles in the management of oculomycosis, Am J Ophthalmol, 1975, *79*, 719.

157. Shadomy, S.: *In vitro* studies with 5-fluorocytosine, Appl Microbiol, 1969, *17*, 871.

158. Steer, P. L., Marks, M. I., Klite, P. D., and Eickhoff, T. C.: 5-fluorocytosine: An oral antifungal compound. A report on clinical and laboratory experience, Ann Intern Med, 1972, *76*, 15.

159. Conen, P. E., Walker, G. R., Turner, J. A., and Field, P.: Invasive primary aspergillosis of the lung with cerebral metastasis and complete recovery, Dis Chest, 1962, *42*, 88.

160. Vedder, J. S., and Schoor, W. F.: Primary disseminated pulmonary aspergillosis with metas-

tatic skin nodules: Successful treatment with inhalation nystatin therapy, JAMA, 1969, *209*, 1191.

161. Hammerman, K. J., Christianson, C. S., Huntington, I., Hurst, G. A., Zelman, M., and Tosh, F. E.: Spontaneous lysis of aspergillomata, Chest, 1973, *64*, 697.

162. Gercovich, F. G., Richman, S. P., Rodriguez, V., Luna, M., McCredie, K. B., and Bodey, G. P.: Successful control of systemic *Aspergillus niger* infections in two patients with acute leukemia, Cancer, 1975, *36*, 2271.

163. Atkinson, G. W., and Israel, H. L.: 5-Fluorocytosine treatment of meningeal and pulmonary aspergillosis, Am J Med, 1973, *55*, 496.

164. Davis, B. D., Dulbecco, R., Eisen, H. N., Ginsberg, H. S., and Wood, W. B., Jr.: Microbiology, Harper and Row, New York, 1967.

165. Sorenson, W. G., Bulmer, G. S., and Criep, L. H Airborne fungi from five sites in the continental United States and Puerto Rico, Ann Allergy, 1974, *33*, 131.

166. Sheldon, W. H., and Bauer, H.: The role of predisposing factors in experimental fungus infections, Lab Invest, 1962, *11*, 1184.

167. Corbel, M. J., and Eades, S. M.: Factors determining the susceptibility of mice to experimental phycomycosis, J Med Microbiol, 1975, *8*, 551.

168. Barturm, R. J., Watnick, M., and Herman, P. G.: Roentgenographic findings in pulmonary mucormycosis, Am J Roentgenol Radium Ther Nucl Med, 1973, *117*, 810.

169. Meyer, R. D., Rosen, P., and Armstrong, D.: Phycomycosis complicating leukemia and lymphoma, Ann Intern Med, 1972, *77*, 871.

170. Beathard, G. A., Sarles, H. E., Remmers, A. R., Jr., Fish, J. C. Lindley, J. D., and Ritzmann, S. E.: Pulmonary phycomycosis associated with lymphocyte depletion, Texas Rep Biol Med, 1970, *28*, 509.

171. Gale, A., and Kleitsch, W. P.: Solitary pulmonary nodule due to phycomycosis (mucormycosis), Chest, 1972, *62*, 752.

172. Addlestone, R. B., and Baylin, G. J.: Rhinocerebral mucormycosis, Radiology, 1975, *115*, 113.

173. Baker, R. D.: The phycomycoses, Ann NY Acad Sci, 1970, *174*, 592.

174. Baker, R. D.: Leukopenia and therapy in leukemia as factors predisposing to fatal mycoses, Am J Clin Pathol, 1962, *37*, 358.

175. Medoff, G., and Kobayashi, G. S.: Pulmonary mucormycoses, N Engl J Med, 1972, *286*, 86.

176. Hughes, W. T.: The deep mycoses, in *Practice of Pediatrics*, vol. 11, V. C. Kelly, ed., Harper and Row, Hagerstown; 1974, chap. 55B.

177. Lombardi, D. L., Mason, J. O., and Hughes, R. K.: Pneumocystis and mucormycosis pneumonitis, Chest, 1970, *57*, 318.

178. Meyer, R. D., Kaplan, M. H., Ong, M., and Armstrong, D.: Cutaneous lesions in disseminated mucormycosis, JAMA, 1973, *225*, 737.

179. Bogard, B. M.: Pulmonary mucormycosis, N Engl J Med, 1972, *286*, 606.

180. Straatsma, B. R., Zimmerman, L. E., and Gass, J. D. M.: Phycomycosis: A clinicopathologic study of fifty-one cases, Lab Invest, 1962, *11*, 963.

181. Landau, J. W., and Newcomer, V. D.: Acute cerebral phycomycosis (mucormycosis): Report of a pediatric patient successfully treated with amphotericin B and cycloheximide and review of pertinent literature, J Pediatr, 1962, *61*, 363.

182. Bennett, J. E.: Chemotherapy of systemic mycoses, N Engl J Med, 1974, *290*, 30, 320.

183. Hammer, G. S., Bottone, E. J., and Hirschman, S. Z.: Mucormycosis in a transplant recipient, Am J Clin Pathol, 1975, *64*, 389.

184. Kahanpää, A.: Yeast fungus flora in patients in a geriatric hospital, Acta Pathol Microbiol Scand [B], 1974, *82*, 81.

185. Somerville, D. A.: Yeasts in a hospital for patients with skin diseases, J Hyg (Camb), 1972, *70*, 667.

186. Pennington, J. E., Block, E. R., and Reynolds, H. Y.: 5-Fluorocytosine and amphotericin B in bronchial secretions, Antimicrob Agents Chemother, 1974, *6*, 324.

187. Ahearn, D. G.: Identification and ecology of yeasts of medical importance, in *Opportunistic Pathogens*, J. E. Prier, and H. Friedman, ed., University Park Press, Baltimore, 1974, pp. 129–146.

188. Bodey, G. P., and Rosenbaum, B.: Effect of prophylactic measures on the microbial flora of patients in protected environment units, Medicine (Baltimore), 1974, *53*, 209.

189. Schimpff, S. C., Young, V. M., Greene, W. H., Vermeulen, G. D., Moody, M. S., and Wiernik, P. H.: Origin of infection in acute nonlymphocytic leukemia: Significance of hospital acquisition of potential pathogens, Ann Intern Med, 1972, *77*, 707.

190. Clayton, Y. M., and Nobel, W. C.: Observations on the epidemiology of *Candida albicans*, J Clin Pathol, 1966, *19*, 76.

191. Louria, D. B., and Brayton, R. G.: Behaviour of candida cells within leukocytes, Proc Soc Exp Biol Med, 1964, *115*, 93.

192. Lehrer, R. I.: Measurement of candidacidal activity of specific leukocyte types in mixed cell populations. I. Normal myeloperoxidase-deficient and chronic granulomatous disease neutrophils, Infect Immun, 1970, *2*, 42.

193. Lehrer, R. I.: Measurement of candidacidal activity of specific leukocyte types in mixed cell populations. II. Normal and chronic granulomatous disease eosinophils, Infect Immun, 1971, *3*, 800.

194. Lehrer, R. I.: The fungicidal mechanism of human monocytes. I. Evidence for myeloperoxidase-linked and myeloperoxidase-independent candidacidal mechanism, J Clin Invest, 1975, *55*, 338.

195. Lehrer, R. I., and Cline, M. J.: Interaction of *Candida albicans* with leukocytes and serum, J Bacteriol, 1969, *98*, 996.

196. Oh, M-H. K., Bodey, G. E., Good, R. A., Chilgren, R. A., and Quie, P. G.: Defective candidacidal capacity of polymorphonuclear leukocytes in chronic granulomatous disease of childhood, J Pediatr, 1969, *75*, 300.

197. Lehrer, R. I.: Functional aspects of a second mechanism of candidacidal activity by human neutrophils, J Clin Invest, 1972, *51*, 2566.

198. Lehrer, R. I., and Cline, M. J.: Leukocyte myeloperoxidase deficiency and disseminated candidiasis: The role of myeloperoxidase in resistance to candida infection, J Clin Invest, 1969, *48*, 1478.

199. Lehrer, R. I., and Cline, M. J.: Leukocyte candidacidal activity and resistance to systemic candidiasis in patients with cancer, Cancer, 1971, *27*, 1211.

200. Dobias, B.: Specific and Nonspecific Immunity in Candida Infections. Experimental Studies of the Role of Candida Cell Constituents and Review of the Literature, Kungl, Boktryckeriet P. A., Norstedt & Söner, Stockholm, 1964.

201. LaForce, F. M., Mills, D. M., Iverson, K., Cousins, R., and Everett, E. D.: Inhibition of leukocyte candidacidal activity by serum from patients with disseminated candidiasis, J Lab Clin Med, 1975, *86*, 657.

202. Pearsall, N. N., and Lagunoff, D.: Immunological responses to *Candida albicans*. I. Mouse-thigh lesion as a model for experimental candidiasis, Infect Immun, 1974, *9*, 999.

203. Sher, N. A., Chapara, S., Greenberg, L. E., and Bernard, S.: Effects of BCG, *Corynebacterium parvum*, and methanol-extraction residue in the reduction of mortality from *Staphylococcus aureus* and *Candida albicans* infections in immunosuppressed mice, Infect Immun, 1975, *12*, 1325.

204. Pearsall, N. N., Sundsmo, J. S., and Weiser, R. S.: Lymphokine toxicity for yeast cells, J. Immunol, 1973, *110*, 1444.

205. Bird, D. C., and Sheagren, J. N.: Evaluation of reticuloendothelial system phagocytic activity during systemic *Candida albicans* infection in mice, Proc Soc Exp Biol Med, 1970, *133*, 34.

206. Baine, W. B., Koenig, M. G., and Goodman, J. S.: Clearance of *Candida albicans* from the bloodstream of rabbits, Infect Immun, 1974, *10*, 1420.

207. Stanley, V. C., and Hurley, R.: The growth of candida species in cultures of mouse peritoneal macrophages, J Pathol, 1969, *97*, 357.

208. Ozato, K., and Vesaka, I.: The role of macrophages in *Candida albicans* infection *in vitro*, Jap J Microbiol, 1974, *18*, 29.

209. Marra, S., and Balish, E.: Immunity to *Candida albicans* induced by *Listeria monocytogenes*, Infect Immun, 1974, *10*, 72.

210. Morelli, R., and Rosenberg, L. T.: Role of complement during experimental candida infection in mice, Infect Immun, 1971, *3*, 521.

211. Hurley, D. L., Balow, J. E., and Fauci, A. S.: Experimental disseminated candidiasis. II. Administration of glucocorticosteroids, susceptibility to infection and immunity, J Infect Dis, 1975, *132*, 393.

212. Ashcraft, K. W., and Leape, L. L.: Candida sepsis complicating parenteral feeding, JAMA, 1970, *212*, 454.

213. Curry, C. R., and Quie, P. G.: Fungal septicemia in patients receiving parenteral hyperalimentation, N Engl J Med, 1971, *285*, 1221.

214. Louria, D. B., Stiff, D. P., and Bennett, B.: Disseminated moniliasis in the adult, Medicine (Baltimore), 1962, *41*, 307.

215. Quie, P. G., and Children, R. A.: Acute disseminated and chronic mucocutaneous candidiasis, Semin Hematol, 1971, *8*, 227.

216. Steinberg, D., Gold, J., and Brodin, A.: Necrotizing enterocolitis in leukemia, Arch Intern Med, 1973, *131*, 538.

217. Myerowitz, R. L., Allen, C. M., and Pazin, G. J.: Disseminated candidiasis: Changes in incidence, underlying diseases, and organ involvement, Abstracts of the Fourteenth Interscience Conference on Antimicrobial Agents and Chemotherapy, submitted for presentation, 1975.

218. Childs, A. J.: Effect of nystatin on growth of *Candida albicans* during antibiotic therapy, Lancet, 1956, *1*, 660.

219. Fitzpatrick, J. J., and Topley, H. E.: Ampicillin therapy and candida outgrowth, Am J Med Sci, 1966, *252*, 310.

220. Ramirez, G., Shuster, M., Kozub, W., and Pribor, H. C.: Fatal acute *Candida albicans* bronchopneumonia: Report of a case, JAMA, 1967, *199*, 340.

221. Lau, H. S., Reiber, C. D., and Dale, C. L.: *Candida albicans* in acute pneumonitis following surgery, Antimicrob Agents Chemother, 1967, 173.

222. Law, E. J., Kim, O. J., Stieritz, D. D., and MacMillan, B. G.: Experience with systemic candidiasis in the burned patient, J Trauma, 1972, *12*, 543.

223. Weekly clinicopathological exercises, Case 24–1972, N Engl J Med, 1972, *286*, 1309.

224. Rosenbaum, R. B., Barber, J. V., and Stevens, D. A.: *Candida albicans* pneumonia: Diagnosis by pulmonary aspiration, recovery without treatment, Am Rev Respir Dis, 1974, *109*, 373.

225. Gaines, J. D., and Remington, J. S.: Dissemi-

nated candidiasis in the surgical patient, Surgery, 1972, *72*, 730.

226. Haley, L. D., and McCabe, A.: A mycologic study of seventy-one autopsies, Am J Clin Pathol, 1950, *20*, 35.

227. Taschdjian, C. L., Kozinn, P. J., and Toni, E. F.: Opportunistic yeast infections with special reference to candidiasis, Ann N Y Acad Sci, 1970, *174*, 606.

228. Kozinn, P. J., and Taschdjian, C. L.: *Candida albicans*: Saprophyte or pathogen, JAMA, 1966, *198*, 170.

229. Eilard, T., Alestig, K., and Wahlen, P.: Treatment of disseminated candidiasis with 5-fluorocytosine, J Infect Dis, 1974, *130*, 155.

230. Ellis, C. A., and Spivack, M. L.: The significance of candidemia, Ann Intern Med, 1967, *67*, 511.

231. Toala, P., Schroeder, S. A., Daly, A. K., and Finland, M.: Candida at Boston City Hospital: Clinical and epidemiological characteristics and susceptibility to eight antimicrobial agents, Arch Intern Med, 1970, *126*, 983.

232. Gantz, N. M., Swain, J. L., Medeiros, A. A., and O'Brien, T. F.: Vacuum blood-culture bottles: Inhibiting growth of candida and fostering growth of bacteroides, Lancet, 1974, 2, 1174.

233. Komorowski, R. A., and Farmer, S. G.: Rapid detection of candidemia, Am J Clin Pathol, 1973, *59*, 56.

234. Bodey, G. P., and Luna, M.: Skin lesions associated with candidiasis, JAMA, 1974, *229*, 1466.

235. Fishman, L. S., Griffin, J. R., Sapico, F. L., and Hecht, R.: Hematogenous candida endophthalmitis: A complication of candidemia, N Engl J Med, 1972, *286*, 675.

236. Edwards, J. E., Jr., Foos, R. Y., Montgomerie, J. Z., and Guze, L. B.: Ocular manifestations of candida septicemia: Review of seventy-six cases of hematogenous candida endophthalmitis, Medicine (Baltimore), 1974, *53*, 47.

237. Robertson, D. M., Riley, F. C., and Hermans, P. E.: Endogenous candida oculomycosis: Report of two patients treated with flucytosine, Arch Ophthalmol, 1974, *91*, 33.

238. Everett, E. D., LaForce, F. M., and Eickhoff, T. C.: Serologic studies in patients with suspected visceral candidiasis, Arch Intern Med, 1975, 135, 1075.

239. Gaines, J. D., and Remington, J. S.: Diagnosis of deep infection with candida. A study of candida precipitins; Arch Intern Med, 1973, *132*, 699.

240. Preisler, H. D., Hasenclever, H. F., and Henderson, E. S.: Anticandida antibodies in patients with acute leukemia: A prospective study, Am J Med, 1971, *51*, 352.

241. Dee, T. H., and Rytel, M. W.: Clinical application of counterimmunoelectrophoresis in detection of candida serum precipitins, J Lab Clin Med, 1975, *85*, 161.

242. Jones, S. A., Brennan, M., and Kundsin, R. B.: Candida serology: An aid in diagnosis of deep-organ candidiasis, J Surg Res, 1973, *14*, 235.

243. Kozinn, P. J., Galen, M. D., Goldberg, P. K., Protzman, W., and Kozinn, M. A.: The precipitin test in systemic candidiasis, JAMA, 1976, *235*, 628.

244. Hellwege, H. H., Fischer, K., and Bläker, F.: Diagnostic value of candida precipitins, Lancet, 1972, 2, 386.

245. Remington, J. S., Gaines, J. D., and Gilmer, M. A.: Demonstration of candida precipitins in human sera by counterimmunoelectrophoresis, Lancet, 1972, *1*, 413.

246. Marier, R., and Andriole, V. T.: Usefulness of CIE in detection of *Candida albicans* antigen and antibody, Clin Res, 1975, *23*, 588A.

247. Weiner, M., Yount, W., and Reisner, H.: Immunopathogenesis of systemic candidiasis: Characterization of purified antibodies and factor B activation by cell wall mannan, Clin Res, 1976, *24*, 27A.

248. Miller, G. G., Witwer, M. W., Braude, A. I., and Davis, C. E.: Rapid identification of *Candida albicans* septicemia in man by gas-liquid chromatography, J Clin Invest, 1974, *54*, 1235.

249. Weinstein, A. J., Johnson, E. H., and Moellering, R. C., Jr.: Candida endophthalmitis: A complication of candidemia, Arch Intern Med, 1973, *132*, 749.

250. Montgomerie, J. Z., Edwards, J. E., Jr., and Guze, L.: Synergism of amphotericin B and 5-fluorocytosine for candida species, J Infect Dis, 1975, *132*, 82.

251. Woods, R. A., Bard, M., Jackson, I. E., and Drutz, D. J.: Resistance to polyene antibiotics and correlated sterol changes in two isolates of *Candida tropicalis* from a patient with an amphotericin B-resistant funguria, J Infect Dis, 1974, *129*, 53.

252. Utz, J. P., and Shadomy, S.: Fungal infections, Clin Pharmacol Ther, 1974, *16*, 912.

253. Hill, H. R., Mitchell, T. G., Matsen, J. M., and Quie, P. G.: Recovery from disseminated candidiasis in a premature neonate, Pediatrics, 1974, *53*, 748.

254. Hoeprich, P. D., Ingraham, J. L., Kleker, E., and Winship, M. J.: Development of resistance to 5-fluorocytosine in *Candida parapsilosis* during therapy, J Infect Dis, 1974, *130*, 112.

255. Vandevelde, A. G., Mauceri, A. A., and Johnson, J. E., III: 5-Fluorocytosine in the treatment of mycotic infections, Ann Intern Med, 1972, *77*, 43.

256. Greene, W. H., and Wiernik, P. H.: Candida endophthalmitis: Successful treatment in a patient with acute leukemia, Am J Ophthalmol, 1972, *74*, 1100.

257. Medoff, G., Comfort, M., and Kobayashi, G. S.: Synergistic action of amphotericin B and 5-fluorocytosine against yeast-like organisms, Proc

Soc Exp Biol Med, 1971, *138*, 571.

258. Hoeprich, P. D., and Finn, P. D.: Activity of combination of antifungal agents against *Candida albicans* and *Cryptococcus neoformans*, Proc Am Soc Microbiol, Washington, 1972, p. 135.

259. Rifkind, D., Marchiaro, T. L., Schneck, S. A., and Hill, R. B.: Systemic fungal infections complicating renal transplantation and immunosuppressive therapy, Am J Med, 1967, *43*, 28.

260. Watson, J. I., Mandl, M. A., and Rose, B.: Disseminated histoplasmosis occurring in association with systemic lupus erythematosis, Can Med Assoc J, 1968, *99*, 958.

261. Cox, F., and Hughes, W. T.: Disseminated histoplasmosis and childhood leukemia, Cancer, 1974, *33*, 1127.

262. Kobayashi, G. S., Medoff, G., Schlessinger, D., Kwan, C. N., and Musser, W. E.: Amphotericin B potentiation of rifampicin as an antifungal agent against the yeast phase of *Histoplasma capsulatum*, Science, 1972, *177*, 709.

263. Deresinski, S. C., and Stevens, D. A.: Coccidioidomycosis in compromised hosts: Experience at Stanford University Hospital, Medicine (Baltimore), 1975, *54*, 377.

264. Pappagianis, D.: Opportunism in coccidioidomycosis, in *Opportunistic Fungal Infections*, E. Chick, A. Balows, and M. L. Furcolow, ed., Charles C Thomas, Springfield, 1975, chap. 20.

265. Onal, E., Lopata, M., and Lourenço, R. V.: Disseminated pulmonary blastomycosis in an immunosuppressed patient, Am Rev Respir Dis, 1976, *113*, 83.

266. Aisner, J., Schimpff, S. C., Sutherland, J. C., Young, V. M., and Wiernik, P. H.: *Torulopsis glabrata* infections in patients with cancer: An increasing incidence, Am J Med, in press.

267. Aisner, J., Sickles, E. A., Schimpff, S. C., Young, V. M., Greene, W. H., and Wiernik, P. H.: *Torulopsis glabrata* pneumonitis in patients with cancer: Report of three cases, JAMA, 1974, *230*, 584.

268. Marks, M. I., Langston, C., and Eickhoff, T. C.: *Torulopsis glabrata*: An opportunistic pathogen in man, N Engl J Med, 1970, *283*, 1131.

269. Pankey, G. A., and Daloviso, J. R.: Fungemia caused by *Torulopsis glabrata*, Medicine (Baltimore), 1973, *52*, 395.

270. Stenderup, A., and Pederson, G. T.: Yeasts of human origin, Acta Pathol Microbiol Scand, 1962, *54*, 462.

271. Huang, S., and Harris, L. S.: Acute disseminated penicillosis: Report of a case and review of pertinent literature, Am J Clin Pathol, 1963, *39*, 167.

272. Murray, J. F., Finegold, S. M., Froman, S., and Will, D. W.: The changing spectrum of nocardiosis, Am Rev Respir Dis, 1961, *83*, 315.

273. Rifkind, D., Marchioro, T. L., Schneck, S. A., and Hill, R. B., Jr.: Systemic fungal infections complicating renal transplantation and immunosuppressive therapy, Am J Med, 1967, *43*, 28.

274. Goodman, J. S., and Koenig, M. G.: Nocardia infections in a general hospital, Ann NY Acad Sci, 1970, *174*, 552.

275. Young, L. S., Armstrong, D., Blevins, A., and Lieverman, P.: *Nocardia asteroides* infection complicating neoplastic disease, Am J Med, 1971, *50*, 356.

276. Bach, M. C., Adler, J. L., Breman, J., P'eng, F. K., Sahyoun, A., Schlesinger, R. M., Madras, P., and Monaco, A. P.: Influence of rejection therapy on fungal and nocardial infections in renal transplant recipients, Lancet, 1973, *1*, 180.

277. Krick, J. A., Stinson, E. B., and Remington, J. S.: Nocardia infection in heart transplant patients, Ann Intern Med, 1975, *82*, 18.

278. Diamond, R. D., and Bennett, J. E.: Disseminated *Nocardia brasiliensis* infection, Arch Intern Med, 1973, *131*, 735.

279. Holm, P.: Seven cases of human nocardiosis caused by *Nocardia farcinica*, Sabouraudia, 1975, *13*, 161.

280. Causey, W. A.: *Nocardia caviae*: A report of 13 new isolations with clinical correlation, Appl Microbiol, 1974, *28*, 193.

281. Kurup, P. V., Randhawa, H. S., Sandhu, R. S., and Abraham, S.: Pathogenicity of *N. caviae*, *N. asteroides* and *N. brasiliensis*, Mycopathol Mycol Appl, 1970, *40*, 113.

282. Cox, F., and Hughes, W. T.: Contagious and other aspects of nocardiosis in the compromised host, Pediatrics, 1975, *55*, 135.

283. Frazier, A. R., Rosenow, E. C., III., and Roberts, G. D.: Nocardiosis: A review of 25 cases occurring during 24 months, Mayo Clin Proc, 1975, *50*, 657.

284. Bujack, J. S., Ottensen, E. A., Dinarello, C. A., and Brenner, V. J.: Nocardiosis in a child with chronic granulomatous disease, J Pediatr, 1973, *83*, 98.

285. Neu, H. C., Silva, M., Hazen, E., and Roseheim, S. H.: Necrotizing nocardial pneumonitis, Ann Intern Med, 1967, *66*, 274.

286. Palmer, D. L., Harvey, R. L., and Wheeler, J. K.: Diagnostic and therapeutic consideration in *Nocardia asteroides* infection, Medicine (Baltimore), 1974, *53*, 391.

287. Pinkhas, J., Izhak, O., deVries, A., Spitzer, S. A., and Heniz, E.: Pulmonary nocardiosis complicating malignant lymphoma successfully treated with chemotherapy, Chest, 1973, *63*, 367.

288. Grossman, C. B., Bragg, D. G., and Armstrong, D.: Roentgen manifestations of pulmonary nocardiosis, Radiology, 1970, *96*, 325.

289. Cohen, M. L., Weiss, E. B., and Monaco, A. P.: Successful treatment of *Pneumocystis carinii* and *Nocardia asteroides* in a renal transplant patient, Am J Med, 1971, *50*, 269.

290. Ruebush, T. K., III., and Goodman, J. S.: *No-*

cardia asteroides bacteremia in an immunosuppressed renal-transplant patient, Am J Clin Pathol, 1975, *64*, 537.

291. Roberts, G. D., Brewer, N. S., and Hermans, P. E.: Diagnosis of nocardiosis by blood culture, Mayo Clin Proc, 1974, *49*, 293.

292. Hamal, P. B.: Primary pulmonary nocardiosis: Case report, Thorax, 1974, *29*, 382.

293. Pier, A. C., Thurston, J. R., and Larsen, A. B.: A diagnostic antigen for nocardiosis: Comparative tests in cattle with nocardiosis and mycobacteriosis, Am J Vet Res, 1968, *29*, 397.

294. Ortiz-Ortiz, L., Contreras, M. F., and Bojalil, L. F.: Cytoplasmic antigens from nocardia eliciting a specific delayed hypersensitivity, Infect Immun, 1972, *5*, 879.

295. Ortiz-Ortiz, L., and Bojalil, L. F.: Delayed skin reactions to cytoplasmic extracts of nocardia organisms as a means of diagnostic and epidemiological study of nocardia infection, Exp Immunol, 1972, *12*, 225.

296. Nelson, E., and Henrici, A. T.: Immunologic studies of actinomycetes, with special reference to the acid-fast species, Proc Soc Exp Biol Med, 1922, *19*, 351.

297. Bourgeouis, L., and Beaman, B. L.: Probable L-forms of *Nocardia asteroides* included in cultured mouse peritoneal macrophages, Infect Immun, 1974, *9*, 576.

298. Krick, J. A., and Remington, J. S.: Resistance to infection with *Nocardia asteroides*, J Infect Dis, 1975, *131*, 665.

299. Krick, J. A., and Remington, J. S.: Effect of human blood polymorphonuclear leukocytes and monocytes on *Nocardia asteroides*, unpublished.

300. Langevin, R. W., and Katz, S.: Fulminating pulmonary nocardiosis, Dis Chest, 1964, *46*, 310.

301. Robboy, S. J., and Vickery, A. L.: Tinctorial and morphologic properties distinguishing actinomycosis and nocardiosis, N Engl J Med, 1970, *282*, 593.

302. Goldman, A. L., and Light, L.: Anterior cervical infections: Complications of transtracheal aspirations (letter to the editor), Am Rev Respir Dis, 1975, *111*, 707.

303. Hosty, T. S., McDurmont, C., Ajello, L., Brumfield, G. L., Georg, L. K., and Caliz, A. A.: Prevalence of *Nocardia asteroides* in sputa examined by a tuberculosis diagnostic laboratory, J Lab Clin Med, 1961, *58*, 107.

304. Raich, R. A., Casey, F., and Hall, W. H.: Pulmonary and cutaneous nocardiosis, Am Rev Respir Dis, 1961, *83*, 505.

305. Krick, J. A., and Remington, J. S.: *Nocardia asteroides* infections, West J Med, 1974, *121*, 235.

306. Humphreys, D. W., Crowder, J. G., and White, A.: Serological reactions to nocardia antigens, Am J Med Sci, 1975, *269*, 323.

307. Peabody, J. W., and Seabury, J. H.: Actinomycosis and nocardiosis: A review of basic differences in therapy, Am J Med, 1960, *28*, 99.

308. Lerner, P. I., and Baum, G. L.: Antimicrobial susceptibility of nocardia species, Antimicrob Agents Chemother, 1973, *4*, 85.

309. Bach, M. C., Sabath, L. D., and Finland, M.: Susceptibility of *Nocardia asteroides* to 45 antimicrobial agents in vitro, Antimicrob Agents Chemother, 1973, *3*, 1.

310. Epstein, E.: Treatment of a cutaneous *Nocardia asteroides* infection with minocycline hydrochloride, West J Med, 1974, *120*, 497.

311. Epstein, E.: Letter to the editor, West J Med, 1974, *121*, 236.

312. Maderazo, E. G., and Quintiliani, R.: Treatment of nocardial infection with trimethoprimsulfamethoxazole, Am J Med, 1974, *57*, 671.

State of the Art ─────────────

Pulmonary Infection in the Compromised Host

Part II[1, 2]

D. M. WILLIAMS, J. A. KRICK, and J. S. REMINGTON

Contents

Viruses

Deoxyribonucleic acid viruses, the cause of latent infection in a significant segment of the normal population, are a cause of significant morbidity and mortality in the compromised population.

Herpes Simplex

Both type 1 and type 2 herpes simplex viruses (HSV) are capable of producing disease in the compromised host. Confirmation of type is only occasionally available in the clinical literature in cases of bronchopulmonary infection (313); however, most cases are presumptively due to type 1 infection because of presumed oropharyngeal origin.

Immunopathologic aspects. Many investigators have attempted to define mechanisms of immunity to this virus, well known for its tendency to produce recurring localized lesions in the normal host. Bastian and associates (314), Barin-

1 From the Department of Medicine, Division of Infectious Diseases, Stanford University School of Medicine, Stanford, Calif.; the Division of Allergy, Immunology and Infectious Diseases, Palo Alto Medical Research Foundation, Palo Alto, Calif.; and the Alamo Medical Clinic, Alamo, Calif.

2 This work was supported by grant no. AI04717 from the National Institutes of Health.

ger and Swoveland (315), and Baringer (316) have provided evidence that nerve ganglia may serve as a reservoir of infection in the asymptomatic host, and Stevens and co-workers (317) have shown in mice that pneumococcal pneumonia can activate virus dormant in ganglia. Aspects of immunity to HSV infection that have been studied include the role of interferon and antibodies, parameters of lymphocyte function, and the role of macrophages.

Hirsch and co-workers (318) observed increased resistance to HSV challenge in suckling mice given stimulated macrophages compared to unstimulated macrophages, and this resistance correlated positively with the greater interferon production by the stimulated macrophages *in vitro*. Interestingly, interferon produced by macrophages was ineffective in protecting other macrophages from HSV infection. Ennis (319) found no apparent association in mice between interferon production and survival after HSV challenge. Lodmell and Notkins (320), using rabbit kidney monolayers and sensitized leukocytes and antigen, found production of an interferon-like mediator and inhibition of viral spread *in vitro*. Fujibayashi and associates (321) have shown in the rabbit that immune lymphocytes produce interferon in response to both HSV antigen alone and to HSV antigen-antibody complexes, whereas control nonimmune lymphocytes do not. This provides evidence that even in the "immune" host, with antibody present, interferon production might be possible. Rasmussen and co-workers (322) looked serially at apparently normal adults during primary or recurrent infection with HSV. Lymphocyte production of interferon, induced by HSV antigen-specific stimulation, peaked at 2 to 6 weeks after clinical disease, thereby making its role in providing protection difficult to explain. Subjects who failed to produce it, however, had more frequent recurrences. This relationship to protection was not true of lymphocyte transformation to HSV antigen; interferon production appeared to be a better prognostic indicator. These investigators also found interferon production a better indicator of active disease than prior sensitization (indicated by lymphocyte transformation).

Other workers have also looked at lymphocyte function in humans with HSV infection. Wilton and associates (323) studied 6 patients with primary HSV infection and 13 with recurrent disease, all of whom were otherwise normal, and reported that whereas antigen-specific lympho-

cyte transformation was similar in patients and control subjects, specific (HSV) induced lymphocyte cytotoxicity and antigen-specific macrophage migration inhibition were impaired in patients. Rosenberg and co-workers (324) studied 41 normal persons, 13 with active herpetic lesions, 21 with neutralizing antibodies but no clinical disease, and 7 without positive serology or clinical history of disease. They found that lymphocytes of seronegative patients did not transform to specific antigen or produce lymphokines, whereas lymphocytes from seropositive persons did; however, lymphocyte transformation was slightly depressed at 7 to 10 days and 28 to 31 days after onset of herpetic lesions in patients with active disease compared to seropositive control subjects without clinical disease. Russell (325) similarly noted antigen-specific lymphocyte transformation in all patients with a history of occasional or frequent "cold sores" and in only 4 of 37 control patients. Response to other antigens or mitogens was similar in the two groups. Starr and co-workers (326) found that lymphocytes from 3 seronegative subjects transformed to specific antigen at a low level, but that seropositive persons had a higher mean stimulation index. Thus, evidence exists for virus-specific, lymphocyte-dependent cell-mediated immunity. The nature of specific defects leading to recurrent disease is less clear. Notkins (327) has noted that antigen, induced by HSV on cell surfaces, could make the cells vulnerable to attack by cytotoxic lymphocytes; what role this plays in controlling virus spread has not yet been determined.

Ennis (319) demonstrated that spleen cells could transfer resistance to HSV challenge when transferred to syngeneic mice and stated that sensitized spleen cells could limit spread of HSV infection in cell cultures. Allison (328) noted that thymectomy and antilymphocyte serum aggravated HSV infections in mice. Oakes (329), also using a murine model, found that immunosuppressive doses of antilymphocyte serum or antithymocyte serum allowed spread of subcutaneously injected HSV from the local site to the central nervous system. No neutralizing antibody could be found in the sera of these mice, and passive transfer of neutralizing antibody to mice treated with antithymocyte serum did not restore resistance to HSV. On the other hand, transfer of HSV-sensitized spleen cells did provide protection if the spleen cells were not treated with antithymocyte serum before transfer.

As alluded to above, macrophages were studied by Hirsch and associates (318) in relation to age-dependent resistance to HSV in a murine model. Peritoneal macrophages of adult mice could protect suckling syngeneic mice from intraperitoneal challenge with HSV, and nonspecifically activated macrophages produced by protease-peptone stimulation were more effective than normal macrophages. As previously stated, interferon did not protect other macrophages from viral infection, but resistance was associated with greater interferon production as well as "more efficient" phagocytosis by macrophages and greater intracellular destruction of virus. Despite these various results, the actual role of the macrophage as well as the lymphocyte in preventing spread of extracellular virus remains to be defined (327).

The role of antibody in HSV infection is similarly unclear. Allison (328) has stated that antibody plays no significant role in prevention of HSV spread once infection is estab.ished. Oakes (329), as previously mentioned, passively transferred neutralizing antibody to antithymocyte-treated mice that could not produce their own and found it was not protective even though passively transferred neutralizing antibody remained in the circulatory system during the period required for HSV to spread from the site of injection to the central nervous system. The concentrations of antibody obtained were comparable to those physiologically produced in normal mice after subcutaneous inoculation of virus. These results suggested that under these circumstances antibody was not an important defense mechanism in preventing spread of virus to the central nervous system in mice. Rosenberg and Notkins (330) demonstrated in the rabbit that virus inocula in combination with antibody did not lead to either antibody production or cell-mediated immunity measured by lymphocyte transformation, perhaps owing to viral aggregation. Stevens and Cook (331) found that viral reactivation in syngeneic mice after transplantation of latently infected ganglia could be prevented by a circulating factor whose effect was mimicked by the administration of anti-HSV antibody (IgG). This suggested that antibody might affect intraneural viral activity (although a cytotoxic effect on neurons was not excluded). Douglas and Couch (332), in a prospective study in humans with chronic HSV infection and recurrent herpes labialis, found no relationship of frequency of isolation of virus or number of lesions to serum neutralizing antibody concentrations. They commented that se-

rum antibody concentrations in adults have tended to be high and constant regardless of disease activity and, in these studies, did not vary with antigenic stimulation. Local IgA antibody in oral secretions did not appear to be important. Similarly, Rasmussen and co-workers (322) did not find any correlation between serum antibody concentrations and disease activity in patients with recurrent HSV infection.

Lodmell and Notkins (320) and Lodmell and associates (333) have suggested 2 phases in the immune response. The first is antigen-specific and involves antibody, complement, and immune leukocytes with mediator production to attract inflammatory cells. The second phase involves cytotoxicity and interferon production designed to inhibit cell-to-cell viral spread. Several investigators have demonstrated that this cell-mediated cytotoxicity may be dependent on the presence of anti-HSV antibody (334, 335).

Thus, although data exist concerning multiple parameters of cellular and humoral immunity in animal and human infection with HSV, the interplay of these factors in preventing and containing HSV infection remains to be clarified.

It is of note that dexamethasone may increase *in vitro* yields of virus (Type 2) and increase plaquing efficiency with some cells *in vitro* (336). In general, however, the reason for the predisposition to recurrent or disseminated infection in the immunosuppressed host remains to be determined.

An interesting clinical example of the interrelationships of parameters of cellular and humoral immunity in defense to this infection is provided by the case reported by Douglas and co-workers (337), in which HSV pneumonia developed in the transplanted lung but not in the patient's own lung. The patient had a prior history of HSV infection, and, therefore, humoral antibody bathed both lungs. This one example seems to indicate the importance of local cellular immunity in resistance to HSV infection.

Pathology. Disease has ranged from tracheobronchitis (313) to pneumonia (337). Nash and Foley (338), in a study of 6 burn patients, described necrosis of alveolar walls, much necrotic debris, a sparse neutrophilic response, and intra-alveolar proteinaceous exudate with or without hemorrhage. Intranuclear inclusions were found within alveolar lining cells. Most lesions were near involved bronchi and bronchioles, but one patient had only pulmonary lesions without tracheobronchial involvement, probably owing to hematogenous spread. The histologic changes were often focal and multiple. Douglas and co-workers (337), in a lung transplant patient with diffuse pneumonia, similarly found hemorrhagic necrosis, destruction of alveolar septae, neutrophils with few mononuclear cells, and an exudate consisting of fibrin plus protein. Intranuclear inclusions that were eosinophilic were also noted, and intranuclear "herpesvirus-like" particles were seen by electron microscopy.

Clinical manifestations. Infection of the respiratory tract with HSV has been reported in alcoholics (313) and in patients with burns (338, 339) and immunosuppression (337, 340, 341). Disease, as noted previously, has varied from tracheobronchitis (313) to pneumonia (337). Pneumonia has been associated with involvement of the upper airway with HSV (342), suggesting aspiration as a mechanism of spread of virus to the lungs (338); it has also occurred without tracheobronchial disease in the setting of disseminated infection and hemotogenous spread (338). Infection with HSV has been reported in conjunction with infection with other opportunistic pathogens (343), frequently making diagnosis difficult (338). Most reported cases have been found at autopsy. Several investigators have emphasized that associated facial, oral, or esophageal herpetic lesions may be a useful clinical clue to the diagnosis (337, 338, 342). Unfortunately, the presence of lesions in these areas also makes interpretation of virus identification in sputum more difficult. The pulmonary disease may be focal (338) or more generalized (337), and except for the possible clue given by associated herpetic lesions, as noted above, diagnosis cannot be made on clinical grounds alone.

There have been too few cases to determine whether any laboratory values are typical of HSV pneumonia. Leukocytosis has been present in several cases. Chest roentgenograms have shown a nonspecific bronchopneumonia or interstitial pneumonia (337, 341, 342).

Diagnosis. Demonstration of HSV involvement of the lungs depends on viral isolation in material not contaminated by oral or upper airway herpetic infection or indirect fluorescent antibody techniques. Electron microscopy may provide a suggestive but not a definitive diagnosis. Tracheal aspiration may reveal intranuclear inclusions (337), and a diagnosis may be established by the methods mentioned previously. Demonstration of cells with intranuclear inclusions is not necessarily diagnostic of HSV

because of similar findings in other viral infections. Needle biopsy of the lung has been successful (341), but because of the morbidity associated with this procedure we prefer lung aspiration or open lung biopsy.

A 4-fold rise in serum neutralizing antibody (337, 341) or complement-fixing or indirect hemagglutinating antibody (344) may be of confirmatory aid, but "nonspecific" rises occur in other febrile illnesses and a titer rise is not by itself diagnostic of HSV as the cause of the pulmonary infection. Detection of specific IgM antibodies has been described (345), but its usefulness in establishing the diagnosis has not yet been clarified.

Prevention and treatment. Idoxuridine therapy at this time seems unacceptable because of its toxicity and lack of proof of effectiveness (346). Cytosine arabinoside has also been toxic (337, 341, 347) and is of unproved effectiveness (347). Adenine arabinoside (15 mg per kg per day, given in 2 equally divided doses during a 12-hour period) is relatively nontoxic and is considered by some investigators to be the current therapy of choice (348). The drug is currently available only on protocol. Interferon (349) has had only limited trials and is available in only a few centers in the United States. Live virus vaccines are unlikely to be tried because of their possible oncogenic effects (350) and there are no data on the use of killed vaccines.

Cytomegalovirus

Cytomegalovirus (CMV) was first isolated approximately 20 years ago (351–353) and is believed to consist of multiple strains. An excellent recent review dealing with this agent was done by Weller (354).

Immunopathologic aspects. Extensive investigation of CMV infection has been performed using the murine model. Because strains of the virus are host specific, extrapolation of results obtained in the mouse to human disease must be done with caution (354). Investigations have been performed to attempt to determine the role of interferon in immunity to CMV. Osborn and Medearis (355) observed mouse strains of CMV to be relatively resistant to the effects of interferon whereas Oie and associates (356) concluded that sensitivity to interferon was related to the viral dose used as a challenge, small doses being sensitive but higher doses very resistant. The ability of CMV to induce interferon production has been a subject of extensive investigation. Henson and Smith (357) found evidence for interferon production by cells infected with the murine strain, recently confirmed by Oie and co-workers (356). Osborn and Medearis (355), on the other hand, did not observe interferon production either in the intact mouse or *in vitro*. Limited studies have been performed using a human system. Recently, Glasgow (358) observed the production of an "interferon-like mediator" in human embryo fibroblast cultures using the AD 169 strain of CMV, and Lang and co-workers (359) showed protection of human cells by interferon against cell-free CMV, but not against the cell-associated virus. Rabson and associates (360) demonstrated marked reduction of plaque formation in human fibroblasts by human CMV when human interferon was present. The role of interferon in resistance to human infection clearly requires further investigation.

The role of macrophages in resistance to CMV is also of interest. Tegtmeyer and Craighead (361) demonstrated that adult mouse peritoneal macrophages could be uniformly infected and produce large amounts of virus. Selgrade and Osborn (362) attempted to infect murine macrophages with the virus but could recover only small amounts of CMV virus and could find no correlation between differences in macrophage resistance to CMV multiplication and strain differences in susceptibility. Suckling mice given syngeneic adult macrophages, however, did show increased resistance to CMV infection, and mice pretreated with silica to depress reticuloendothelial function did have an increased mortality rate when infected with CMV. These results led Selgrade and Osborn to conclude that although the macrophage was important in resistance to CMV in the mouse, its effect probably was in the induction phase of immunity rather than as a site of control of viral replication.

Lymphocyte function has also been examined in relation to immunity to CMV. Treatment of mice, naturally infected with CMV, with antithymocyte serum leads to histopathologic evidence of dissemination of this virus (363). Selgrade and Osborn (362) showed that lymphocytes from nonimmune adult mice increased resistance of suckling mice to CMV. Brody and Craighead (364) were able to produce pulmonary infection in mice using antiserum to murine lymphocytes. Of interest is the fact that electron microscopy studies of pulmonary tissue from these mice revealed viral particles within monocytes (and occasionally in alveolar macrophages), prompting the suggestion that the monocyte might act as a vehicle for dissemination of CMV in the immunosuppressed host. Simmons and associates (365) in a study of renal transplant patients observed that lymphocyte transformation to phytohemagglutinating antibody remained low in 4 patients who died (even when immunosuppression was reduced or stopped) compared to values in "patients who had recovered from viral infection." The values in the patients who recovered did not differ from those found in 61 control immunosuppressed patients. These data suggest that suppression of lymphocyte function might be of pathogenetic and prognostic significance.

The role of antibody in immunity to CMV is less clear. Antibody does not prevent virus shedding in urine or oral secretions (366). *In vitro,* neutralizing antibody prevented development of viral cytopathic effect in human tissue culture when mixed with the viral inoculum (358). If antibody was added after cell infection, initial cytopathic effects were not prevented, but viral spread to other cells was decreased at late time periods (358). Simmons and associates (365) noted that antibody response to the virus in renal transplant patients was decreased in 6 patients who died, only one of whom had a 4-fold titer rise. (The fact that antibody rises can be late even in normal subjects must be considered.) In their renal transplant series, Ho and co-workers (367) reported that most clinically recognizable disease due to CMV occurred in seronegative recipients of kidneys from seropositive donors, suggesting the possibility of some protective effect in terms of development of symptoms in patients who already had positive titers before receiving transplants.

Because of the increase in symptomatic human infections coincident with immunosuppressive treatment (368), animal studies have been performed using immunosuppressive therapy. Cortisone treatment in the mouse model led to disseminated disease (369). Irradiation similarly led to more extensive and often fatal infection (370).

Because of the possibility that in transplant patients host-versus-graft reactions (365, 367, 371) or graft-versus-host reactions (372) may enhance disease, the effect of histoincompatability has been studied in mice. Adult mice chronically infected just after birth or *in utero* carry virus that can be activated by co-cultivating spleen lymphocytes with histoincompatible mouse embryo cells (373). Wu and co-workers (374) demonstrated increased CMV titers in spleen and kidneys of chronically infected mice after they were given histoincompatible skin allografts, suggesting a role of the host-versus-graft reaction in reactivation of this virus.

Pathology. Craighead (366) has described the typical pathologic findings in pulmonary CMV infection in the adult. He divided the pathology into 3 groups : (*1*) diffuse panlobar interstitial disease, (*2*) focal interstitial pneumonia, and (*3*) scattered alveolar macrophages showing inclusions but unaccompanied by inflammation. In the first type, extensive filling by alveoli by interstitial fluid is seen along with protein accumulation with mononuclear cell infiltration. Occasional hyaline membranes are seen and, in contrast to the mouse model, inclusions are found in pneumocytes as well as macrophages. The focal disease has a similar histologic appearance with apparent random distribution. Lungs were also described from which CMV was cultured but that failed to show typical haloed "owl-eyed" intranuclear inclusions, making the significance of the culture unclear.

Clinical manifestations. Clinical disease associated with CMV infection has been commonly reported in organ transplant patients (365, 367, 368, 371, 375–380), in patients with leukemia, Hodgkin's disease, and lymphosarcoma (381–383), in bone marrow transplant recipients (372, 384, 385), and in association with administration of immunosuppressive drugs (386) and has varied clinically from a mild course to fulminant disease and death.

The difficulties in diagnosis will be discussed below, but it is necessary to mention here the special problem of diagnosis of CMV infection in renal transplant patients because much of the clinical data we will discuss is from that group. Rifkind and associates (371) found CMV in urine cultures in 65 per cent of 26 patients without clinical disease. Coulson and associates (377) noted similar serologic rises after transplant in patients with and without clinical disease, and observed CMV complement-fixing (CF) titers of greater than 1:16 in 50 to 73 per cent of their dialyzed population at any one time. These observations, coupled with the uncertainty of the significance of positive CMV cultures from pulmonary tissues mentioned above (366), mean that in many cases presented as CMV pneumonitis in the literature the diagnosis is tenuous. Increasing serologic titers to CMV after renal transplantation may represent asymptomatic reactivation of latent virus. Symptomatic disease may be more common in cases of pri-

mary infection, but further investigation of this point is needed.

Coulson and co-workers (377) described 13 cases of what they considered to be CMV pneumonitis in renal transplant patients. Fever characteristically began 40 days after transplant and lasted 4 to 6 weeks and was associated with bilateral interstitial pneumonia. All patients had dyspnea and relative hypoxemia and 5 died of respiratory failure, usually with suprainfection with other organisms. Nonproductive cough was common. Actual inclusion bodies in pulmonary tissue, however, were demonstrated in only 2 of their patients; the data leading to the diagnosis of pulmonary infection with CMV were indirect: by urine and throat cultures or by liver biopsy. Fine and associates (378) described 9 renal allograft recipients who also developed fever on the mean post-operative day 40, persisting 8 to 19 days, with pulmonary infiltrates and pulmonary symptoms in 3 patients. Cough and tachypnea were associated with rales on physical examination and eventual death in one of the 3 patients with pneumonitis. Fine and co-workers described hematologic findings that included leukopenia in 8 patients with significant lymphocytosis in 6, thrombocytopenia in 4 patients, and anemia in 8 patients. Simmons and co-workers (365) studied 46 patients after transplant in whom they believed the time of onset of CMV infection could be documented (365). Thirty-three had fever. Thirty developed a white blood cell count of < 5,000 per mm³ that preceded seroconversion by an average of 30 days. The peak incidence (by serologic diagnosis and viral isolation) was 30 to 70 days after transplant. Six patients died. Roentgenographic evidence of interstitial pneumonia was seen in "about half" of the fatal cases in the third week of symptoms, and "irreversible pulmonary edema" was the terminal event with autopsy evidence of pneumonitis and CMV inclusion bodies. CMV was most easily isolated from urine, but sputum and bronchoscopy specimens were also frequently positive. A correlation of disease was also found with clinical rejection. Fiala and associates (380) observed that symptoms usually occurred 1 to 3 months after renal transplantation in their series. In their series, 11 of 61 transplanted patients developed pulmonary infiltrates believed most likely to be due to CMV. These investigators also noted an association of disease with rejection; initial rejection was followed by evidence of active CMV infection in 94 per cent of patients. In at least 2 of 18 patients, viremia preceded clinical rejection, suggesting a viral cause of rejection rather than the reverse. Ninety-six per cent of patients had evidence of CMV infection within 7 months of transplantation.

Rifkind and co-workers (371) identified CMV-like cells in the lungs of 27 of 51 transplant patients who came to autopsy. In 7 (26 per cent) of these 27 patients, multiple 2- to 4-mm bilateral lung nodules were noted by chest roentgenogram. The facts that lung nodules were seen on roentgenogram in only 26 per cent of their cases and that one patient with this radiographic finding but without evidence of pulmonary CMV was found suggest limited diagnostic usefulness of this sign. Goodman and co-workers (387) noted that in 2 patients with this radiographic picture, CMV was the only pulmonary pathogen found and that the nodules were seen in the outer one third of the lung field. That recovery in the immunosuppressed host might occur even with severe pulmonary involvement (diagnosed by aspiration biopsy of the lung) is suggested by the case report of Jeffery and associates (375). Recovery in their patient may have been associated with discontinuance of immunosuppressive drugs.

CMV pneumonia in patients with leukemia, Hodgkin's disease, and lymphosarcoma has had pathologic features and symptoms (when described) similar to those just mentioned.

Although some compromised patients probably acquire CMV disease through extensive blood transfusions (388–390), reactivation of latent infection is also frequent (367, 378, 391). Recent data have implicated latent infection in donor kidneys as a source of the infection (367).

Recent interest has developed in interstitial pneumonia believed to be due to CMV after human marrow transplantation (372, 384). Meyers and associates (372) described 33 patients who developed interstitial pneumonia after marrow transplantation. Signs and symptoms included tachypnea, nonproductive cough, dyspnea, and unilateral or bilateral rales. Development of pneumonia was associated with allogenic grafts and graft-versus-host disease. No association was found with blood transfusions, but, as in renal transplant patients, there was an association with positive serologic test titers in the donor. Typical histologic changes (intranuclear inclusion bodies) were found in alveolar epithelial cells in 9 of 17 autopsy cases. Cultures of the lungs for virus were positive in 7 of the 9. The cause in the other cases is less clear. Both

cases and "non-cases" had similar serologic changes and similar rates of positive antemortem viral cultures from a variety of sources including sputum, urine, and blood, again emphasizing the difficulty of relating these findings to diagnosis.

The severity of the pneumonia in this population may be inversely related to the immunocompetence of the recipient (384).

Diagnosis. The diagnosis of CMV pneumonia is complicated by all of the findings alluded to previously. Serology has frequently been used as a diagnostic tool, and the CF test has been employed most widely. Waner and co-workers (393), performing serial measurements of CF antibodies in 20 blood donors, found great variations in titer results over time; 11 persons had titers ranging between $\geq$1:8 and <1:4 at least once, thus casting doubt on the significance of titer rises, at least in some cases (393). However, in a study of hospital employees and nurses during a 4- to 5-year period, Yeager (394) found that when CMV CF titers were all run against the same antigen at the same time, no 4-fold rises or falls occurred in 71 persons with chronic positive titers and no titer changes from >1:8 to <1:8 were found. Reliability and reproducibility in sera with titers of <1:8 were believed to be poor. These latter observations increase confidence in the CF test; however, it remains indirect at best in terms of diagnosis of pulmonary infection. Craighead (366) in a pathology study observed that the correlation between CF titers and extent of pulmonary involvement was poor. Detection of CF antibody may require a battery of CMV antigens owing to antigenic variation, and heterologous rises with varicella-zoster may occur (384). Neutralizing antibodies can also be measured (354, 391), but tests for these are difficult to perform and have been less widely used, although they may be more sensitive than those for CF antibodies (391). Measurement of indirect hemagglutinating antibody is considered by some to be the most satisfactory serologic method for diagnosis (384). It is important to recognize that in the transplant population IgM antibody may persist for years and does not necessarily indicate primary infection (391, 392).

The most direct means of diagnosis is examination of pulmonary tissue stained with hematoxylin and eosin to demonstrate intranuclear inclusions with concurrent viral culture. Because obtaining lung tissue may not be feasible in many patients, bronchial brushing with tissue examination may be useful and should be considered (395). Bronchoscopy with bronchial washings submitted for cytology and culture has also been used successfully (396). These procedures avoid the necessity for lung aspiration or biopsy; however, as noted by Behrens and Quick (396), care must be used in interpreting inclusion bodies in this material because of similar changes produced by herpesvirus and adenovirus infections.

Interpretation of positive cultures in the absence of conclusive histologic changes might be aided by the application of indirect immunofluorescent techniques to detect CMV antigen in tissues (384). Molecular hybridization or *in situ* cyto-hybridization have also been considered (384).

Cox and Hughes (397) did not find viremia useful in diagnosing active CMV infection in children with lymphatic leukemia, and Simmons and co-workers (365) found it difficult to detect in patients after renal transplant. Fiala and associates (380), on the other hand, observed viremia in 42 per cent of renal transplant patients during the first 7 months after transplantation. This viremia persisted for 1 to 13 weeks. Viruria was present in 68 per cent of the cases and chronic. Viremia, therefore, seemed more likely to indicate active infection (386). CMV titers were 2.3 to 7.7 times greater in polymorphonuclear than mononuclear leukocytes when both were positive (386). The reasons for the discrepancies in these studies of viremia are not known.

Hematologic and hepatic function tests may suggest infection but are not diagnostic. Cold agglutinins, rheumatoid factor, and other immunologic abnormalities have been described (354) but are similarly nonspecific. Inclusion bodies have not been found commonly in cells in urine in adult cases (381, 382), and thus examination for these is not a useful diagnostic test.

The finding of the "classical" retinouveitis associated with cytomegalovirus infection or ophthalmologic examination is considered to be diagnostic (398, 399).

Prevention and treatment. At present there is no effective therapy for infection with CMV. Interferon (400), idoxuridine (401, 402), cytosine arabinoside (403, 404), and adenine arabinoside (405, 406) have all been considered for treatment of CMV infection, but none has been proved effective in large-scale trials in the adult compromised host. Adenine arabinoside, in a limited study in this population, was disap-

pointing, with no effect on CMV viremia and only a slight reduction in viruria being found (405). In a second study in renal allograft recipients, no clinical improvement with adenine arabinoside was observed and hematologic toxicity led to discontinuation of therapy in 2 of the 3 patients (406). Use of hyperimmune globulin has also been discussed (384) but remains of unproved efficacy.

Varicella-Zoster

Varicella-zoster is a pathogen of concern in immunosuppressed patients, both those with malignancies (407) and those immunosuppressed for other reasons, e.g., to prevent organ graft rejection (408) or as treatment for the nephrotic syndrome (409). Infection is usually considered primary in cases of varicella and due to reactivation in those of zoster (410), but epidemics of zoster considered by some investigators to be due to reexposure have been described (407, 411), so that the distinction is not complete.

Immunopathologic aspects. Various aspects of immunity to varicella-zoster infection have been examined, including studies of lymphocyte transformation, the role of interferon, and antibody.

In a study involving otherwise healthy patients recovering from herpes zoster and seronegative control subjects (children), Jordan and Merigan (412) found that antigen (varicella-zoster viral antigen)–specific lymphocyte transformation could be demonstrated in 7 of 8 patients with recent zoster but in none of the control subjects (whose lymphocytes could, however, transform to phytohemagglutinating antibody). The degree of transformation did not correlate with disease activity. Evidence of depression of cell-mediated immunity, possibly leading to the evolution of herpes zoster infection, was provided by Russell and co-workers (413), who studied 14 adult patients within 3 days of onset of the varicella-zoster rash and found a significant depression of antigen-specific lymphocyte transformation in 12. Further evidence of impairment of cellular function in varicella-zoster was provided by Twomey and associates (414), who found that monocytes obtained from patients during the period of early cutaneous disease were functionally defective in the mixed leukocyte reaction. Stevens and Merigan (415) and Stevens and associates (416) examined various immunologic parameters with regard to dissemination of varicella-zoster in 151 patients with herpes zoster. They failed to find any correlation of dissemination with presence or absence of delayed hypersensitivity to multiple skin test antigens, lymphocyte transformation to phytohemagglutinating antibody, or circulating lymphocyte counts. Schimpff and associates (407), on the other hand, stated that patients unreactive to dinitrochlorobenzene were more likely to disseminate varicella-zoster virus.

In their studies of lymphocyte transformation, Jordan and Merigan (412) found *in vitro* lymphocyte interferon production to be dependent on the method of lymphocyte preparation and unrelated to varicella-zoster disease activity or the immune status of the patients studied. The interferon thus produced may have been induced nonspecifically by non-antigenic components of the varicella-zoster preparation used. Stevens and Merigan (415), in an attempt to define the factors influencing dissemination, measured vesicle interferon serially in patients with herpes zoster. They noted that development of peak vesicle interferon levels was followed by arrest of dissemination within 48 hours in all of the 21 patients in whom appropriate data were available to make this determination. This was true regardless of the number of days after onset of infection or the number of days of dissemination that had elapsed. No patients with localized disease and high vesicle interferon levels had evidence of subsequent dissemination of virus (415). More recently, Stevens and associates (416) reported studies in 30 patients with varicella-zoster; 4 were normal and 26 had malignancies (including 5 patients with Hodgkin's disease) or were receiving immunosuppressive therapy. Vesicles were examined during the disease course. Polymorphonuclear leukocytes were the earliest and predominant cells noted in vesicle fluid. Small numbers of lymphocytes and monocytes were also found with macrophagelike cells at the vesicle base. Increases of cells and interferon occurred at approximately the same time in the disease. In 17 of 18 patients with disseminated varicella-zoster infection in whom a sharp rise in these parameters could be demonstrated, the rise in cells and interferon preceded the cessation of dissemination, indicating the probable importance of these parameters in controlling dissemination. These results were somewhat surprising in view of the small numbers of lymphocytes found in the fluid because this cell type had been considered necessary for interferon production and cytotoxicity. The investigators concluded that vesicle interferon levels correlated better with the clinical

course than did other parameters, including vesicle fluid cell count.

The role of antibody in protection against dissemination is unclear. Schimpff and associates (407) found that the frequency of herpes zoster development in patients with lymphoma but not in patients with leukemia correlated with absence of antibody titers to the virus. However, they did not attempt to relate this to dissemination. Stevens and Merigan (415) reported relatively slower development of CF antibody in patients with dissemination. However, development of complement-fixing antibody definitely followed development of peak interferon levels and did not occur until after the end of dissemination in 9 of 25 patients specifically observed for this. Five patients experienced dissemination despite the fact that they began to form antibody before dissemination began (415). More recently, Stevens and co-workers (416) reported cessation of dissemination in 11 of 18 patients before CF antibody production occurred. Uduman and co-workers (418), in a study of 14 patients with dissemination in a group of 55 patients with herpes zoster, measured both CF antibody and fluorescent antibody against the membrane antigen of varicella-zoster and found no significant difference in antibody concentrations in patients with disseminated and localized disease up to 10 days after onset of herpes zoster. Titers in both tests were actually somewhat higher in the disseminated cases. High concentrations of antibody did not prevent dissemination. These studies as a whole clearly indicate that antibody alone is not the major factor in prevention or control of dissemination of varicella-zoster virus. In contrast are the observations in chickenpox. In a study by Gershon and associates (419) in 21 immunocompromised children, 15 of whom had no pre-existing antibody, administration of antibody before onset in the exposed compromised host seemed to modify the disease course favorably.

Among the recognized predisposing factors to activation or spread of varicella-zoster are Hodgkin's disease in advanced stages (407, 420, 421), and recent irradiation (407, 408, 420, 422).

The role of cytotoxic drugs and corticosteroids is less clear, but in some cases they may have been a predisposing factor (407, 420, 422). Prior involvement of the dermatome with disease or prior irradiation seemed significant to its future involvement with varicella-zoster (407, 420).

Splenectomy correlated positively with an increased incidence in one series (420) but not in others (407, 421). In renal transplant patients receiving immunosuppressive therapy, Rifkind (408) found normal antibody responses to varicella-zoster in patients without underlying malignancy and noted no complications in 6 patients with varicella-zoster infection. He interpreted his data as suggesting that the increased severity of varicella-zoster infection that occurs in patients with malignancy might relate to their underlying disease rather than to the therapy they are receiving.

Pathology. The pulmonary pathology has been most extensively studied in patients with varicella pneumonia without known underlying disease. Triebwasser and co-workers (423) described histopathologic features ranging from focal necrosis to complete consolidation. The most striking changes followed a peribronchiolar distribution. Intranuclear inclusion bodies were seen in septal cells along with edema, mononuclear cell invasion, septal cell proliferation, and occasional lining of alveoli and bronchioles with a hyaline membrane. Exudate may be found in the bronchioles. Eventual development of pulmonary fibrosis and nodular calcification has also been described (424).

Pik and Gikas (425) in a review of varicella-zoster pneumonia have described autopsy findings in a patient with Hodgkin's disease and varicella-zoster pneumonia. Diffuse consolidation and edema were found involving multiple lobes of the lung. Sections of the lungs revealed pneumonitis with macrophages, neutrophils, fibrin, and hyaline membranes in alveolar spaces as well as focal areas of interstitial necrosis. A few alveolar lining cells contained intranuclear inclusions. These investigators described a second patient (with chronic lymphocytic leukemia) whose lungs post mortem contained hemorrhagic necrotic zones with fibrin precipitation. Many alveolar cells contained prominent eosinophilic intranuclear inclusion bodies.

Clinical manifestations. The incidence of varicella-zoster infection has varied with the underlying disease. In one study, it was 25 per cent in patients with Hodgkin's disease, 8.7 per cent in patients with other lymphomas, 1.8 per cent in patients with solid tumors, and 1.2 per cent in patients with acute leukemia (407). The incidence was 8.2 per cent in renal transplant recipients (408). The incidence of varicella-zoster pneumonia in immunocompromised patients is more difficult to evaluate. It was 3 per cent in a group of 101 children with herpes zoster and cancer (421). One autopsy-proved death due to pneumonia occurred among 129 cases of varicella-zoster in the Stanford series (420). In normal adults with varicella pneumonia (423, 426), the roentgenogram typically shows peribronchiolar bilateral nodular infiltrate (<0.5 cm in diameter) with sparing of the apices. Pleural effusion and hilar adenopathy have also been described but are uncommon. The severity of the roentgenographic pattern is often out of proportion to the physical findings, which included rales, rhonchi, wheezing, evidence of consolidation (423), and less frequently, pleural rubs (425). Such signs, although most often minimal, have been reported in 50 to 60 per cent of patients with varicella pneumonia (423). All patients with pulmonary involvement had the typical rash (423). Patients may be minimally symptomatic. In one series, 4 of 26 cases were found only by roentgenogram (427). Symptoms that usually developed 1 to 3 days after the onset of rash included dyspnea, cough, tachypnea, and, not infrequently, hemoptysis and chest pain, mimicking pulmonary embolism and infarction (423, 428). The frequency of unexpected sudden death has been emphasized (426, 429). Clinical findings in immunosuppressed patients with varicella-zoster pneumonia tend to be similar to those observed in normal persons with varicella pneumonia and include rash, dry cough, wheezing, dyspnea, chest pain, eventual sputum production, rales, and consolidation (425, 429, 430). Spontaneous recovery does occur (430). Cyanosis and high fever may develop. Roentgenographic findings mimic those seen in primary varicella pneumonia (425). Hematologic studies in the otherwise normal host with varicella pneumonia usually show a normal to slightly elevated white blood cell count with a predominance of polymorphonuclear leukocytes and normal hematocrit and platelet counts (423). In the compromised host, of course, these factors will be influenced by the patient's underlying disease and therapy. Blood gas determinations frequently reveal hypoxia.

Diagnosis. The combination of varicella-zoster rash and pneumonitis is suggestive of pneumonia due to varicella-zoster. Although other microbial causes of pneumonia such as *Pneumocystis carinii* have been found in this setting (421), the incidence of dual infection is low. Complement-fixing antibodies (431), neutralizing antibodies (432), and antibodies to varicella-zoster membrane antigens can be measured (433). The latter may be positive in disseminated infection when the CF antibody test is equivocal (418, 433). The diagnosis of varicella-zoster infections may be supported by the appearance of or rising titers of antibody and isolation of virus from lesions. Fluorescence microscopy using fluorescein tagged antisera specific for varicella-zoster has been of great value in our institutions in identification of virus in scrapings of the base of vesicles (434), but definitive diagnosis of the etiology of the pulmonary infection requires more direct evidence. Intranuclear inclusion bodies have been found in sputum (435), and sputum examination is obviously desirable, although care must be taken because intranuclear inclusions are not specific for this disease. Transtracheal aspiration can assist in ruling out other causes of pneumonia in these cases and in looking for intranuclear inclusions. The decision whether to undertake further invasive procedures must be based on an assessment of the risks of the procedure in a given patient versus the potential gain in a setting in which dual infection is uncommon. Clearly, the most definitive evidence is provided by demonstration of typical histologic features and isolation of virus from lung tissue itself.

Prevention and treatment. At present, the best therapy is probably directed toward prevention of infection. Gershon and associates (419) have shown that varicella can be significantly modified in high-risk immunocompromised children by the prophylactic use of zoster-immune globulin within 72 hours of exposure to varicella. Use of zoster-immune globulin to treat established infection or to prevent herpes zoster in adults cannot now be recommended (418) but has been used in small numbers of patients in an uncontrolled manner with equivocal results (407).

Cytosine arabinoside has been disappointing. Davis and associates (436), in a small trial performed in a double blind manner in 8 patients with a history of recent chemotherapy or radiation therapy, found that 150 mg per m² of body surface per 36 hours had no effect on the clinical course of the disease. Stevens and co-workers (437), using 100 mg per m² per 24 hours given within 48 hours of the onset of the dissemination in a randomized double blind controlled study involving 39 patients, most of whom had Hodgkin's disease or other lymphoma (31 patients), noted that cytosine arabinoside did not shorten the dissemination phase of herpes zoster and significantly prolonged dissemination in some

patients. A subgroup of patients with Stage III or IV lymphoma was identified whose course was worsened by the drug. These patients had greater hematologic toxicity and a delay of appearance of interferon in vesicles and depression of vesicle cellular response. Schimpff and co-workers (438), using 30 mg per m² per day of cytosine arabinoside in a study of 17 patients, 13 of whom had lymphoma, found in a double blind placebo-controlled trial that this dose was nontoxic but was ineffective in preventing dissemination or reducing local symptoms of herpes zoster. Other results with cytosine arabinoside have been similarly disappointing (417, 436).

Results with adenine arabinoside appear hopeful in early trials (439, 439A). Interferon is also being evaluated (440, 441). Double blind placebo-controlled trials conducted at Stanford to date (T. C. Merigan: Personal communication) have indicated less organ involvement in both patients with varicella and in those with herpes zoster treated with interferon compared to placebo-treated patients if therapy was started early. Less pain and distal cutaneous spread were also found in the interferon recipients with herpes zoster. The patients with herpes zoster primarily had underlying lymphoma, whereas those with varicella had leukemia. Interferon is currently available only on research protocol at a few medical centers. Further trials using higher doses are underway as part of a continuing effort to evaluate the ability of interferon to reduce pain, prevent dissemination, and shorten the duration of the disease.

Adenovirus

Serious infection due to adenoviruses occurs occasionally in immunologically compromised patients (442–444). Myerowitz and associates (444) described a renal transplant recipient who developed progressive nodular pulmonary infiltrates and a diffuse bilateral interstitial pneumonia (444). Although aspergillus was isolated from the lungs and the patient also had herpetic esophagitis, the investigators presented evidence implicating adenovirus as the cause of the interstitial pneumonia. The diagnosis was made post mortem and required electron microscopic and virologic as well as serologic studies.

Mycobacteria: Mycobacterium tuberculosis **and Atypical Mycobacterial Infection**

Infection with *M. tuberculosis* has been a significant problem in the compromised host. Parker and co-workers (445) in 1932 found a prevalence of active M. *tuberculosis* infection of 20 per cent in patients with Hodgkin's disease. Recently, Kaplan and associates (446) found M. *tuberculosis* infection associated with Hodgkin's disease, cancer of the lung, lymphosarcoma, and reticulum cell sarcoma. Previous hospitalization for M. *tuberculosis* was noted in 37 of 201 patients in their study, emphasizing that reactivation of latent disease is an important factor. Atypical mycobacterial infection has more recently been recognized as a significant problem in the compromised population as well (447–456).

Immunopathologic aspects. Because an excellent review of the mechanisms of acquired resistance to mycobacterial infections has recently been published (457), our discussion will cover only limited aspects. The pathogenesis of mycobacterial infections remains an active field of investigation. Although polymorphonuclear leukocytes are seen at the site of the infection at early time periods (458) and ingested virulent organisms reduce the migration of this cell type (459), polymorphonuclear leukocytes are quickly replaced by mononuclear cells as the infection progresses. Monocytes and macrophages are believed to be the most important effector cells of cellular resistance to mycobacteria. Numerous studies have been performed to define the function of these cells in resistance to tuberculosis. In *in vitro* studies, Henderson and associates (460) observed an increase in the percentage of actively phagocytic alveolar macrophages in rabbits naturally resistant to tuberculosis. Others have noted no significant difference in phagocytosis by immune and nonimmune macrophages (461, 462). Lurie (463) infected cell cultures implanted in the anterior chambers of normal rabbit eyes with M. *tuberculosis*. Using this model, he demonstrated that mononuclear phagocytes of rabbits previously immunized with M. *tuberculosis* inhibited multiplication of M. *tuberculosis* to a much greater degree than did normal mononuclear cells. Suter (462) also observed *in vitro* that tubercle bacilli multiplied much more readily in monocytes from normal guinea pigs or rabbits than in those from animals vaccinated with bacille Calmette-Guérin (BCG). Berthrong (461) was able to induce similar resistance in macrophages by airborne infection with attenuated tubercle bacilli. Mackaness and associates (464) studied 4 strains of M. *tuberculosis* and noted a correlation of viru-

lence and growth rate *in vitro* in rabbit monocytes. Patterson and Youmans (465) demonstrated *in vitro* that splenic lymphocytes from specifically immunized mice conferred on normal peritoneal macrophages the ability to inhibit the tubercle bacillus. The induction of resistance was apparently effected by a filterable substance that may have been a lymphokine. Collins and co-workers (466) recently demonstrated a marked exacerbation of BCG infection in mice depleted of T lymphocytes compared to normal control mice (466).

Attempts to transfer immunity to M. *tuberculosis* have been made, and many investigators have reported successful transfer of immunity *in vivo* by means of cells (463, 466–469). Objections have been raised to the design of these studies. Mixed populations of lymphoid cells were used in all; in some, the animals used were outbred. Life of the transferred cells would have been short, and resistance was probably being actively initiated by organisms in the transferred cells rather than by the cells themselves (457, 470). Recently, however, Lefford and co-workers (470) were able adoptively to transfer immunity to tuberculosis to normal rats using syngeneic immune lymphocytes obtained from the thoracic duct (470).

Spencer and associates (471) have used inhibition of macrophage migration as a test of cellular immunity in guinea pigs, using splenic lymphocytes or cells obtained from pulmonary lavage, and have demonstrated a compartmentalization of cell-mediated immunity. In this study, local respiratory cell-mediated immunity was greater after immunization by the respiratory tract than after subcutaneous immunization, and systemic immunization was greater after subcutaneous immunization with BCG or M. *tuberculosis* (471). Yamamoto and associates (472) had previously correlated migration inhibition induced by "lung cells" but not by peritoneal cells with resistance to airborne challenge with M. *tuberculosis* again showing a compartmentalization effect.

Podleski and Podleski (473) have demonstrated circulating lymphocytes cytotoxic to mastocytoma target cells coated with purified protein derivative (PPD) in 16 of 23 tuberculosis patients. The significance of this is unclear.

Immunologic memory in the mycobacterial system does not appear to be dependent on persistence of viable organisms. Lefford and McGregor (474) recently showed in rats that delayed hypersensitivity, resistance to infection, and capacity to transfer resistance by thoracic duct cells persisted long after viable BCG organisms were eliminated by therapy.

The question of the relationship between tuberculin hypersensitivity and resistance to tuberculosis remains a subject of debate (457) and will be only briefly mentioned here. Neiburger and co-workers (475) found a disparity between hypersensitivity and immunity in animals whose lymphocytes could induce migration inhibition in response to antigen and animals protected against virulent challenge with *M. tuberculosis* and believed that this provided evidence against an identity of hypersensitivity and immunity. Some investigators have strongly believed that delayed hypersensitivity and immunity in tuberculosis involve distinctly different immunologic mechanisms (475A). Shapiro and associates (476) found a correlation between level of resistance of vaccinated guinea pigs and hypersensitivity to 100 TU of PPD; they noted a waning of hypersensitivity with time but not a waning of resistance. Collins and Mackaness (457, 477) have stated that "any tuberculous infection of vaccinated but no longer hypersensitive individuals induces an immediate anamnestic response," thus making the clinical significance of the distinction between hypersensitivity and resistance in the person with prior hypersensitivity unclear and perhaps artificial.

The role of serum and antibody factors in resistance to *M. tuberculosis* is unclear. Whereas certain workers (461–463) noted no significant effect of immune sera on the ability of mononuclear cells to deal successfully with tuberculosis infection, others have found a significant effect (478). Hsu (479) noted no effect of immune serum on intracellular multiplication in guinea pig macrophages. Two groups have reported successful transfer of tuberculin sensitivity with serum or plasma in guinea pigs (480, 481). However, Collins and associates (482) observed transfer of immediate but not delayed hypersensitivity by this means, and Lefford and co-workers (470) could not transfer immunity by means of serum. Therefore, the ability to transfer true delayed hypersensitivity or immunity in this manner remains in doubt. Antibody can be demonstrated in the serum of infected patients by a variety of means (483) and, indeed, can be found universally, by some tests, in all persons whether or not they are infected (484). The relationship of antibody to immunity seems unproved and doubtful.

Salvin and co-workers (485), using a murine model, reported a correlation between methods of sensitization with BCG and old tuberculin that resulted in maximal production of lymphokines (including type II interferon) and those that led to protection against aerosol challenge with a virulent strain of *M. tuberculosis*. However, further investigation of this association is required before conclusions can be drawn as to its importance.

The effect of cortisone on macrophage resistance to *M. tuberculosis* has been studied and is of importance in view of the apparent increase of virulence of the infection in the compromised patient (461). Although no significant functional derangement was noted in one study (461), a decreased ability of macrophages to digest bacilli was suggested in another (486). In one study, cortisone did not appear to affect significantly the rate of *M. tuberculosis* multiplication in guinea pig macrophages *in vitro* but led to a greater cytotoxic effect on the macrophages (479).

Pathology. Stead (487) has described well the pathogenesis of pulmonary infection in the normal host. Most infections in adults are due to reactivation of dormant infection, although exogenous reinfection does occur (488). Primary infection usually occurs in the best-ventilated portion of the lungs and produces a solid type of caseation necrosis (487). Because of the higher oxygen tension, chronic tuberculosis most commonly affects the apices and produces a more liquid form of caseation that is more easily aspirated and thereby may lead to spread of the infection (487). Cavity formation has been related to hypersensitivity reactions and can apparently be prevented in rabbits by desensitization procedures (489). *M. tuberculosis* pneumonia, which is unusual in adults, may result from intrabronchial spread of the contents of cavities (446).

Tuberculosis in the compromised host has varied from typical reactivation tuberculosis with upper lobe cavitary or noncavitary disease, to diffuse infiltration involving several lobes (*M. tuberculosis* pneumonia) with or without pleural effusion, to disseminated disease involving other organs as well as the lung (446). Histologic findings have usually not been discussed in detail. In patients dying with atypical mycobacterial infection, caseous pulmonary nodules containing acid-fast organisms, bronchopneumonia, pleural effusion, cavities, and miliary lesions with dissemination have been described, but typical giant cells have been infrequently reported (450, 451, 453, 454). Granuloma formation has been described in disseminated *M. kansasii* infection (8 of 10 cases) (449).

Clinical manifestations. As stated above, infection with *M. tuberculosis* and atypical mycobacteria has been a significant problem in the compromised host. Feld and associates (456) recently reported a study dealing with both types of infection. They found mycobacteriosis in 59 patients with malignant disease in a retrospective study dealing with the years 1968 to 1973 at the M.D. Anderson Hospital and Tumor Institute in Houston. The incidence of mycobacteriosis among cancer patients was 65 per 100,000 compared with a rate of 45 per 100,000 in the same age group in the state of Texas. Forty-five patients were male and 14 were female; the median age at time of diagnosis was 60 years. Twenty-nine patients had infection with *M. tuberculosis* and 30 with atypical mycobacteria. Eighty-six per cent of the infections were considered to be confined to the lung, and only 3 cases of miliary disease were found, all caused by *M. tuberculosis*. The most common associated neoplasm was squamous cell carcinoma of the head and neck. Seven cases were associated with lymphoma and 5 with leukemia. Five of 29 patients with *M. tuberculosis* were receiving chemotherapy at the time they developed their infections, whereas 10 of 30 patients with atypical mycobacterial infections were receiving such therapy. Atypical mycobacterial infections were mostly Runyon groups I and IV, with 12 cases of *M. kansasii,* 7 cases of *M. fortuitum,* and 2 cases each of *M. scrofulaceum, M. aquae,* and *M. avium.* Single cases of infection with *M. vaccae, M. chelonei,* and *M. terrae* were found. Principal symptoms were fever, chills, cough, and hemoptysis. A positive reaction to PPD was demonstrated in 8 of 12 patients with infection caused by *M. tuberculosis* and in 2 of 6 patients with infection caused by atypical mycobacteria. The main source of isolation of the organism was sputum or bronchial washings. Thirty-one of the 59 patients died. Nine autopsies were performed. *M. tuberculosis* was found at autopsy in 3 of the 4 patients believed to be infected by this organism, and it was noted that all died of their infection. In contrast, of the 5 patients believed to be infected with atypical mycobacteria, organisms were found in 3 at autopsy but only "minimal" evidence of infection was noted, e.g., local granulomas. Information about the total dosage of therapy the patients had received was not pro-

vided. Only 2 patients were reported in whom the diagnosis was not established before death; both were infected with *M. tuberculosis.* Cases of atypical mycobacterial infection with more impressive postmortem changes will be discussed subsequently.

The largest reported series devoted to cancer patients infected with *M. tuberculosis* alone is that of Kaplan and associates (446) from Memorial Sloan-Kettering Cancer Center in New York. Their report is of a retrospective study in 201 patients with neoplastic disease who developed tuberculosis discovered at the time the neoplasm was first diagnosed or during therapy for it. Prevalence rates were highest in patients with Hodgkin's disease, cancer of the lung, lymphosarcoma, and reticulum cell sarcoma, ranging from 96 cases per 10,000 to 78 cases per 10,000, respectively. Active disease occurred most frequently after administration of chemotherapy in patients with Hodgkin's disease, lymphosarcoma, and reticulum cell sarcoma. Patients who had tuberculosis diagnosed after they had been treated for their cancer were more likely to have diffuse infiltration of the lung involving more than one lobe or disseminated disease, as opposed to untreated patients who tended to have only upper lobe disease. Infection tended to increase in severity with increasing immunosuppression. Even relatively short-term corticosteroid therapy, e.g., less than 4 months, seemed to produce more severe disease (often in combination with other immunosuppressive therapy). Infection in lymphoma patients was often associated with other opportunistic infections such as herpes zoster or cryptococcosis.

Infection, especially in patients with lymphoproliferative disorders and those with lung cancer, may be fulminant, with rapid development of clinical disease. One case is described that originated in a Ghon complex and developed into devastating pneumonia in 6 days with death due to respiratory failure (446). In the series reported by Kaplan and associates (446), disseminated infection with *M. tuberculosis* developed in 29 of 34 patients after immunosuppressive therapy and was fatal in 91 per cent of them. *M. tuberculosis* pneumonia was uniformly fatal. The over-all mortality rate in their 201 cases was 17 per cent, but in the patients with lymphoproliferative disease it was 48 per cent. No patient developed tuberculosis while taking isoniazid for prophylaxis, and most patients in whom the diagnosis was made and who received treatment did well. In 33 patients with tuberculosis who were tested, skin tests were positive in two-thirds, and skin tests therefore seemed definitely worthwhile as a screening procedure as early as possible for all patients about to undergo immunosuppression. A miliary pattern on chest roentgenogram was not universally seen in disseminated disease. In an earlier report on pulmonary tuberculosis in cancer patients from the same center, it is of note that chest roentgenograms were "positive" for tuberculosis in 88 per cent with a definitely negative roentgenogram in only 5.8 per cent (490). No mention is made of how often they were repeated, however. Sputum smear or culture was positive in about 45 per cent of cases in whom this examination was performed. No mention was made of the number of sputum samples examined for evidence of tuberculosis per patient. The cancers found most frequently in association with *M. tuberculosis* infection in this series were respiratory, oral, digestive, and breast, but information regarding relative therapy or degree of immunosuppression was not provided.

Morrow and Anderson (491), examining 213 cases of reticuloendothelial malignancies at the Atomic Bomb Casualty Commission, Hiroshima, from 1949 to 1962, found an increased rate of disseminated tuberculosis in patients with chronic myelogenous leukemia and myelofibrosis but not in cases of acute leukemia. No cases were found associated with lymphomas. The prevalence of dissemination correlated positively with duration of the clinical course of the underlying disease but did not correlate well with antineoplastic therapy. Oswald (492), in a review of the British literature in 1963, noted an incidence of acute tuberculosis of 3 to 4 per cent in patients with myeloid leukemia, with a tendency to miliary dissemination. Andre and co-workers (493) had previously reported tuberculosis in association with myelosclerosis and myeloid metaplasia and, in a review of the literature to 1961, also noted a tendency for miliary disease in these cases. Glasser and associates (494), in a review of 3,507 patients with tuberculosis, discovered a prevalence of acute leukemia of 2 per 1,000, which they believed was not significantly elevated compared to other groups. In summary, tuberculosis seems to occur with a variety of underlying malignancies and appears to have a tendency for fulminant disease and dissemination in this patient population.

Infection with *M. tuberculosis* has also been a problem in the renal transplant population. Pradhan and associates (495), in a study of 136 chronic dialysis patients on no immunosuppressive therapy, described 5 cases of active tuberculosis, 3 of whom had pulmonary infiltrates. Four of 5 patients did well on antituberculosis drugs. The final case was diagnosed post mortem. Neff and Hudgel (496) noted tuberculosis in only 3 of 400 renal transplant patients from 1962 to 1972. They described one case of miliary tuberculosis diagnosed by positive sputum cultures after renal transplant in a patient who relapsed despite 20 months of 2-drug antituberculosis therapy. The organism developed resistance to isoniazid, leading the investigators to suggest triple drug therapy in this population.

Atypical mycobacterial infection, as previously noted, has also been documented as a significant problem in the compromised patient population. McNutt and Fudenberg (447) described a patient treated with busulfan and chlorambucil for a myeloproliferative disorder who developed a disseminated scotochromogen infection (although this was not confirmed at autopsy 8 months later after antituberculosis therapy). Roentgenographic changes showed only a Ghon complex of uncertain cause (447). The diagnosis was established by liver biopsy and the patient responded to triple drug therapy. Grillo-López and co-workers (450) described a patient with chronic granulocytic leukemia treated with intermittent busulfan and roentgenographic therapy who developed a right upper lobe infiltrate and right pleural effusion. Results of cultures of sputum, pleural fluid, and bone marrow (which were available only after the patient had died) and caseous nodules with acid-fast bacilli seen in the lung post mortem confirmed the diagnosis. McCusker and Green (454) described a patient with chronic granulocytic leukemia and busulfan treatment along with radiation therapy who developed miliary pulmonary lesions as part of a disseminated scotochromogen infection. Post mortem, necrotic material packed with acid-fast bacilli was found in the lungs.

Disseminated atypical infection has also been described in renal homograft recipients (448, 449). Fraser and associates (449) described disseminated *M. kansasii* infection in a transplant recipient who was receiving corticosteroids and azathioprine. The infection appeared to originate with a cellulitis and abscess in a foot. Inflammatory reaction consisted primarily of polymorphonuclear cells; no granulomas were seen. Three nodular densities developed in the lungs. Sputum cultures were negative by stained smear for tuberculosis, but cultures obtained at bronchoscopy were positive for *M. kansasii.* The patient responded to triple drug therapy and change of corticosteroid therapy to alternate-day instead of daily administration.

Other cases of disseminated *M. kansasii* infection with pulmonary involvement in patients receiving corticosteroids have been reported (451–453, 455). Severe leukocytopenia has been noted and seemed, in at least one case (453), to antedate the mycobacterial infection, although in other cases leukopenia was probably secondary to infection (451, 453). PPD skin tests tended to be weakly positive using up to 250 TU, but PPD-Y produced an 18-mm response in one patient in whom it was used (449). It is thus evident that infection with typical and atypical mycobacteria can be a serious problem in the compromised host. In general, atypical mycobacterial infection has appeared to be less fulminant. The first step in diagnosis is the consideration of the mycobacterioses as a cause of disease in this group of patients.

Diagnosis. As noted above, diagnosis has depended on obtaining sputum specimens for smear or culture (at times by bronchoscopy), skin tests (which are often positive, even in immunosuppressed patients), and biopsy and culture of other sites such as liver or bone marrow. Because of its increased sensitivity, fluorescence microscopy may aid in demonstrating organisms in tissue or sputum (497). Feld and associates (456), on the basis of their experience with mycobacteriosis in patients with malignant diseases, stated that one positive sputum culture is sufficient for the diagnosis of infection with *M. tuberculosis,* whereas 2 positive cultures should be obtained before making the diagnosis of atypical mycobacterial infection unless the organism is demonstrated in tissue. No standardized serologic test is in common use. The chest roentgenogram has been useful in indicating a pulmonary abnormality but has not been specific for tuberculosis in this population. Although typical pulmonary disease characteristic of tuberculosis may be present, the chest roentgenogram is often nondiagnostic and may not reveal miliary lesions in patients with disseminated disease (446).

Treatment. Standard tuberculosis therapy has often been successful in this group of patients (446), although emergence of resistance has been noted (496). The fundamental problem is suspecting the diagnosis in time to initiate therapy (446). As previously discussed, prophylaxis in patients believed to be at risk as suggested by Kaplan and associates (446) before immunosuppressive therapy is to be encouraged. A discussion of the specifics of treatment of *M. tuberculosis* and atypical mycobacterial infection is beyond the scope of this review and the reader is referred to other sources for this information (498, 499).

Pneumocystis carinii

P. carinii, first noted as a cause of epidemic pneumonitis in orphanages in Europe, has in more recent years become recognized as a significant pathogen in the compromised host. Indeed, a prospective and retrospective study of interstitial pneumonia in an immunosuppressed population identified *P. carinii* as the most common cause of that entity (500). A recent extensive and superb review of pneumocystosis by Ruskin (501) has appeared.

The taxonomic position of *P. carinii* is currently unclear. The most characteristic form of the organism is the cyst, which may contain up to 8 merozoites. However, a trophozoite form has also been observed and is the form of the organism that replicates. Electron microscopic studies have shown that the trophozoite has pseudopodium-like projections (502–506) that interconnect to form a reticular framework and may fasten organisms to the alveolar wall (507). Pifer and Hughes (508) have reported the cultivation of *P. carinii* obtained from both human and murine sources *in vitro* using embryonic chick epithelial lung cells. The parasite did not seem to enter the lung cells. Instead, the investigators reported that during reproduction, a vegetative form of the *P. carinii* trophozoite attaches to the host cell (probably for the transport of nutrients) until replication has occurred and a mature cyst has formed, at which point excystment occurs and the vegetative cell detaches from the host cell. Further studies of this nature are required to clarify the taxonomy of the organism. Currently, it is usually classified with the protozoa.

Immunopathologic aspects. Extensive experience with animal models and with human cases suggests that disease related to *P. carinii* probably is due more directly to failure of host defense mechanisms than to inherent virulence of the organism. Of the many animal experiments performed in which host defenses have been compromised, among the most illuminating are those of Frenkel and co-workers (509), who studied a group of rats that spontaneously developed pneumocystosis in 6 to 8 weeks when treated with corticosteroids twice weekly. Their findings that the disease regressed spontaneously in rats in which corticosteroid therapy was discontinued after 35 days (whereas rats continued on corticosteroids died) and that cyclophosphamide was the only agent other than corticosteroids that could activate clinical disease when given as a single agent may have relevance to human disease. Irradiation, nitrogen mustard, and 6-mercaptopurine did not result in clinical pneumocystosis. Splenectomy and neonatal thymectomy were also ineffective in predisposing to overt disease. Attempts to transmit infection from rats to mice and hamsters were unsuccessful. Sheldon (510) had similarly shown in a rabbit model that cortisone activates latent pneumocystosis.

Recently, Hughes and associates (511), in a randomized study of 149 children with acute lymphocytic leukemia receiving differing amounts of immunosuppressive therapy, were able to relate the incidence of pneumocytis pneumonia to the intensity of chemotherapy. Previously they had noted that children with cancer who developed pneumocystis pneumonitis had a significantly lower serum albumin and body weight at the onset of disease than a matched group of cancer patients who did not develop pneumocystosis (512). An attempt was made to duplicate this observation in a murine model. They found that rats maintained on a protein-free diet also developed pneumocystosis, whereas control animals fed a 23 per cent protein diet did not. Deaths from pneumonitis (which were rare with protein depletion alone) were precipitated by concomitant cortisone treatment. Survival of animals could be achieved by protein repletion.

Organ transplant recipients develop pneumocystosis only after they receive immunosuppressive therapy (513–516), and patients with malignancy also seem at significant risk only after treatment with chemotherapy or corticosteroids. Robbins (517), in 1967, could find no published case of *P. carinii* infection in patients with untreated Hodgkin's disease, and Burke and Good (518), in a review of 350 cases of pneumocytosis, found only 17 with an underlying lymphoreticular malignancy for which immunosuppressive therapy had not been given. The drugs implicated most frequently, as in the animal model, have been corticosteroids and cyclophosphamide. Rifkind and co-workers (513) in a study of renal transplant patients, noted

that pneumonitis often became clinically apparent only when corticosteroid doses were being tapered. Others have noted a similar phenomenon in children with malignancy during steroid tapering (519, 520). Frenkel and co-workers (509) noted that in rats, pneumonia increased when corticosteroids were withdrawn, presumably because as immunosuppression was removed, exudate and inflammation appeared in the alveoli and respiratory function deteriorated until the organisms were cleared. It may well be, therefore, that host immune response mechanisms play a major role in determining the severity of signs and symptoms of pneumocystis pneumonitis (521).

That antibody formation may be important in defense against the organism is suggested by the observations that many case histories of pneumocystosis have occurred in children with hypogammaglobulinemia (522–535). Walzer and associates (536), in a review of the disease in children, concluded that humoral immunologic dysfunction is important in the pathogenesis of the disease. Infected children often exhibited low concentrations of IgG, although no characteristic pattern of immunoglobulin abnormality could be found. Pneumocystis infection was frequently associated with disease, producing pronounced defects in both humoral and cellular immunity. Although only a single report of a patient with a pure T cell deficiency disease and pneumocystosis has been published (537), immunoglobulin concentrations have been normal in many children with pneumocystosis (538), and data obtained in animal models clearly indicate that derangement of cellular immunity is likely to play a major role in the production of clinical disease in the compromised human adult.

Little is known regarding the epidemiology of this infection. Person-to-person transfer of the organism may be important in some cases. Hendley and Weller (539) observed that corticosteroid-treated, cesarean-section originated, barrier-sustained rats developed patent infections with pneumocystis if housed in direct contact with or exposed to a common air supply from standard infected rats, whereas control corticoid-conditioned animals remained free of infection. There are 2 published reports of development of the disease in immunosuppressed patients in beds adjoining an index case (540, 541). Singer and associates (542) suggested person-to-person spread as a possible cause of a clustering of cases they observed among 11 patients during a 3-

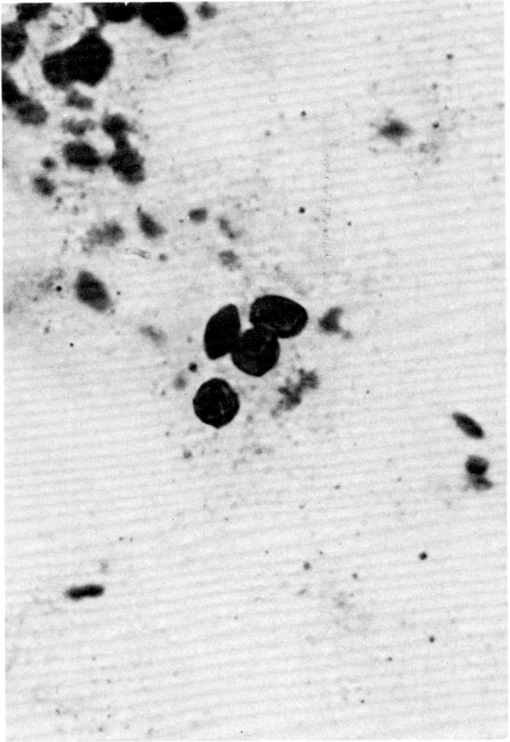

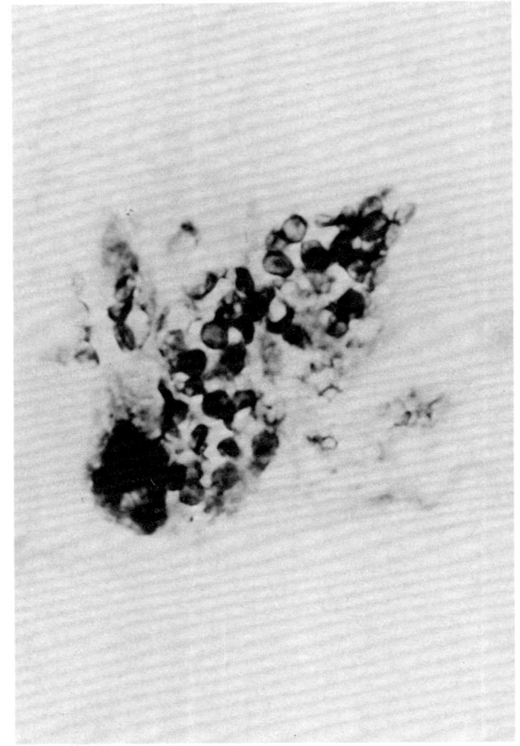

Fig. 1. *Pneumocystis carinii* pulmonary infection.

A. An example of *P. carinii* cysts in a biopsy specimen of lung tissue stained with silver.

B. An alveolus filled with *P. carinii* cysts (silver stained).

month period. Ten of the patients had lymphoma or leukemia. Corticosteroid therapy in 7 of the 11 patients was decreased or stopped 5 days to 3 weeks before diagnosis. Six of the patients were in the pediatric age group and all of these had had extensive contact in the outpatient department. Three of the pediatric patients shared the same room. A physician who had an indirect immunofluorescent titer to pneumocystis of 1:16 cared for 3 adult patients. Another physician involved in the care of 6 patients had a similar titer. There is also a report of the development of infection in 3 members of one household: a leukemic husband, his apparently normal wife, and their child (543). Although all of these reports suggest that the infection is contagious, this has not been proved.

Pathology. The most characteristic finding after hematoxylin and eosin staining of pulmonary tissue is a foamy eosinophilic material of high carbohydrate content filling the alveoli. This is composed largely of *P. carinii*. Price and Hughes (544) regard the exudate as consisting of coalesced macrophages in which remnant organisms are seen (based on a study of children with malignant disease). Thickened septa caused by hyperplasia of alveolar lining cells are present, but extensive cellular infiltrates, especially plasma cells noted in epidemic disease in children, are infrequent in the disease in the compromised host (524, 545, 546). As previously noted, the most characteristic form of the organism is the cyst, although a trophozoite form has also been observed. Organisms vary from oval to crescentic in shape and are frequently seen in groups within the alveolus (figure 1). As stated above, the trophozoites appear to have pseudopodium-like projections that interact with other organisms to form a reticular framework and may also help to fasten the organisms to the alveolar wall. Interstitial fibrosis is a rare but recognized sequela of pneumocystis pneumonia (although effects of drugs and concurrent infection with other agents often cannot be completely excluded as a cause of the fibrosis) (518, 547, 548). Granulomatous reactions (549) and calcification of lung tissue (518- 550) have also been described. Involvement of thoracic lymph nodes and hilar nodes has also been noted (518, 551) and systemic dis-

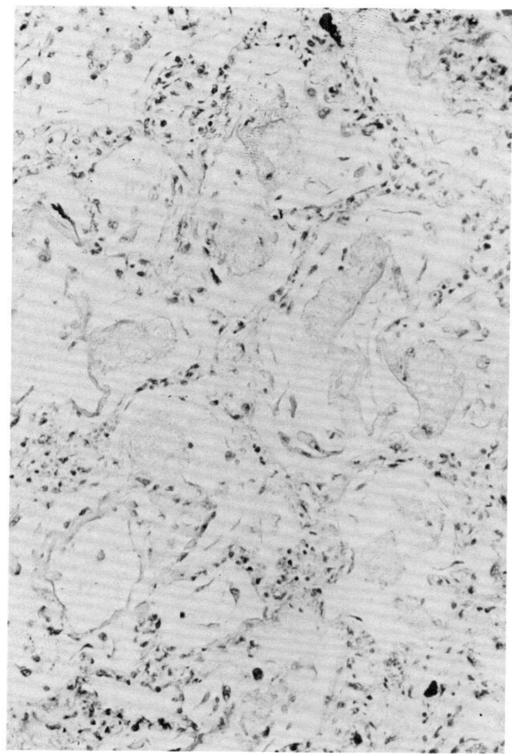

C. A specimen stained with periodic acid-Schiff stain under low power, showing foamy exudate in the alveoli.

semination has been reported in several cases (552, 553). Such instances, however, are rare (551).

Clinical manifestations. Walzer and associates (554), in a summary of cases of *P. carinii* pneumonia reported to the Center for Disease Control from 1967 to 1970, noted that the highest incidence was in children less than one year of age (554). The next highest incidences were in the age groups 1 to 9 and 50 to 59 years. Sixty-three per cent of patients were male, 92 per cent were white, and 5 per cent were black. Almost all had a serious underlying condition. Leukemia was the most common condition and lymphatic leukemia the most frequent type among these. Primary immunodeficiency diseases, Hodgkin's disease, and organ transplantation were also frequent predisposing conditions. The latter were the most common associations in early and middle adulthood, and chronic lymphatic leukemia was the most common underlying condition in the age group over 50. Interestingly, Simon and associates (555) have described a case of chronic localized pulmonary pneumocy-

tosis in an immunologically hyperresponsive host, a 20-year-old man with allergic bronchopulmonary aspergillosis.

There are no pathognomonic clinical signs of the infection. Focal infection may be asymptomatic (556, 557). Onset may be gradual or abrupt (518), although rapid development of fever, dyspnea, and nonproductive cough is more common (538, 545, 554). In the series of patients reported in the summary from the Center for Disease Control, dyspnea was the most common symptom (91 per cent of cases). Physical findings were usually not impressive; rales and cyanosis were described most frequently. Forrest (558) noted that a bilateral perihilar distribution with sparing of peripheral lung fields has been thought typical of early disease, but many exceptions occur. He stated that radiologically the infection may appear to be interstitial or alveolar. Pleural effusions, although rare, do not exclude the disease (although other coincident causes for the effusions remain difficult to rule out). Paramediastinal sparing and consolidation have also been noted attesting to the wide spectrum of radiologic findings in this infection. Friedman and associates (559) described 2 cases with hypoxia in which *P. carinii* was demonstrated in a specimen obtained by bronchial brush biopsy; these patients initially had normal or nearly normal chest roentgenograms. Unilateral infiltrates occur and may be segmental (558, 560). Cross and Steigbigel (561) reported a case with nodular densities. Thus, there is no diagnostic radiographic presentation and, in view of the possible changes produced by the underlying disease or concomitant infection, no radiographic picture that excludes the diagnosis.

Eosinophilia has been described in infants (518, 556, 562, 563) but is not a common finding in adults. Cold agglutinins have been found by some (513, 514), but others have not substantiated this finding (545, 564) and it may have been that they were due to coexisting viral infection. Arterial blood gas measurements may show early hypoxemia and hypocapnia, but hypercapnia has also been noted (565). Pulmonary function measurements have shown an increase in both the alveolar-arterial P_{O_2} difference and dead space and reduced compliance without evidence of obstruction (566, 567). Most patients had a slight leukocytosis, mild anemia, and normal platelet counts. Leukopenia was a significant negative prognostic factor.

Twenty-four per cent of cases have been noted to have concurrent infections, most commonly bacterial (554). Cytomegalovirus is the most common recognized concurrent viral infection (554). The apparent high frequency of pneumocystis and CMV suggests the possibility of symbiosis between the 2 organisms (502, 567–569).

It has also been noted, especially in patients with lymphatic leukemia, that pneumocystosis often occurs when the patient is in remission, suggesting above all that recognition of *P. carinii* infection in such patients is critical because treatment may be life saving.

Diagnosis. Diagnosis requires demonstration of the organisms in sputum or pulmonary tissue. Demonstration of the organism in sputum is difficult because spontaneous sputum production in patients infected with *P. carinii* is usually minimal. Sputum production may be increased by nebulization techniques (570). At best, sputum examination has been a low yield procedure with estimated positive results of 6 per cent in the series of cases summarized by Walzer and associates (554). Yields may be increased by adding the material obtained directly to a special fixative (571). Recent experience at UCLA and Stanford has suggested that transtracheal aspiration results may be better than had been previously realized. Transtracheal aspiration yielded material containing pneumocystis organisms in 8 of 60 attempts (572). Three additional patients had pneumocystis organisms in expectorated sputum and one patient had organisms in both expectorated sputum and transtracheal aspirate. The procedures that have proved most helpful for diagnosis in immunosuppressed patients are percutaneous needle aspiration or needle biopsy of the lung and open lung biopsy (573). We no longer use needle biopsy of the lung because it results too frequently in diagnostic failures in subsequently proved cases and excessive complications, including significant pneumothorax and intrapulmonary hemorrhage in nearly half the cases (574). In 2 of our patients, this procedure clearly led to their demise. We have had more success with percutaneous needle aspiration (575) using a thin-walled 18-gauge needle. This procedure is used in children and adults who are not thrombocytopenic and who are not severely dyspneic and tachypneic, thus allowing them to cooperate during the procedure. We generally advocate the use of open lung biopsy, especially in patients with potential bleeding problems and in the more critically ill. This procedure offers less chance of sampling error, more tissue for histologic examination, and better control of potential bleeding. It is remarkably well tolerated even by the most severely ill patients (574). In the Center for Disease Control report, no false-negatives resulted from this procedure, and similar results have been reported by others (576). Because of the risks of general anesthesia in patients with respiratory embarrassment (554, 571, 577), however, bronchopulmonary lavage (578) and endobronchial or transbronchial brush biopsy are being used with greater frequency (554, 559, 571, 579–581).

CF tests used in Europe for investigation of epidemic cases have not been successful in diagnosis in compromised hosts (513, 582). Norman and Kagan (583), using the indirect fluorescent antibody test, found the sensitivity low, with positive results in only one third of cases in immunosuppressed patients and apparent false-positive results in cases of disease due to CMV and fungi.

To provide maximal potential therapeutic benefit in this disease, we believe that early and aggressive diagnostic measures are mandatory when the diagnosis of pneumocystis pneumonia is entertained (508). If sputum or transtracheal aspirate fails to reveal an etiologic agent in an immunosuppressed patient suspected of having pneumocystis pneumonia, a more definitive diagnostic procedure must be undertaken without hesitation before deterioration of the patient's condition occurs and invasive diagnostic procedures become more hazardous (573).

It should be emphasized that a pulmonary infiltrate is not a requirement for consideration of this diagnosis, and in this patient population unexplained fever and hypoxia alone may be an indication for a vigorous diagnostic approach such as bronchial brush biopsy in an attempt to secure an early diagnosis of this treatable infection before further clinical deterioration occurs.

Treatment. Pentamidine isethionate is the chemotherapeutic agent that has been used most extensively in this disease. It is generally administered as a single daily intramuscular injection of 4 mg per kg for 14 days. It can be administered intravenously also, but this route has been associated with most of the serious anaphylactic and hypotensive reactions reported. Other side effects are merely annoying and rarely require discontinuing therapy. The most common are hypoglycemia, azotemia, elevation of serum glutamic oxaloacetic transaminase, pain, and sterile abscess formation at injection sites (584). In a case treated at Stanford, an extensive abscess developed with myonecrosis of most of one buttock requiring extensive plastic surgery. Several patients have had megaloblastic bone marrow changes and low serum folate concentrations. This may be alleviated by the administration of folinic acid, apparently without impairing the therapeutic effect of the drug (518).

In the Stanford series, 21 patients were treated with the drug through 1973. Thirteen (62 per cent) of these recovered or died of other causes (573). Forty-one children were treated with this agent at St. Jude's Hospital with a recovery rate of 68 per cent (538). In the Center for Disease Control summary of cases in the United States, 42 per cent of 163 patients recovered with pentamidine therapy, with 63 per cent recovering if therapy was given for at least 9 days, indicating the need for early diagnosis and treatment (554). The mortality rate in untreated patients who are immunosuppressed is estimated to be virtually 100 per cent (560).

Difficulty may be encountered in eradication of viable organisms. Richman (585), for example, found pneumocystis organisms in a lung aspirate 3 days after 14 days of pentamidine therapy at a time when the patient seemed clinically cured. An initial course of pentamidine therapy was followed by relapse in 14 per cent of 28 children at St. Jude's Hospital (538).

Because of the drug side effects described above, especially local reaction and abscess formation (518, 538, 584, 586, 587), other medications have been tried. Pyrimethamine and a sulfonamide (sulfadiazine or triple sulfonamides) have been shown to be as effective as pentamidine by Frenkel and associates (509) in the rat model. Ten proved cases of *P. carinii* pneumonia have been reported that were treated with this combination (513, 518, 540, 558, 588). Six responded to therapy, 3 died after inadequate therapy, and there was one indeterminant response. The dosage schedule was that given in the section on toxoplasmosis. Folinic acid may be given in conjunction with these drugs to allay bone marrow toxicity and does not antagonize their effectiveness against *P. carinii*. There are no comparative studies on the efficacy of pyrimethamine and sulfadiazine versus pentamidine.

Recently, Hughes and co-workers (589) have reported effective use of trimethoprim-sulfamethoxazole in the cortisone-treated rat model. They also used this drug combination in children with *P. carinii* pneumonitis (590). Fourteen children were treated with 20 mg per kg of

trimethoprim and 100 mg per kg of sulfamethoxazole per day. Eleven of 14 recovered completely with trimethoprim-sulfamethoxazole alone. Clinical defervescence occurred in a median of 3 days, and chest roentgenograms were normal in 5 to 15 days with a median of 8 days. Pentamidine therapy was added in 3 cases because of progressive disease. One of these patients recovered completely; the other 2 died. In one of these, *P. carinii* pneumonitis of "moderate severity" was discovered at autopsy; in the other, no organisms were seen. Side effects were minimal. Maculopapular rash was noted in one patient and nausea and vomiting in 3, possibly drug related. In no case did side effects demand the discontinuance of therapy. Lau and Young (591) recently treated 5 adults with *P. carinii* pneumonia with trimethoprim-sulfamethoxazole using a dosage schedule of 3 to 6 tablets (80 mg of trimethoprim and 400 mg of sulfamethoxazole per tablet) orally every 8 to 12 hours for 10 to 16 days. Four of the 5 patients had a clinical response with rapid improvement and clearing of the pulmonary infiltrates. A slight decrease in white blood count and platelets, unresponsive to folinic acid, was seen in one patient. The investigators found a dose of 12 to 15 tablets per day necessary to achieve therapeutic blood concentrations in this population. No relapses occurred. Although further experience is needed, these results are definitely encouraging. Trimethoprim-sulfamethoxazole is currently under study as a prophylactic agent in high-risk situations, and initial results appear very promising (Hughes, W. T.: Personal communication).

Protozoa: Toxoplasma gondii

T. gondii, an obligate intracellular protozoan is a common cause of latent infection of man (592) and can persist in tissues throughout the life of its host (593). It is capable of producing devastating illness in the compromised host (594, 595). The major method of spread of the organism is from cat feces and ingestion of undercooked meats. However, in the compromised host, it has been transmitted by leukocyte transfusion (596, 597). Although *T. gondii* is a relatively infrequent cause of pulmonary disease in this population, we believe it merits detailed discussion because it is treatable and, in some cases, preventable.

Immunopathologic aspects. Antibody, which is neutralizing for *T. gondii* in the presence of the complement-properdin system, appears early in infection in humans and animals. Such antibody is protective in some animal model studies (598) but does not alone appear to be effective in preventing exacerbation *in vivo* in humans.

In most reported cases of disseminated toxoplasmosis in the compromised host, the disease appears to be due to activation of a previous latent infection (599). Animal models have been developed to study factors that affect reactivation and spread of infection. Frenkel (600), in 1957, first showed that ionizing radiation and cortisone in a hamster model exacerbate latent *T. gondii* infection and lead to multifocal central nervous system lesions. Stahl and associates (601) found that cortisone, 6-mercaptopurine, or splenectomy in chronically infected mice led to the production of a lethal encephalitis. Metzger and co-workers (602), in a rat model, demonstrated prolongation of parasitemia by cortisone.

Several investigators have performed studies to examine the importance of cell-mediated immunity and the macrophage as an effector cell in resistance to *T. gondii*. Strannegard and Lycke (603) demonstrated that antilymphocyte serum leads to exacerbation of infection in mice with a decrease in survival time. More recent work by Stahl (Personal communication, 1975) has shown that thymectomy, but not bursectomy, predisposes to lethal toxoplasma infection in chickens, pointing to the importance of cell-mediated immunity in this infection. Other studies have been performed to examine more closely the role of the macrophage in this infection. Normal human monocytes and monocyte-derived macrophages from normal or *T. gondii*–infected persons are unable to kill *T. gondii in vitro* (604, 605). Such phagocytic cells may thus serve as a transport mechanism for the parasites, thereby providing a means of dissemination of the infection. However, when monocytes or macrophages are incubated in the presence of lymphokines (605), killing or inhibition of multiplication results (605, 606). Which of these observations are relevant to control or spread of infection in humans awaits demonstration, but it is of note that Hodgkin's disease, which may compromise "cellular" immunity to a greater degree than other malignancies (607), was the underlying disease in more than one third of patients severely infected with *T. gondii* in a recent review of 81 cases of toxoplasmosis in patients with neoplasia, connective tissue disorders, or transplant recipients (608).

Investigations of other parameters of cellular immunity during infection with *T. gondii* in humans have demonstrated antigen-specific lymphocyte transformation as long as 19 years after initial infection (609) as well as leukocyte migration inhibition (610).

Pulmonary toxoplasmosis has been produced in animal models using subcutaneous, intravenous, intranasal, or aerosol challenge (611). In sheep, 5 days after intravenous inoculation, *T. gondii* was found in the lungs, liver, and spleen. By the fourteenth day, only the lungs contained organisms, and by the twenty sixth day after infection these were negative as well. After intranasal challenge in mice, an acute pulmonary infection ensues, with production of peribronchiolar inflammatory nodules and a hemmorrhagic alveolitis with death of the animals (611). The relevance of this model to the human infection, which probably is initiated from the gastrointestinal tract, has been questioned (611). Couvreur (611) has postulated, on the basis of the human and animal pathophysiologic data, that immunologic reactions are important in the production of the interstitial pulmonary disease.

Pathology. Lung tissue at autopsy in cases of *T. gondii* pneumonitis in both normal and compromised hosts has shown a diffuse interstitial pneumonitis with a fibrinopurulent exudate in the bronchioles and alveoli (612, 613). In some cases, inflammatory cells were not prominent (612), and in others alveolar walls contained fibroblasts, macrophages, plasma cells, lymphocytes, and occasional polymorphonuclear leukocytes (611, 613). Occasional hyaline membrane formation has also been noted (612). Intracellular protozoa are noted in alveolar macrophages (612) and pseudocysts, cysts, and proliferative forms are seen in the alveolar lining cells and the alveoli themselves. Focal bronchopneumonia has also been described (614, 615), as well as pulmonary fibrosis and granulomas (611).

Clinical manifestations. Although *T. gondii* is infrequently recognized in postmortem lung tissue, this parasite is a definite cause of pneumonia in the immunosuppressed host. A retrospective survey of immunocompromised patients with diffuse interstitial pneumonia from the National Cancer Institute and National Institutes of Health indicated that one of 22 patients with this diagnosis had *T. gondii* as the probable cause (500). Because *T. gondii* is frequently found associated with other pathogens in lung material from compromised hosts (614–616), to define better the manifestations of toxoplasma infection in the lungs it is probably useful to examine the clinical disease as reported in more normal hosts. Hooper (613) described a 43-year-old white man with panhypopituitarism who died with respiratory symptoms and in whom proliferative forms of *T. gondii* were seen in lung tissue. Pinkerton and Henderson (612) reported 2 cases of adult pulmonary toxoplasmosis proved histologically and by animal inoculation. One patient, a 50-year-old white man, had associated portal cirrhosis. The other, a 43-year-old white woman, had no known underlying disease. Symptoms included a prodrome of malaise followed by the sudden onset of chills and fever with development of a dry, nonproductive cough and dyspnea. Physical examination of the chest revealed coarse bibasilar rales in both cases and dullness to percussion. A chest roentgenogram showed prominent hilar shadows with increased "lung markings" in the lower lobes bilaterally suggesting "pulmonary congestion" with possible areas of consolidation. The patients became cyanotic and died in respiratory failure. Each had an associated maculopapular rash. Postmortem examination confirmed the diagnosis of interstitial pneumonitis with marked congestion and accumulation of frothy fluid; intracellular *T. gondii* were seen in alveolar cells and macrophages. Couvreur (611) stated that chest roentgenographic findings commonly include signs of interstitial disease, edema, or multiple foci of bronchopneumonia.

As stated above, cases of pneumonitis associated with malignancy or organ transplantation are in general more complicated clinically because of multiple infection (614–616). Luna and Lichtiger (615) described a typical case in a 24-year-old man with Hodgkin's disease receiving chemotherapy who had a clinical picture similar to that described in the cases of Pinkerton and Henderson (612) and Hooper (613). The patient died in respiratory failure, and "free organisms consistent with *T. gondii*" were seen in necrotic areas of the lung. However, many inclusion bodies consistent with CMV were also present in alveolar cells. Electron microscopic studies were consistent with both of these diagnoses.

Many other cases have been reported in immunologically compromised patients in which the diagnosis of toxoplasmic pneumonitis is more circumstantial and indefinite, being based on identification of the organism in nonpulmonary tissues or serologic criteria (617–619). Evidence from these less well documented cases suggests that resolution of the pulmonary infection may be quite slow and that disease may recur several years later (618). These cases also emphasize that the combination of pulmonary disease with evidence of central nervous system infection or rash in a compromised host should lead to a consideration of *T. gondii* as the etiologic agent, the diagnosis all too frequently being made post mortem because it was never suspected.

Diagnosis. Strict criteria for diagnosis (573, 620) demand the demonstration of trophozoites of *T. gondii* in tissues or body fluids or the detection of specific type and titer of antibodies in the serum. Cysts may persist in tissue for years (593), and demonstration of this form or demonstration of organisms by animal inoculation is not sufficient to establish a causal relationship to acute pulmonary infection. Although isolation from enlarged lymph nodes does not necessarily imply recent infection (621), such isolation most likely suggests the presence of the trophozoite form because cysts are rarely found in lymph nodes (620). Pathologic diagnosis is much more difficult because the proliferating intracellular organisms often do not stain well with hematoxylin and eosin, and inflammatory cell response may be suppressed by immunosuppressive medication (622). However, evidence for acute infection may be gained from histologic studies of lymph node biopsy material (623) and lung tissue, and refinements such as immunofluorescent staining for *T. gondii* antigen (624) may make this method even more useful in determination of the cause of an acute pulmonary disease.

Serodiagnosis has proved useful and practical, but interpretation is complicated by the fact that 35 to 70 per cent of adults in the United States have antibodies to this organism (625, 626), and even in acute infection IgG antibodies measured by the standard Sabin-Feldman dye test (627) or conventional immunofluorescent antibody test (628) may have already reached a peak by the time the diagnosis is considered and the tests run. Furthermore, a serologic diagnosis does not conclusively prove the cause of the pulmonary disease in any given patient. To make a diagnosis of acute toxoplasmosis by serologic methods, it is necessary to demonstrate a rising titer (from negative to a high titer or from a low titer to a high titer, 1:1,000 to ≧ 1:16,000). The IgM-fluorescent antibody test (620, 629) has proved most useful in the diagnosis of acute toxoplasmosis in the adult. At present, we consider dye test or immunofluorescent antibody test titers of ≧ 1:1,000, even if stable, when combined with positive IgM-fluorescent antibody titers of ≧ 10 and a consistent clinical picture, to be compatible with a diagnosis of acute toxoplasmosis. A very high dye test or immunofluorescent antibody test titer of ≧ 1:16,000, combined with an IgM-fluorescent antibody test titer of ≧ 1:160, is probably diagnostic of acute infection, even without associated clinical evidence. A positive IgM-fluorescent antibody test does not necessarily mean, however, that the infection is still in the acute stage. Although in most cases IgM-fluorescent antibody titers rise rapidly and thereafter fall to low titers (1:10 or 1:20) within a few weeks or months, in some patients they remain elevated for a year or longer. Although immunosuppressed patients in general are able to produce antibody (630), occasionally a fall in titer associated with immunosuppression or specific anti-toxoplasma therapy has been observed (596, 629). We are familiar with cases in which death resulted from disseminated toxoplasmosis in which no antibodies could be detected. Because of the frequently encountered difficulty in serologic diagnosis of toxoplasmosis in immunosuppressed patients, it is suggested that banks of serum from such patients be established as early as possib'e in the disease course before immunosuppressive therapy is begun. These sera can later be run in parallel with those obtained after infectious complications have occurred (620).

Prevention and treatment. The combination of pyrimethamine and sulfonamides is synergistic against the proliferative form and remains the recommended treatment regimen. It appears to be effective in compromised patients (608). Sulfadiazine and a trisulfapyrimidine mixture (e.g., equal parts of sulfadiazine, sulfamerazine, and sulfamethazine) are the most active sulfonamides against *T. gondii*. The suggested maintenance dose of pyrimethamine is a total of 1 mg per kg of body weight per day by mouth, with a maximal dose of 25 mg per day. A loading dose of 100 to 200 mg may be given in the first 24 hours of treatment in adults to obtain high blood concentrations rapidly. In young children, twice the daily recommended dose can be given for the first 3 to 4 days of treatment. Sulfonamides should be given in a dose of 100 to 150 mg per kg of body weight per day as 4 equal portions every 6 hours. The optimal duration of therapy has not been established, and no data exist concerning treatment of pulmonary infection, but a minimum of 1-month should be considered adequate in most cases.

Irreversible bone marrow aplasia has been reported with this combination when used with immunosuppressive drugs in myeloblastic leukemia (631). Folinic acid (leucovorin calcium) can be used in conjunction with pyrimethamine to prevent this complication. It should be noted that folic acid is believed by some paradoxically to exacerbate underlying hematologic malignancy (632). Clindamycin has proved effective in a mouse model (633, 634) but has not been adequately tested in human cases. It should be noted that the fixed drug combination of trimethoprim-sulfamethoxazole cannot be considered a substitute for pyrimethamine plus sulfadiazine (or triple sulfonamides) because trimethoprim has no significant activity against *T. gondii* (635, 636).

Although most cases in the compromised host are believed to be due to exacerbation of latent infection, it seems advisable to recommend certain guidelines for prevention of infection because primary infection in such patients can result in fulminant disease and death (637). This topic has been discussed in detail in a recent publication (599).

Helminths: Strongyloides stercoralis

Infection with *S. stercoralis* can be a significant problem in the immunocompromised host, including patients with malignancies and patients receiving steroids or cytotoxic drugs (638–643). Although gastrointestinal involvement has been the most prominent feature in these cases (with production of enterocolitis) (639, 642), extensive pulmonary disease with diffuse involvement of the lung and pneumonia (alveolar or nodular) on chest roentgenogram has been described (641, 642). Larvae of *S. stercoralis* have been found in sputum (642) and bronchial washings (641). Gastric aspirates and stool samples have been positive as well, and it has been suggested that examination of stool for this infection should be performed in all patients before immunosuppression is undertaken, even those exposed to the parasite many years earlier (644). In some patients, eosinophilia may be a useful diagnostic clue (642). Treatment of pulmonary infection with thiabendazole has led to improvement (642), and cure of significant gastrointestinal disease in the compromised host has been achieved with doses of 1 g per day for 2 days (642).

Acknowledgment

The writers thank Dr. Joel Ruskin, Dr. David Stevens, and Dr. Stanley Deresinski for their helpful suggestions.

References

313. Jordan, S. W., McLaren, L. C., and Crosby, J. H.: Herpetic tracheobronchitis, Arch Intern Med, 1975, *135*, 784.

314. Bastian, F. O., Rabson, A. S., Yee, C. L., and Tralka, T. S.: *Herpesvirus hominis*: Isolation from trigeminal ganglion, Science, 1972, *178*, 306.

315. Baringer, J. R., and Swoveland, P.: Recovery of herpes simplex virus from human trigeminal ganglia, N Engl J Med, 1973, *288*, 648.

316. Baringer, J. R.: Recovery of herpes simplex virus from human sacral ganglions, N Engl J Med, 1974, *291*, 828.

317. Stevens, J. G., Cook, M. L., and Jordan, M C.: Reactivation of latent herpes simplex virus after pneumococcal pneumonia in mice, Infect Immun, 1975, *11*, 635.

318. Hirsch, M. S., Zisman, B., and Allison, A. C.: Macrophages and age-dependent resistance to herpes simplex virus in mice, J Immunol, 1970, *104*, 1160.

319. Ennis, F. A.: Host defense mechanisms against herpes simplex virus. II. Protection conferred by sensitized spleen cells, J Infect Dis, 1973, *127*, 632.

320. Lodmell, D. L., and Notkins, A. L.: Cellular immunity to herpes simplex virus mediated by interferon, J Exp Med, 1974, *140*, 764.

321. Fujibayashi, T., Hooks, J. J., and Notkins, A. L.: Production of interferon by immune lymphocytes exposed to herpes simplex virus-antibody complexes, J Immunol, 1975, *115*, 1191.

322. Rasmussen, L. E., Jordan, G. W., Stevens, D A., and Merigan, T. C.: Lymphocyte interferon production and transformation after herpes simplex infections in humans, J Immunol, 1974, *112*, 728.

323. Wilton, J. M. A., Ivanyi, L., and Lehner, T.: Cell mediated immunity in *Herpesvirus hominis* infections, Br Med J, 1972, *1*, 723.

324. Rosenberg, G. L., Snyderman, R , and Notkins, A.: Production of chemotactic factor and lymphotoxin by human leukocytes stimulated with herpes simplex virus, Infect Immun, 1974, *10*, 111.

325. Russell, A. S.: Cell-mediated immunity to herpes simplex virus in man, J Infect Dis, 1974, *129*, 142.

326. Starr, S. E., Karatela, S. A., Shore, S. L., Duffey, A., and Nahmias, A. J : Stimulation of human lymphocytes by herpes simplex virus antigens, Infect Immun, 1975, *11*, 109.

327. Notkins, A. L.: Immune mechanisms by which the spread of viral infections is stopped, Cell Immunol, 1974, *11*, 478.

328. Allison, A. C.: Immunity and immunopathology in virus infections, Ann Inst Pasteur Lille, 1972, *123*, 585.

329. Oakes, J. E.: Role for cell-mediated immunity in the resistance of mice to subcutaneous herpes simplex virus infection, Infect Immun, 1975, *12*, 166.

330. Rosenberg, G. L., and Notkins, A L.: Induction of cellular immunity to herpes simplex virus: Relationship to the humoral immune response, J Immunol, 1974, *112*, 1019.

331. Stevens, J. G., and Cook, M. L.: Maintenance of latent herpetic infections: An apparent role for anti-viral IgG, J Immunol, 1974, *113*, 1685.

332. Douglas, R. G., Jr., and Couch, R. B.: A prospective study of chronic herpes simplex virus infection and recurrent herpes labialis in humans, J Immunol, 1970, *104*, 289.

333. Lodmell, D L., Niwa, A., Hayashi, K., and Notkins, A. L.: Prevention of cell-to-cell spread of herpes simplex virus by leukocytes, J Exp Med, 1973, *137*, 706.

334. Shore, S. L., Nahmias, A. J., Starr, S. E., Wood, P. A., and McFarlin, D. E.: Detection of cell-dependent cytotoxic antibody to cells infected with herpes simplex virus, Nature, 1974, *251*, 350.

335. Rager-Zisman, B., and Bloom, B. R.: Immunological destruction of herpes simplex virus infected cells, Nature, 1974, *251*, 542.

336. Costa, J., Yee, C., Troost, T., and Rabson, A. S.: Effect of dexamethasone on herpes simplex virus type two infection *in vitro*, Nature, 1974, *252*, 745.

337. Douglas, R. G., Jr., Anderson, M. S., Weg, J. G., Williams, T., Jenkins, D. E., Knight, V., and Beall, A. C.: Herpes simplex virus pneumonia, JAMA, 1969, *210*, 902.

338. Nash, G., and Foley, F. D.: Herpetic infection of the middle and lower respiratory tract, Am J Clin Pathol, 1970, *54*, 857.

339. Foley, F. D., Greenawald, K. A., Nash, G., and Pruitt, B. A., Jr.: Herpesvirus infection in burned patients, N Engl J Med, 1970, *282*, 652.

340. Cheever, A W., Valsamis, M. P., and Rabson, A. S.: Necrotizing toxoplasmic encephalitis and herpetic pneumonia complicating treated Hodgkin's disease, N Engl J Med, 1965, *272*, 26.

341. Beall, A. C., Jenkins, D. E., Weg, J. G., Stevens, P. M., Noon, G. P., Johnson, P. C., Bell, R. L , Knight, J. V., Rossen, R. D., Butler, W. T., Douglas, R. G., Jr., Williams, T. W., Lewis, J. M., Murgen, F. D., McIntire, R. S., Anderson, M. S., Balsauer, A. M., and DeBakey, R. M. E.: Human lung allotransplantation: Report of

two cases, Am J Surg, 1970, *119*, 300.

342   Herout, V., Vortel, V., and Vondrackova, A.: Herpex simplex involvement of the lower respiratory tract, Am J Clin Pathol, 1966, *46*, 411.

343. Case records of the Massachusetts General Hospital. Case 15-1973, N Engl J Med, 1973, *288*, 780.

344. Back, A. F., and Schmidt, N. J.: Indirect hemagglutinating antibody response to *Herpesvirus hominis* types one and two in immunized laboratory animals and in natural infections of man, Appl Microbiol, 1974, *28*, 392.

345. Skaug, K., and Tjotta, E.: Diagnosis of recent herpes simplex infections. A modified immunofluorescent test, Acta Pathol Microbiol Scand [B], 1974, *82*, 323.

346. Boston Interhospital Virus Study Group and the NIAID-Sponsored Cooperative Antiviral Clinical Study: Failure of high dose 5-iodo-2'-deoxy-uridine in the therapy of herpes simplex virus encephalitis, N Engl J Med, 1975, *292*, 599.

347. Chow, A. W., Ronald, A., Fiala, M., Hryniuk, W., Weil, M. L., St. Geme, J., Jr., and Guze, L. B.: Cytosine arabinoside therapy for herpes simplex encephalitis. Clinical experience with six patients, Antimicrob Agents Chemother, 1973, *3*, 412.

348. Ch'ien, L. T., Whitley, R. J., Nahmias, A. J., Lewin, E. B., Linneman, C. C., Jr., Frenkel, L. D., Ballanti, J. A., Buchanan, R. A., and Alfred, C. A., Jr.: Antiviral chemotherapy and neonatal herpes simplex virus infection: A pilot study, Pediatrics, 1975, *55*, 678.

349. Kobza, K., Emodi, G., Jest, M., Hilti, E., Leuenberger, A., Binswanger, U., Thiel, G., and Brunner, F. P.: Treatment of herpes infection with human exogeneous interferon (letter to the editor), Lancet, 1975, *1*, 1343.

350. Vaccination against an oncogenic herpes virus (editorial), Lancet, 1975, *1*, 504.

351. Rowe, W. P., Hartley, J. W., Waterman, S., Turner, H. C., and Huebner, R. J.: Cytopathogenic agent resembling human salivary gland virus recovered from tissue cultures of human adenoids, Proc Soc Exp Biol Med, 1956, *92*, 418.

352. Smith, M. G.: Propagation in tissue cultures of a cytopathogenic virus from human salivary gland virus (SGV) disease, Proc Soc Exp Biol Med, 1956, *92*, 424.

353. Weller, T. H., Macaulay, J. C., Craig, J. M., and Wirth, P.: Isolation of intranuclear inclusion producing agents from infants with illnesses resembling cytomegalic inclusion disease, Proc Soc Exp Biol Med, 1957, *94*, 4.

354. Weller, T. H.: The cytomegaloviruses: Ubiquitous agents with protean clinical manifestations, N Engl J Med, 1971, *285*, 203.

355. Osborn, J. E., and Medearis, D. N., Jr.: Status of relationship between mouse cytomegalovirus and interferon, Proc Soc Exp Biol Med, 1966, *121*, 819.

356. Oie, H. K., Easton, J. M., Ablashi, D. V., and Baron, S.: Murine cytomegalovirus: Induction of and sensitivity to interferon in vitro, Infect Immun, 1975, *12*, 1012.

357. Henson, D., and Smith, R. D.: Interferon production *in vitro* by cells infected with the murine salivary gland virus, Proc Soc Exp Biol Med, 1964, *117*, 517.

358. Glasgow, L. A.: Cytomegalovirus interference *in vitro*, Infect Immun, 1974, *9*, 702.

359. Lang, D. J., Thomas, M. T., and Gresser, I.: Protection par l'interféron de cellules embryonnaires humaines contre l'infection par le virus cytomegalique, C R Acad Sci [D] (Paris), 1969, *268*, 3137.

360. Rabson, A. S., Tyrrell, S. A., and Levy, H.: Inhibition of human CMV *in vitro* by double-stranded polyribocytidylic-inosinic acid, Proc Soc Exp Biol Med, 1969, *131*, 495.

361. Tegtmeyer, P. J., and Craighead, J. E.: Infection of adult mouse macrophages *in vitro* with CMV, Proc Soc Exp Biol Med, 1968, *129*, 690.

362. Selgrade, M. K., and Osborn, J. E.: Role of macrophages in resistance to murine CMV, Infect Immun, 1974, *10*, 1383.

363. Gardner, M. B., Officer, J. E., Parker, J., Estes, J. D., and Rongey, R. W.: Induction of disseminated virulent cytomegalovirus infection by immunosuppression of naturally chronically infected wild mice, Infect Immun, 1974, *10*, 966.

364. Brody, A. R, and Craighead, J. E.: Pathogenesis of pulmonary cytomegalovirus infection in immunosuppressed mice, J Infect Dis, 1974, *129*, 677.

365. Simmons, R. L., Lopez, C., Balfour, H., Jr., Kalis, J., Rattazzi, L. C., and Najarian, J. S.: Cytomegalovirus: Clinical virological correlations in renal transplant recipients, Ann Surg, 1974, *180*, 623.

366. Craighead, J. E.: Pulmonary cytomegalovirus infection in the adult, Am J Pathol, 1971, *63*, 487.

367. Ho, M., Suwansirikul, S., Dowling, J. N., Youngblood, L. A., and Armstrong, J. A.: The transplanted kidney as a source of cytomegalovirus infection, N Engl J Med, 1975, *293*, 1109.

368. Kanich, R. E., and Craighead, J. E.: Cytomegalovirus infection and cytomegalic inclusion disease in renal homotransplant recipients, Am J Med, 1966, *40*, 874.

369. Henson, D., Smith, R. D., Gehrke, J., and Neopolitan, C.: Effect of cortisone on nonfatal mouse cytomegalovirus infection, Am J Pathol, 1967, *51*, 1001.

370. Henson, D., Smith, R. D., and Gehrke, J.: Nonfatal mouse cytomegalovirus hepatitis: Combined morphologic, virologic, and immunologic observations, Am J Pathol, 1966, *49*, 871.

371. Rifkind, D., Goodman, N., and Hill, R. B.: The clinical significance of CMV infection in renal transplant recipients, Ann Intern Med, 1967, *66*, 1116.

372. Meyers, J. D., Spencer, H. C., Watts, J. C., Gregg, M. B., Stewart, J. A., Troupin, R. H., and Thomas, E. D.: Cytomegalovirus pneumonia after human marrow transplantation, Ann Intern Med, 1975, *82*, 181.

373. Olding, L. B., Jensen, F. C., and Oldstone, M. B. A.: Pathogenesis of cytomegalovirus infection, J Exp Med, 1975, *141*, 561.

374. Wu, B. C., Dowling, J. N., Armstrong, J. A., and Ho, M.: Enhancement of mouse cytomegalovirus infection during host versus graft reaction, Science, 1975, *190*, 56.

375. Jeffery, J. R., Guttmann, R. D., Becklake, M. R. Beaudoin, J. G., and Morehouse, D. D.: Recovery from severe cytomegalovirus pneumonia in a renal transplant patient, Am Rev Respir Dis, 1974, *109*, 129.

376. Anderson, H. K., and Spencer, E. S.: Cytomegalovirus infection among renal allograft recipients, Acta Med Scand, 1969, *186*, 7.

377. Coulson, A. S., Lucas, Z. J., Condy, M., and Cohn, R.: An epidemic of cytomegalovirus disease in a renal transplant population, West J Med, 1974, *120*, 1.

378. Fine, R. N., Grushkin, C. M., Malekzadeh, M., and Wright, H. T., Jr.: Cytomegalovirus syndrome following renal transplantation, Arch Surg, 1972, *105*, 564.

379. Craighead, J. E., Hanshaw, J. B., and Carpenter, C. B.: Cytomegalovirus infection after renal allotransplantation, JAMA, 1967, *201*, 725.

380. Fiala, M., Payne, J. E., Berne, T. V., Moore, T. C., Henle, W., Montgomerie, J. Z., Chatterjee, S. N., and Guze, L. B.: Epidemiology of CMV infection after transplantation and immunosuppression, J Infect Dis, 1975, *132*, 421.

381. Gottmann, A. W., and Beatty, E. C., Jr.: Cytomegalic inclusion disease in children with leukemia or lymphosarcoma, Am J Dis Child, 1962, *104*, 180.

382. Rosen, P., and Hajdu, S.: Cytomegalovirus inclusion disease at autopsy of patients with cancer, Am J Clin Pathol, 1971, *55*, 749.

383. Bodey, G. P., Werleake, P. T., Douglas, G., and Levin, R. H.: Cytomegalic inclusion disease in patients with acute leukemia, Ann Intern Med, 1965, *62*, 899.

384. Neiman, P., Wasserman, P. B., Wentworth, B. B., Kao, G. F., Learner, K. G., Storb, R., Buckner, C. D., Clift, R. A., Fefer, A., Fass, L., Glucksberg, H., and Thomas, E. D.: Interstitial pneumonia and cytomegalovirus infection as complications of human marrow transplantation, Transplantation, 1973, *15*, 478.

385. Infections with cytomegalovirus in bone marrow transplantation: Report of a workshop, J Infect Dis, 1975, *132*, 114.

386. Evans, D. J., and Williams, E. D.: Cytomegalic inclusion disease in the adult, J Clin Pathol, 1968, *21*, 311.

387. Goodman, N., Daves, M. L., and Rifkind, D.: Pulmonary roentgen findings following renal transplantations, Radiology, 1967, *89*, 621.

388. Stevens, D. P., Barker, L. F., Ketcham, A. S., and Myer, H. M., Jr.: Asymptomatic cytomegalovirus infection following blood transfusion in tumor surgery, JAMA, 1970, *211*, 1341.

389. Prince, A. M., Szmuness, W., Millian, S. J., and David, D. S.: A serologic study of CMV infections associated with blood transfusions, N Engl J Med, 1971, *284*, 1125.

390. Kane, R. C., Rousseau, W. E., Noble, G. R., Tegtmeier, G. E., Wulff, H., Herndon, H. B., Chin, T. D. .W, and Bayer, W. L.: Cytomegalovirus infection in a volunteer blood donor population, Infect Immun, 1975, *11*, 719.

391. Nagington, J.: Cytomegalovirus antibody production in renal transplant patients, J Hyg (Camb), 1971, *69*, 645.

392. Langenhuysen, M. M. A. C., The, T. H., Nieweg, H. O., and Kapsenberg, J. G.: Demonstration of IgM cytomegalovirus-antibodies as an aid to early diagnosis in adults, Clin Exp Immunol, 1970, *6*, 387.

393. Waner, J. L., Weller, T. H., and Kevy, S. V.: Patterns of cytomegaloviral complement-fixing antibody activity: A longitudinal study of blood donors, J Infect Dis, 1973, *127*, 538.

394. Yaeger, A. S.: Longitudinal serological study of cytomegalovirus infections in nurses and in personnel without patient contact, J Clin Microbiol, 1975, *2*, 448.

395. Jain, U., Mani, K., and Frable, W.: Cytomegalic inclusion disease: Cytologic diagnosis from bronchial brushing material, Acta Cytol (Baltimore), 1973, *17*, 467.

396. Behrens, H. W., and Quick, C. A.: Bronchoscopic diagnosis of cytomegalovirus infections, J Infect Dis, 1974, *130*, 174.

397. Cox, F., and Hughes, W. T.: Cytomegaloviremia in children with acute lymphocyte leukemia, J Pediatr, 1975, *87*, 190.

398. Chumbley, L. C., Robertson, D. M., Smith, T. F and Campbell, R. J.: Adult cytomegalovirus inclusion retino-uveitis, Am J Ophthalmol, 1975, *80*, 807.

399. Cox, F., Meyer, D., and Hughes, W. T.: Cytomegalovirus in tears from patients with normal eyes and with acute cytomegalovirus chorioretinitis, Am J Ophthalmol, 1975, *80*, 817.

400. Falcoff, E., Falcoff, R., Fournier, F., and Chany, C.: Production en masse, purification partielle, et caracterisation d'un interféron destiné a des essais thérapeutiques humaines, Ann Inst Pasteur (Paris), 1966, *111*, 562.

401. Barton, B. W., and Tobin, J. O.: The effect of

idoxuridine on the excretion of cytomagalovirus in congenital infection, Ann NY Acad Sci, 1970, *173*, 90.

402. Conchie, A. F., Barton, B. W., and Tobin, J. O.: Congenital cytomegalovirus infection treated with idoxuridine, Br Med J, 1968, *4*, 162.

403. Kraybill, E. N., Sever, J. L., Avery, G. B., and Movassaghi, N.: Experimental use of cytosine arabinoside in congenital cytomegalovirus infection, J Pediatr, 1972, *80*, 485.

404. McCracken, G. H., Jr., and Luby, J. P.: Cytosine arabinoside in the treatment of congenital cytomegalic inclusion disease, J Pediatr, 1972, *80*, 488.

405. Ch'ien, L. T., Cannon, N. J., Whitley, R. J., Diethelm, A. G., Dismukes, W. E., Scott, C. W., Buchanan, R. A., and Alfred, C. A., Jr.: Effect of adenine arabinoside on cytomegalovirus infections, J Infect Dis, 1974, *130*, 32.

406. Rytel, M. W., and Kauffman, H. M.: Clinical efficacy of adenine arabinoside in therapy of cytomegalovirus infections in renal allograft recipients, J Infect Dis, 1976, *133*, 202.

407. Schimpff, S., Serpick, A., Stoler, B., Rumack, B., Mellin, H., Joseph, J. M., and Block, J.: Varicella-zoster infection in patients with cancer, Ann Intern Med, 1972, *76*, 241.

408. Rifkind, D.: The activation of varicella-zoster virus infections by immunosuppressive therapy, J Lab Clin Med, 1966, *68*, 463.

409. Resnick, J., and Schanberger, J. E.: Varicella reactivation in nephrotic syndrome treated with cyclophosphamide and adrenal corticosteroids, J Pediatr, 1973, *83*, 451.

410. Pagano, J.: Diseases and mechanisms of persistent DNA virus infection: Latency and cellular transformation, J Infect Dis, 1975, *132*, 209.

411. Rado, J. P., Tako, J., Geder, L., and Jeney, E.: Herpes zoster house epidemic in steroid-treated patients, Arch Intern Med, 1965, *116*, 329.

412. Jordan, G. W., and Merigan, T. C.: Cell-mediated immunity to varicella-zoster virus: *In vitro* lymphocyte responses, J Infect Dis, 1974, *130*, 495.

413. Russell, A. S., Maini, R. A., Bailey, M., and Dumonde, D. C.: Cell-mediated immunity to varicella-zoster antigen in acute herpes zoster (shingles), Clin Exp Immunol, 1973, *14*, 181.

414. Twomey, J. J., Gyorkey, F., and Norris, S. M.: The monocyte disorder with herpes zoster, J Lab Clin Med, 1974, *83*, 768.

415. Stevens, D. A., and Merigan, T. C.: Interferon, antibody, and other host factors in herpes zoster, J Clin Invest, 1972, *51*, 1170.

416. Stevens, D. A., Ferrington, R. A., Jordan, G. W., and Merigan, T. C.: Cellular events in zoster vesicles: Relation to clinical course and immune parameters, J Infect Dis, 1975, *131*, 509.

417. Betts, R. F., Zaky, D. A., Douglas, R. G., Jr., and Royer, G.: Ineffectiveness of subcutaneous cy

tosine arabinoside in localized herpes zoster, Ann Intern Med, 1975, *82*, 778.

418. Uduman, S. A., Gershon, A. A., and Brunell, P. A.: Should patients with zoster receive zoster immune globulin?, JAMA, 1975, *234*, 1049.

419. Gershon, A. A., Steinberg, S., and Brunell, P. A.: Zoster immune globulin: A further assessment, N Engl J Med, 1974, *290*, 243.

420. Goffinet, D. R., Glatstein, E. J., and Merigan, T. C.: Herpes zoster-varicella infections and lymphoma, Ann Intern Med, 1972, *76*, 235.

421. Feldman, S., Hughes, W. T., and Kim, H. Y.: Herpes zoster in children with cancer, Am J Dis Child, 1973, *126*, 178.

422. Schimpff, S. C., O'Connell, M. J., Greene, W. H., and Wiernik, P. H.: Infections in 92 splenectomized patients with Hodgkin's disease, Am J Med, 1975, *59*, 695.

423. Triebwasser, J. H., Harris, R. E., Bryant, R. E., and Rhoades, E. R.: Varicella pneumonia in adults, Medicine, 1967, *46*, 409.

424. Raider, L.: Calcification in chickenpox pneumonia, Chest, 1971, *60*, 504.

425. Pek, S., and Gikas, P. W.: Pneumonia due to herpes zoster, Ann Intern Med, 1965, *62*, 350.

426. Burton, G. G., Sayer, W. J., and Lillington, G. A: Varicella pneumonitis in adults: Frequency of sudden death, Dis Chest, 1966, *50*, 179.

427. Mermelstein, R. H., and Freireich, A. W.: Varicella pneumonia, Ann Intern Med, 1961, *55*, 456.

428. Glick, N., Levin, S., and Nelson, K.: Recurrent pulmonary infarction in adult chickenpox pneumonia, JAMA, 1972, *222*, 173.

429. Chelius, C. J.: Herpes zoster generalisatus, Wis Med J, 1960, *59*, 565.

430. Kain, H. K., Feldman, C. A., and Cohn, L. H.: Herpes zoster generalisatis pneumonia, Arch Intern Med, 1962, *110*, 98.

431. Brunell, P. A., and Casey, H. L.: Crude tissue culture antigen for determination of varicella-zoster complement-fixing antibody, Public Health Rep. 1964, *79*, 839.

432. Count, A. E., and Shaw, D. G.: Neutralization tests with varicella-zoster virus, J Hyg (Camb), 1969, *67*, 343.

433. Williams, V., Gershon, A., and Brunell, P. A.: Serologic response to varicella-zoster membrane antigens measured by indirect immunofluorescence, J Infect Dis, 1974, *130*, 669.

434. Schmidt, N. J., Lennette, E. H., Woodie, J. D., and Ho, H. H.: Immunofluorescent staining in the laboratory diagnosis of varicella-zoster virus infections, J Lab Clin Med, 1965, *66*, 403.

435. Williams, B., and Capers, T. H.: The demonstration of intranuclear inclusion bodies in sputum from a patient with varicella pneumonia, Am J Med, 1959, *27*, 836.

436. Davis, C. M., Van Dersarl, J. W., and Coltman, C. A., Jr.: Failure of cytarabine in varicella-

zoster infections, JAMA, 1973, *224*, 122.

437. Stevens, D. A., Jordan, G. W., Waddell, T. F., and Merigan, T. C.: Adverse effect of cytosine arabinoside on disseminated zoster in a controlled trial, N Engl J Med, 1973, *289*, 873.

438. Schimpff, S. C., Fortner, C. L., Greene, W. H., and Wiernik, P. H.: Cytosine arabinoside for localized herpes zoster in patients with cancer: Failure in a controlled trial, J Infect Dis, 1974, *130*, 673.

439. Johnson, M. T., Luby, J. P., Buchanan, R. A., and Mikulec, D.: Treatment of varicella-zoster virus infections with adenine arabinoside, J Infect Dis, 1975, *131*, 225.

439A. Whitley, R. J., Ch'ien, L. T., Dolin, R., Galasso, G. J., and Alford. C. A., Jr.: Adenine arabinoside therapy of herpes zoster in the immunosuppressed, N Engl J Med, 1976, *294*, 1193.

440. Emodi, G., Rufli, T., Just, M., and Hernandez, R.: Human interferon therapy for herpes zoster in adults, Scand J Infect Dis, 1975, 7, 1.

441. Merigan, T. C., Rand, K. H., Abdallah, P. S., Jordan, G. W., Feldman, S., and Fried, R. P.: Administration of human leukocyte interferon in varicella-zoster infections. II. Preliminary controlled trials to establish effective dosage in patients with malignancy, Session VIId, Antivirals with clinical potential; A symposium at Stanford University, Calif., Aug. 26–27, 1975, J Infect Dis, in press.

442. Wigger, H. J., and Blanc, W. A.: Fatal hepatic and bronchial necrosis in adenovirus infection with thymic alymphoplasia, N Engl J Med, 1966, *275*, 870.

443. Roos, R., Chou, S. M., Rogers, N. G., Basnight, M., and Gajdusek, D. C.: Isolation of an adenovirus 32 strain from human brain in a case of subacute encephalitis, Proc Soc Exp Biol Med, 1972, *139*, 636.

444. Myerowitz, R. L., Stalder, H., Oxman, M. N., Levin, M. J., Moore, M., Leith, J. D., Gautz, N. W., and Pellegrini, J.: Fatal disseminated adenovirus infection in a renal transplant recipient, Am J Med, 1975, *59*, 591.

445. Parker, F., Jr., Jackson, H., Jr., Bethea, J. M., and Otis, F.: Studies of diseases of the lymphoid and myeloid tissues: The coexistence of tuberculosis with Hodgkin's disease and other forms of malignant lymphoma, Am J Med Sci, 1932, *184*, 694.

446. Kaplan, M. H., Armstrong, D., and Rosen, P.: Tuberculosis complicating neoplastic disease, Cancer, 1974, *33*, 850.

447. McNutt, D. R., and Fudenberg, H. H.: Disseminated scotochromogen infection and unusual myeloproliferative disorder, Ann Intern Med, 1971, *75*, 373.

448. Graybill, J. R., Silva, J., Jr., Fraser, D. W., Lordon, R., and Rogers, E.: Disseminated mycobacteriosis due to *Mycobacterium abscessus* in two recipients of renal homografts, Am Rev Respir Dis, 1974, *109*, 4.

449. Fraser, D. W., Buxton, A. E., Naji, A., Barker, C. F., Rudnick, M., and Weinstein, A. J.: Disseminated *Mycobacterium kansasii* infection presenting as cellulitis in a recipient of a renal homograft, Am Rev Respir Dis, 1975, *112*, 125.

450. Grillo-López, A. J., Rivera, E., Castillo-Staab, M., and Maldonado, N.: Disseminated *M. kansasii* infection in a patient with chronic granulocytic leukemia, Cancer, 1971, *28*, 476.

451. Buhler, V. B., and Pollak, A.: Human infection with atypical acid fast organisms, Am J Clin Pathol, 1953, *23*, 363.

452. Wood, L. E., Buhler, V. B., and Pollak, A.: Human infection with the "yellow" acid-fast bacillus, Am Rev Tuberc, 1956, *73*, 917.

453. Kilbridge, T. M., Gonnella, J. S., and Bolan, J. T.: Pancytopenia and death. Disseminated anonymous mycobacterial infection, Arch Intern Med, 1967, *120*, 38.

454. McCusker, J. J., and Green, R. A.: Generalized nontuberculous mycobacteriosis, Am Rev Respir Dis, 1962, *86*, 405.

455. Hagmar, B., Kutti, J., Lundin, P., Norlin, M., Weinfeld, A., and Wahlén, P.: Disseminated infection caused by *Mycobacterium kansasii*, Acta Med Scand, 1969, *186*, 93.

456. Feld, R., Bodey, G. P., and Groschel, D.: Mycobacteriosis in patients with malignant disease, Arch Intern Med, 1976, *136*, 67.

457. Collins, F. M.: Acquired resistance to mycobacterial infections, Adv Tuberc Res, 1972, *18*, 1.

458. Vorwald, A. J.: The early cellular reaction in the lungs of rabbits injected intravenously with human tubercle bacilli, Am Rev Tuberc, 1932, *25*, 74.

459. Allgower, M., and Bloch, H.: The effect of tubercle bacilli on migration of phagocytes *in vitro*, Am Rev Tuberc, 1949, *59*, 562.

460. Henderson, J. J., Dannenberg, A. M., Jr., and Lurie, M. G.: Phagocytosis of tubercle bacilli by rabbit pulmonary alveolar macrophages and its relation to native resistance to tuberculosis, J Immunol, 1963, *91*, 553.

461. Berthrong, M.: The macrophage-tubercle bacillus relationship and resistance to tuberculosis, Ann NY Acad Sci, 1968, *154*, 157.

462. Suter, E.: Multiplication of tubercle bacilli within mononuclear phagocytes in tissue culture derived from normal animals and animals vaccinated with BCG, J Exp Med, 1953, *97*, 235.

463. Lurie, M.: Studies on the mechanisms of immunity in tuberculosis, J Exp Med, 1942, *75*, 247.

464. Mackaness, G. B., Smith, N., and Wells, A. Q.: The growth of intracellular tubercle bacilli in relation to their virulence, Am Rev Tuberc, 1954, *69*, 479.

465. Patterson, R. J., and Youmans, G. P.: Demonstration in tissue culture of lymphocyte-mediated immunity to tuberculosis, Infect Immun, 1970, *1*, 600.

466. Collins, F. M., Congdon, C. C., and Morrison, N. E.: Growth of *Mycobacterium bovis* (BCG) in T lymphocyte-depleted mice, Infect Immun, 1975, *11*, 57.

467. Suter, E.: Passive transfer of acquired resistance to infection with *Mycobacterium tuberculosis* by means of cells, Am Rev Respir Dis, 1961, *83*, 535.

468. Sever, J. L.: Passive transfer of resistance to tuberculosis through the use of monocytes, Proc Soc Exp Biol Med, 1960, *103*, 326.

469. Millman, I.: Passive transfer of resistance to tuberculosis, Am Rev Respir Dis, 1962, *85*, 30.

470. Lefford, M. J., McGregor, D. D., and Mackaness, G. B.: Immune response to *Mycobacterium tuberculosis* in rats, Infect Immun, 1973, *8*, 182.

471. Spencer, J. C., Waldman, R. H., and Johnson, J. E., III.: Local and systemic cell-mediated immunity after immunization of guinea pigs with live or killed *M. tuberculosis* by various routes, J Immunol, 1974, *112*, 1322.

472. Yamamoto, K., Anacker, R. L., and Ribi, E.: Relationship between inhibitory activity of lung cells and resistance to airborne challenge with *M. tuberculosis* H37Rv, Infect Immun, 1970, *1*, 595.

473. Podleski, W. K., and Podleski, U. G.: Circulating cytotoxic lymphocytes in human tuberculosis, Am Rev Respir Dis, 1973, *108*, 791.

474. Lefford, M. J., and McGregor, D. D.: Immunological memory in tuberculosis, Cell Immunol, 1974, *14*, 417.

475. Neiburger, R. G., Youmans, G .P., and Youmans, A. S.: Relationship between tuberculin hypersensitivity and cellular immunity to infection in mice vaccinated with viable attenuated mycobacterial cells or with mycobacterial ribonucleic acid preparations, Infect Immun, 1973, *8*, 42.

475A. Youmans, G. P.: Relation between delayed hypersensitivity and immunity in tuberculosis, Am Rev Respir Dis, 1975, *111*, 109.

476. Shapiro, C. D. K., Harding, G. E., and Smith, D. W.: Relationship of delayed-type hypersensitivity and acquired cellular resistance of experimental airborn TB, J Infect Dis, 1974, *130*, 8.

477. Collins, F. M., and Mackaness, G. B.: The relationship of delayed hypersensitivity to acquired antituberculous immunity, Cell Immunol, 1970, *1*, 253.

478. Fong, J., Schneider, P., and Elberg, S. S.: Studies on tubercle bacillus-monocyte relationship, J Exp Med, 1956, *104*, 455.

479. Hsu, H. S.: Cellular basis of cortisone-induced host susceptibility to tuberculosis, Am Rev Respir Dis, 1969, *100*, 677.

480. Kochan, I., and Bendel, W. L., Jr.: Passive transfer of tuberculin hypersensitivity in guinea pigs, J Allergy, 1966, *37*, 284.

481. Dupuy, J. M., Kalpaktosoglou, P., and Good, R. A.: Transfer with a plasma fraction of delayed hypersensitivity to PPD in guinea pigs, J Immunol, 1970, *104*, 1384.

482. Collins, F. M., Volkman, A., and McGregor, D. D.: Transfer of delayed and arthus sensitivity with blood plasma from x-irradiated guinea pigs, Immunology, 1970, *19*, 501.

483. Minden, P., and Farr, R. S.: Binding between components of the tubercle bacillus and humoral antibodies, J Exp Med, 1969, *130*, 931.

484. Bardana, E. J., Jr., McClatchy, J. K., Farr, R. S., and Minden, P.: Universal occurrence of antibodies to tubercle bacilli in sera from nontuberculous and tuberculous individuals, Clin Exp Immunol, 1973, *13*, 65.

485. Salvin, S. B., Ribi, E., Granger, D. L., and Younger, J. S.: Migration inhibitory factor and type II interferon in the circulation of mice sensitized with mycobacterial components, J Immunol, 1975, *114*, 354.

486. Lurie, M. B., Zappasodi, P., Dannenberg, A. M., Jr., and Swartz, I. B.: Constitutional factors in resistance to infection: The effect of cortisone on the pathogenesis of tuberculosis, Science, 1951, *113*, 234.

487. Stead, W. W.: Pathogenesis of a first episode of chronic pulmonary tuberculosis in man: Recrudescence of residuals of the primary infection or exogenous reinfection?, Am Rev Respir Dis, 1967, *95*, 729.

488. Raleigh, J. W., and Wichelhausen, R.: Exogenous reinfection with *Mycobacterium tuberculosis* confirmed by phage typing, Am Rev Respir Dis, 1973, *108*, 639.

489. Yamamura, Y., Yasaka, O., Hideo, M., and Yamamura, Y.: Prevention of tuberculous cavity formation by desensitization with tuberculin-active peptide, Am Rev Respir Dis, 1974, *109*, 594.

490. Cliffton, E. E., and Irani, B. B.: Pulmonary tuberculosis in cancer, NY State J Med, 1970, *70*, 274.

491. Morrow, L. B., and Anderson, R. E.: Active tuberculosis in leukemia, Arch Pathol, 1965, *79*, 484.

492. Oswald, N. C.: Acute tuberculosis and granulocytic disorders, Br Med J, 1963, *2*, 1489.

493. Andre, J., Schwartz, R., and Dameshek, W.: Tuberculosis and myelosclerosis with myeloid metaplasia, JAMA, 1961, *178*, 1169.

494. Glasser, R. M., Waler, R. I., and Herion, J. C.: The significance of hematologic abnormalities in patients with tuberculosis, Arch Intern Med, 1970, *125*, 691.

495. Pradhan, R. P., Katz, L. A., Nidus, B. D., Matalon, R., and Eisinger, R. P.: Tuberculosis in dialyzed patients, JAMA, 1974, *229*, 798.

496. Neff, T. A., and Hudgel, D. W.: Miliary tuberculosis in a renal transplant recipient, Am Rev Respir Dis, 1973, *108*, 677.

497. Wellmann, K. F., and Teng, K. P.: Demonstration of acid-fast bacilli in tissue sections by fluorescence microscopy, Can Med Assoc J, 1962, *87*, 837.

498. Fox, W., and Mitchison, D. A.: State of the art. Short-course chemotherapy for pulmonary tuberculosis, Am Rev Respir Dis, 1975, *111*, 325.

499. Johnston, R. F., and Wildrick, K. H.: State of the art review. The impact of chemotherapy on the care of patients with tuberculosis, Am Rev Respir Dis, 1974, *109*, 636.

500. Goodell, B., Jacobs, J. B., Powell, R. B., and DeVita, V. T.: *Pneumocystis carinii*: The spectrum of diffuse interstitial pneumonia in patients with neoplastic diseases, Ann Intern Med, 1970, *72*, 337.

501. Ruskin, J.: *Pneumocystis carinii*, in *Infectious Diseases of the Fetus and Newborn Infant*, J. S. Remington, and J. O. Klein, ed., W. B. Saunders, Philadelphia, 1976.

502. Barton, F. G., Jr., and Campbell, W. G., Jr.: Further observations on the ultrastructure of the pneumocystis, Arch Pathol, 1967, *83*, 527.

503. Huang, S. N., and Marshall, K. G.: *Pneumocystis carinii* infection. A cytologic, histologic and electron microscopic study of the organisms, Am Rev Respir Dis, 1970, *102*, 623.

504. Campbell, W. G., Jr.: Ultrastructure of pneumocystis in human lung. Life cycle in human pneumocystosis, Arch Pathol, 1972, *93*, 312.

505. Van der Meer, G., and Brug, S. L.: Infection par pneumocystis chez l'homme et chez les animaux, Ann Soc Belg Med Trop, 1942, *22*, 301.

506. Barton, E. G., and Campbell, W. G.: *Pneumocystis carinii* in lungs of rats treated with cortisone acetate, Am J Pathol, 1969, *54*, 209.

507. Ham, E. K., Greenberg, S. D., Reynolds, R. C., and Singer, D. B.: Ultrastructure of *Pneumocystis carinii*, Exp Mol Pathol, 1972, *14*, 362.

508. Pifer, L. L., and Hughes, W. T.: Cultivation of *Pneumocystis carinii in vitro* (abstract), Pediatr Res, 1975, *9*, 344.

509. Frenkel, J. K., Good, J. T., and Shultz, J. A.: Latent pneumocystis infection of rats, relapse and chemotherapy, Lab Invest, 1966, *15*, 1559.

510. Sheldon, W. H.: Experimental pulmonary *Pneumocystis carinii* infection in rabbits, J Exp Med, 1959, *110*, 147.

511. Hughes, W. T., Feldman, S., Aur, R. J. A., Verzosa, M. S., Hustu, O., and Simone, J. V.: Intensity of immunosuppressive therapy and the incidence of *Pneumocystis carinii* pneumonitis, Cancer, 1975, *36*, 2004.

512. Hughes, W. T., Price, R. A., Sisko, F., Havron, W. S., Kafatos, A. G., Schonland, M., and Smythe, P. M.: Protein-calorie malnutrition, a host determinant for *Pneumocystis carinii* infection, Am J Dis Child, 1974, *128*, 44.

513. Rifkind, D., Faris, T. D., and Hill, R. B.: *Pneumocystis carinii* pneumonia. Studies on the diagnosis and treatment, Ann Intern Med, 1966, *65*, 943.

514. Rifkind, D., Starzl, T. E., Marchioro, T. L., Waddell, W. R., Rowlands, D. T., and Hill, R. B. Transplantation pneumonia, JAMA, 1964, *189*, 808.

515. Fulginiti, V. A., Scribner, R., Groth, C. G., Putnam, C. W., Brettschneider, L., Gilbert, S., Porter, K. A., and Starzl, T. E.: Infections in recipients of liver homografts, N Engl J Med, 1968, *279*, 619.

516. LeClair, R. A.: Transplantation pneumonia associated with *Pneumocystis carinii* among recipients of cardiac transplant, Am Rev Respir Dis, 1969, *100*, 874.

517. Robbins, J. B.: *Pneumocystis carinii* pneumonitis: A review, Pediatr Res, 1967, *1*, 131.

518. Burke, B. A., and Good, R. A.: *Pneumocystis carinii* infection, Medicine, 1973, *52*, 23.

519. Kossel, A.: Interstitielle plasmazellulare pneumonie beim älteren kind als folge lang dauernder corticosteroidbehanglung, Disch Med Wochenschr, 1962, *87*, 1133.

520. Johnson, H. D., and Johnson, W. W.: *Pneumocystic carinii* pneumonia in children with cancer. Diagnosis and treatment, JAMA, 1970, *214*, 1067.

521. DeVita, V. T., and Goodell, B. W.: *Pneumocystis carinii* pneumonia (letter to the editor), Ann Intern Med, 1970, *73*, 343.

522. Burke, E. C., Brown, A. L., and Weed, L. A.: *Pneumocystis carinii* pneumonia: Report of case in infant with hypogammaglobulinemia, Proc Staff Meet Mayo Clin, 1962, *37*, 129.

523. Becroft, D. M. O., and Costello, J. M.: *Pneumocystis carinii* pneumonia in siblings: Diagnosis by lung aspiration, NZ Med J, 1965, *64*, 273.

524. Burke, B. A., Korovetz, L. J., and Good, R. A.: Occurrence of *Pneumocystis carinii* pneumonia in children with agammaglobulinemia, Pediatrics, 1961, *28*, 196.

525. Robbins, J. B., Miller, R. H., Arean, V. M., and Pearson, H. A.: Successful treatment of *Pneumocystis carinii* pneumonitis in a patient with congenital hypogammaglobulinemia, N Engl J Med, 1965, *272*, 708.

526. Bird, T., and Thompson, J.: *Pneumocystis carinii* pneumonia, Lancet, 1957, *1*, 59.

527. Hutchison, J. H.: Congenital agammaglobulinemia (letter to the editor), Lancet, 1955, *2*, 1196.

528. McKay, E., and Richardson, J.: *Pneumocystis carinii* pneumonia associated with hypogammaglobulinemia, Lancet, 1959, *76*, 299.

529. Russell, J. G. B.: Pneumocystis pneumonia associated with agammaglobulinemia, Arch Dis Child, 1959, *34*, 338.

530. Hendry, W. S., and Patrick, R. L.: Observations

on thirteen cases of *Pneumocystis carinii* pneumonia, Am J Clin Pathol, 1962, *38*, 401.

531. Marshall, W. C., Weston, H. J., and Bodian, M.: *Pneumocystis carinii* pneumonia and congenital hypogammaglobulinemia, Arch Dis Child, 1964, *39*, 18.

532. Rodgers, T. S., and Haggie, M. H. K.: *Pneumocystis carinii* pneumonia associated with hypogammaglobulinemia responding to pentamidine (letter to the editor), Lancet, 1964, *1*, 1042.

533. Allboné, E. C., Goldie, W., and Marmion, B. P.: *Pneumocystis carinii* pneumonia and progressive vaccinia in siblings, Arch Dis Child, 1964, *39*, 26.

534. Patterson, H. H., Lindsey, I. L., Edwards, E. S., and Logan, W. D.: *Pneumocystis carinii* pneumonia and altered host resistance: Treatment of one patient with pentamidine isethionate, Pediatrics, 1966, *38*, 388.

535. Roberts, F. B., and Nielsen, H. S.: *Pneumocystis carinii* pneumonia. An unsuccessfully treated case, Can Med Assoc J, 1966, *94*, 1235.

536. Walzer, P. D., Schultz, M. G., Western K. A., and Robbins, J. B.: *Pneumocystis carinii* pneumonia and primary immune deficiency diseases of infancy and childhood, J Pediatr, 1973, *82*, 416.

537. DiGeorge, A. M.: Congenital absence of the thymus and its immunologic consequences: Occurrence with congenital hypoparathyroidism, in *Immunologic Deficiency Diseases in Man,* R. A. Good and D. Bergsma ed. Birth Defects, Original Article Series, National Foundation Press, New York, 1968.

538. Hughes, W. T., Price, R. A., Kim, H. K., Coburn, T. P., Grigsby, D., and Feldman, S.: *Pneumocystis carinii* pneumonitis in children with malignancies, J Pediatr, 1973, *82*, 404.

539. Hendley, J. O., and Weller, T. H.: Activation and transmission in rats of infection with pneumocystis, Proc Soc Exp Biol Med, 1971, *137*, 1401.

540. Ruskin, J., and Remington, J. S.: The compromised host and infection. I. *Pneumocystis carinii* pneumonia, JAMA, 1967, *202*, 1070.

541. Brazinsky, J. H., and Phillips, J. E.: Pneumocystis pneumonia transmission between patient with lymphoma (letter to the editor), JAMA, 1969, *209*, 1527.

542. Singer, C., Armstrong, D., Rosen, P. P., and Scholtenfeld, D.: *Pneumocystis carinii* pneumonia: A cluster of eleven cases, Ann Intern Med, 1975, *82*, 772.

543. Watanabe, J. M., Chinchiniam, J., Weitz, C., and McIlvanie, S. K.: *Pneumocystis carinii* pneumonia in a family, JAMA, 1965, *193*, 685.

544. Price, R. A., and Hughes, W. T.: Histopathology of *Pneumocystis carinii* infestation and infection in malignant disease in childhood, Hum Pathol, 1974, *5*, 737.

545. Vogel, C. L., Cohen, M. H., Powell, R. D., Jr., and DeVita, V. T.: *Pneumocystis carinii* pneumonia, Ann Intern Med, 1968, *68*, 97.

546. Rubin, E., and Zak, F. G.: *Pneumocystis carinii* pneumonia in the adult, N Engl J Med, 1960, *262*, 1315.

547. Whitcomb, M. E., Schwarz, M. I., Charles, M. A., and Larson, P. H.: Interstitial fibrosis after *Pneumocystis carinii* pneumonia, Ann Intern Med, 1970, *73*, 761.

548. Hughes, W. T., and Johnson, W. W.: Recurrent *Pneumocystis carinii* pneumonia following apparent recovery, J Pediatr, 1971, *79*, 755.

549. Schmid, K. O.: Studien zur Pneumocystis-erkrankung des Menschen. I. Mitteilung, das weschselnde Erscheinungsbild der Pneumocystis Pneumonie beim Säugling; konkordante und discordante Form. Pneumocystosis granulamotose, Frankf Z Pathol, 1964, *74*, 121.

550. Minielly, J. A., Mills, S. D., and Holley, K. E.: *Pneumocystis carinii* pneumonia, Can Med Assoc J, 1969, *100*, 846.

551. Barnett, R. N., Hull, J. G., Vortel, V., and Schwarz, J.: *Pneumocystis carinii* in lymph nodes and spleen. Arch Pathol, 1969, *88*, 175.

552. Jarnum, S., Rasmussen, E. F., Ohlsen, A. S., and Sorensen, A. W. S.: Generalized *Pneumocystis carinii* infection with severe idiopathic hypoproteinemia, Ann Intern Med, 1968, *68*, 138.

553. Awen, C. F., and Balzan, M. A.: Systemic dissemination of *Pneumocystis carinii* pneumonia, Can Med Assoc J, 1971, *104*, 809.

554. Walzer, P. D., Perl, D. P., Krogstad, D. J., Rawson, P. G., and Schultz, M. G.: *Pneumocystis carinii* pneumonia in the United States: Epidemiologic, diagnostic and clinical features, Ann Intern Med, 1974, *80*, 83.

555. Simon, H. B., Guerry, D., IV, Breslow, A., and Kirkpatrick, C. H.: Opportunistic pathogens in the immunologically hyperresponsive host, Am J Med, 1973, *55*, 856.

556. Sheldon, W. H.: Pulmonary *Pneumocystis carinii* infection, J Pediatr, 1962, *61*, 780.

557. Sheldon, W. H.: Subclinical pneumocystis pneumonitis, Am J Dis Child, 1959, *97*, 287.

558. Forrest, J. V.: Radiographic findings in *Pneumocystis carinii* pneumonia, Radiology, 1972, *103*, 539.

559. Friedman, B. A., Wenglin, B. D., Hyland, R. H., and Rifkind, D.: Roentgenographically atypical *Pneumocystis carinii* pneumonia, Am Rev Respir Dis, 1975, *111*, 89.

560. Luna, M. A., Bodey, G. P., Goldman, A. M., and Lichtiger, B.: *Pneumocystis carinii* pneumonitis in cancer patients, Tex Rep Biol Med, 1972, *30*, 41.

561. Cross, A. S., and Steigbigel, R. T.: *Pneumocystis carinii* pneumonia presenting as localized nodular densities, N Engl J Med, 1974, *291*, 831.

562. Feinberg, S. B., Lester, R. G., and Burke, B. A.:

The Roentgen findings in *Pneumocystis carinii* pneumonia, Radiology, 1961, *76*, 594.

563. Jose, D. G., Gatti, R. A., and Good, R. A.: Eosinophilia with *Pneumocystis carinii* pneumonia and immune deficiency syndromes, J Pediatr, 1971, *79*, 748.

564. Rosen, P., Armstrong, D., and Ramos, C.: *Pneumocystis carinii* pneumonia. A clinicopathologic study of 20 patients with neoplastic diseases, Am J Med, 1972, *53*, 428.

565. Kerpel-Fronius, E., Varga, F., and Bata, G.: Blood gas and metabolic studies in plasma cell pneumonia and in newborn prematures with respiratory distress, Arch Dis Child, 1964, *39*, 473.

566. Lyons, H. A., Vinijchaikul, K., and Hennigar, G. R.: *Pneumocystis carinii* pneumonia unassociated with other disease, Arch Intern Med, 1961, *108*, 929.

567. Doak, P. B., Becroft, D. M. O., Harris, E. A., Hitchcock, G. C., Leeming B. W. A., North, J. D. K., Montgomerie, J. Z., and Whitlock, R. M. I.: *Pneumocystis carinii* pneumonia-transplant lung, Q J Med, 1973, *165*, 59.

568. Russell, H. T., and Nelson, B. M.: Pneumocystis pneumonitis in American infants, Am J Clin Pathol, 1956, *26*, 1334.

569. Pliess, G., and Seifert, K.: Elektronenoptische Untersuchung bei experimenteller Pneumocystose, Beitr Pathol, 1959, *120*, 399.

570. Fortuny, I. E., Tempero, K. F., and Amsden, T. W.: *Pneumocystis carinii* pneumonia diagnosed from sputum and successfully treated with pentamidine isethionate, Cancer, 1970, *26*, 911.

571. Bradshaw, M., Myerowitz, R. L., Schneerson, R., Whisnant, J. K., and Robbins, J. B.: *Pneumocystis carinii* pneumonitis, Ann Intern Med, 1970, *73*, 775.

572. Lau, W. K., Young, L. S., and Remington, J. S.: Diagnosis of *Pneumocystis carinii* pneumonia by examination of pulmonary secretions, JAMA, in press.

573. Remington, J. S., and Anderson, S. E., Jr.: Diagnosis and treatment of pneumocystosis and toxoplasmosis in the immunosuppressed host, Transplant Proc, 1973, *5*, 1263.

574. Gentry, L. O., Ruskin, J., and Remington, J. S.: *Pneumocystis carinii* pneumonia. Problems in diagnosis and therapy in 24 cases, Calif Med, 1972, *116*, 6.

575. Johnson, H. D., and Johnson, W. W.: *Pneumocystis carinii* pneumonia in children with cancer, JAMA, 1970, *214*, 1067.

576. Rosen, P. P., Martini, N., and Armstrong, D.: *Pneumocystis carinii* pneumonia. Diagnosis by lung biopsy, Am J Med, 1975, *58*, 794.

577. Gaensler, E. A., Moister, M. V. B., and Hamm, J.: Open-lung biopsy in diffuse pulmonary disease, N Engl J Med, 1964, *270*, 1319.

578. Drew, W. L., Finley, T. N., Mintz, L., and Klein, H. Z.: Diagnosis of *Pneumocystis carinii* pneumonia by bronchopulmonary lavage, JAMA, 1974, *230*, 713.

579. Fennessey, J. J.: A technique for the selective catheterization of segmental bronchi using arterial catheters, Am J Roentgenol Radium Ther Nucl Med, 1966, *96*, 936.

580. Finley, R., Kieff, E., Thomsen, S., Fennessey, J., Beem, M., Lerner, S., and Morello, J.: Bronchial brushing in the diagnosis of pulmonary disease in patients at risk for opportunistic infection, Am Rev Respir Dis, 1974, *109*, 379.

581. Andersen, H. A.: Lung biopsy via the bronchoscope, Ann Otol Rhinol Laryngol, 1970, *79*, 933.

582. Smith, E., and Gaspar, I. A.: Pentamidine treatment of *Pneumocystis carinii* pneumonitis in an adult with lymphatic leukemia, Am J Med, 1968, *44*, 626.

583. Norman, L., and Kagan, I. G.: Some observations on the serology of *Pneumocystis carinii* infections in the United States, Infect Immun, 1973, *8*, 317.

584. Western, K. A., Perera, D. R., and Schultz, M. G.: Pentamidine isethionate in the treatment of *Pneumocystis carinii* pneumonia, Ann Intern Med, 1970, *73*, 695.

585. Richman, D. D., Zamvil, L., and Remington, J. S.: Recurrent *Pneumocystis carinii* pneumonia in a child with hypogammaglobulinemia, Am J Dis Child, 1973, *125*, 102.

586. Charles, M. A., and Schwarz, M. I.: *Pneumocystis carinii* pneumonia, Postgrad Med, 1973, *53*, 86.

587. DeVita, V. T., Emmer, M., Levine, A., Jacobs, B., and Berard, C.: *Pneumocystis carinii* pneumonia. Successful diagnosis and treatment of two patients with associated malignant processes, N Engl J Med, 1969, *280*, 287.

588. Kirby, H. B., Kenamore, B., and Guckian, J. C.: *Pneumocystis carinii* pneumonia treated with pyrimethamine and sulfadiazine, Ann Intern Med, 1971, *75*, 505.

589. Hughes, W. T., McNabb, P. C., Makres, T. D., and Feldman, S.: Efficacy of trimethoprim and sulfamethoxazole in the prevention and treatment of *Pneumocystis carinii* pneumonitis, Antimicrob Agents Chemother, 1974, *5*, 289.

590. Hughes, W. T., Feldman, S., and Sanyal, S. K.: Treatment of *Pneumocystis carinii* pneumonitis with trimethoprim-sulfamethoxazole, Can Med Assoc J, 1975, *112*, 47S.

591. Lau, W. B., and Young, L. S.: Co-trimaxazole treatment of *Pneumocystis carinii* pneumonia in adults, Clin Res, 1976, *24*, 113A.

592. Feldman, H. A.: Toxoplasmosis, N Engl J Med, 1968, *279*, 1370, 1431.

593. Remington, J. S., and Cavanaugh, E. N.: Isolation of the encysted form of *Toxoplasma gondii* from human skeletal muscle and brain, N Engl J Med, 1965, *273*, 1308.

594. Remington, J. S.: Toxoplasmosis: Recent developments, Annu Rev Med, 1970, *21*, 201.

595. Remington, J. S.: Toxoplasmosis in the adult, Bull NY Acad Med, 1974, *50*, 211.

596. Roth, J. A., Siegel, S. E., and Levine, A. S.: Fatal recurrent toxoplasmosis in a patient initially infected via a leukocyte transfusion, Am J Clin Pathol, 1971, *56*, 601.

597. Siegel, S. E., Lunde, M. N., Gelderman, A. H., Halterman, R. H., Brown, J. A., Levine, A. S., and Graw, R. G., Jr.: Transmission of toxoplasmosis by leukocyte transfusions, Blood, 1971, *37*, 388.

598. Krahenbuhl, J. L., Ruskin, J. ,and Remington, J. S.: The use of killed vaccines in immunization against an intracellular parasite: *Toxoplasma gondii*, J Immunol, 1972, *108*, 425.

599. Swartzberg, J. E., and Remington, J. S.: Transmission of toxoplasma, Am J Dis Child, 1975, *129*, 777.

600. Frenkel, J. K.: Effects of cortisone, total body radiation, and nitrogen mustard on chronic latent toxoplasmosis, Am J Pathol, 1957, *33*, 618.

601. Stahl, W., Matsubayashi, H., and Akao, S.: Modifications of subclinical toxoplasmosis in mice by cortisone, 6-mercaptopurine, and splenectomy, Am J Trop Med Hyg, 1966, *15*, 869.

602. Metzger, M., Przerwa-Tetmajer, A., and Wojciechowski, A.: The Influence of zymosan, cortisone, and x-rays on the course of experimental toxoplasmosis in white rats, Arch Immunol Ther Exp, 1963, *11*, 227.

603. Strannegard, O., and Lycke, E.: Effect of antithymocyte serum on experimental toxoplasmosis in mice, Infect Immun, 1972, *5*, 769.

604. Anderson, S. E., Jr., and Remington, J. S.: Effect of normal and activated human macrophages on *Toxoplasma gondii*, J Exp Med, 1974, *139*, 1154.

605. Borges, J. S., and Johnson, W. D., Jr.: Inhibition of multiplication of *Toxoplasma gondii* by human monocytes exposed to T-lymphocyte products, J Exp Med, 1975, *141*, 483.

606. Anderson, S. E., and Remington, J. S.: Unpublished observations.

607. Miller, D. G.: Immunologic Diseases, Little, Brown and Co., Boston, 1965.

608. Ruskin, J., and Remington, J. S.: Toxoplasmosis in the compromised host, Ann Intern Med, 1976, *84*, 173.

609. Krahenbuhl, J. L., Gaines, J. D., and Remington, J. S.: Lymphocyte transformation in human toxoplasmosis, J Infect Dis, 1972, *125*, 283.

610. Gaines, J. D., Araujo, F. G., Krahenbuhl, J. L., and Remington, J. S.: Simplified *in vitro* method for measuring delayed hypersensitivity to latent intracellular infection in man (toxoplasmosis), J Immunol, 1972, *109*, 179.

611. Couvreur, J.: Le poumon et la toxoplasmose, Rev Fr Mal Respir, 1975, *3*, 525.

612. Pinkerton, H., and Henderson, R. G.: Adult toxoplasmosis, JAMA, 1941, *116*, 807.

613. Hooper, A. D.: Acquired toxoplasmosis, Arch Pathol, 1957, *64*, 1.

614. Vietzke, W. M., Gelderman, A. H., Grimley, P. M., and Valsamis, M. P.: Toxoplasmosis complicating malignancy, Cancer, 1968, *21*, 816.

615. Luna, M. A., and Lichtiger, B.: Disseminated toxoplasmosis and cytomegalovirus infection complicating Hodgkin's disease, Am J Clin Pathol, 1971, *55*, 499.

616. Stinson, E., Bieber, C. P., Griepp, R. B., Clark, D. A., Shumway, N. E., and Remington, J. S.: Infectious complications after cardiac transplantation in man, Ann Intern Med, 1971, *74*, 22.

617. Carey, R. M., Kimball, A. C., Armstrong, D., and Lieberman, P. H.: Toxoplasmosis. Clinical experiences in a cancer hospital, Am J Med, 1973, *54*, 30.

618. Kennedy, B. J., and Theologides, A. T.: Pulmonary infiltrate, initial manifestation of toxoplasmosis, Minn Med, 1971, *54*, 321.

619. Ludlam, G. B., and Beattie, C. P.: Pulmonary toxoplasmosis?, Lancet, 1963, *2*, 1136.

620. Anderson, S. E., Jr., and Remington, J. S.: Current concepts in diagnosis: The diagnosis of toxoplasmosis, South Med J, 1975, *68*, 1433.

621. Siim, J. C.: Toxoplasmosis aquisitia lymphonodosa: Clinical and pathologic aspects, Ann NY Acad Sci, 1956, *64*, 185.

622. Frenkel, J. K., Nelson, B. M., and Arias-Stella, J.: Immunosuppression and toxoplasmic encephalitis. Clinical and experimental aspects, Hum Pathol, 1975, *6*, 97.

623. Dorfman, R. F., and Remington, J. S.: Value of lymph node biopsy in the diagnosis of acute acquired toxoplasmosis, N Engl J Med, 1973, *289*, 878.

624. Tsunematsu, Y., Shioiri, K., and Kusano, N.: Three cases of lymphadenopathica toxoplasmotica. With special reference to the application of fluorescent antibody technique for detection of toxoplasma in tissues, Jap J Exp Med, 1964, *34*, 217.

625. Feldman, H. A., and Miller, L. T.: Serologic study of toxoplasmosis prevalence, Am J Hyg, 1956, *64*, 320.

626. Feldman, H. A.: Toxoplasma and toxoplasmosis, Hosp Pract, 1969, *4*, 64.

627. Sabin, A. B., and Feldman, H. A.: Dyes as microchemical indicators of a new immunity phenomenon affecting a protozoan parasite (toxoplasma), Science, 1948, *108*, 660.

628. Walton, B. C., Benchoff, B. M., and Brooks, W. H.: Comparison of the indirect fluorescent antibody test and methylene blue dye test for detection of antibodies to *T. gondii*, Am J Trop Med Hyg, 1966, *15*, 149.

629. Remington, J. S., Miller, M. J., and Brownlee,

I.: IgM antibodies in acute toxoplasmosis. II. Prevalence and significance in acquired cases, J Lab Clin Med, 1968, *71*, 855.

630. Vogel, C. L., and Lunde, M. N.: Toxoplasma serology in patients with malignant disease of the reticuloendothelial system, Cancer, 1969, *23*, 614.

631. Rose, M. S., Black, P. J., and Barkhan, P.: Fatal outcome after combined therapy for myeloblastic leukemia and toxoplasmosis (letter to the editor), Lancet, 1973, *1*, 600.

632. Helmer, R. E.: Hazard of folinic acid with pyrimethamine and sulfadiazine (letter to the editor), Ann Intern Med, 1975, *82*, 124.

633. McMaster, P. R. B., Powers, K. G., Finerty, J. F., and Lunde, M. N.: The effect of two chlorinated lincomycin analogues against acute toxoplasmosis in mice, Am J Trop Med Hyg, 1973, *22*, 14.

634. Araujo, F. G., and Remington, J. S.: Effect of clindamycin on acute and chronic toxoplasmosis in mice, Antimicrob Agents Chemother, 1974, *5*, 647.

635. Feldman, H. A.: Effects of trimethoprim and sulfisoxazole alone and in combination on murine toxoplasmosis, J Infect Dis, 1973, *128* (Supplement, p. 774).

636. Remington, J. S.: Trimethoprim-sulfamethoxazole in murine toxoplasmosis, Antimicrob Agents Chemother, 1976, *9*, 222.

637. Swartzberg, J. E., and Remington, J. S.: Transmission of toxoplasma, Am J Dis Child, 1975, *129*, 777.

638. Civantos, F., and Robinson, M. J.: Fatal strongyloidiasis following corticosteroid therapy, Am J Dig Dis, 1969, *14*, 643.

639. Cruz, T., Reboucas, G., and Rocha, H.: Fatal strongyloidiasis in patients receiving corticosteroids, N Engl J Med, 1966, *275*, 1093.

640. Fagundes, L. A., Busato, O., and Bretano, L.: Strongyloidiasis: Fatal complication of renal transplantation (letter to the editor), Lancet, 1971, *2*, 439.

641. Rassiga, A. L., Lowry, J. L., and Forman, W. B.: Diffuse pulmonary infection due to *Strongyloides stercoralis*, JAMA, 1974, *230*, 426.

642. Rivera, E., Maldonado, N., Vélez-García, E., Grillo, A. J., and Malaret, G.: Hyperinfection syndrome with *Strongyloides stercoralis*, Ann Intern Med, 1970, *72*, 199.

643. Rogers, W. A., Jr., and Nelson, B.: Strongyloidiasis and malignant lymphoma. Opportunistic infection by a nematode, JAMA, 1966, *195*, 685.

644. Brown, H. W., and Perna, V. P.: An overwhelming strongyloides infection, JAMA, 1958, *168*, 1648.

The Use of Radioisotope Techniques for the Evaluation of Patients with Pulmonary Disease[1]

HENRY N. WAGNER, JR.

Contents

Introduction

Cardiopulmonary Nuclear Medicine

Nuclear Instrumentation

Measurement of Regional Lung Function

Pulmonary Embolism

How Perfusion Lung Scans Are Interpreted

Parenchymal Lung Disease

Radioactive Tracers in Preoperative Assessment of Regional Lung Function

Early Detection of Obstructive Lung Disease

Pulmonary Venous Hypertension

Cor Pulmonale

Differential Diagnosis of Cyanosis

Inhalation of Aerosols

Summary

Introduction

Radioactive tracer studies of the lung began in 1955 when Knipping and associates (1) first used xenon-133 as a possible aid in the early diagnosis of carcinoma of the lung. They were not successful, but their work is of historic interest. Subsequently, West and co-workers (2) at Hammersmith Hospital in London began to use cyclotron-produced radioactive gases, including oxygen-15 and radioactive carbon dioxide in physiologic studies of the lungs. These studies

provided important information about the effects of gravity and other factors on the distribution of ventilation and perfusion and documented the regional character of involvement in many patients with obstructive lung disease. It was not until 1963, however, that a radioactive tracer procedure began to achieve widespread clinical usefulness in studies of the lungs (3).

Cassen and associates (4) invented the rectilinear scanner in 1951, and shortly thereafter this device began to be used in hospitals throughout the world in the diagnosis of thyroid and brain disorders, setting the stage for its use in the study of the distribution of pulmonary arterial blood flow. The impetus to the development of lung scanning was the emphasis in the 1960s on the emergency surgical treatment of acute massive pulmonary embolism. Lung scanning and pulmonary arteriography developed hand in hand in the late 1960s and were given momentum by the Urokinase Pulmonary Embolism Trial (5), which increased our understanding of the role of these procedures and the natural history of pulmonary embolic disease.

Today, lung scanning is widely used in medical practice, and research studies of the use of radioactive tracers in diseases of the heart as well as the lungs are proceeding at a rapid pace. It is beyond the scope of this article to describe the use of radioactive tracers in cardiovascular disease in detail (6–10), but the advances being made in nuclear medicine procedures in coronary and valvular heart disease are being extended to the diagnosis of cor pulmonale (11). In cardiovascular nuclear medicine, the distinction between the pulmonary and the cardio-

---

[1] From the Divisions of Nuclear Medicine and Radiation Health, The Johns Hopkins Medical Institutions, Baltimore, Md. 21205.

vascular systems is becoming less emphasized and it is useful to consider them together.

Cardiopulmonary Nuclear Medicine

A half century ago, Blumgart and Weiss (11) conceived the idea that radioactive tracers would be useful for the study of the circulation. They measured the velocity of the circulation by injecting solutions of radium salts intravenously and monitoring the time of arrival of the tracer at the opposite antecubital fossa in a group of normal persons and patients with cardiac diseases. The instrument they used was a cloud chamber, one of the earliest radiation detection devices. Their concepts became a reality with the advent of safe, efficient radioactive tracers, the invention of sensitive detection instruments, and application of modern data processing. The latter has made possible the achievement of a quantitative capability not previously present. Although still in the process of evolution, such quantitative studies are rapidly achieving widespread use in the study of the heart and lungs. As Pierson and Van Dyke (8) stated recently, "One of the important developments of instrumentation which enables nuclear medicine to become quantitative is the development of the digital computer to the stage where it is fast enough, small enough, cheap enough and responsive enough for ordinary mortals to deal with on a friendly basis." They proposed further that "the seventies should be the decade of calibration and validation of these techniques, to the satisfaction of the critical scientist."

As with radiographs, the great value of radioactive tracer studies lies in their capability for nondestructive, simple measurements. But whereas radiographs provide information primarily about body structures, radioactive tracers make their greatest contribution in permitting measurement of *regional function*. Although it is true that contrast angiography and other radiographic techniques also provide functional information, the ability to employ hundreds of safe and potentially useful radioactive tracers in nuclear medicine makes it theoretically possible to study nearly every function of the body.

Let us consider first the measurement of regional pulmonary arterial blood flow. There are 300 million pulmonary arterioles of diameter 15 to 30 μm and 280 billion capillaries of diameter 5 to 7 μm in the lungs. Because pulmonary blood vessels are temporarily occluded by particles of a larger size, lung perfusion imaging is based on the intravenous injection of radioactive particles or microspheres of human serum albumin of diameter 15 to 30 μm. Because the density of the microspheres is comparable to that of red blood cells, their distribution throughout the lungs is determined by the distribution of pulmonary arterial blood flow. During injection the patient is in the supine position and breathing normally; forced inspiration or expiration changes the distribution of particles in the lungs. Patients suspected of having pulmonary venous hypertension are often injected while in an erect position. The perfusion of the apices, normally less than to the bases in this position, is increased in patients with this problem because the pulmonary vascular resistance is increased in the lower regions of the lung with diversion of blood flow to the upper regions. In a patient with right-to-left shunt some of the microspheres will reach the systemic arterial circulation; therefore, care must be taken not to inject more than 50,000 microspheres.

Regional ventilation is determined by imaging with a scintillation camera the initial distribution and washout of the inhaled radioactive gas, ^{133}Xe. The patient lies in a supine position with the detector beneath him and inhales the ^{133}Xe, which is mixed with air. Regional ventilation is determined after an initial single breath, after 5 min of equilibration of rebreathing ^{133}Xe from a closed system, and during the clearance of the gas from the lungs. Regional ventilation is estimated from the image by visual assessment of the retention of the gas or by quantification of regional clearance rates with a computer. Bronchoconstriction, bronchial obstruction, or tissue destruction cause decreased regional concentrations of the radioactive gas. The supine position is selected to facilitate correlation of ventilation and perfusion. It is essential that the patient be in the same position during both types of examination.

Nuclear Instrumentation

In looking at a problem in medical diagnosis, the physiologically oriented physician asks himself or herself what functions should be measured to help solve the patient's problems and what degree of spatial and temporal resolution is required in the measurements. Will it be necessary to measure only pulmonary perfusion, or must both perfusion and ventilation be measured? Will it suffice to measure the function of the lungs as a whole, or will it be necessary to compare the functions of one region with another? Will it suffice to measure the distribution of blood flow with intravenously injected microspheres, or will it be necessary to make rapid measurements of the distribution of a radioactive gas throughout the lungs or of the changes in the volumes of the cardiac chambers as they fill and empty? Individual counting intervals of as little as one-fiftieth of a second must be examined for certain studies such as the ejection fraction of the ventricles (8, 12). These factors determine the types of radiation detection instruments that can be used and the types of measurements that can be made.

The most widely used instrument in nuclear medicine today for measurement of the distribution of activity *in vivo* is the γ scintillation camera, invented by Anger (13) and subsequently greatly improved by the addition of data processing equipment (14). When we consider that the γ camera can create images with 10,000 or more image cells (picture elements), each of which may be made up of 256 or even more counts per min, we can appreciate the large amount of data generated and the impossibility of quantification without the use of a computer. Although video instrumentation has been used by some for analysis of γ camera data, most prefer the use of digital computer systems (15).

The maximal spatial resolution of the scintillation camera using the highest resolution collimator is about one centimeter at the face of the detector with considerable falloff at greater depths. Usually a computer matrix of 64 × 64 is used, although a 128 × 128 picture element matrix is better. The temporal resolution requirement depends on the type of study being performed. For studies such as the washout of ^{133}Xe from the lungs, cardiac output, intracardiac shunt measurement, and transit time analyses from one cardiac chamber to another, 0.5 or 1.0 sec frames will suffice. If the time activity curve of the right or left ventricle is to be obtained, 48 or more frames per sec are desirable. With high degrees of temporal or spatial resolution, there are statistical limitations imposed by the limitation in the amount of radioactive tracer that is administered. In such cases, a compromise must be made between temporal and spatial resolution. The addition of a digital computer greatly expands the usefulness of the scintillation camera, particularly in quantification of the results. Special purpose (hardwired) devices are also being developed and applied at a rapid rate and help increase the value of the studies, although with less flexibility than the digital systems.

Measurement of Regional Lung Function

The application of physiologic principles to the study of lung function has greatly improved both our understanding of the pathophysiology of lung disease and the care of the patients. Pulmonary functional evaluation includes measurement of vital capacity, inspiratory and expiratory reserve volumes, inspiratory capacity, functional residual capacity, residual volume, and total lung capacity. These measure the function of the lungs as a whole and are performed with a spirometer or a body plethysmograph.

Radioactive tracers are most widely used to measure regional function. Even in normal persons, all parts of the lung are not uniformly ventilated and perfused. In certain lung diseases, the hallmark is the abnormal distribution of function. Tracer studies supplement the information obtained in procedures such as maximal voluntary ventilation, peak flow rates, lung compliance, airway resistance, and dead space/volume measurements. Let us next consider specific diseases.

Pulmonary Embolism

The most widely used radioactive tracer procedure in the study of the lungs is the perfusion lung scan. Although not a specific test for pulmonary embolism, it is a sensitive test because it gives an accurate depiction of the distribution of regional pulmonary arterial blood flow (16–18). The physician is often faced with the problem of a patient who has pain in the calf or pleuritic chest pain. It is likely that in more than 80 per cent of patients who are previously healthy and ambulatory, pain in the calf or pleuritic-type chest pain is not caused by deep vein thrombosis or pulmonary embolism. Often leg pain is nothing more serious than a pulled muscle, inflammation of varicose veins, mild trauma, or cramp. Less commonly, a ruptured Baker's cyst may simulate the pain and swelling of venous thrombosis. Of course, marked swelling of the calf and thigh with unequivocal signs should lead to hospitalization of the patient and heparinization, but because this can cause bleeding in up to 20 per cent of patients, the decision to anticoagulate the patient should not be made without adequate evidence (19).

A normal 4-view lung scan makes it exceedingly unlikely that pulmonary embolism is present. One of the reasons for the popularity of lung scanning is that it provides information useful in making important decisions concerning anticoagulation of the patient. In the pres-

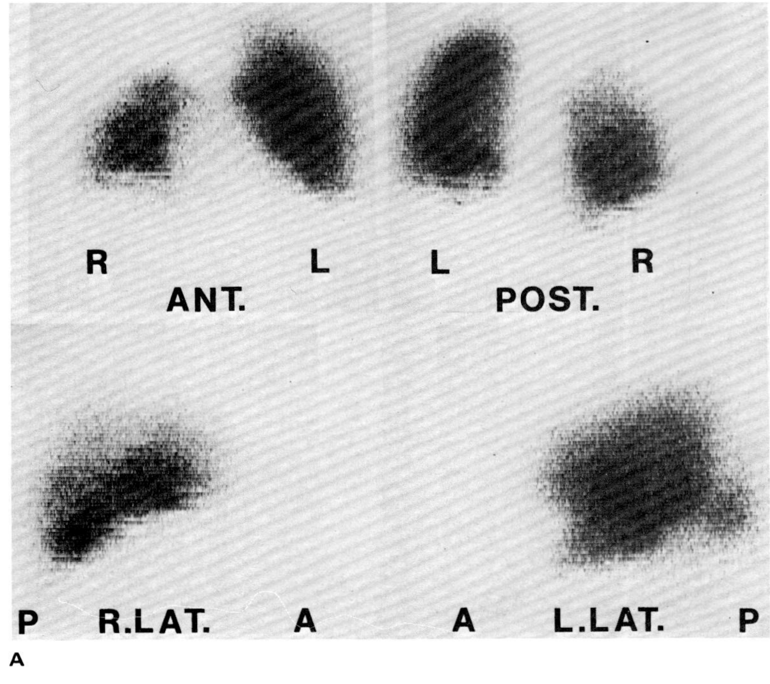

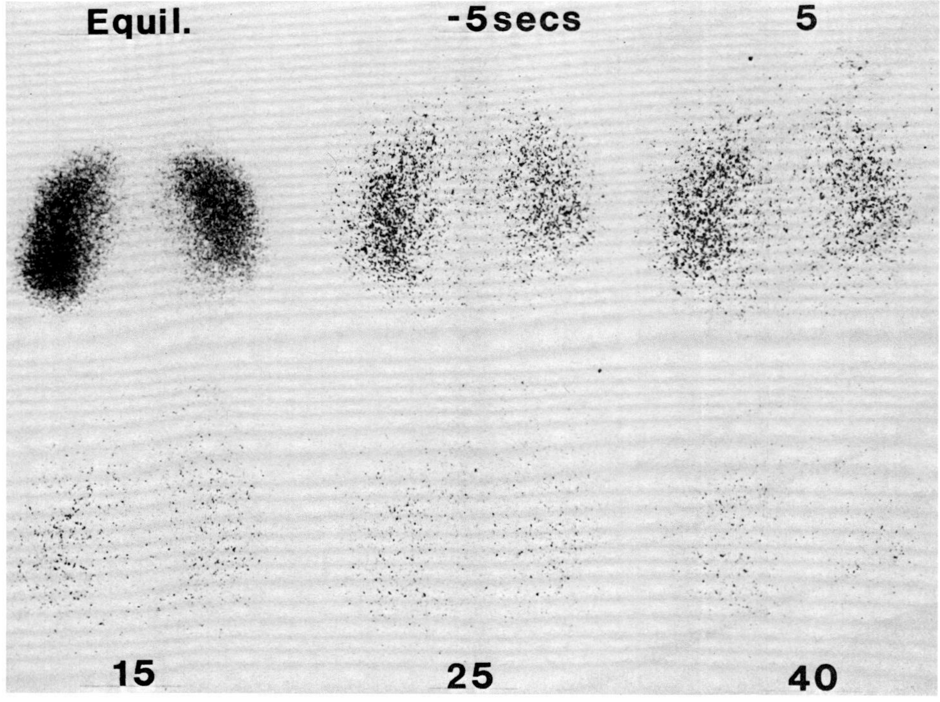

Fig. 1. A. (*Top*) Bilateral perfusion defects are noted on this 4-view scan of a patient with pulmonary emboli. R = right, L = left, A = anterior, P = posterior, Ant. = anterior, Post. = posterior, L. Lat. = left lateral, R. Lat. = right lateral. B. (*Bottom*) A normal xenon-133 ventilation study of the same patient. Both lungs are well ventilated and there is no delay noted in the washout phase. Equil. = equilibration view.

ence of a negative lung scan, no further pursuit of the diagnosis of pulmonary embolism is necessary.

In pulmonary embolism there are usually one or more segmental perfusion defects noted in the lung, the regional ventilation study is normal, and an accompanying chest radiograph is often normal (figure 1A, B). Most emboli occur in the lower lobes of the lungs and involve the superior and posterior segments. A lobar defect or lack of perfusion to one entire lung may be noted if a large vessel is occluded. It is often helpful to repeat a positive lung scan in 4 to 5 days to observe the characteristic changing pattern or perfusion defects in pulmonary embolism. This is due to partial resolution of original emboli, new emboli, or fragmentation of a large embolus into smaller emboli. The probability of acute pulmonary emboli is increased when on a repeat scan new perfusion defects appear, whereas some defects clear. Usually the perfusion defects resolve significantly within the first 2 weeks and then to a lesser extent during the next 3 months.

In 1967 Tow and Wagner (20) examined the rate of recovery of pulmonary arterial blood flow in a series of patients with pulmonary embolism. Of the patients with small lesions (less than 15 per cent), 4 per cent recovered completely, the lung scan being interpreted as normal within 2 weeks. After 4 months 67 per cent had recovered and an additional 8 per cent had improved. Thirty per cent of the patients with moderate-sized lesions (15 to 30 per cent) recovered within 3 weeks, whereas 38 per cent recovered after 4 months and another 13 per cent improved. Twenty per cent of the patients with severe lesions (greater than 30 per cent) recovered within 4 weeks, 20 per cent recovered after 4 months, and an additional 50 per cent improved. Thirty-three per cent of the patients with major emboli had persistent perfusion defects on the lung scan for more than a year. The resolution of pulmonary emboli was slower in the presence of cardiovascular disease and with increasing age of the patient. New emboli occurred in less than 10 per cent of cases of pulmonary embolism and in such patients new segmental defects were noted on the scan.

How Perfusion Lungs Scans Are Interpreted

The characteristics of perfusion defects help increase the diagnostic specificity as follows (21):

(1) The interpretation of "no evidence of pulmonary embolism" may be made if a 4-view lung scan (anterior, posterior, and both laterals) is normal.

(2) If the blood flow to the apices is greater than to the bases of the lungs and there is no evidence of focal perfusion defects, the interpretation should be "probable pulmonary venous hypertension without evidence of pulmonary embolism."

(3) Pulmonary congestion or pleural effusion is suggested if there is no evidence of segmental perfusion defects and if the regions of decreased perfusion correspond to one or more fissures, often with increased blood flow to the upper portions of the lungs.

(4) If on the posterior but not the anterior view one lung has a decrease in perfusion, there is a high probability of pleural effusion (figure 2).

(5) Symmetric perfusion defects at the apices

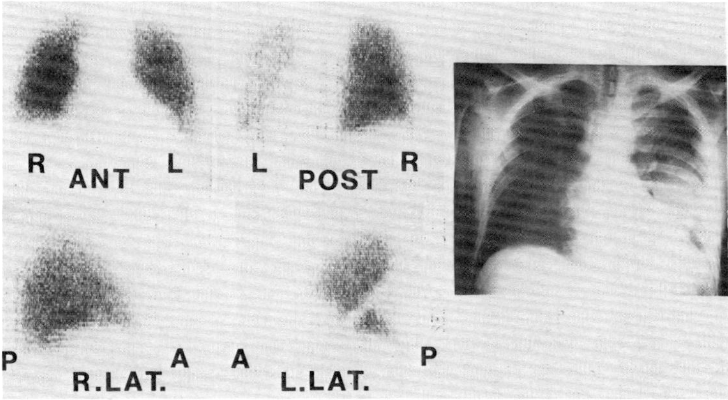

Fig. 2. A marked decrease in perfusion is noted in the posterior and right lateral views of this 4-view lung scan. This patient has a left-sided pleural effusion, as noted on the chest radiography. For definition of abbreviations, see figure 1.

indicate parenchymal lung disease rather than pulmonary embolism.

(*6*) A high probability of pulmonary embolism is suggested when one or more perfusion defects correspond with segmental arteries. An accompanying radiograph may be normal. In the presence of chronic obstructive pulmonary disease, arteriography will determine superimposed pulmonary embolism.

(*7*) It is frequently noted in young adults with tetralogy of Fallot or other causes of right-to-left shunts that there is an increased concentration of radioactivity in the kidneys, denoting a right-to-left shunt (figure 3). Regional perfusion defects are observed in patients with congenitally hypoplastic pulmonary arteries. An extreme example is shown in figure 4.

(*8*) Pulmonary infection is indicated when the perfusion defects correspond to areas of consolidation on the radiograph.

(*9*) There is a high probability of neoplasm when an entire lung lacks perfusion. Hilar bronchogenic carcinoma is more likely to produce this effect than pulmonary embolism.

(*10*) Pulmonary edema is indicated when there are nonsegmental perfusion defects noted on the scan together with decreased perfusion of the medial aspects of the lung and along the fissures. Increased perfusion may be observed in the apices of the lungs in such patients.

Parenchymal Lung Disease

One of the important contributions of radioactive tracer studies of the lungs has been to document that all lung diseases have decreased pulmonary arterial blood flow to the involved regions. This does not mean that they are totally ischemic, because the blood flow is provided in most cases by the bronchial circulation. It does mean that intravenously injected particles fail to accumulate in these regions in the absence of a right-to-left intracardiac shunt. These findings

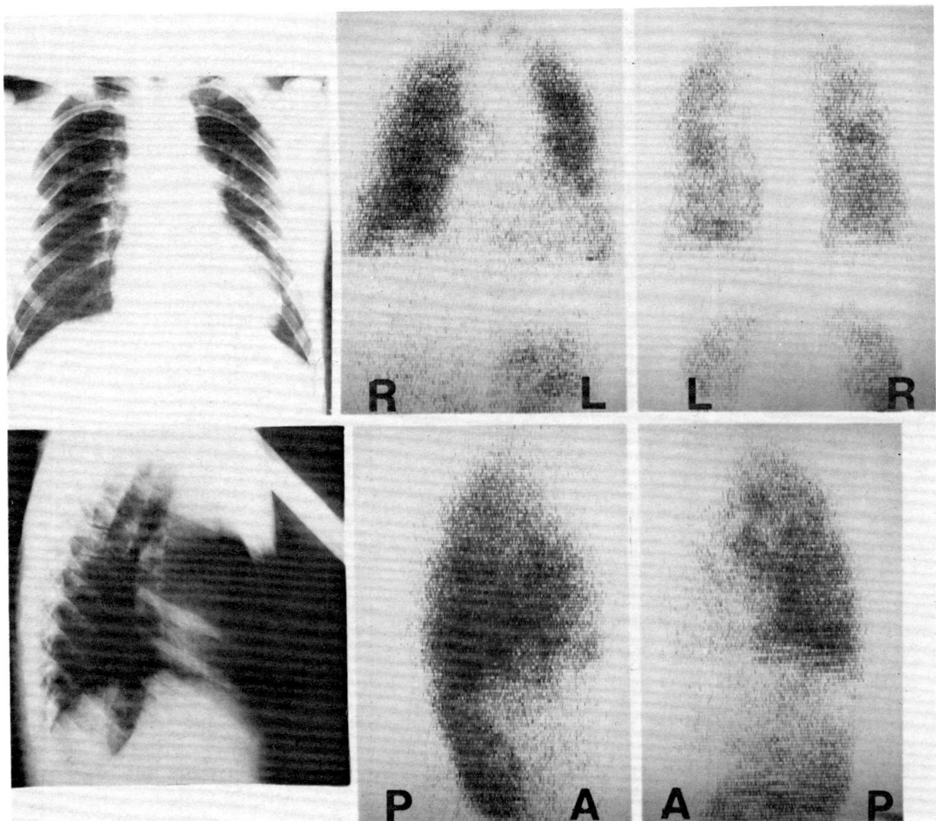

Fig. 3. There are multiple subsegmental perfusion defects noted bilaterally in this patient with Eisenmenger's disease. The activity noted in the kidneys indicates a right-to-left shunt, which is associated with this disease. For definition of abbreviations, see figure 1.

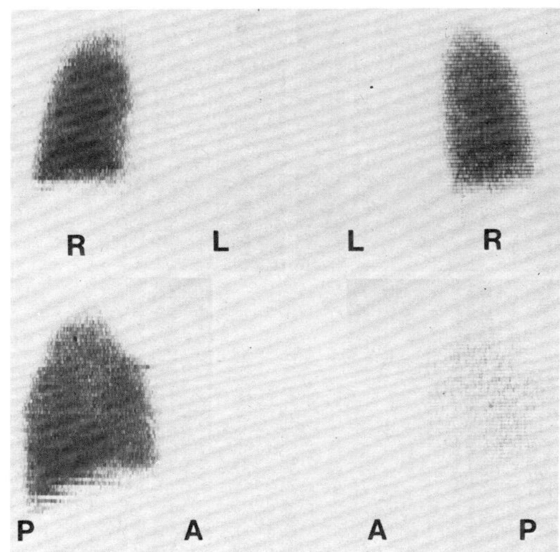

Fig. 4. This patient with a hypoplastic left pulmonary artery has minimal perfusion to the left, as noted in the lung scan. For definition of abbreviations, see figure 1.

complicate the interpretation of perfusion lung scans, but are at times valuable in the assessment of the degree of regional involvement by disease processes.

Combined measurement of both regional ventilation and perfusion greatly improves the diagnostic specificity. It is now common practice to perform ^{133}Xe ventilation studies together with anterior, posterior, and both lateral views of the distribution of perfusion. The use of multiple views permits characterization of lesions according to their size, shape, and position. The technique of radiospirometry with ^{133}Xe requires the use of either the scintillation camera or multiple radiation detectors (14). The latter permit the use of smaller administered doses of ^{133}Xe, but one does not obtain the spatial resolution that can be obtained with the scintillation camera. The use of the scintillation camera permits closer correlation of perfusion and ventilation defects. With the scintillation camera, the first step is to have the patient inhale radioactive ^{133}Xe from a spirometer. The patient takes a deep breath, and the initial distribution of the activity is determined in the form of a single image. The second step consists of having the patient rebreathe the ^{133}Xe for a period of 3 to 5 min. An image is obtained at the time that reveals the ^{133}Xe space or alveolar air space. This image is particularly suitable for comparison with the single breath inhalation study, so that

the relationship between ventilation and lung volume can be ascertained. After the equilibration image, the patient is allowed to breathe into a collection system and the rate of clearance of the xenon from the various zones of the lung is measured. In most cases, this is done by serial images at 5-sec intervals, but in many laboratories the data are recorded in some storage system so that the clearance rate constants can be measured mathematically.

In patients with parenchymal lung disease, such as infections (22) or chronic obstructive pulmonary disease (23, 24), the perfusion defects are accompanied by regional ventilation defects. The chest radiograph of a patient with sarcoidosis is shown in figure 5A; in 5B is the distribution of perfusion defects in the same patient. Lobar perfusion defects are noted in the perfusion lung scans of patients with lobar pneumonia with consolidation. Patchy nonsegmental perfusion defects are noted in the case of bronchopneumonia. Because there is reduced ventilation to the affected area, there is absence of ^{133}Xe noted on the ventilation study. Either diminished ventilation or lack of ventilation, which corresponds to discrete perfusion defects, are noted in patients with bullae (figure 6A, B).

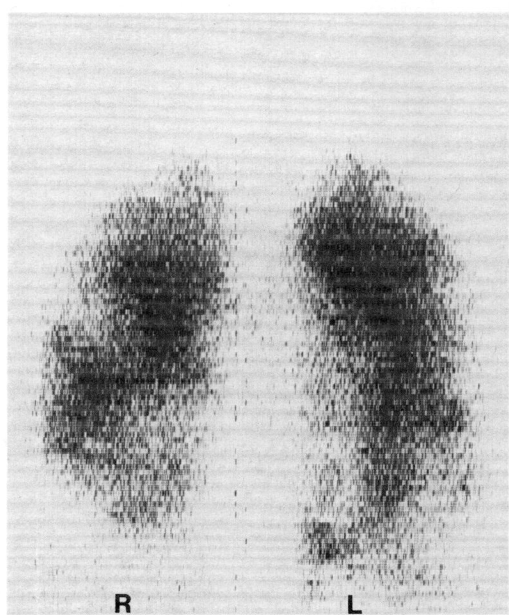

Fig. 5. A. This anterior view of the lung scan reveals a nonhomogeneous distribution of radioactivity throughout both lungs. The diagnosis of this patient was sarcoidosis.

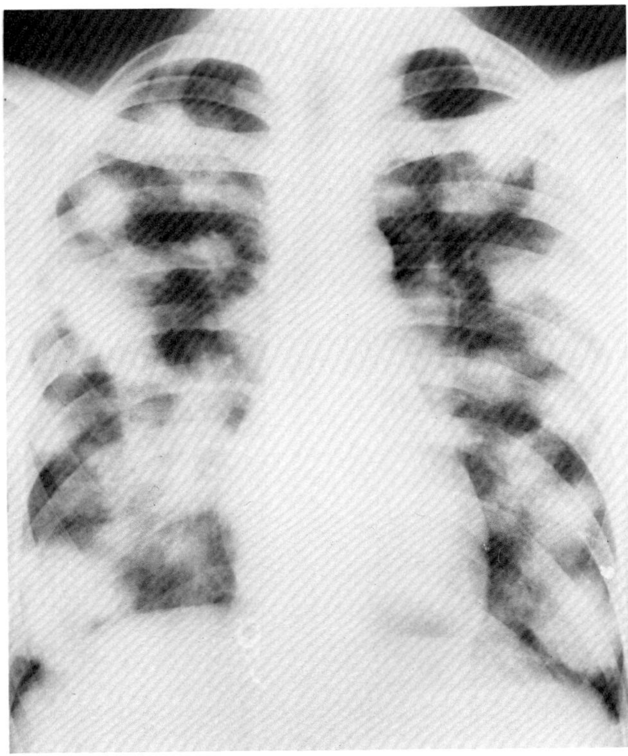

Fig. 5. B. A chest radiograph shows diffuse involvement of the disease bilaterally. R = right; L = left.

A lung scan performed in patients during an asthmatic attack often reveals large, irregular, segmental and nonsegmental defects (25). A changing pattern is noted on repeated studies during several days. A normal lung scan may be obtained between attacks (figures 7A–C).

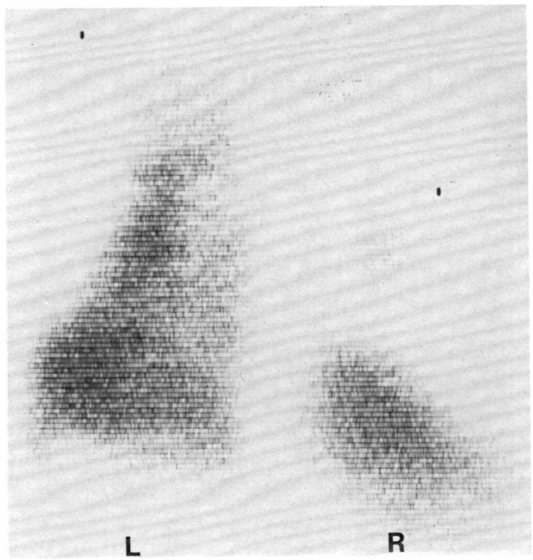

Fig. 6 A. This anterior view of the lung scan of a patient with bullous emphysema shows marked decrease in perfusion to the right lung and upper lobes of the left lung. R = right; L = left.

Diminished ventilation corresponding to the perfusion defects is noted in the ventilation study.

In patients with carcinoma of the lung the perfusion defect is often massive, often involving the entire lung. This may result from extrinsic obstruction of the main pulmonary artery. Regional ventilation is diminished when there is bronchial obstruction (figure 8).

Radioactive Tracers in Preoperative Assessment Of Regional Lung Function

The classic method for examination of differential lung function before pulmonary resection has been bronchospirometry (26, 27). More recently radioactive tracer techniques have provided a useful, noninvasive alternative (28–31). Both regional perfusion and ventilation have proved useful. Such studies have been found useful in the localization of roentgenologically occult cancer (30, 32), in providing information about the extent of involvement of the lungs (31), and in predicting the pulmonary functional loss after resection.

A number of radioactive tracers that concentrate in neoplasms have been evaluated in patients with lung cancer. About 80 per cent of patients with bronchial neoplasms accumulated gallium-67 (33). Mercury-197 has also been used for this purpose. Lesions smaller than 2 cm in diameter could not be visualized with the use of

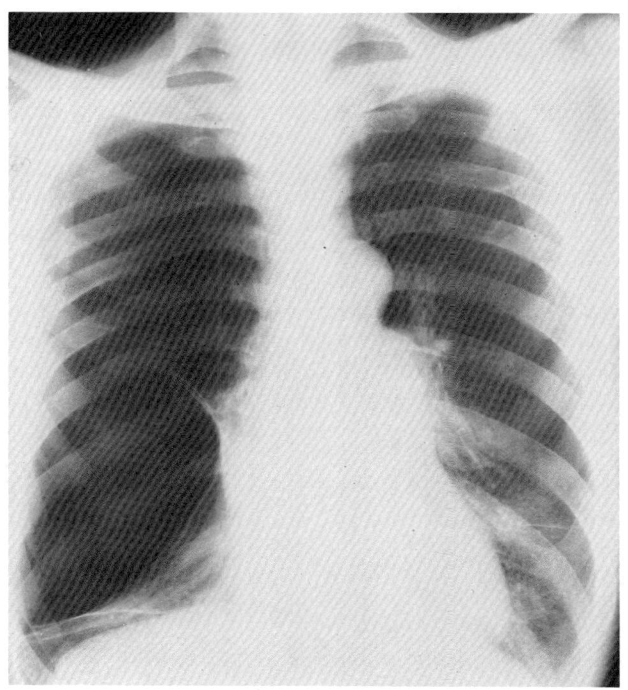

Fig. 6. B. The chest radiograph reveals a massive bulla in the right lung and bullae in the upper and middle lobes of the left lung.

[197]Hg scintigraphy. Arborelius and associates (34) combined the use of [197]Hg scintigraphy in radiospirometry and found an accuracy of 80 per cent.

Tracer studies have been used preoperatively in patients with tuberculosis (22) and bullous emphysema as well as in carcinoma of the lung.

Early Detection of Obstructive Lung Disease

It is well accepted that the chest radiograph is an insensitive means of detecting early obstructive lung diseases as well as pulmonary embolism. This has led to the increasing interest in techniques such as closing volume measurements and regional measurements with radioactive tracers to provide more sensitive tests.

After the pioneering physiologic investigations of Dollery and co-workers (35), Ball and associates (36) in 1962 used ^{133}Xe and observed regional ventilation abnormalities in patients with

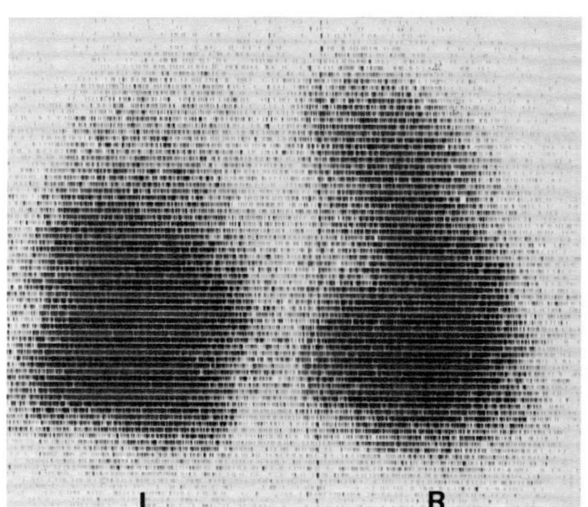

Fig. 7. A. This patient's lung scan was performed during an acute asthmatic attack. The posterior view shows bilateral perfusion defects more marked in the right upper lobe.

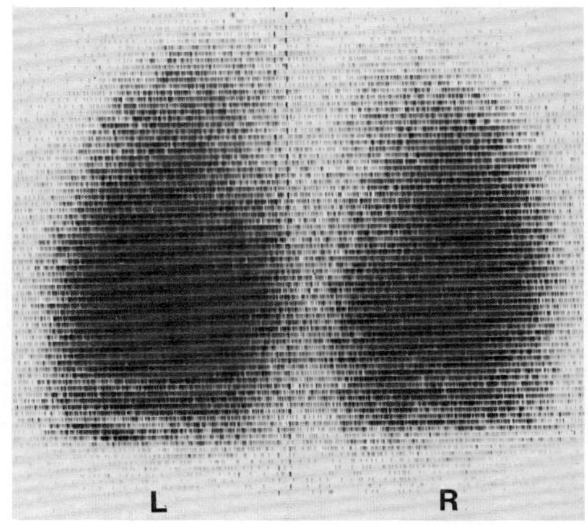

Fig. 7. B. A scan performed the following day revealed perfusion to the originally poorly perfused regions. R = right; L = left.

chronic obstructive lung disease. Since then, regional abnormalities have been found in asthma, chronic bronchitis, and emphysema.

Perfusion and ventilation images in a patient with emphysema are shown in figures 9A and B. For comparison, figure 10 is an example of a ^{133}Xe ventilation study with the scintillation camera in a person with normal ventilation.

Of particular interest is the finding of Anthonisen and associates (23) that symptomatic patients with chronic obstructive pulmonary disease and nearly normal spirometric pulmonary function tests have clear-cut regional abnormalities. Two subsequent reports suggest that regional lung function measurements can detect abnormalities in asymptomatic subjects at a time when measurement of whole lung function including closing volumes is still within the variation observed among healthy persons. In the first study (37), radioisotopic regional lung function measurements using both albumin microspheres labeled with technetium-99m and inhaled ^{133}Xe were compared to measurement of total lung function in a population of 30 participants in an epidemiologic study of the causative factors of obstructive pulmonary disease. Five of the 8 asymptomatic subjects who had no evidence of obstructive lung disease by the tests of total function had abnormal regional function measurements. The closing volume was abnormal in 3 of these 5, suggesting the presence of peripheral airways disease. Regional lung function was abnormal in all subjects who were symptomatic, who had a forced expiratory volume in 1 sec/forced vital capacity ratio < 75 per cent, or who had an elevated closing volume or residual volume. The data suggested that measurement of regional lung function may be a highly sensitive test for the early diagnosis of chronic obstructive lung disease. A long-term prospective study would be required to determine the significance of these regional abnormalities.

A second study (38) suggesting the sensitivity of regional function measurements was a study of 18 narcotics addicts without any symptoms of respiratory disease. Thirteen had regional abnormalities of perfusion of the lungs; 5 had abnormal zones of ventilation as well.

Only time will tell the ultimate usefulness of regional pulmonary function measurements in the early diagnosis of obstructive airways disease.

Pulmonary Venous Hypertension

Left ventricular failure and disease of the mitral valve frequently cause pulmonary venous hypertension. Redistribution of pulmonary arterial blood flow can be demonstrated in patients with congestive cardiac failure when tracers are injected in the supine position, resulting in increased perfusion to the upper lung fields. A

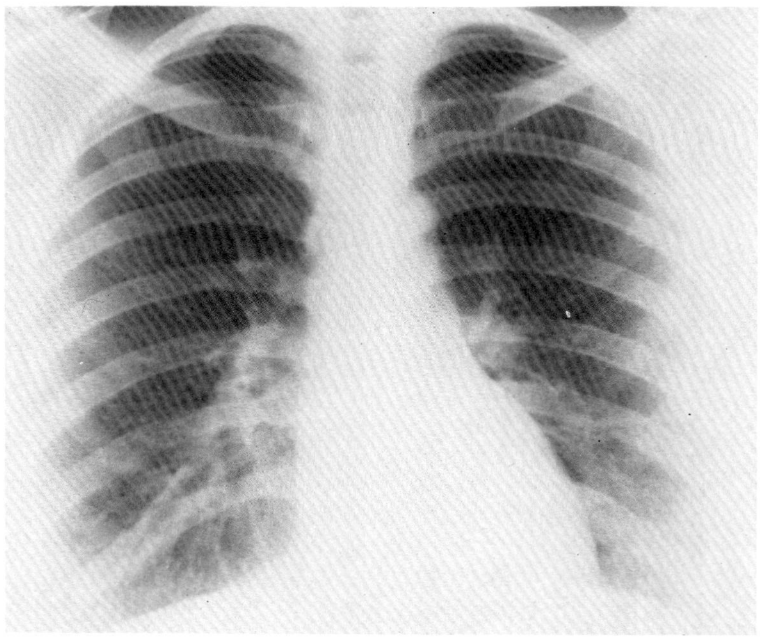

Fig. 7. C. A chest radiograph of the same patient.

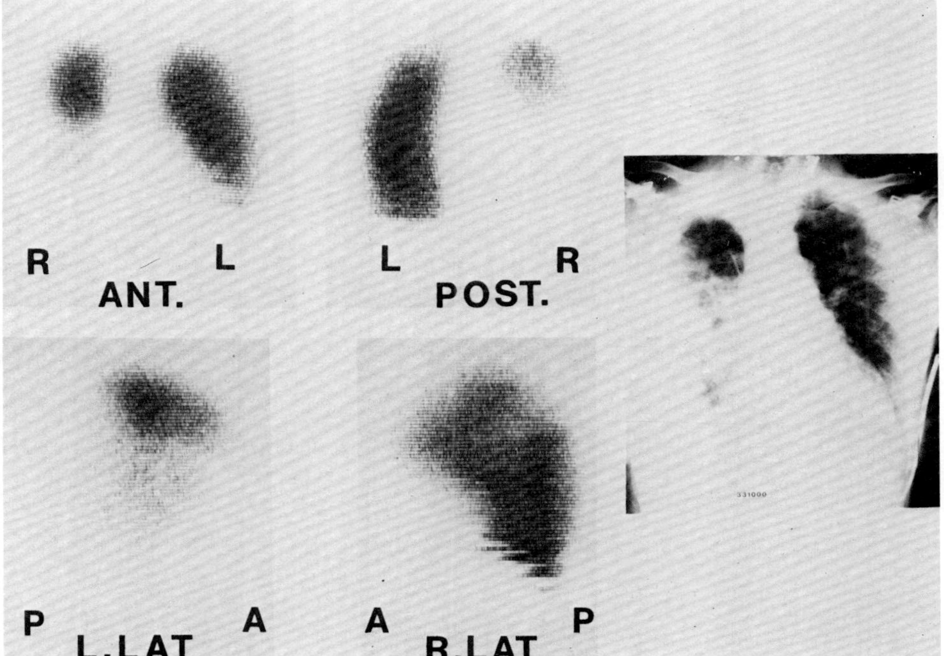

Fig. 8. The 4-view lung scan and chest radiograph reveal extensive involvement of carcinoma of the right lung. There is a marked decrease in perfusion to the middle and lower lobes of the right lung. For definition of abbreviations, see figure 1.

perfusion defect may be noted in the right middle lung field as a result of an enlarged atrium. In patients with cardiac failure the ventilation study is usually normal. A decrease in volume will be noted on the equilibration study with a normal washout if the patient has edematous lungs.

Cor Pulmonale

A recent use of radioactive tracers in patients with lung disease is in the study of the heart. Although these techniques are used today primarily in patients with coronary heart disease, they are beginning to be used in patients with lung disease. There are 3 types of procedures: (1) Distribution of regional myocardial blood flow can be depicted with the use of potassium analogues, such as ionic thallium-201 or rubidium-81. (2) Radionuclide angiocardiography is based on imaging the passage of an intravenously injected dose of [^{99m}Tc] albumin as it passes through the heart, lungs, and great vessels. The size of the intracardiac chambers, transit times from one region of the circulation to another, and the presence of left-to-right intracardiac chambers can be detected. (3) Regional and general contractility of both ventricles can be determined after the [^{99m}Tc] albumin has become distributed in the vascular compartment. This is accomplished by "gating" or activating the scintillation camera by means of the patient's electrocardiogram. Several hundred beats can be examined during the end of systole and diastole. Comparison of the scintillation camera images of the heart can reveal the end-systolic and end-diastolic volumes, stroke volume, and ejection fraction. Validation studies to date have been limited to the study of the left ventricle, but initial results indicate that important information can be obtained about the right ventricle as well. The position of the patient that is most useful is the left anterior oblique position in which the right and left ventricles can be viewed separately. The intraventricular septum can be viewed to permit proper positioning of the patient.

The types of information that can be obtained in these studies are dilatation and hypertrophy of the right and left ventricles and the relative performance of these 2 structures. In many patients to date, the differential diagnosis of cor pulmonale and the latter condition complicated

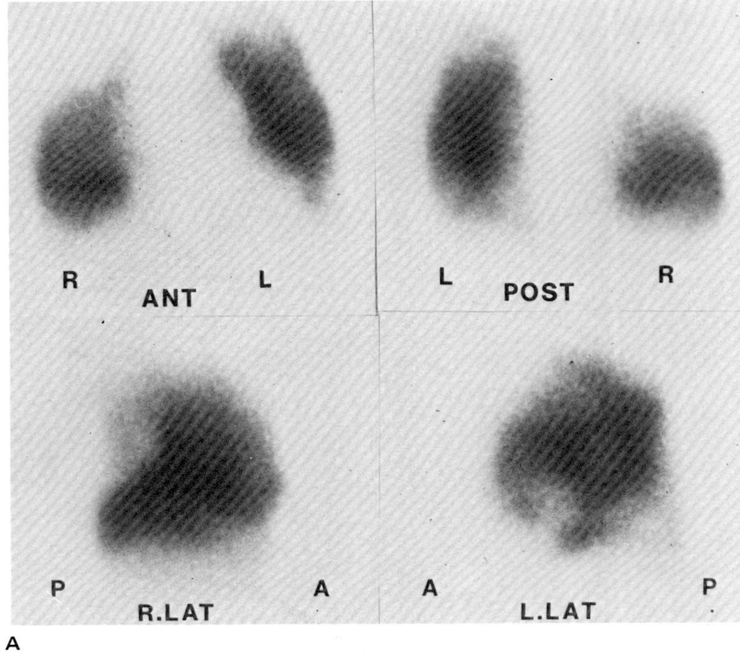

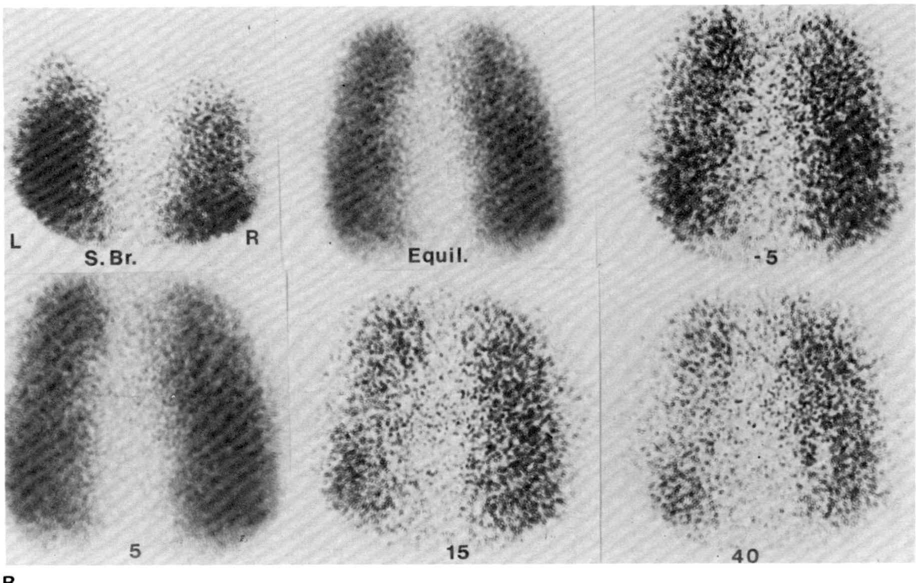

Fig. 9 A. (*Top*) In this patient with emphysema, the 4-view lung scan reveals nonsegmental perfusion defects bilaterally. There is decreased perfusion to both apices, more marked on the right. B. (*Bottom*) Decreased ventilation of both apices is noted in the single breath (S. Br.) view of the xenon-133 ventilation study. Delayed washout of the ^{133}Xe from both lungs is noted bilaterally. Equil. = equilibration view; for definition of other abbreviations, see figure 1.

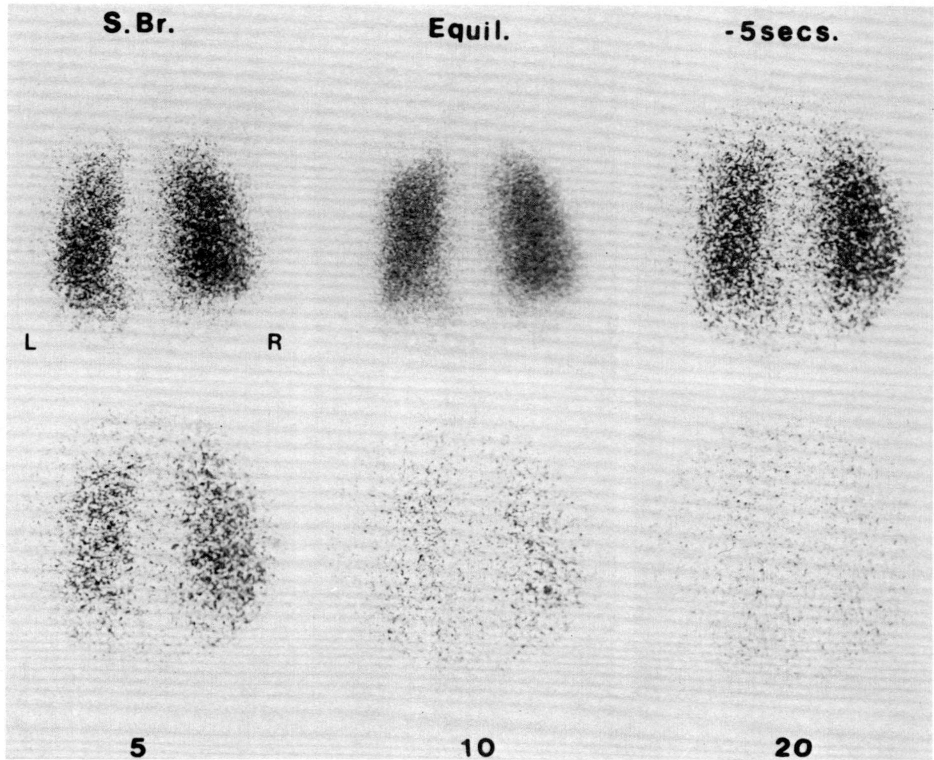

Fig. 10. This normal ventilation study shows a uniform distribution of the xenon-133 gas in both lungs, in the single breath (S. Br.) and equilibration (Equil.) views. The 133Xe is expelled rapidly and uniformly as noted in the washout phase of the study (bottom row). R = right; L = left.

by coronary heart disease and left ventricular dysfunction have been aided by these procedures. Only time will tell their eventual role, but initial results have been encouraging.

Differential Diagnosis of Cyanosis

Another area of usefulness of radioactive tracers is the study of patients with suspected respiratory problems is the diagnosis of right-to-left intracardiac shunts. In 1970 Hurley and associates (39) reported the use of radionuclide angiocardiography in the differential diagnosis of patients with congenital cyanotic heart disease. In all 30 patients with congenital cyanotic heart disease, the radionuclide angiocardiogram indicated an intracardiac right-to-left shunt. There were 3 false positives among the 46 other patients, none of whom had shunts. The principal indication was the appearance of the tracer in the left heart or abdominal aorta before the lungs were fully perfused. These results were confirmed and extended by Wesselhoeft and associates (40) in 43 children 3 years of age or less,

26 of whom had congenital heart disease. The criteria were improved and all 26 patients were correctly diagnosed as having congenital heart disease. There were no false positives. In many patients, the type of abnormality, such as transposition of the great arteries and truncus arteriosus, was correctly diagnosed before cardiac catheterization. Further validation and improvements were made by Kriss (7), and by others.

In normal subjects the pulmonary mean transit time, which can be measured or estimated subjectively by inspection of the serial images of the radionuclide angiocardiogram, averaged 6.5 ± 1.0 sec. Interpretation of transit times involves estimation of cardiac chamber sizes, because the reciprocal of the mean transit time in a given region is the ratio of blood flow through the region to the volume of the region the tracer is crossing.

Inhalation of Aerosols

For almost a decade, aerosolized droplets incorporating a radioactive tracer, such as ^{99m}Tc or indium-113m, have been used in experimental and clinical studies of the lungs (41, 42). The goal has been to facilitate measurement of the relative perfusion and ventilation to regional lesions as an aid in the differential diagnosis of pulmonary thromboembolism. In this method, the patient is connected to a nebulizer, the nostrils are occluded by means of a clip, and the patient breathes normally with a mouthpiece connected to a nebulizer. About 1.5 mCi of [^{99m}Tc] albumin or 3.0 mCi of ^{113m}In solution are retained by the lung parenchyma. The droplet size must be optimized so that the particles are small enough to reach the alveoli. Lung imaging is begun immediately and 4 views are obtained. Characteristic patterns have been observed in patients with chronic obstructive pulmonary disease, including bullous emphysema and chronic bronchitis.

The distribution of the aerosol is related both to bronchial mucous deposits and other obstructions as well as to the distribution of ventilation. The measurement is not purely regional ventilation but is determined to a large degree by deposition of the aerosol by impaction. An important advantage of the use of inhaled aerosols rather than ^{133}Xe is that multiple views can be obtained. In the case of ^{133}Xe, only one view can be obtained unless the ^{133}Xe is administered several times. On the other hand, the advantage of ^{133}Xe is that ventilation rather than ventilation plus impaction is measured. An advantage of the use of ^{113m}In is that the aerosol inhalation study can be performed immediately after the perfusion study with ^{99m}Tc microspheres. The higher energy photon emission (390 kev) from ^{113m}In can be easily distinguished from the lower photon energy (140 kev) of ^{99m}Tc.

An advantage of the inhaled aerosol technique is that mucociliary activity can be investigated, although only preliminary studies of this type have been performed to date. It is likely that inhaled particle studies will become more prevalent in the future. Most laboratories still use ^{133}Xe for measurement of regional ventilation and ^{99m}Tc microspheres or particles for regional perfusion.

Summary

Although it is true that pulmonary perfusion scanning is generally accepted primarily in the differential diagnosis of pulmonary embolism, the introduction of regional ventilation studies with radioactive ^{133}Xe, the use of the computer to provide quantitative data, and the advances being made in cardiovascular nuclear medicine indicate that nuclear medicine procedures will be used more and more in the evaluation of patients with a variety of lung and heart diseases. They have already proved of value in the following circumstances: (1) differential diagnosis of pulmonary embolism; (2) assessment of regional involvement in pulmonary parenchymal disease, including degenerative, neoplastic, and infectious diseases; (3) detection of bullous disease and the determination of the possible effectiveness of surgery; (4) assessment of the response to radiation therapy in patients with carcinoma of the lung; (5) detection of pulmonary venous hypertension in patients with mitral valve or left ventricular disease; (6) detection of cor pulmonale; (7) differential diagnosis of cyanosis in newborn infants.

References

1. Knipping, H. W., Bolt, W., Vernath H., Valentin, H., Ludes, H., and Endler, P.: Ein neue methode zur prufung der herz und lungen funktion. Die regionale funktion analyse in der lungen und herzklinik mit hilfe der radioactiven endelgases xenon-133, Dtsch Med Wochenschr, 1955, *80*, 1146.
2. West, J. B., Dollery, C. T., and Hugh-Jones, P.: The use of radioactive carbon dioxide to measure regional blood flow in the lungs of patients with pulmonary disease, J Clin Invest, 1961, *40*, 1.
3. Wagner, H. N., Sabiston, D. C., McAfee, J. G., Tow, D., and Stern, H. S.: Diagnosis of massive pulmonary embolism in man by radioisotope scanning, N Engl J Med, 1964, *271*, 377.
4. Cassen, B., Curtis, L., Reed, C., and Libby, R.: Instrumentation of I-131 used in medical studies, Nucleonics, 1951, *9*, 46.
5. Urokinase pulmonary embolism trial, A national cooperative study, Circulation, 1973, Supplement II; AHA Monograph 39.
6. Jones, R. H., and Anderson, P. A. W.: Congenital heart disease: Imaging and analytic methods, in *Quantitative Nuclear Medicine Cardiography*, R. N. Pierson, Jr., J. P. Kriss, R. H. Jones, and W. J. MacIntyre, ed., John Wiley and Sons, New York, 1975, p. 32.
7. Kriss, J. P.: Acquired cardiovascular disease, in *Quantitative Nuclear Medicine Cardiography*, R. N. Pierson, Jr., J. P. Kriss, R. H. Jones, and W. J. MacIntyre, ed., John Wiley and Sons, New York, 1975, p. 66.
8. Pierson, R. N., Jr., and Van Dyke, D. C.: Analysis of left ventricular function, in *Quantitative Nuclear Medicine Cardiography*, R. N. Pierson, Jr., J. P. Kriss, R. H. Jones, and W. J. MacIntyre, ed., John Wiley and Sons, New York, 1975, p. 123.

9. Wagner, H. N., Jr.: The heart and circulation, in *Nuclear Medicine*, H. N. Wagner, Jr., ed., Hospital Practice Publishing Co., New York, 1975, p. 112.

10. Wagner, H. N., Jr., and Rhodes, B. A.: Radioactive tracers in diagnosis of cardiovascular disease, Prog Cardiovasc Dis, 1972, *15*, 1.

11. Blumgart, H. L., and Weiss, S.: Studies on the velocity of blood flow. VII. The pulmonary circulation time in normal resting individuals, J Clin Invest, 1927, *4*, 399.

12. Zaret, B. L., Strauss, H. W., Hurley, P. J., Natarajan, T. K., and Pitt, B.: A noninvasive scintiphotographic method for detecting regional ventricular dysfunction in man, N Engl J Med, 1971, *284*, 1165.

13. Anger, H. O.: Instruments: Specific devices, in *Nuclear Medicine*, H. N. Wagner, Jr., ed., Hospital Practice Publishing Co., Inc., New York, 1975, p. 29.

14. Natarajan, T. K., and Wagner, H. N., Jr.: Functional Images of the Lungs in Dynamic Studies with Radioisotopes in Medicine, International Atomic Energy Agency, Vienna, SM-185/15, vol. II, 1974.

15. Wagner, H. N., Jr., and Natarajan, T. K.: Computers, in *Nuclear Medicine*, H. N. Wagner, Jr., ed., Hospital Practice Publishing Co., Inc., New York, 1975, p. 41.

16. Gilday, D. L., Poulose, K. P., and Deland, F. H.: Accuracy of detection of pulmonary embolism by lung scanning correlated with pulmonary angiography, Am J Roentgenol Radium Ther Nucl Med, 1972, *115*, 732.

17. Greenspan, R. H.: Does a normal isotope perfusion scan exclude pulmonary embolism?, Invest Radiol, 1974, *9*, 44.

18. Tow, D. E., and Simon, A. L.: Comparison of lung scanning and pulmonary angiography in the detection and follow-up of pulmonary embolism. The urokinase pulmonary embolism trial experience, Prog Cardiovasc Dis, 1975, *17*, 239.

19. Sasahara, A. A., McIntyre, K., Criss, A. J., and Belko, J. S.: Aggressive approach to the management of pulmonary embolism, Cardiovasc Clin, 1969, *1*, 261.

20. Tow, D. E., and Wagner, H. N., Jr.: Recovery of pulmonary arterial blood flow in patients with pulmonary embolism, N Engl J Med, 1967, *276*, 1063.

21. Wagner, H. N., Jr., and Strauss, H. W.: Radioactive tracers in the differential diagnosis of pulmonary embolism, in *Cardiovascular Nuclear Medicine*, H. W. Strauss, B. Pitt, and A. E. James, ed., C. V. Mosby Co., St. Louis, 1974, p. 278.

22. Lopez-Majano, V., Wagner, H. N., Jr., Tow, D. E., and Chernick, V.: Radioisotope scanning of the lungs in pulmonary tuberculosis, JAMA, 1965, *194*, 1053.

23. Anthonisen, N. R., Bass, H., Oriol, A., Place, R. E. G., and Bates, D. V.: Regional lung function in patients with chronic bronchitis, Clin Sci, 1968, *35*, 495.

24. Bentivoglio, L. G., Beerel, F., Stewart, P. B., Bryan, A. C., Ball, W. C., Jr., and Bates, D. V.: Studies of regional ventilation and perfusion in pulmonary emphysema using xenon 133, Am Rev Respir Dis, 1963, *88*, 315.

25. Heckscher, T., Bass, H., Oriol, A.: Regional lung function in patients with bronchial asthma, J Clin Invest, 1968, *47*, 1063.

26. Gaensler, E. A., Patton, W. E., and Frank, N. R.: Bronchospirometry. VII. Indications, J Lab Clin Med, 1953, *41*, 456.

27. Snider, G. L.: A critical evaluation of bronchospirometric measurement in predicting loss of ventilatory function due to thoracic surgery, J Lab Clin Med, 1964, *64*, 321.

28. Maynard, C. D.: Role of the scan in bronchogenic carcinoma, Semin Nucl Med, 1971, *1*, 195.

29. Tauxe, W. N., Carr, D. J., and Thorsen, H. C.: Perfusion lung scans in patients with inoperable primary lung cancer, Mayo Clin Proc, 1970, *45*, 337.

30. Wagner, H. N., Jr., Lopez-Majano, V., Tow, D. E., and Langan, J. K.: Radioisotope scanning of lungs in early diagnosis of bronchogenic carcinoma, Lancet, 1965, *1*, 344.

31. Arborelius, M., Jr., Kristersson, S., Lindell, S. E., Miorner, G., and Svanberg, L.: Xenon-133 radiospirometry and extension of lung cancer, Scand J Respir Dis, 1971, *52*, 145.

32. Lindell, L., Lindell, S. E., and Svanberg, L.: Regional lung function in roentgenologically occult lung cancer, Scand J Respir Dis, 1972, *53*, 109.

33. Larson, S. M., Milder, M. S., and Johnston, G. S.: Tumor-seeking radiopharmaceuticals: Gallium-67, in *Radiopharmaceuticals*, G. Subramanian, ed., Society of Nuclear Medicine, Inc., New York, 1975, p. 413.

34. Arborelius, M., Nosslin, B., and Lindell, S. E.: 197Hg-scintigraphy and 133Xe-radiospirometry in the diagnosis of pulmonary tumor, Scand J Respir Dis, 1974, *85* (Supplement, p. 119).

35. Dollery, C. T., Hugh-Jones, P., and Matthews, C. M. E.: Use of radioactive xenon for studies of regional lung function, Br Med J, 1962, *2*, 1006.

36. Ball, W. C., Jr., Stewart, P. B., Newsham, L. G., and Bates, D. V.: Regional pulmonary function studied with xenon 133, J Clin Invest, 1962, *41*, 519.

37. McKusick, K., Wagner, H. N., Jr., Soin, J. S., Benjamin, J. J., Cooper, M., and Ball, W. C.: Measurement of regional lung function in the early detection of chronic obstructive pulmonary disease, Scand J Respir Dis, 1974, *85* (Supplement, p. 51).

38. Soin, S. S., McKusick, K. A., and Wagner, H. N., Jr.: Regional lung function in narcotic addicts,

JAMA, 1973, *224*, 1717.
39. Hurley, P. J., Strauss, H. W., and Wagner, H. N., Jr.: Radionuclide angiocardiography in the diagnosis of congenital heart disease in infants, Circulation, 1972, *45*, 77.
40. Wesselhoeft, H., Hurley, P. J., Wagner, H. N., Jr., and Rose, R. D.: Nuclear angiocardiography in the diagnosis of congenital heart disease in infants, Circulation, 1972, *45*, 77.
41. Taplin, G. V., Poe, N. D., Dore, E. K., and Greenberg, A.: Bronchial patency and aerated space assessment by scintiscanning, LCFB, 1967, *16*, 297.
42. Taplin, G. V., Poe, N. D., Dore, E. K., Greenberg, A., and Isawa, T.: Radioaerosol inhalation scanning, in *Pulmonary Investigation with Radionuclides*, A. J. Gilson and W. M. Smoak, ed., Charles C Thomas, Springfield, Ill., p. 296.

The Connective Tissue of Lung[1]

ALLAN J. HANCE and RONALD G. CRYSTAL

Contents

[1] From the Section on Pulmonary Biochemistry, National Heart and Lung Institute, Bethesda, Md. 20014.

Introduction

In the past decade, there has been an explosion of interest in the connective tissue of the body. We know now that the 3 general categories of connective tissue, collagen, elastic fibers, and proteoglycans, are all heterogeneous, with multiple types and substructures. In addition, numerous enzyme systems have been discovered that are critical for preparing each connective tissue component for its structural function. Connective tissue is vital to the structure and function of every tissue; it gives blood vessels viscoelastic properties; skin and tendon, toughness; bone, a matrix to calcify.

The lung, of course, is no exception. Connective tissue comprises approximately 25 per cent of the adult human lung and is an intimate part of all lung structures. The lung is the one organ of the body in which we can estimate the contribution of connective tissue to mechanical behavior *in vivo* and in which abnormalities in connective tissue very quickly appear as abnormalities in function. The purpose of this review is multifold: (*1*) to define the components of connective tissue in general terms and, specifically, as related to lung; (*2*) to describe the mechanisms controlling the presence of connective tissue in lung; (*3*) to summarize the current concepts of how connective tissue influences lung structure and function in both health and disease; (*4*) to discuss some possible future directions for the study of lung connective tissue and approaches to the therapy of lung disease.

Collagen

Because of the abundance and wide distribution of collagen, its biochemistry has received considerable attention, and it is the best characterized of the connective tissue proteins. In the adult human lung, collagen represents 15 to 20 per cent of the total tissue mass and 60 to 70 per cent of the total connective tissue mass (1, 2).

To provide a general background for understanding the function of collagen in the lung, this section will briefly review the molecular structure of collagen and will emphasize aspects of collagen metabolism that are important for understanding the control of lung collagen homeostasis. Where applicable, we will detail what is known about the composition, localization, biosynthesis, and degradation of lung collagen. In later sections, we will describe the alterations in quality, quantity, and localization of lung collagen in development and disease. Finally, these concepts will be combined with information on other lung connective tissue components to try to summarize the relationships of connective tissue to lung function and how these relationships can be modified to normalize the disordered connective tissue in certain lung diseases.

Structure

Collagen is an important structural component throughout the lung, including the tracheobronchial tree, vascular tree, parenchyma, and pleura. The fundamental unit of collagen is the tropocollagen molecule, which, by its capacity to copolymerize with other tropocollagen molecules and to interact with a variety of other connective tissue elements, is capable of forming structures such as cartilage, basement membrane, and various fibrils that form the pleura and the skeleton of the lung parenchyma.

Tropocollagen is a rod-shaped molecule (1.5 $\times$ 300 nm) composed of 3 α chains in a right-handed helical arrangement (3). The right-handed "triple helical" tropocollagen is, in turn, wound in a left-handed "super coil" during fibril formation (4). Tropocollagen is heterogeneous; the 4 types found in the body are distinguishable by the α chains composing them. Type I tropocollagen contains two $\alpha 1$ (I) chains and one $\alpha 2$ chain, and thus has the structure $[\alpha 1\ (I)]_2 \alpha 2$. Each of the other tropocollagens, Type II, Type III, and Type IV, is composed of 3 identical α chains of the appropriate type; the structures are $[\alpha 1\ (II)]_3$, $[\alpha 1\ (III)]_3$, and $[\alpha 1\ (IV)]_3$, respectively. The 5 known α chains, $\alpha 1$ (I), $\alpha 2$, $\alpha 1$ (II), $\alpha 1$ (III), and $\alpha 1$ (IV), have different primary amino acid sequences and thus are the products of different structural genes (5, 6). Lung contains all 4 tropocollagens, and thus is the most heterogeneous of all tissues studied with regard to collagen composition (1).

Although the 4 tropocollagens are clearly distinguishable by their α chain composition, they do share certain structural features. Every α chain has a molecular weight (MW) of 95,000 to 100,000 daltons; each is composed of approximately 1,050 amino acids (3). More than 1,000 of these amino acids occur in repetitive triplets of the form, (glycine-X-Y)$_n$. Although the amino acids represented by X and Y are variable, there is a high content of alanine, proline, lysine, hydroxyproline, and hydroxylysine (5). The latter 2 amino acids are especially characteristic of collagen; their formation will be discussed in the section on biosynthesis. Although elastin (5), the Clq component of complement (7), and perhaps other noncollagen structural proteins also contain hydroxyproline (8), the content of hydroxyproline in collagen is considerably higher. Hydroxylysine is even more characteristic of collagen; it is not present in elastin, although there are small amounts in Clq (7). The α chains are also unique proteins in that they have low tyrosine and methionine contents, and no tryptophan (5).

At the N- and C-terminal ends of each α chain, there are regions of approximately 20 amino acids that do not have the glycine-X-Y sequence (3). These regions, known as "teleopeptides," do not take part in helix formation, but they do have an important role in crosslink formation both within and between tropocollagen molecules (4) (see below).

Not all of these common features have been studied in tropocollagen isolated from lung, but from what is known, there is nothing to suggest that there will be tissue-specific differences.

Interestingly, although all tropocollagens share these characteristics, the structure of each type of tropocollagen can vary beyond that attributable to the differences in primary amino acid sequence. These differences will be discussed below in relation to each tropocollagen type; they include the degree of hydroxylation of lysyl and prolyl residues, the number and type of carbohydrates attached to the tropocollagen, and the number, type, and location of crosslinks that are formed during and after fibril formation. It is probably the uniqueness of each tropocollagen that allows it to perform its structural function in a different way, depending on the requirements of a given tissue.

Type I ([α1 (I)]$_2$α2). Type I collagen is the most ubiquitous collagen in the body, being the most abundant type in skin, bone, tendon, and a number of other tissues (9–11). Large amounts of Type I collagen are also present in lung; pre-sumably, Type I collagen constitutes a significant proportion of the collagen in the large bronchi and blood vessels. In addition, Type I collagen is also synthesized by lung parenchyma, indicating a role in support of the interstitium (12–14). *In vitro*, Type I collagen readily forms fibrils that have high tensile strength. These fibrils are tightly packed, leaving little room for ground substance (15).

Because of the ubiquity of Type I collagen, it is not surprising that more than one cell type is capable of its synthesis. Because the interstitial cell, fibroblast, and pericyte have the same general morphologic features in lung, the general term "mesenchymal cell" will be used to describe them all. A very large proportion of adult lung cells are mesenchymal (16). The lung mesenchymal cell is capable (in tissue culture) of synthesizing Type I collagen (Hance, A. J., Bradley, K., and Crystal, R. G.: J Clin Invest, in press); and in addition, a cell isolated from cat lung of apparent parenchymal epithelial origin has been shown to synthesize this collagen type (17, 18). In other tissues, a wide variety of nonmesenchymal cells, including cells of epithelial and neural origin, have been shown to be capable of collagen synthesis (19–21). Therefore, it is not unlikely that a number of other nonmesenchymal cell types in lung will also be shown to be capable of collagen synthesis. The current assessment of lung cells capable of collagen synthesis is given in table 1.

Type II [α1 (II)]$_3$. Type II collagen has been identified only in cartilagenous tissue (6). This is also true in lung, where Type II has been found only in trachea and bronchi; it is the major collagen synthesized by these structures maintained in explant culture (13) (table 1). Type II collagen does not form prominent fibrils within these tissues, but rather is found in association with large amounts of proteoglycan (22) (see below for a discussion of these compounds). These proteoglycan-collagen complexes are maintained by strong ionic interactions that may be fostered by the presence of a considerable amount of carbohydrate attached to Type II collagen (23).

The cell responsible for the synthesis of Type II collagen in lung has not been identified. In other tissues, chondroblasts are the only cells that synthesize Type II collagen in adult tissues (24), and chrondroblasts in tracheal and bronchial cartilage are probably responsible for its synthesis in lung.

TABLE 1

RELATIONSHIP OF LUNG CELLS TO LUNG CONNECTIVE TISSUE SYNTHESIS AND DEGRADATION*

Structure	Specific Cell Type	Collagen Synthesis[†]				Elastic Fiber Synthesis**	Proteoglycan Synthesis	Collagenase	Elastase	Glycosamino-glycan Degradative Enzymes
		Type I	Type II	Type III	Type IV					
Parenchyma		Yes	No	Yes	?	Yes	Yes[††]	Probable	?	Probable***
	Alveolar Types I and II	Probable[†††]	?	Probable[†††]	?	?	?	?	?	?
	Endothelial	Probable***	?	Probable***	?	?	Yes	?	?	?
	Mesen-chymal****	Yes	No	Yes	?	Probable***	Probable***	Probable***	?	Probable***
	Macrophage	No	No	No	No	?	?	Yes	Yes	Yes
Blood vessels		Yes	No	Probable	?	Probable***	?	?	?	?
	Smooth muscle cell	Probable***	?	Probable***	?	Probable***	?	?	?	?
Tracheo-bronchial tree		Probable	Yes	?	?	Probable[††††]	Probable[††††],*****	?	?	?
	Chondroblast	No	Probable***	?	?	?	Probable*****	?	?	?

*References to the literature are given in the text.

[†]Type I = Type I tropocollagen, etc.

**In most cases, only the elastin component has been demonstrated to be synthesized.

[††]Hyaluronic acid, chondroitin sulfates, dermatan sulfate, heparin, and heparan sulfate.

***Shown in cells derived from tissue other than lung. It is probable that lung cells behave similarly.

[†††]Epithelial cells derived from fetal cat lung and maintained in culture make Types I and III; it is unknown whether alveolar Type II cells isolated directly from lung will make collagen.

****"Mesenchymal" cell is a general term including the fibroblast, the interstitital cell, and the pericyte. These cells are indistinguishable morphologically.

[††††]The tracheobronchial tree contains cells (smooth muscle and mesenchymal) that probably synthesize elastic fibers and proteoglycans.

*****Probably chondroitin sulfates and keratan sulfate.

Type III [α1 (III)]$_3$. The structure of Type III collagen differs from that of Type I and Type II in that Type III has a higher hydroxyproline content and contains cysteine (25). Type III is more difficult to solubilize from adult tissues than Type I, although digestion of tissues with pepsin (which digests the teleopeptide, but not the helical, regions of tropocollagen), markedly increases its recovery (25, 26). Type III collagen constitutes a major percentage of fetal, but not adult, skin and has been found to be a constituent of a number of other tissues, including lung (11, 25–27). So far, it has been found only in tissues that also contain Type I collagen and that also support epithelium or endothelium. The localization of Type III collagen to specific structures in lung has not, as yet, been accomplished.

Lung mesenchymal cells grown in tissue culture are capable of synthesizing Type III collagen in addition to Type I (Hance, A. J., Bradley, K., and Crystal, R. G.: J Clin Invest, in press). Interestingly, preliminary work indicates that certain cultured lung cells of epithelial origin also synthesize both Type I and Type III collagen (17, 18) (table 1).

Type IV [α1 (IV)]$_3$. Type IV, or basement membrane, collagen has been difficult to isolate from lung, because it is closely associated with a number of proteoglycans and other glycoproteins through ionic and disulfide bonds (28). Type IV collagen investigated in other tissues appears to have a number of distinctive characteristics (29–31). It has a high content of cysteine and hydroxylysine and contains a large amount of carbohydrate, including mannose and hexosamine, neither of which is found in other collagens. In addition, the unusual amino acid 3-hydroxyproline is found in abundance in Type IV collagen (31); 4-hydroxyproline is common in other collagen types. Type I contains a single 3-hydroxyproline residue (32), making it the only collagen other than Type IV to have this amino acid. Collagen isolated from rabbit lung does contain small amounts of 3-hydroxyproline, but its source has not been identified (12).

Collagenous protein has been extracted from lung parenchyma using techniques that solubilize basement membrane in other tissues (29), but amino acid analysis suggested considerable contamination with noncollagen proteins. Notably, this "alveolar basement membrane" collagen did not contain significant 3-hydroxyproline, raising the possibility that alveolar Type IV collagen is different from the better-studied renal and lens capsule basement membrane collagen. The cell type(s) responsible for synthesis of basement membrane collagen in lung are currently unknown (table 1). It is interesting to speculate that lung epithelial and endothelial cells synthesize their own basement membrane, analogous to synthesis of basement membrane by chick lens epithelial cells (33).

Biosynthesis of Collagen

Collagen is synthesized in a precursor form termed protropocollagen, which is composed of 3 precursor proα chains. Between the synthesis of component proα chains and the formation of the mature collagen fibril, a complex series of events must take place, including (*1*) hydroxylation of prolyl and lysyl residues; (*2*) glycosylation; (*3*) alignment of component proα chains and triple helix formation; (*4*) secretion; (*5*) selected proteolytic digestion at both the ends of the protropocollagen molecule; (*6*) fibril formation; and (*7*) crosslinking (figures 1 and 2). Each of these steps, and their importance in determining the nature of the final collagen product, will be discussed briefly.

Translation of collagen messenger ribonucleic acid (mRNA). Nothing is known concerning the transcription of collagen mRNA or the mechanism of its transcriptional control. Collagen mRNA is known to be translated on ribosomes found to the membranes of the rough endoplasmic reticulum (34–37), as is typical for proteins destined for secretion (38) (figure 1). The large collagen mRNA (MW > 1.6 × 10^6 daltons) (39) is capable of accommodating many ribosomes, and therefore, the polysomes directing its synthesis are large (37, 40). Translation of collagen mRNA has been studied in a cell-free system derived from lung; the requirements for translation are similar to those of other proteins (37, 41).

Although all somatic cells have the same complement of genetic material, the differences manifested by specific cell types presumably are secondary to the restriction of different genes in different cells. Thus, all cells do not have collagen mRNA available to be translated, and those that do may have different collagen mRNAs coding for individual collagen types. For example, it is assumed, but not proved, that the mesenchymal cell probably has α1 (I), α2, and α1 (III) mRNA; the chrondoblast, α1 (II) mRNA; the alveolar macrophage, which does not synthesize collagen (17), no collagen mRNA.

The translation product of collagen mRNA is

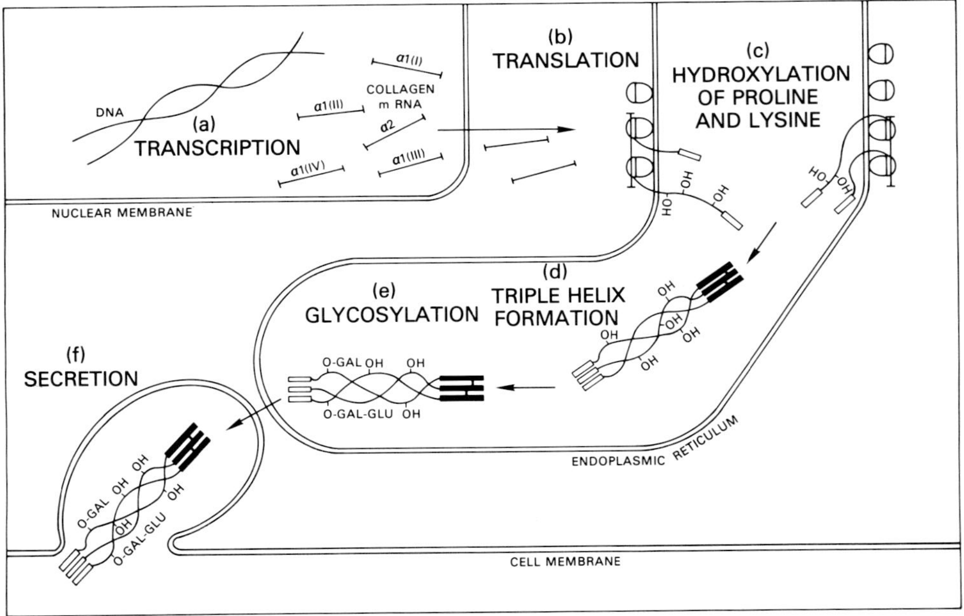

Fig. 1. Schematic representation of the biosynthesis of collagen. (a) Transcription of collagen structural genes results in synthesis of collagen messenger ribonucleic acid (mRNA). Each α chain type is translated from a distinct mRNA. It is assumed, but not proved, that each differentiated cell transcribes only the collagen mRNAs specific for the collagen type characteristic for that cell. DNA = deoxyribonucleic acid. (b) Collagen mRNAs are transported from the nucleus to the ribosomes lining the rough endoplasmic reticulum. As the precursor proα chains are synthesized, they move into the cisternae of the endoplasmic reticulum, where (c) some prolyl and lysyl residues are enzymatically hydroxylated (−OH). Proα chains contain an N-terminal noncollagen peptide (▢—), a middle collagen α chain (————), and a C-terminal non-collagen peptide (—■). (d) Three proα chains are aligned into protropocollagen (probably, in part, through disulfide bonds in the C-terminal noncollagen peptide), and the middle α chains coil into a triple helix. (e) Before secretion, some hydroxylysyl residues are glycosylated by enzymatic addition of the monosaccharide, galactose (GAL), or the disaccharide, glucosylgalactose (GLU-GAL-). Glycosylation takes place before proα chains are released from the ribosome, but may continue after helix formation. (f) The completed tropocollagen is secreted from the cell.

not the α chain, but rather, a large precursor (MW: 150,000 daltons) called the proα chain (42) (figure 1). Translation time for an intact proα chain is probably 7 to 8 min *in vivo* (43). The proα chain contains 3 regions: an N-terminal noncollagenous region (MW: 20,000 daltons); a middle α chain region (MW: 95,000 daltons), and a C-terminal noncollagenous region (MW: 35,000 daltons). The amino acid sequences of the N- and C-terminal noncollagenous regions are very different from those of the α chain region in that they do not contain the repeating glycine-X-Y sequences, and tryptophan is present in the C-terminal region (42, 44–47). The importance of these N- and C-terminal regions and the conversion of the proα chain to its final α chain form will be discussed later. Before this conversion takes place, there are 3 important

alterations to the middle α chain "collagenous" region of the proα chain: (*1*) conversion of selected prolyl residues to hydroxyproline; (*2*) conversion of selected lysyl residues to hydroxylysine; (*3*) glycosylation of some hydroxylysyl residues (figure 1).

Hydroxylation of proline. As the proα chain is being synthesized on the collagen mRNA, certain prolyl residues are enzymatically converted to hydroxyproline by prolyl hydroxylase (15). This enzyme is bound to the membranes lining the cisternae of the rough endoplasmic reticulum (48–50) and is dependent on the cofactors Fe^{++}, atmospheric O$_2$, α-ketogluterate, and ascorbic acid (or a substitute reducing agent) for activity (51, 52). The enzyme hydroxylates in the 4-position only prolyl residues that are in the sequence, glycine-X-proline-glycine (42). Formation of the collagen triple helix limits further action of the enzyme (53). A separate enzyme may be required to form 3-hydroxyproline (found only in α1 (I) and α1 (IV) chains), which can be formed from prolyl residues only in the sequence, glycine-proline-Y-glycine.

Under normal circumstances, most prolyl hydroxylation occurs while the proα chain is still a nascent chain (before translation has been completed), although it is possible to hydroxylate prolyl residues in completed chains (54); however, not all prolyl residues in the appropriate sequence need be hydroxylated, and differences have been described in the hydroxylation of the same prolyl residue in different tissues from the same species (5, 55). In addition, the degree of hydroxylation varies greatly among the various collagen α chain types; α1 (IV) is hydroxylated most completely (ratio of hydroxyproline to proline = 1.5), followed by Type III (1.2) (25), Type II (0.9) (23), and Type I (0.7 to 0.8) (5).

Prolyl hydroxylase activity is easily detected in lung tissue; in one study, the level of activity (per mg of tissue protein) was higher in lung than any other tissue studied (50). The degree of hydroxylation of Type I collagen in lung is similar to that in other tissues (12). The hydroxylation of individual prolyl residues or degree of hydroxylation of other lung collagen types has not been examined.

Hydroxylation of prolyl residues appears to

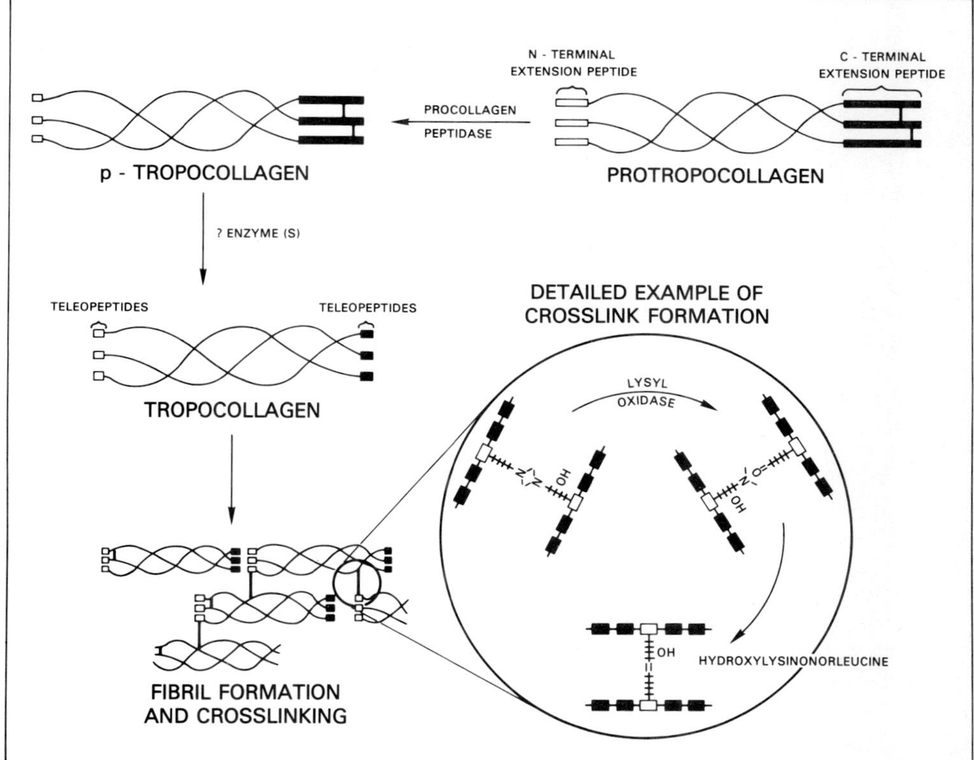

Fig. 2. Extracellular steps in collagen fibril formation. Newly secreted protropocollagen (upper right) consists of 3 coiled collagen α chains plus N-terminal (▢—) and C-terminal (——■) noncollagen peptides. Proteolytic action of procollagen peptidase cleaves the N-terminal noncollagen peptides, producing the intermediate p-tropocollagen (upper left). Further proteolytic activity removes the C-terminal noncollagen peptides, leaving tropocollagen (center left), composed of a helical region of 3 α chains with short, nonhelical teleopeptides (▢— and —■) at either end. Tropocollagens then polymerize to form the collagen fibril (lower left), which is reinforced by crosslinks (heavy lines). The circle at lower right illustrates the steps in formation of the crosslink, hydroxylysinonorleucine. First, lysyl oxidase converts lysine to the aldehyde, allysine. Then, the allysine residue and a hydroxylysine in an adjacent chain interact to form the final crosslink. In the presence of β-aminopropionitrile, lysyl oxidase is inhibited, and crosslinking does not occur.

be important for forming and stabilizing the collagen triple helix, although it may serve other functions (42). Hydroxylation can be inhibited severely by removing necessary cofactors or by using proline analogues that are incorporated into α chains, but cannot be hydroxylated. In several systems, underhydroxylation has been shown to result in delayed triple helix formation and inhibition of secretion (42, 56–59). These underhydroxylated proα chains may be more susceptible to intracellular degradation. This could be a vulnerable step in collagen biosynthesis, where therapeutic intervention might slow the process of pathologic collagen accumulation.

Whether or not hydroxylation of prolyl residues by prolyl hydroxylase is an important control mechanism in normal collagen synthesis remains unknown.

Tissue culture experiments have shown that the concentration of prolyl hydroxylase need not correlate with the rate of collagen synthesis (60, 61). In some cases, however, prolyl hydroxylase activity does correlate with increased collagen formation; activity in silicotic rat lung increased to 250 per cent more than the control value, and the increased activity preceded histologically apparent collagen accumulation (62).

Hydroxylation of lysine. In many respects, the hydroxylation of lysyl residues is analogous to prolyl hydroxylation; lysyl residues are hydroxylated as translation proceeds, and only residues in the glycine-X-lysine-glycine sequence are hydroxylated. The necessary enzyme, lysyl hydroxylase, requires the same cofactors and is membrane-bound, and triple helix formation inhibits further lysyl hydroxylation (42, 63–65). Lysyl hydroxylase activity has been detected in chick lung; in the 15-day-old chick embryo, the concentration was lower than that found in skin and bone, but similar to that in heart and kidney (66).

Hydroxylation of lysine appears to be important in several respects. Lysyl and hydroxylysyl residues are the sites of crosslink formation between tropocollagens. Whether or not a lysyl residue involved in crosslink formation is hydroxylated changes the nature and strength of the crosslink formed (5, 67). Hydroxylysyl residues are also important sites at which carbohydrate is attached to tropocollagen (42). Although the precise function of these carbohydrate moieties is unknown, a number of functions have been postulated (see below).

As with hydroxylation of proline, all lysyl residues in the correct sequence need not be hydroxylated. Changes in the degree of hydroxylation of a single type of collagen in different tissues have been described. In addition, the degree of hydroxylation can change with age (68–70). Type I collagen isolated from 4-month-old rabbit lung has twice the hydroxylysine content as newborn rabbit lung Type I; the sum of lysyl and hydroxylysyl residues remains constant (12). How this change modifies subsequent glycosylation, crosslink formation, or otherwise affects collagen structure is unknown, as are the mechanisms by which lysyl hydroxylase activity is regulated. The degree of hydroxylation is also different in the different collagen types; the lysyl residues are more fully hydroxylated in Type II and Type IV collagen than in Type I and Type III (5, 23, 25, 29).

Glycosylation. During biosynthesis of collagen, certain hydroxylysyl residues in the α chain portion of the proα chain are altered by the addition of either the monosaccharide, galactose, or the disaccharide, glucosylgalactose (5). These saccharide units are added sequentially. First, the enzyme, uridine diphosphate (UDP)-galactose:galactosyl transferase, links galactose to collagen through the hydroxyl group of hydroxylysine. Subsequently, some, but not all, of the galactosyl residues are glucosylated by a separate enzyme, UDP-glucose: glucosyl transferase (71, 72). The site of glycosylation is uncertain, although hydroxylysine-linked mono- and disaccharides have recently been identified in nascent proα chains still attached to the ribosome (73). The fact that glycosylation enzymes are capable of acting on native protropocollagen suggests that further glycosylation could take place later. Other types of carbohydrate are attached to Type IV collagen (31) and may be present in the nonhelical peptide regions of other procollagen types (74).

The enzymes necessary for glycosylation have been identified in lung microsomes and can use native tropocollagen as a substrate (75). The level of activity was very high in 10-day-old rat lung (only cartilage contained more activity), and the relative activities of the 2 enzymes were nearly equal. The level of activity of both enzymes decreased with aging, which correlates with the rates of collagen synthesis in lung (see below).

The function of glycosylation remains uncertain, although a number of possible functions have been suggested, including identifying the proα chain as a protein destined for secretion

(42), partially regulating crosslink formation (67, 76), and inducing collagen-mediated platelet aggregation (77). Glycosylated hydroxylysine residues do participate in crosslink formation, but how the rate of formation or stability of these crosslinks is modified remains unknown (67, 76).

Differences in the degree of glycosylation have been found between tissues, and at different ages in the same tissue, analogous to differences in the hydroxylation of prolyl and lysyl residues (78, 79). Differences in glycosylation of different collagen types is also considerable. Hydroxylysyl residues in Type IV collagen are more than 80 per cent glycosylated, almost entirely with glucosylgalactose. Hydroxylysyl residues in Type II collagen are approximately 40 per cent glycosylated, with an equal distribution of mono- and disaccharides (23). The degree of glycosylation of lung collagens has not been studied.

Procollagen and helix formation. The importance of the N- and C-terminal noncollagenous "pro" regions of the proα chain is just beginning to be understood. Near the time of release the newly synthesized proα chains from the ribosome, but before helix formation, 3 proα chains of the appropriate type are aligned, probably through interaction of the noncollagenous regions. This association is further stabilized by disulfide bonds in the C-terminal region (42, 46, 47, 80–83). Subsequent triple helix formation of the middle α chain "collagenous" region results in the formation of protropocollagen, the form in which collagen is probably secreted from the cell (42). Other functions that have been suggested for the "pro" regions include (*1*) ensuring solubility of collagen during cellular and extracellular transport (80, 83, 84); (*2*) facilitating proper orientation of tropocollagen during fibrillogenesis (85); and (*3*) inhibiting premature crosslink formation (86).

Secretion. Optimal secretion requires protropocollagen to be in the triple helical configuration (42) (figure 1). The mechanism by which the newly synthesized protropocollagen is secreted by the cell remains uncertain. A merocrine pattern of secretion, typical of many proteins, has been suggested; protropocollagen moves from the smooth endoplasmic reticulum to the Golgi apparatus, to Golgi-derived vacuoles, and eventually to the extracellular space (87, 88). Other patterns of secretion have been suggested, such as secretion of protropocollagen in vesicles that bypass the Golgi apparatus, or secretion by exocytosis of protropocollagen released from the endoplasmic reticulum into the cell cytoplasm

(6). The mechanism of secretion of collagen in lung cells has not been investigated.

Fibril formation and crosslinking. The ultimate ability of collagen to serve its supportive function requires the formation of strong collagen fibrils, which, together with associated proteoglycans and noncollagen connective tissue glycoproteins, form the matrix for individual tissues. This requires cleavage of the "pro" region, polymerization of tropocollagen in a specific orientation, and stabilization of the fibril through intra- (between α chains within tropocollagen) and intermolecular (between tropocollagen molecules) crosslinks (figure 2).

Before completion of extracellular fibrillogenesis, the N- and C-terminal "pro" regions are cleaved in a series of steps (protropocollagen → p-tropocollagen → tropocollagen) that requires at least 2 distinct proteolytic enzymes (46, 47). Under normal circumstances, the N-terminal peptide is cleaved first, and subsequently, the disulfide-linked C-terminal peptide is removed. All 5 types of α chain are first synthesized in precursor form. The rate at which the N- and C-terminal "pro" regions are cleaved may differ for the different types of collagen, and in the case of basement membrane collagen, cleavage may never be complete (89).

In the types of collagen in which it has been studied (Types I and II), the polymerization of tropocollagen molecules during fibrillogenesis occurs in a specific fashion, with a staggered arrangement, each tropocollagen overlapping its neighbor by 67 nm or a multiple of that distance (3).

Crosslinking is not necessary for fibril formation, but without crosslinking, the fibrils lack high tensile strength. Crosslinks are derived through lysyl or hydroxylysyl residues on neighboring chains, and their formation begins with the oxidation of the ε-amino group of lysine or hydroxylysine to the corresponding δ-semialdehyde, allysine or hydroxyallysine (5). This step requires lysyl oxidase, a Cu⁺⁺-requiring enzyme that acts on tropocollagen primarily after the onset of fibril formation (90, 91). The enzyme can be inhibited by copper deficiency and by β-aminoproprionitrile (BAPN) (92). Lysyl oxidase activity has been demonstrated in lung; the enzyme appears to have the same properties as that described in other tissues (93).

After aldehyde formation, crosslinks form either through aldol condensation of 2 allysine aldehydes (intramolecular crosslinks) or by the Shiff base reaction between allysine (or hydroxyallysine) and a lysyl (or hydroxylysyl) residue on an adjacent tropocollagen (5, 67). This second step in crosslink formation can be inhibited by semicarbazide or penicillamine, both of which react with the newly formed aldehyde groups and prevent subsequent crosslinks (92). Several important crosslink types have been described in collagen, but their contents in various tissues differ widely (5, 94). After crosslink formation, subsequent reduction or rearrangement of the crosslink region can form even more stable links (67, 94, 95). Both Types III and IV tropocollagen contain cysteine residues, suggesting that disulfide-bonded crosslinks can occur in certain collagen types in addition to the covalent aldehyde-mediated crosslinks.

Crosslink formation is undoubtedly of great importance in determining lung structure, and changes in crosslink formation may play a role in the molecular basis of development, aging, and lung disease. Currently, little information is available concerning collagen crosslinking in lung, although lysyl-derived aldehydes have been found in lung collagen (96). Because inhibitors of crosslink formation increase the solubility of lung collagen, intermolecular crosslinks are probably present (12). The location, amount, stability, and changes in aging and disease of lung collagen crosslinks has not been explored directly.

Degradation of Collagen

As will be discussed later, the adult lung continually synthesizes collagen; yet, on the average, the concentration of collagen in the adult lung does not change (12). To preserve the constancy of collagen per unit lung mass, there must be a continual destruction of collagen at a rate that matches the synthetic rate. The mechanisms by which this takes place are just beginning to be understood.

In the triple helical form, collagen is very resistant to proteolytic attack, thus placing considerable restriction on possible mechanisms of collagen proteolysis (97–101). The source of collagenolytic enzymes, their mechanisms of action, and their interaction with proteolytic inhibitors are important determinants of collagen homeostasis.

Once the α chains are in triple helical form, only 3 known classes of enzymes can disrupt them under physiologic conditions: microorganism collagenase, cathepsin B1, and vertebrate collagenase (101). In the lung, the first could be important in certain infections, whereas the lat-

ter 2 are probably important in normal collagen catabolism.

Microorganism collagenase. Certain bacteria (*Clostridium histolyticum, Pseudomonas aeruginosa, Bacteroides melaninogenicus,* and *Mycobacterium tuberculosis*) and fungi (*Streptomyces madurae, Trichophyton schoenleinii,* and *Aspergillus oryzae*) produce an extracellular collagenase that can cleave any form of collagen into small pieces (98). (Except for cathepsin B1, the "collagenases" attack only the α chain portions of collagen, not the N-terminal or C-terminal precursor peptides.) For example, Clostridial peptidase A, the best studied of these enzymes, cleaves a single α chain into 150 to 200 fragments (98); it can hydrolyze lung α1 (I), α2, α1 (II), and α1 (III) collagens (12, 13; Hance, A. J., Bradley, K., and Crystal, R. G.: J Clin Invest, in press). It attacks collagen chains at -Y↓glycine-X- bonds, requires Ca^{++}, and is inhibited by ethylenediaminetetra acetate (EDTA), cysteine, and serum α-globulins (98). It is not known what role bacterial collagenases play in the destruction of lung tissue in parenchymal infection.

Cathepsin B1. This is a protease that has been described in lysosomes of rat liver (101–103). In purified form, it is capable of degrading collagen fibrils at acid pH (optimal pH: 3 to 5 units) and, in contrast to microorganism or vertebrate collagenases, it is activated by EDTA and cysteine. It attacks tropocollagen molecules at the N-terminal nonhelical region and then cleaves at multiple sites in the helical region. Other cathepsins (e.g., cathepsin D) do not affect helical collagen (101). Although cathepsin B1 has not been specifically isolated from lung (102), it should be looked for, because it is possibly an important determinant of the catabolism of lung collagen that has been phagocytosed while still in the fibrillar form (figure 3). It is not likely that this enzyme has any role in the extracellular milieu, because it requires a pH found only in lysosomes.

Vertebrate collagenase. As with the collagenase produced by microorganisms, these enzymes are secreted and attack collagens in the extracellular space (figure 3). They have been found in explant culture systems of the tadpole tail, skin, carrageenin granuloma, bone, postpartum uterus, and rheumatoid synovium, and in cell cultures of fibroblasts, polymorphonuclear leukocytes, and peritoneal macrophages (97–101, 104–106). In preliminary experiments in our laboratory, Horwitz has demonstrated collagen-

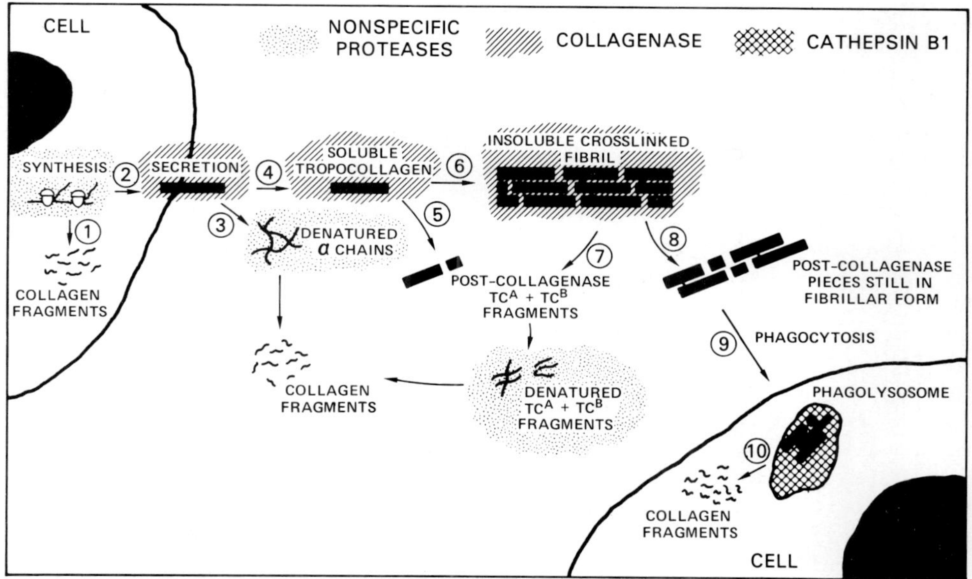

Fig. 3. Schematic representation of collagen degradation. (*1*) Intracellular degradation can occur before triple helix formation. This process does not require collagenase; numerous nonspecific proteases can hydrolyze collagen when it is in the nonhelical form. (*2*) Once the α chains are in the triple helix, and under normal physiologic extracellular conditions, the α chains can be degraded only by vertebrate collagenase or microorganism collagenase (presumably, the latter is not normally present). (*3*) If the triple helix is denatured (e.g., underhydroxylated collagen will denature under physiologic conditions), the α chains can be attacked by nonspecific proteases. (*4*) The conversion of protropocollagen to soluble tropocollagen leaves 3 α chains in helical form; they can be degraded only by collagenase. (*5*) Proteolysis by vertebrate collagenase leaves tropocollagen in 2 helices, and N-terminal TCᴬ fragment, and a smaller C-terminal TCᴮ fragment. Under physiologic conditions, these fragments denature and can be attacked by nonspecific proteases. (*6*) If the tropocollagen is incorporated into the insoluble crosslinked fibril, proteolysis can occur with (*7*) collagenase, or (*8*) if the intermolecular crosslinks leave the postcollagenase pieces still in fibrillar form, the partially degraded fibril can be (*9*) phagocytized. In the resulting phagolysosome, enzymes such as cathepsin B1 can degrade the fibril at acid pH.

ase secretion from explants of rabbit lung parenchyma and cultured rabbit alveolar macrophages. As with the microorganism collagenases, these collagenases require Ca^{++}, and are inhibited by EDTA, cysteine, and serum α-globulins (97–101). A precursor form of the enzyme ("procollagenase" or "zymogen") has been described (107–109). Although vertebrate collagenase will attack denatured collagen, it is most active against the tropocollagen molecule, whether in solution or in the fibrillar form (97–101). This enzyme has extraordinary specificity; it cleaves the tropocollagen at one site three-fourths of the distance from the N-terminus of the molecule, always between a glycine-isoleucine (or leucine) bond (110). Whereas intact tropocollagen remains helical at 37°C, the 2 helical fragments resulting from vertebrate collagenase attack will denature at body temperature. Once collagen is in a nonhelical form, it can be degraded nonspecifically by a large number of enzymes active at neutral pH (e.g., extracellular) or acid pH (e.g., within phagolysosomes) (101) (figure 3).

Lung collagen catabolism. There are 2 known sources of vertebrate collagenase that can attack lung collagen, the polymorphonuclear leukocyte and the alveolar macrophage. We do not know which cells are responsible for the production of the enzyme secreted by rabbit parenchyma, although by analogy to other tissues, it is probable that lung mesenchymal cells synthesize and secrete collagenase (table 1). The fact that the ubiquitous serum α-globulins inhibit collagenases makes the study of these enzymes in lung very difficult, because the α-globulins are present in parenchyma (111, 112).

Although there is clearly a collagenase present

in the azurophilic granules of the human poly-morphonuclear leukocyte, certain aspects of this enzyme suggest that it may be different from oth-er vertebrate collagenases (101, 104, 105, 109). It is not inhibited by serum α-globulins, and in purified form it will not attack collagen fibrils unless an "assistor enzyme," also from the gran-ulocyte, is added; however, a pure collagenase isolated from human leukemic granulocytes can be inhibited by $α_1$-antitrypsin and $α_2$-macro-globulin (113). The role the leukocyte collagen-ase plays in lung collagen destruction is not clear at this time.

Although collagenase is required to initiate the degradation of helical collagen, there are non-collagenase enzymes that degrade nonhelical collagen. Collagen is in this form in 2 circum-stances: (1) newly synthesized proα chains be-fore normal helix formation; (2) when post-synthetic modifications (e.g., proline hydroxyla-tion) have not been completed, the proα or α chains may be unable to maintain a helical con-figuration. This type of collagen degradation, including at least some intracellular degrada-tion, has been demonstrated in *in vitro* systems, including parenchymal explants of lung (114).

Although proteolysis of newly synthesized col-lagen (e.g., before fibril formation) appears, at first glance, to be a wasteful mechanism to con-trol net collagen secretion (i.e., it expends en-ergy to synthesize and then to degrade a signifi-cant amount of that which is synthesized), it is a well-described characteristic of both mammali-an and bacterial cells (115). It may be useful in several ways: (1) it allows the cell to remove abnormal proteins arising by mutations, errors in synthesis, denaturation, or modification (e.g., underhydroxylation of collagen secondary to as-corbic acid deficiency); (2) the ability to "turn over" newly synthesized proteins continuously gives the cell an additional rapid means of con-trolling the quantity of that protein. Regard-less of its role in control of net collagen synthesis, reduction of collagen overproduction could be approached therapeutically by increasing in-tracellular degradation.

In summary, if lung collagen is not degraded early by noncollagense mechanisms, it may be degraded in the helical (soluble or fibrillar) form by macrophage, leukocyte, or (possibly) parenchymal collagenase. A cleavage by any of these enzymes could result in 2 subsequent mechanisms to complete proteolysis (figure 3): (1) denaturation and attack by nonspecific pro-teases in the extracellular milieu; (2) phago-cytosis and intracellular degradation (116) in the phagolysosome by an enzyme analogous to liver cathepsin B1. Both are potential sites for therapeutic intervention in human lung disor-ders involving collagen.

Morphology of Lung Collagen

Approximately 30 to 40 per cent of collagen in the lung is in the large airways, large blood ves-sels, and septae dividing major lung segments (16). The remainder is present in the various sub-compartments of parenchyma, including alveo-lar interstitium, basement membrane, small blood vessels, and transitional airways. Although differences exist in the morphologic organization of collagen in each location, certain anatomic generalizations are possible.

The terminology used to describe collagen morphologically is confusing. We will use the term "fibers" to refer to structures seen with the light microscope; "fibrils," for structures with crossbanding; "nonbanded fibrils," for fibrils < 40 nm in diameter. The term "microfibrils," sometimes used to describe the smallest collagen fibrils, should be avoided because of confusion with the term "microfibrils" or "microfibrillar component" used to describe a specific substruc-ture of the elastic fiber. "Reticulin" is a light mi-croscopic term that has no clear electron micro-scopic counterpart, although "reticular fila-ments" are described in electron micrographs (116).

Collagen fibers are distinguishable by light microscopy with a number of stains (118); none of these methods is specific for one collagen type. In the lung, collagen fibers are seen in all struc-tures, although they are not prominent in the interstitium. Electron microscopic views of col-lagen fibers show that the fibers consist of a large number of densely packed fibrils. The fibrils have prominent cross striations occurring with a reg-ular periodicity of 68 nm, with finer banding in between (3, 15). The major 68 nm bands result from the staggered packing of tropocollagen dur-ing fibrillogenesis. As a result, the N-terminal end of one tropocollagen does not closely abut the C-terminal end of the adjacent tropocolla-gen; instead, a space is left in the fibril that stains intensely as the major band. The minor cross striations result from the alignment of po-lar amino acids in tropocollagens that overlap in the fibril. Fibrils have a wide spectrum (40 to 200 nm) of diameters and can exist together or alone.

So-called "reticulin" or "reticulin fibers" were

first defined by a silver methionine stain; reticulin stains intensely black, whereas collagen fibers stain yellow (119). Reticulin is widely distributed in lung. It is probably a complex structure composed of several classes of connective tissue; their exact compositions are unknown. It has been suggested that they contain collagen, proteoglycans, lipid, and noncollagen protein (119–120). The resistance of reticulin to trypsin and its sensitivity to collagenase suggest that the collagenous portion (of unknown type) is an important constituent (100).

Tracheal and bronchial cartilage. A distinctive feature of the larger airways is the presence of cartilagenous support within the walls. In the trachea and first-order bronchi, cartilage is present as irregular plates that do not encircle the airway. Once the airways penetrate the parenchyma, cartilage is present as irregular rings that are part of the bronchial walls down to the ninth-order branches (121). The appearance of bronchial cartilage has not received detailed study, but it appears similar to hyaline cartilage found elsewhere in the body. The cartilage contains collagen (Type II) in the form of fine, nonbanded fibrils associated with an amorphous proteoglycan matrix. The perichondrium contains, in part, Type I collagen that appears as banded fibrils. These fibrils fuse with the continuous bronchovascular framework, firmly attaching cartilage within the walls of the airway (121).

The structural importance of cartilage is underscored by the consequences of congenital absence of cartilage, a finding frequently confined to individual lung segments. Without the added support given by cartilage, airway closure produces tension emphysema in the affected segments (122).

Bronchovascular framework. Large collagen fibers traverse the lung in association with the subdividing bronchial and vascular trees. These fibers are present in both longitudinal and circular arrays, both of which branch and fuse with each other. The fibers supporting the smaller branches of the airways and vasculature become progressively smaller in diameter. Reticulin is a more prominent feature of the bronchovascular parenchyma (121). Within the parenchyma, collagen fibrils are arranged in a helical fashion as they encircle respiratory bronchioles and alveolar ducts. Finally, the fibrils circle the alveolar openings and spread out as a thin net within the individual walls of the polygonal alveoli (123).

Alveolar interstitium. At the level of the alveolar interstitium, collagen fibrils and elastic fibers may be found in close association; but frequently, they are individually grouped (figure 4). Considerable attention has been directed toward understanding the precise arrangement of collagen fibrils that allows maximal support without interference with the primary function of gas exchange. Within the interstitium, fibrils are present in a central "sheet" or "meshwork" along with cellular elements (macrophages, mesenchymal cells, and mast cells) and other connective tissue components (125–130). On each side of this central supporting layer is the extensive capillary network composed of capillaries that weave their way through the interstitium, appearing first on one side of the alveolar septum and then on the other. Thus, the capillaries seem to have a polarity, with 50 per cent or less of the capillary basement membrane embedded in the central fibrillar meshwork; the remaining capillary basement membrane fused with the alveolar basement membrane (126, 128) (figure 4). Thus, the pathway traversed by gases is reduced to a minimum; gases have only to penetrate the epithelial cell layer and the fused alveolar-capillary basement membrane to reach blood within the pulmonary circulation. In disease states, this orientation can be destroyed, but early thickening of the central interstitial sheet (e.g., in edema or fibrosis) need not lengthen the path for gas diffusion (130, 131).

Basement membrane is a prominent structural feature of the alveolar interstitium, serving as the site of attachment of epithelial lining cells to the alveolar walls and surrounding the capillaries of the pulmonary vasculature. The composition of pulmonary basement membrane has received little study, but probably contains a specialized collagen type (Type IV) and associated proteoglycans and noncollagen glycoproteins. Usually, basement membrane appears amorphous, although small (< 10-nm) nonbanded fibrils have been described (116); the collagen composition of these nonbanded fibrils is unknown. Fibrils from the interstitial sheet merge with the alveolar basement membrane, especially in areas where capillaries are not closely applied to the alveolar basement membrane (figure 4).

Pleura. The pleura also contains substantial amounts of connective tissue. The parietal pleura consists of a pleural cell layer, a thin layer of reticulin, and a dense, collagenous layer, but no elastic fibers (132). The visceral pleura also has a laminated construction. The outer cellular layer rests on a thin, connective tissue layer under

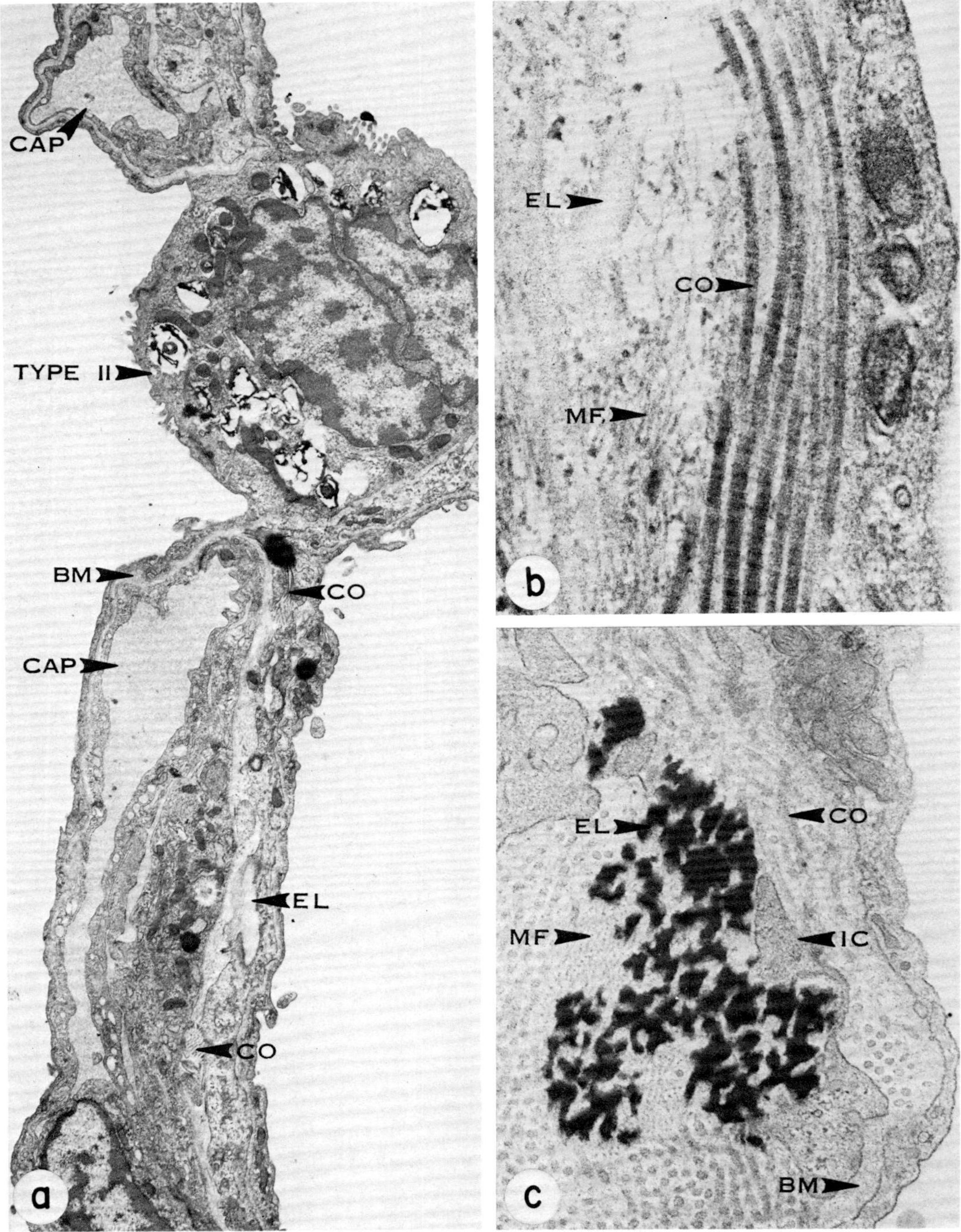

Fig. 4. Connective tissue in the adult rabbit lung parenchyma. The lung from a 1-year-old rabbit was inflated to a pressure of 15 cm H_2O with 3 per cent glutaraldehyde in 0.1 M phosphate buffer (pH 7.2). (a) Epithelial, capillary, and interstitial structures in the parenchyma. Alveolar type II cell (TYPE II), capillary (CAP), basement membrane (BM), collagen (CO), and elastin (EL) are labeled. The basement membrane surrounding the capillary merges with the collagen and elastin in the interstitium. Mesenchymal cells are seen throughout the interstitium (uranyl acetate and lead citrate stains; original magnification: × 7,500). (b) Higher-power view of collagen (CO) and elastic fibers in the interstitium. Crossbanding of the collagen fibrils is apparent. The

which lies the "chief layer." The latter contains both collagen and elastic fibers, which lie parallel to the lung surface, but which often turn abruptly, penetrating the parenchyma to join the fibers of the bronchovascular framework. The visceral pleura is therefore firmly attached to the underlying lung. Plaques of collagen have been described lying on the parietal pleura, especially in association with asbestos exposure (133). The collagen types composing the pleura are unknown.

Elastic Fibers

The presence of elastic fibers in the lung was demonstrated histologically more than 70 years ago. A knowledge of the general mechanical properties of lung *in vivo* led to the natural assignment of lung "elastic" properties to the presence of these fibers in lung parenchyma, airways, blood vessels, and pleura. Although this association seems obvious, the actual assignment of lung mechanical behavior to specific biochemically defined components of the elastic fiber was only begun in the past 10 years. There have been 2 major problems to overcome: (*1*) until recently, the actual composition of elastic fibers was not known; (*2*) the complex anatomic and biochemical interactions among the various components of connective tissue have prevented the development of simple models of connective tissue determinants of lung mechanical properties. This section will detail the current knowledge of elastic fiber morphology, composition, synthesis, and degradation in general, and as specifically related to lung. In a later section, we will combine these data with comparable information on other lung connective tissue components in order to interpret studies relating lung composition to lung mechanical properties in normal and diseased lungs.

Morphology

Classic morphologic stains used to define elastic fibers include resorcinol-iron-basic fuchsin (Weigert), orecein-iron hematoxylin (Verhoeff), and aldehyde-fuchsin (Gomori) (118, 134). Some are not specific for elastic fibers (e.g., the Gomori-aldehyde fuchsin method stains both elastic fibers and mucopolysaccharides deep purple), whereas others do differentiate connective tissue elements (e.g., the Weigert method stains elastic fibers blue-black to black; collagen, pink to red, and other connective tissue components, yellow) (134). Other stains commonly used for light microscopy either do not stain elastic fibers (e.g., acidophilic dyes, including eosin, fast green, and orange G; basic dyes, including hematoxylin, methylene blue, and safranin) or variably stain elastic fibers (e.g., periodic acid-Schiff, metachromic dyes, or the colloidal iron stain) (134). The mechanisms of action of these stains are, in general, not known. In lung, these stains demonstrate elastic fibers in all structures, including visceral pleura (121). The elastic fibers appear in the parenchyma as a continuum, complexly intertwined with collagen and ground substance elements (123).

Early observations with the electron microscope demonstrated that the elastic fibers were heterogeneous, with both amorphous and fibrillar components being visualized (135). The consensus is that the fibrillar constituents (termed "microfibrils" or "microfibrillar component") are each 10 to 12 nm in diameter, with a denser periphery than center, giving a tubular appearance (135–138). The second component of the elastic fiber is amorphous to the limits of resolution of the electron microscope (figure 4). One of the problems in studying these 2 components is that they both cannot be well stained with the same method, and thus, electron micrographs usually demonstrate the microfibrillar component with "holes" in place of the amorphous component, or vice versa. Anionic stains (phosphotungstic acid and silver tetraphenylporphine solfonate) are used for the positively charged amorphous component, whereas cationic stains (uranyl acetate, lead tartrate, or lead citrate)

---

elastic fibers are composed of amorphous elastin (EL) and a microfibrillar component (MF) (uranyl acetate and lead citrate stains; original magnification: × 75,000). With this stain, the microfibrils are well seen, but the elastin is not (see text). (c) Interstitium stained with Verhoeff's hematoxylin and lead citrate (124). The elastin (EL) is densely stained; the microfibrils (MF) are seen on end as tubular structures. Collagen (CO), basement membrane (BM), and the cytoplasm of an interstitial cell are seen (IC). At the lower left corner, surrounding the elastic fiber, collagen fibrils are seen on end. Note that the elastic fiber is in close association with the interstitial cell and that the fiber is composed of central elastin and more peripheral microfibrils (original magnification: × 36,000). These electron micrographs were kindly done by V. Ferrans, section on Pathology, National Heart and Lung Institute.

                                   HANCE AND CRYSTAL

are used for the negatively charged microfibrillar component (135) (table 2). Studies of aortic elastic fibers have shown that portions of the elastic fibers stain with ruthenium red, suggesting a carbohydrate component (139). This is probably in the microfibrillar component of the fibers.

Electron microscopic observation of tissues at various ages has shown that the ratio of microfibrillar to amorphous component appears to decrease with maturation (137). In the developing fetal bovine ligamentum nuchae, elastic fibers are almost entirely composed of the microfibrils. When the microfibrils first appear outside a cell, they remain in close intimacy, occupying infoldings of the cell surface. With advancing age, the microfibrils appear to be invested with the amorphous component within the preformed cylinder of the microfibrils. With maturation, almost the entire center of the fiber is amorphous, with the microfibrils moved peripherally (135, 137) (figure 4).

The differential staining characteristics and changes in relative abundance during maturation led to the proposal that the microfibrillar and amorphous components were distinct macromolecules, although until these components were defined biochemically, it was believed that the microfibrils might be precursors of the amorphous component. Given the classic work of Ross and Bornstein (137), however, we now know that they are distinct, with no precursor-product relationship. Elastic fibers have not been investigated thoroughly in lung, although numerous studies have demonstrated their presence. With Verhoeff's iron hematoxylin stain (124), both components can be seen in the alveolar interstitium of the adult rabbit lung, although the more peripheral microfibrils stain less intensely (figure 4).

Composition, Biosynthesis, and Crosslinks of Elastic Fibers

The extraordinary insolubilty of elastic fibers has been the major reason for the delay in their biochemical definition. The methods generally used to isolate elastic fibers consist of a series of harsh biochemical extraction techniques, with the elastic fibers defined as "the residue." Most of the biochemical definition of elastic fibers has been accomplished using bovine ligamentum nuchae, because of its high (approximately 70 to 80 per cent) elastic fiber content (140). When the 2 morphologic components of the fetal bovine ligamentum nuchae were "biochemically"

TABLE 2

COMPOSITION AND PROPERTIES OF THE MATURE ELASTIC FIBER AND ITS COMPONENTS

Component	Electron Microscopic Stains		Molecular Weight (daltons)	Distinguishing Amino Acids					
	Phosphotungstic Acid	Uranyl Acetate		Nonpolar*	Polar†	Cysteine	Methionine	Hydroxyproline	Crosslinks**
Elastic fiber††	Yes	Yes	↑↑	Yes††	Yes††	Yes††	Yes††	Yes††	Yes††
Tropoelastin	?	?	40–70,000	↑	↓	No	No	Yes	Yes
Elastin	Yes	No	↑↑	↑	↓	No	No	Yes	Yes
Microfibrils	No	Yes	270,000	↓	↑	Yes	Yes	No	No***

*The most prevalent nonpolar amino acids include glycine, alanine, valine, proline, leucine, and isoleucine.

†Polar amino acids include aspartic acid, glutamic acid, lysine, arginine, and histidine.

**Desmosine, isodesmosine, and lysinonorleucine.

††The mature elastic fiber is more than 90 per cent elastin, with the remainder the microfibrillar component; the amino acid composition of the elastic fiber reflects this mixture.

***Microfibrils may contain disulfide crosslinks.

dissected (135–138), it was shown that the microfibrils were rich in polar amino acids (e.g., aspartic and glutamic acids), contained significant amounts of cysteine and methionine, and had no hydroxyproline or crosslinks (table 2). Quite distinctly, the amorphous component was rich in nonpolar amino acids (alanine, valine, leucine, and isoleucine), contained no cysteine or methionine, but did have small amounts of hydroxyproline and crosslinks (table 2). Neither the amorphous component nor the microfibrillar component contains hydroxylysine, thus distinguishing them from collagen. The amino acid composition of the amorphous component was identical to that previously described for "elastin," a protein classically isolated from ligamentum nuchae as the residue not solubilized in the Lansing "hot alkali" procedure (141).

These findings have been confirmed by other investigators, and current terminology holds that the elastic fiber is composed of both components, with "elastin" being the amorphous compo-

nent. Although these biochemical studies are just beginning to be applied to lung, it is important to keep in mind that the "elastic fiber" is a variably heterogeneous mixture of elastin and microfibrils, whereas "elastin" is only one of the protein components of the elastic fiber.

Elastin. The fact that elastin is an insoluble polymer severely hampered the development of the technology necessary to understand its composition and synthesis. The discoveries of a soluble elastin precursor (142–150), elastin crosslinks (5, 140, 151, 152), and the enzyme necessary to begin the process of crosslinking the precursor into insoluble elastin (90, 153) have resulted in a generally cohesive story of elastin biosynthesis and composition (figure 5).

The precursor to elastin, tropoelastin, is synthesized on the rough endoplasmic reticulum of mesenchymal cells. Two cell types, the fibroblast and the smooth muscle cell, have now been been shown to participate in tropoelastin synthesis, although it is probable that other cells

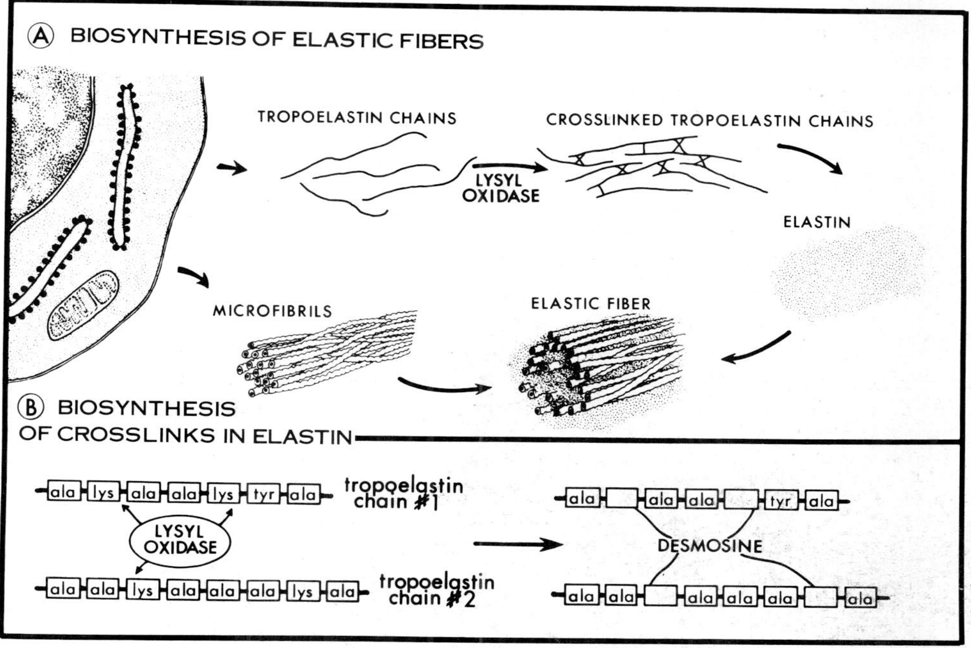

Fig. 5. Biosynthesis of the elastic fiber and elastin crosslinks. (A) A mesenchymal cell first synthesizes the microfibrils. These are elongated, beaded structures lying in semiparallel array. At some later point, the cell synthesizes tropoelastin chains. The enzyme, lysyl oxidase, converts selected lysyl residues in the tropoelastin to aldehydes that subsequently form crosslinks. The crosslinked amorphous component (elastin) invests the microfibrils to form the mature elastic fiber. It is not known whether the conversion of tropoelastin to elastin occurs before or after the association with the microfibrils. (B) An example of the formation of a desmosine crosslink between 2 tropoelastin chains. The lysyl residues are surrounded by alanine residues. Although it has been proposed that as many as 4 tropoelastin chains could be held together by a single desmosine crosslink, only the configuration shown here has, as yet, been demonstrated (140, 154–156).

have this capacity (135, 157, 158) (table 1). Tropoelastin has an MW of 40,000 to 70,000 daltons, depending on the method used in its isolation (145, 147, 149). The disparity in MW values found by different investigators suggests the possibility that tropoelastin is not the actual protein synthesized by the cell, but that a larger protein, protropoelastin, is the original form synthesized (analogous to proα chains of collagen). Such a precursor has not been found as yet. Tropoelastin is predominantly composed of amino acids that are nonpolar, so the molecule is not very soluble in water. Tropoelastin has not been completely sequenced, but it is known to have a primary structure very different from that of collagen, including repetitious sequences of the peptides glycine-glycine-valine-proline, proline-glycine-valine-glycine-valine, and proline-glycine-valine-glycine-valine-alanine (159). It is known that, like collagen, some of the prolyl residues in tropoelastin are hydroxylated, forming hydroxyproline. There is no methionine, cysteine, or hydroxylysine in tropoelastin, but there are significantly larger amounts of lysine in tropoelastin than in elastin (135) (table 2).

The excess of lysine residues in tropoelastin compared to elastin is due to the conversion of some lysyl residues into covalent crosslinks that hold together the tropoelastin molecules (140). Although there are many intermediates in the formation of elastin crosslinks, the 3 major final crosslinks (desmosine, isodesmosine, and lysinonorleucine) have been identified (140, 151, 152) (figure 6). The crosslinking process begins with a copper-dependent extracellular enzyme, lysyl oxidase, that catalyzes the oxidative deamination of the ε-amino group of lysine to an aldehyde (90, 153). This is the same enzyme that is responsible for aldehyde formation in collagen crosslinking. Once formed, these aldehydes unite with neighboring lysine-derived aldehydes or other lysine residues to form the crosslinks. For example, the crosslink, desmosine, can be derived from 4 lysine residues contained in 2 tropoelastin sequences, as shown in figure 5 (154–156). It is speculated that other crosslink arrangements possibly join up to 4 tropoelastin chains (140). Thus elastin, the amorphous part of the elastic fiber, is converted from tropoelastin by the crosslinking process. It is known that these crosslinks form outside of the cell, but the temporal and physicial relationship of elastin crosslinking to the association of elastin with the microfibrillar component of elastic fibers is not known.

A great deal of insight into the process of elastin maturation has come from methods used to prevent the crosslinking process. The key enzyme, lysyl oxidase, depends on Cu^{++}, and thus animals made copper deficient have severe abnormalities in elastin because of an inability of this enzyme to function normally (142). Because lysyl oxidase is also the key enzyme in collagen crosslinking, any abnormality in elastin due to inhibition of lysyl oxidase should also result in collagen crosslink abnormalities. For example, the muscular arteries of copper-deficient swine have breaks in the internal elastic membrane,

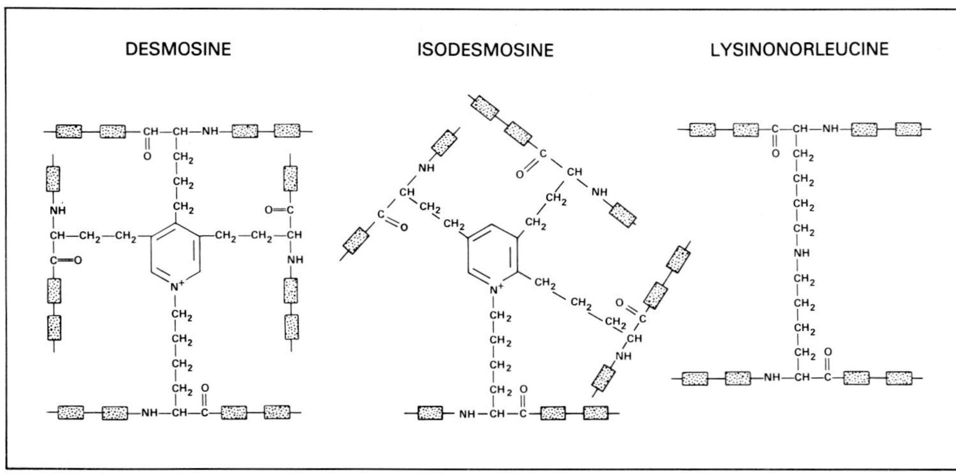

Fig. 6. Examples of elastin crosslinks. The chemical composition of the crosslink region is shown; the other amino acids in the linked tropoelastin chains are represented as (—▨—). All crosslinks are derived from lysyl residues in the tropoelastin chains. Theoretically, desmosine or isodesmosine can link 2, 3, or 4 tropoelastin chains. Lysinonorleucine can link only two (140, 151, 152).

and the animals often die of aortic rupture (142). Analysis of elastin extracted from these animals yields relatively higher amounts of tropoelastin and lower amounts of the crosslinks (143–146).

When animals are fed BAPN, they develop a disease (osteolathyrism) characterized by major alterations in elastin and collagen crosslinking (92). This compound inhibits lysyl oxidase and thus, as with copper deficiency, results in reduced crosslink formation and inhibition of the normal maturation of connective tissue proteins.

There is also a striking inhibition of desmosine formation when penicillamine is given to laboratory animals. Although the tropoelastin does not become crosslinked, the action of lysyl oxidase is undisturbed, and lysine-derived aldehydes (ϵ-aminoadipic acid-δ-semialdehyde) are formed. Thus, penicillamine blocks the maturation of elastin crosslinks at a step beyond the initial deamination of lysine (160).

These crosslink inhibitors are important not only in the experimental study of the maturation of connective tissue, but may also be useful prototypes in the development of drugs designed to inhibit the process of connective tissue deposition in certain lung disorders.

The presence of elastin in the elastic fiber is presumably responsible for giving the fiber mechanical properties similar to those of rubber (140). Both rubber and elastin have high extensibility, a low Young's modulus, and low tensile strength (compared to collagen). At low loads, purified elastin has a low modulus, linear stress-strain curve. At moderate loads, the stress-strain curve is also linear, but with a higher modulus. At high loads, stretching becomes irreversible, and elastin ruptures. The mechanical properties of the microfibrillar component and the complete elastic fiber are not known.

Microfibrils. Compared to elastin, much less is known about the composition, synthesis, and maturation of the microfibrils. The microfibrils are susceptible to proteolytic digestion by trypsin, chymotrypsin, or pepsin, whereas elastin is not. Dithiothreitol, a reducing agent, is useful in solubilizing microfibrils away from elastin in the elastic fiber, presumably by reducing the large number of cystine disulfide bonds in the microfibrils. In contrast to elastin, the microfibrils contain, in addition to cysteine, methionine and large amounts of polar amino acids; they do not contain hydroxyproline, desmosine, isodesmosine, or lysinonorleucine (137, 138) (table 2). Recent studies have demonstrated that chick lung microfibrillar component has an amino acid composition similar to that of microfibrils isolated from ligamentum nuchae (161; Rosenbloom, J.: Personal communication). The fact that the microfibrils contain no hydroxylysine definitively proves that they do not contain any of the known types of collagen. The microfibrils probably do contain a number of sugar moieties, including hexose and hexosamine, whereas elastin does not (138, 146). It is not clear, however, whether the microfibrils are composed of a single glycoprotein or are a heterogeneous group of glycoproteins. Recent studies with smooth muscle cultures have demonstrated a cysteine-containing protein of MW 270,000 daltons (reduced) that may be a precursor of at least a portion of the microfibrils (Muir, L., Ross, R.; Bornstein, P.: Unpublished data).

The relationship of the microfibrillar component of the elastic fiber to the amorphous (elastin) component is not yet clear. Because the ratio of microfibrils to elastin in ligamentum nuchae elastic fiber decreases with development, it has been suggested that the microfibrils play roles in orienting growth and in polymerizing the elastic fiber (135, 136). It is assumed that the microfibrils and elastin are not covalently crosslinked, because the former can be removed from the elastic fiber without proteolytic agents (137, 138).

Analysis of Elastic Fibers

An understanding of the composition, synthesis, and maturation process of elastic fibers is necessary to understand the specificities of assays used in the measurement of "elastic fiber" content and synthesis in lung. Although it may be possible to quantify "mature elastin" by measuring crosslink content (96), most methods used to quantify elastic fibers rely on its insolubility. There are 3 basic variations on this theme: (*1*) exposure of the tissue to "hot alkali" (e.g., the Lansing procedure, 0.1 M sodium hydroxide at 100°C for 1 hour) (141); (*2*) exposure to denaturing "solvents" (e.g., 6 M guanidine) (135, 162); (*3*) exposure to enzymes (163). The methods are often combined (162, 164). These techniques do not detect tropoelastin, and a variable amount of intermediate forms (not fully crosslinked) of elastin are probably lost during extraction. Hot alkali extraction of lung leaves predominantly elastin, but it contains higher concentrations of polar amino acids than expected, a hallmark of contamination with the microfibrillar component (165–167). This suggests that the identical procedure may quantify variable amounts of elastic fiber components, depending on the structure examined and the age of the tissue.

Collagenase treatment has also been used to isolate "elastic fibers" from crude connective tissue (168). In contrast to alkali extraction, collagenase treatment leaves intact elastic fibers, but, unfortunately, fails to solubilize numerous nonelastic structural proteins.

Recently, an elastin assay that takes advantage of the high content of valine-proline dipeptides in the amino acid sequence of tropoelastin has been described (169). Although this method has not been fully proved, it is a prototype of an important conceptual approach to the quantification of all elastin present, independent of its stage in the maturation process and the nature of the associated structural elements. At this time, there is no method available to quantify the content of the microfibrillar component of the elastic fiber, although it may be possible to develop an assay using an antibody against purified microfibrils (Rosenbloom, J.: Personal communication). Except for the valine-proline dipeptide assay, no method has been developed that accurately quantifies the synthesis of either component of the elastic fiber in lung.

Degradation of Elastic Fibers

There have been very few studies of the degradation of elastic fibers. Studies in which [14C]-glycine was injected into adult rats to label aortic elastin showed that there was no significant decrease in the specific activity of [14C]glycine in elastin during a period of 9 days, suggesting that elastin turnover is probably very slow (170). A similar study with [14C]lysine came to the same conclusion (171). Pierce and associates (172) followed the disappearance of radioactively labeled elastin in rats for more than 1 year and suggested that skin elastin turned over faster than lung elastin; but in both, turnover was very slow. More recent investigations have shown that mature elastin turns over very slowly, if at all, although elastin synthesis is active (173). This suggests that there is relatively more degradation of newly synthesized (not fully crosslinked) elastin, because the tissues studied synthesized, but did not accumulate, elastin. In experimental animals, it can be demonstrated that circulating elastin antibodies are present; this has led to the suggestion that newly synthesized elastin may be broken down, and peptides released into the circulation (173).

Although most studies of elastin degradation have been confined to the aorta, it must be assumed, from current knowledge, that the mature elastin component of elastic fibers is degraded very slowly. In the adult animal, if there is not continued accumulation of lung elastin, there must be continued degradation of at least the newly synthesized elastin in order to maintain this balance. This is crucially important for considering the mechanism of "elastolysis." Whereas enzymes, such as trypsin, do not attack mature elastin, it has been well documented that they hydrolyze peptide bonds in tropoelastin (159). Thus, although the major focus of attention on elastin degradation is on the enzyme elastase, it should be kept in mind that if a large bulk of elastoylsis is of immature elastin forms (e.g., noncrosslinked tropoelastin), a host of proteolytic enzymes could be involved, and it is not necessary to invoke the action of a specific "elastase" to explain elastolysis. This susceptibility of newly synthesized elastin may be particularly important in disease states of lung involving activation of inflammatory responses. The situation may be similar to collagen degradation, in which the single proα or α chain is susceptible to a variety of proteolytic enzymes, whereas the triple helical forms of collagen are susceptible only to collagenases.

When mature elastin is degraded, it is most probably degraded by an "elastase"; this group of enzymes is characterized by the ability to hydrolyze this insoluble polymer. Elastase has been found in pancreas, leukocytes, macrophages, plants, microorganisms, and, perhaps, platelets (174). Several different assays are available, using varied substrates, including congo red-elastin, orcein-elastin, elastin itself (assaying for amino acids released colorimetrically or with radioactive label), and several artificial N-blocked alanine methyl esters (174). Amino acid analysis of purified pancreatic elastase suggests that it is a compact globular protein of approximately 240 amino acids (MW: approximately 25,000 daltons). Proelastase, an inactive precursor of elastase, is found in pancreas; it is activated to elastase by tryptic cleavage of a single peptide bond near the N-terminus. The proelastase will specifically bind to elastin, but will not cleave it. Pancreatic elastase is readily soluble in water and is quite stable. It has a pH optimum of 8.8 (174).

The elastolytic activity of elastase can be inhibited by sodium chloride (NaCl) (50 mM NaCl causes 50 per cent inhibition) and by serum α-globulins (174, 175). The α_1-antitrypsin type Pi MM completely inhibits human leukocyte elastase, whereas type Pi ZZ only partially inhibits, if at all (176). Interestingly, there is an inhibitor of elastase present in the cytosol fraction of human granulocytes; this inhibitor is distinct from α_1-antitrypsin (176). Although this inhibitor is probably less significant than serum antiproteinases, it may be important in the local milieu; a similar inhibitor has also been found in the cytosol fraction of human alveolar macrophages (177). There has been a great deal of interest in elucidating the structure and mechanism of action of the active site of inhibitors of elastase. Once understood, it might be possible to develop small molecules (e.g., short polypeptide chains) that would bind to the active site and inhibit elastolytic activity (178). Such inhibitors may prove to be useful clinically in the α_1-antitrypsin disorders.

There is often confusion in the lung literature regarding elastase for several reasons. (*1*) Unlike vertebrate and microorganism collagenases, which are specific for collagen in the helical form, purified elastase is not specific for elastin. For example, it has been shown to degrade ribonuclease and the A and B fractions of oxidized insulin. A recent review points out that the physiologic activity of elastase should be viewed as that of a broad-specificity protease (174).

(*2*) Many studies using elastase, including those studying the effects of elastase on lung, assay its activity on substrates other than purified elastin. This is done principally for convenience, and assays using orcein-elastin or ester-linked substrates may not truly reflect the enzyme's activity against native elastic fibers (179).

(*3*) There are several sources of "elastase," including pancreas, leukocytes, and macrophages. It has not been demonstrated that these enzymes are identical.

(4) Many "elastase" preparations have not been purified and may contain a variety of proteolytic enzymes. The most persistent contaminants of pancreatic elastase are the other pancreatic endopeptidases, trypsin and the chymotrypsins (174).

These characteristics of "elastase" should be kept in mind in interpreting experiments of elastase-induced emphysema, especially when the elastase is of pancreatic origin, as are most commercially available elastase preparations.

Elastic Fibers in Lung

Although it is widely accepted that elastic fi-bers are of crucial importance in the maintenance of lung structure and mechanical properties, there have been very few studies of lung elastic tissue. One of the first morphologic descriptions was by Fisher (180), who described elastic fibers in the airways of birds. Modern morphologic studies have demonstrated elastic fibers in all major lung structures, including airways, blood vessels, parenchyma, and pleura (181–185). Unfortunately, none of these studies has systematically examined the amorphous and microfibrillar components of the elastic fiber in individual lung structures during lung development or aging, so there has been no definitive morphologic baseline established of the normal elastic fiber in animal or human lung.

The terminology used to describe elastic fibers in the older electron microscopic morphologic literature is quite confusing in terms of current definitions of elastic fiber composition; however, numerous investigators pointed out that lung elastic tissue has 2 components. In 1955, Rhodin and Dalhamn (183) demonstrated 2 components in the elastic fiber of the lamina propria of the rat tracheal mucosa. Their "fine fibrils" are the microfibrillar component, and the "dense, non-fibrous cement substance" is elastin. A study of the tunica propria of mouse bronchioles noted "elastic fibers" (elastin) and 11-nm "filaments" (microfibrillar component) (184). Low (185) found 4- to 12-nm "microfibrils" in the parenchyma and trachea; these microfibrils had a dense outer shell and lucid core and were associated with elastin.

The most complete study of lung elastic fibers has been done in the developing chick. Elastogenesis in chick lung parenchyma is almost identical to that in the ligamentum nuchae. It starts at day 14 to 16, with sparse bundles of microfibrils appearing among smooth muscle cells. With increasing maturity, the newly formed elastic fibers develop an amorphous core with a peripheral mantle of microfibrils. As in the ligamentum nuchae, there is differential staining of the elastin and microfibrils, and an age-related change in the ratio of the 2 components in the elastic fibers (181).

Elastin has been purified from lung by a variety of methods, including hot alkali (165–167), denaturing reagents (162), enzymes (163), and by a combination of all these methods (164). Whereas homogeneous tropoelastin has not yet been isolated from lung, the elastin obtained from lung has an amino acid composition similar to that of elastin in other tissues and contains the characteristic residues, desmosine and isodesmosine. The active enzyme necessary for elastin crosslinking has been isolated from hamster lung (93, 186); it appears to have the same characteristics as skin and bone lysyl oxidase. The microfibrillar component of lung elastic fibers has recently been isolated from embryonic chick lung (Rosenbloom, J.: Personal communication). In addition, the amino acid composition studies of John and Thomas (166) and Evans and associates (165) leave little doubt that the microfibrillar component is present at all stages of lung development. Thus, both morphologic and biochemical investigations make it seem likely that lung elastic fibers are similar, if not identical to, elastic fibers from other tissues.

The Proteoglycans

General Characteristics

All tissues contain amorphous, acellular, poorly described material termed "ground substance." This amorphous matrix generally invests the extracellular space surrounding other connective tissue elements. Ground substance contains serum constituents (e.g., proteins, glucose, urea, amino acids, electrolytes, and hormones), cell metabolites, degradative products of collagen and elastic fibers, enzymes, proteoglycans, and other glycoproteins (187, 188). The "other glycoproteins" are poorly defined, but probably include elastic fiber microfibrils and are clearly distinct from the 7 known proteoglycans. Considerably more is known about the composition, synthesis, and function of proteoglycans.

The proteoglycans are composed of both protein and glycosaminoglycan (GAG). The latter are well-defined complex polysaccharides that used to be called acid mucopolysaccharides (187). The GAG are covalently linked to the protein portion of the proteoglycan (except, perhaps, in hyaluronic acid, for which there is a controversy concerning whether hyaluronic acid exists alone or as a polysaccharide-protein complex) (187, 188).

Very little is known of the composition of the protein portion of the proteolgycans, except that they are large proteins in which serine is usually the amino acid to which the linkage to the GAG is formed by an ester bond. In some proteoglycans, such as the keratan sulfate-protein, linkage of the GAG to the protein can occur through threonine residues as well (187, 189, 190). There are variable numbers of GAG chains attached to each protein, but the number is large, usually 30 to 100. In most cases, all of the GAG chains attached to the protein are identical; thus, the proteoglycans are named for the specific GAG component. The exception is the chondroitin sulfate-keratan sulfate-protein complex found in cartilage (191). Except for heparin, which is stored in mast cells, all of the proteoglycans are extracellular, unless they are in the process of secretion or degradation.

The 7 types of GAG include hyaluronic acid, chondroitin-4-sulfate, chondroitin-6-sulfate, dermatan sulfate, heparin, heparan sulfate, and keratan sulfate (187). They are all composed of repeating disaccharides; each disaccharide contains an amino sugar (termed, hexosamine) and an uronic acid sugar (table 3). In all cases, the hexosamine is basically glucosamine or galactosamine with side groups such as sulfate-, acetyl-, or sulfamino- attached; the uronic acid is glucuronic or iduronic, except for keratan sulfate, in which galactose is substituted for the uronic acid. There are a varying number of these repeating disaccharide units in each GAG chain, usually 10 to 60, except in hyaluronic acid, which has as many as 2,500 (187, 189, 190). All 7 types of GAG are found in lung (2, 192), with keratan sulfate being confined to the tracheobronchial tree, presumably in the cartilage (2).

By several criteria, the connective tissue proteoglycans are clearly distinguishable from mucin glycoproteins secreted by the tracheobronchial tree. (1) The mucin glycoproteins have much shorter carbohydrate side chains on the protein. (2) The mucin glycoproteins have a large proportion of N-acetylglucosamine, glucose, galactose, and fucose, but lack uronic acid. (3) Some of the mucin glycoproteins are acidic secondary to the presence of sialic acid (and, occasionally, sulfate), but most are neutral (compared to most proteoglycans, which are acidic because of the high sulfate content). (4) Newly synthesized tracheal glycoproteins are resistant to hyaluronidase (the same enzyme cleaves several GAG) (2, 193).

Histologically, there are no specific stains for GAG. Methods such as periodic acid-Schiff, alcian blue, and toluidine blue staining for light microscopy, and ruthenium red for electron microscopy all positively stain GAG; however, other acidic materials (e.g., nucleic acids and other acidic glycoproteins) may stain with these methods (118). There are no methods that specifical-

TABLE 3

STRUCTURAL FEATURES OF THE GLYCOSAMINOGLYCAN
COMPONENT OF PROTEOGLYCANS*

GLYCOSAMINOGLYCAN	AMINO SUGAR (HEXOSAMINES)	URONIC ACID	APPROXIMATE NUMBER OF DISACCHARIDES
HYALURONIC ACID 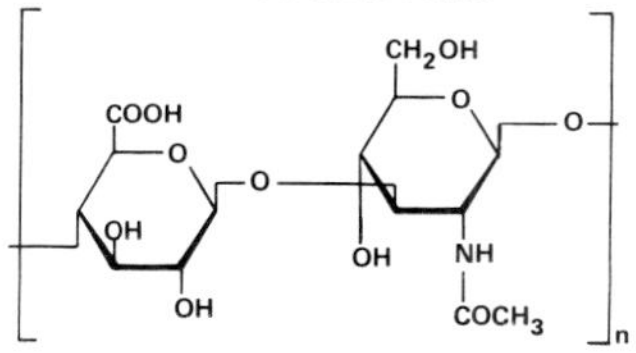	N-acetylglucosamine	Glucuronic	500-2500
CHONDROITIN 4-SULFATE 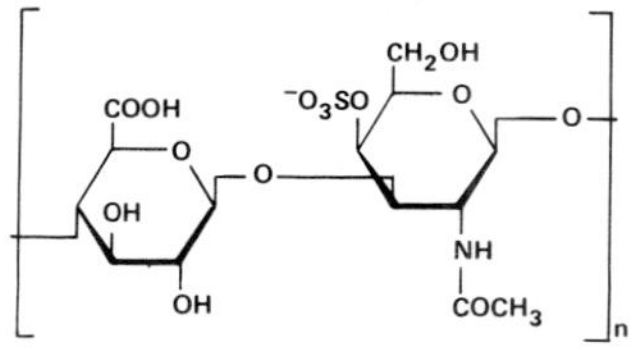	N-acetylgalactosamine 4-sulfate	Glucuronic	60
DERMATAN SULFATE 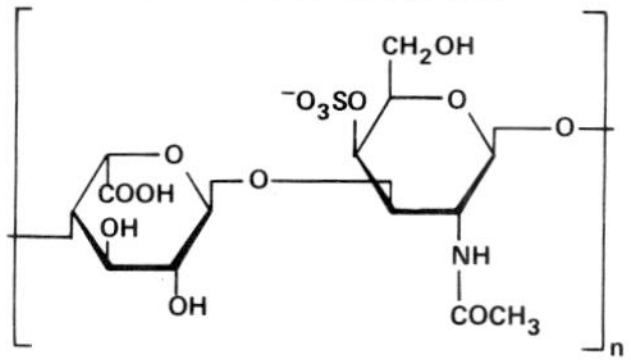	N-acetygalactosamine 4 or 6-sulfate	Iduronic	40-60
KERATAN SULFATE 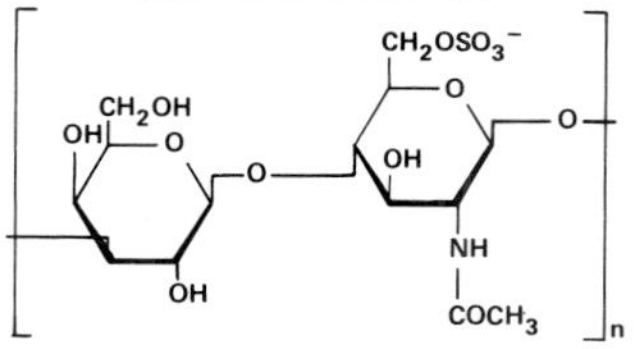	N-acetylglucosamine 6-sulfate	(Galactose)	10-20
HEPARAN SULFATE AND HEPARIN 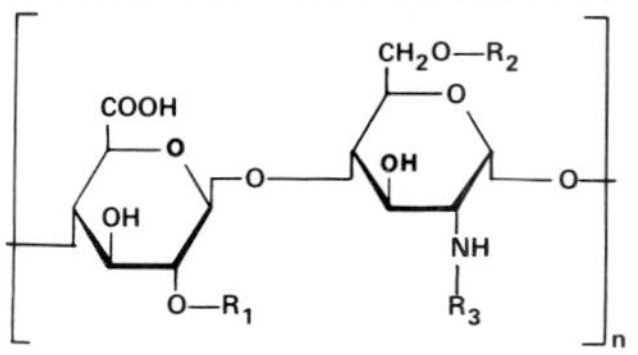	Heparan SO_4 { N-sulfamidoglucosamine or N-acetylglucosamine 6-sulfate } Heparin N-sulfamidoglucosamine 6-sulfate	Glucuronic or Iduronic	10-20

*The left-hand column indicates the structure of the repeating disaccharides that constitute glycosaminoglycan polysaccharide chains. Chondroitin-6-sulfate is identical to chondroitin-4-sulfate, except the former is sulfated at carbon-6. For heparan sulfate, R_1 = hydrogen (H); R_2 = H or sulfate (SO_3^-); R_3 = H, $COCH_3$, or SO_3^-. For heparin, R_1 = H or SO_3^-; R_2 = SO_3^-; R_3 = SO_3^-. The center columns identify the pairs of hexosamines and uronic acids that constitute the repeating disaccharide units. The right-hand column indicates the approximate number of disaccharide units in the polysaccharide chains.

ly identify a specific GAG; however, there are enzymes, e.g., hyaluronidase and chondroitinase ABC, that selectively degrade GAG types, and morphologic studies can be done before and after enzymatic digestion of the tissue to help localize a specific GAG.

There is almost nothing known of the mechanisms of biosynthesis of the protein portion of proteoglycans, although studies with protein synthesis inhibitors suggest that the mechanisms are similar to those of other proteins destined for secretion. The protein probably must be synthesized before GAG synthesis begins (194). To begin GAG synthesis, in general, the first sugar residue is enzymatically linked to the protein through an ester linkage to serine (figure 7). Subsequently, the GAG chain is elongated by sequential addition of individual sugars carried to the end of the growing GAG chain as precursor nucleotide sugars. In the GAG studied, the first few sugar residues added to the protein are different from the alternating sugar residues found in the rest of the chain. The sugar residues in the "linkage region" (e.g., xylose-galactose-glucuronic acid- are the linkage residues in chondroitin-4- and -6-sulfate) require separate enzymes for incorporation. Sulfate is added, where appropriate, after the repeating disaccharide residues are incorporated into the growing GAG chain. Sulfate transferases catalyze this transfer of sulfate groups from "activated sulfate" (3'-phosphoadenlylylsulfate) to the GAG chain (figure 7).

The enzymes responsible for GAG synthesis are not well defined; they are probably an intrinsic part of the membranes of the rough endoplasmic reticulum, smooth endoplasmic reticulum, and Golgi apparatus. A more detailed description of GAG synthesis can be found in several reviews (190, 195).

The elucidation of the genetic defects in the hereditable mucopolyssachaidoses led to a description of the stepwise degradation of GAG by lysosomal enzymes (β-glucuronidase, β-N-acetylhexosaminidase, N-acetylhexosamine-O-sulfatase, N-sulfatase, and iduronidase). Rather than taking place in the extracellular space, most GAG degradation occurs within phagolysosomes (187, 196).

There is limited information defining which cells synthesize GAG (Table 1). At a minimum, mesenchymal cells, i.e., fibroblasts, chondrocytes (195, 197), and endothelial cells (198, 199) are responsible, and it is probable that mast cells synthesize at least heparin (195). In addition, epithelial cells have been implicated in GAG synthesis (200). Mesenchymal cells may be responsible for GAG degradation, and phagocytic cells, such as macrophages, are known to contain enyzmes that cleave GAG (187, 201).

Glycosaminoglycans in Lung

Until recently, there was very little information available concerning the GAG in lung, although for years, lung has been a known source of heparin, heparan sulfate, and dermatan sul-

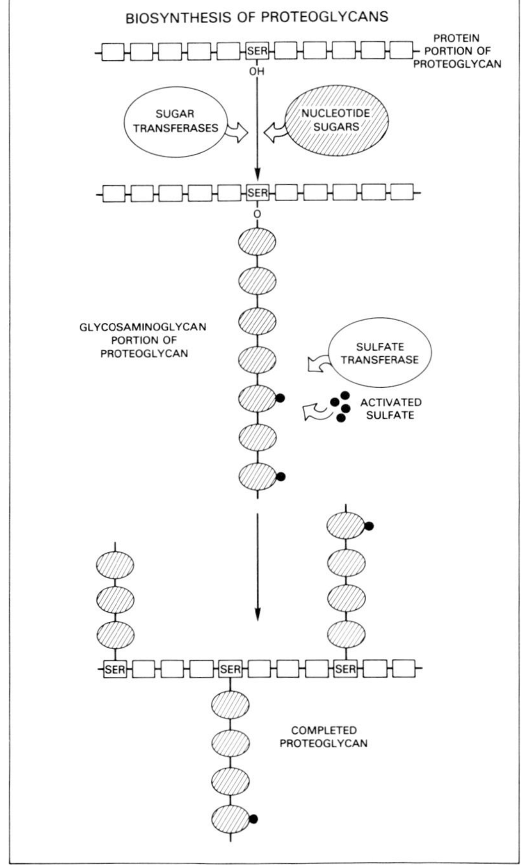

Fig. 7. Biosynthesis of the proteoglycans. The protein portion of the proteoglycan is synthesized first (—☐— = amino acid). Starting with a link to a serine residue (ser), sugar transferases take component nucleotide sugars and add them sequentially to the growing sugar side chain, forming the glycosaminoglycan (GAG) portion of the proteoglycan. Except for the first few sugars added, all of the sugars in the GAG are in repeating disaccharide units (table 3). In the synthesis of sulphated GAG, a sulfate transferase takes activated sulfate (3'-phosphoadenylsulfate) and adds sulfate to the GAG where appropriate. The completed proteoglycan has a single protein and many GAG side chains. See text for details.

fate. For example, a common source of the heparin used clinically is purified from bovine lung. There have been no systematic morphologic studies of lung GAG, although GAG can be seen to be abundant in the trachea and present in parenchyma.

Hyaluronic acid, chondroitin-4- and -6-sulfate, dermatan sulfate, heparin, and heparan sulfate have been found in bovine (202), rat (203) and rabbit (192) parenchyma and in bovine pleura (202). There is no keratan sulfate in the parenchyma or pleura, but it has been described in human tracheobronchial cartilage (204). In the adult, the concentration of the combined GAG represent approximately 0.5 per cent of the dry weight of parenchyma (2). In the next section, we will detail the changes in lung GAG type and quantity with maturation.

Except for endothelial cells, it is not known which cells of the lung synthesize the GAG (199); but rabbit lung parenchyma is active in GAG synthesis *in vitro* (192) (table 1). In the adult, total GAG synthesis includes continued production of each GAG type (hyaluronic acid, heparan sulfate, chondroitin-4- and -6-sulfate, heparin, and dermatan sulfate). This will be discussed later with reference to lung maturation.

Quantification of Connective Tissue in Normal Lung

As detailed by Thurlbeck (205), the development of lung is extraordinarily complex and quite species dependent. The connective tissue components are so important in the control of lung development *in utero* and in the postnatal mechanical properties of lung, that the eventual understanding of the mechanisms controlling the amounts, types, and locations of lung connective tissue will be invaluable in understanding anatomic and physiologic lung maturation. In this discussion, we will arbitrarily divide the discussion by connective tissue component, rather than by age. Morphologic correlates will only be mentioned; they are amply described by Thurlbeck (205).

Collagen

The most detailed data concerning changes in lung collagen with age are from the rabbit (12). In these studies, most of the lung was used, so the values for collagen concentration are average values of parenchyma, small and moderate-sized bronchi, and small and moderate-sized blood vessels, omitting hilar structures and

visceral pleura (figure 8). Although total lung mass of the rabbit increases rapidly from 10 days before birth through the neonatal period, the total amount of collagen in the lung accumulates even faster, so that the average concentration of collagen in lung is constantly increasing until maturity is reached. Once the rabbit passes through the weanling period, lung mass (12) and collagen concentration are stable (figure 8).

Preliminary data from (J. Collins: Unpublished observations) our laboratory indicate that after birth, most age-related changes in lung collagen concentration occur in the parenchyma. By comparison, tracheal, bronchial tree, and vasculature tree collagen concentrations change slowly. These quantitative biochemical measurements parallel what is seen morphologically; by birth, the bronchial and vascular trees are completely developed, yet there is continued alveolar maturation until the weanling period (205).

There are only preliminary data concerning the changes in human lung collagen during lung growth. There is a 12-fold increase in paren-

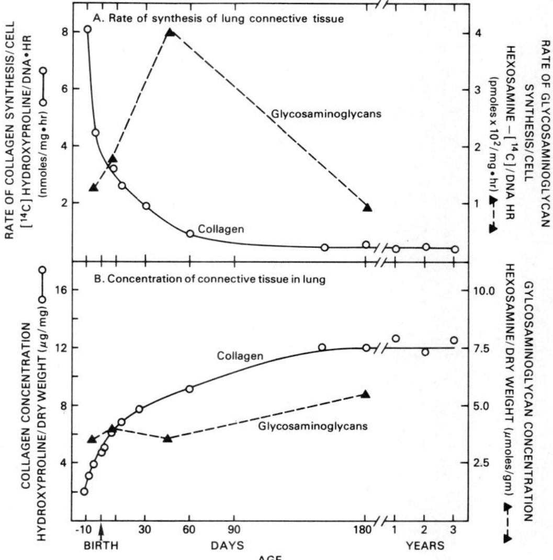

Fig. 8. Rate of synthesis and content of connective tissue elements during development of the rabbit lung. (A) Rate of collagen synthesis per cell (○———○) and rate of glycosaminoglycan synthesis per cell (▲-----▲). The maximal rate of glycosaminoglycan synthesis occurs substantially later than maximal collagen synthesis. (B) Concentration of collagen and glycosaminoglycans in lung at several ages; "−10" refers to 10 days before birth. The collagen data include parenchyma and small- to moderate-sized airways and blood vessels (12). The glycosaminoglycan data are primarily from parenchyma (192). DNA = deoxyribonucleic acid.

chymal collagen concentration as the lung matures from the second-trimester fetal to adult stage (14), but there is no information at intermediate times. It is not clear whether human lung collagen concentration remains stable once maturity is reached (123, 206–213); in general, major changes have not been found. Much of the data is based on older, less specific methods, and differences in site selection (212) and sex (207) make comparisons between studies difficult.

In tissues other than lung, there is increasing evidence that there are age-related changes in the types of collagen present. For example, in skin, the ratio of Type III collagen to Type I collagen probably decreases with age (27). The marked heterogeneity of lung collagen, together with the known age-related differences in the development of lung structures, suggest that significant age-related alterations in the quantity of each collagen type will be found.

Elastic Fibers

It is difficult to summarize the changes in elastic fibers during maturation, because the technology used to quantify elastic tissue is crude, and most older studies used methods in which "elastin" was variably contaminated with other material, including the microfibrillar component. No studies have specifically quantified lung elastic fiber microfibrils.

There are no data quantifying lung elastin concentration in the fetal or neonatal period, except in the chick, in which preliminary studies suggest a 5-fold increase in elastin concentration from 12 to 20 days *in utero* (Rosenbloom, J.: Personal communication). Correlative electron microscopic studies showed that elastic fibers begin to accumulate in peribronchial areas between 17 and 20 days (181, and Rosenbloom, J.: Personal communication). In the human fetus, analysis of elastin crosslinks has not demonstrated any change from 19 to 40 weeks of age (165). In the same study, it was pointed out that the "elastin" had a ratio of nonpolar amino acids (indicative of elastin) to polar amino acids (indicative of microfibrils) that increased with time *in utero*. This is probably because the methods used to isolate "elastin" also included microfibrillar component. Thus, the percentage of microfibrils in lung elastic fibers probably decreases with development, similar to that found in the maturing ligamentum nuchae (137).

There are more data available concerning lung elastic fibers once the lung is fully matured. But here also, the methods used are not specific for either elastin or microfibrils, even though most of the studies purport to quantify "elastin." As a result, data as to whether the elastin concentration in the parenchyma remains stable or increases with age are conflicting. Johnson and Andrews (213), using human parenchyma, found that the percentage of lung connective tissue that was elastin increased during aging. Pierce and Hocott (207) noted an age-related increase in the elastin concentration of the right middle lobe; but it was later found that this increase was probably from the pleura, interlobular septa, bronchi, and blood vessels, not from the parenchyma (123). As with collagen, there are differences in elastin concentration with sex (207), site (apex versus base) (212), and structure (123). In general, available data suggest that in adult human lung, elastin is a major component of pleura and parenchyma, but not of the tracheobronchial tree (123). The ratio of total collagen to total elastin varies from structure to structure. This ratio is 3 to 4:1 in parenchyma, 7 to 10:1 in bronchi, and 2 to 4:1 in blood vessels (123).

As with elastin in fetal life, there is no evidence that elastin becomes more crosslinked with postnatal development.

Proteoglycans

There are no data that quantify the protein moiety of these complex materials in lung. In the rabbit, analysis of total parenchymal glycosaminoglycan concentration shows that it is relatively stable throughout the newborn and weanling periods, but then increases approximately 60 per cent as the parenchyma completes the maturing process (192) (figure 8). In most species, total GAG represents 0.4 to 1.0 per cent of the dry weight of the adult parenchyma (2). There are marked differences in the per cent distribution of the specific types of parenchymal GAG with growth (192) (figure 9); these changes may have significance in relation to changing parenchymal properties during development.

Control of Connective Tissue Accumulation in Normal Lung and Experimental Models of Lung Growth

Collagen

As outlined above, there is a marked increase in collagen concentration as the lung develops from the late fetal stage to full maturity. The increase in average collagen concentration is probably due, at least in part, to the marked differ-

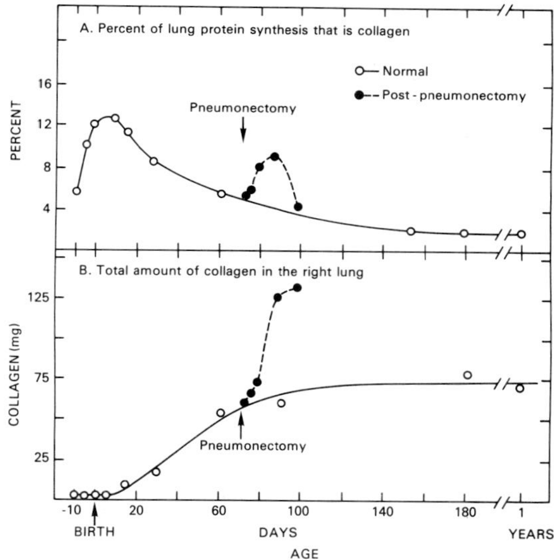

Fig. 9. Control of collagen accumulation in the rabbit lung during development and after pneumonectomy-induced lung growth (12, 214). (A) Shift of the protein-synthesizing capabilities of lung toward, and then away from, collagen synthesis during periods of rapid lung growth; (O———O) = normal; (●----●) = postpneumonectomy. The percentage of amino acids incorporated into collagen compared with total protein is shown. (B) Total amount of collagen in the right lung during normal lung development (O———O) and after left pneumonectomy (●----●) in the 72-day-old rabbit. In both normal and postpneumonectomy lung growth, the accumulation of lung collagen is preceded by a shift of the protein-synthesizing machinery toward collagen. After growth is complete, the relative percentage of protein synthesis that is collagen returns to normal; "−10" = 10 days before birth.

ence in the rate of collagen synthesis found in fetal and newborn lungs compared to the adult lung (12) (figure 8). Whereas the rate of collagen synthesis per cell (averaged over all lung cells) is at a constant low level in the adult, it is 16 times higher in late fetal life and 5 times higher in the newborn. Not only are there higher absolute rates of collagen synthesis in early life, it appears that the lung shifts its protein-synthesizing capabilities toward collagen synthesis during this period (12) (figures 9). In the late fetal and early newborn stage of development, approximately 12 per cent of the amino acids incorporated into protein by lung go into collagen, compared to 4 per cent in the adult. This ability to shift the emphasis of protein synthesis toward collagen appears to be available to the lung whenever it grows.

This concept is dramatically illustrated in the case of postpneumonectomy lung growth. For some time, it has been known that if one lung is removed from the rabbit, cat, dog, or rat, the mass of the remaining lung increases to approximately that of both lungs. In general, the resulting lung is essentially normal, although there is still debate as to whether this growth response reflects primarily an increase in the number or size of individual alveoli. When a left pneumonectomy is performed on a 72-day-old rabbit, total lung mass doubles within 1 month. This growth is accompanied by a shift in the emphasis of protein synthesis toward collagen synthesis (214) (figure 9). As collagen accumulates and reaches a stable state (yielding a normal average collagen concentration for new lung), the protein-synthesizing machinery goes back to synthesizing collagen at a normal rate. Interestingly, these marked shifts in biochemical activity seem to be controlled by mechanical factors, because obliteration of the pleural space remaining after resection of the left lung completely halts the increase in right lung growth and the concomitant changes in collagen synthesis and accumulation that usually occur after pneumonectomy (214).

The rates of collagen synthesis in the midtrimester human fetal lung are approximately the same as those in the adult human lung and the adult rabbit lung (14). Detailed data on the rates of collagen synthesis in the late fetal, newborn, or adolescent human lung are not available. If the situation is analogous to that in the rabbit (either normal or postpneumonectomy lung growth), we would expect higher levels of collagen synthesis during the rapid growth phase of human lung maturation.

Although there is an apparent relationship between a high rate of collagen synthesis and collagen accumulation, it must be kept in mind that an accumulation of any biochemical component is the result of a balance between the relative rates of synthesis and degradation of this component. Because synthesis of collagen is constant in the adult rabbit, the constant collagen concentration throughout maturity demands that there be a constant rate of collagen degradation that will balance this continued synthesis. Preliminary studies by Cowan and associates (114) have shown that throughout postnatal lung maturation of rabbits, there are no significant changes in the rate of degradation of newly synthesized collagen, suggesting that the control of age-related collagen accumulation is through synthetic mechanisms, rather than by a decrease in degradative mechanisms. Nothing is known about collagen degradation in the human lung.

The changes in collagen synthesis and degradation described are average changes, including all lung structures and all collagen types. The relative changes in synthesis and degradation of specific types of collagen during periods of growth are not known. If the normal pattern of synthesis and degradation of each type of collagen in lung can be described for the different stages of lung maturation, it will be possible to compare these parameters in diseased lung as well (215). For example, in pulmonary fibrosis, the lung may revert to a fetal pattern of types of collagen synthesized, in the same way that red cell precursors revert to fetal hemoglobin synthesis in certain adult hematologic disorders.

Elastic Fibers

As pointed out in the section on quantification, there is very little information regarding the amounts of elastic fiber elastin and microfibrillar components during growth. There are no data available concerning age-related changes in the rates of synthesis of either component. Studies have shown that mouse lung synthesizes elastin (169), that embryonic chick lung synthesizes elastin (Rosenbloom, J.: Personal communication), and that lysyl oxidase activity (per unit lung mass) is increased after unilateral pneumonectomy in the rat (93), but no system has as yet yielded quantitative information as to the site or quantity of lung elastin during growth. Because there is increasing evidence that elastic fibers are fundamental to alveolar maturation, future quantification of elastic fibers should be useful in helping to understand these processes.

Proteoglycans

There is no method available to quantify the synthesis of the protein portion of the proteoglycans, but detailed data are now available concerning glycosaminoglycan synthesis in the maturing rabbit parenchyma. The post-weanling increase in GAG concentration found in rabbit parenchyma may, in part, be due to the relative increase in the rate of synthesis of parenchymal GAG per cell (averaged over all parenchymal cells) seen in the weanling period (192) (figure 8); however, the relative changes in the concentration of each type of glycosaminoglycan in the parenchyma cannot be due only to changes in

rates of synthesis, because the rates of synthesis of specific types of GAG do not necessarily parallel the dramatic alterations in concentration of GAG types found with age (192) (figure 10). Presumably, interstitial GAG concentration is controlled by the balance of synthesis and degradation. Although enzymes such as hyaluronidase have been described in lung (201), the general mechanisms and rates of GAG degradation in lung have not been studied.

Studies with lung buds have shown that the composition of the extracellular connective tissue strongly influences primordial lung structure and facilitates bronchial branching (216, 217). For example, when lung buds are placed on one side of a filter, bronchial branching occurs if mesodermal elements are on the other side, but no branching occurs if the mesoderm is removed (217). If lung buds are treated with collagenase and the mesoderm withheld, pre-

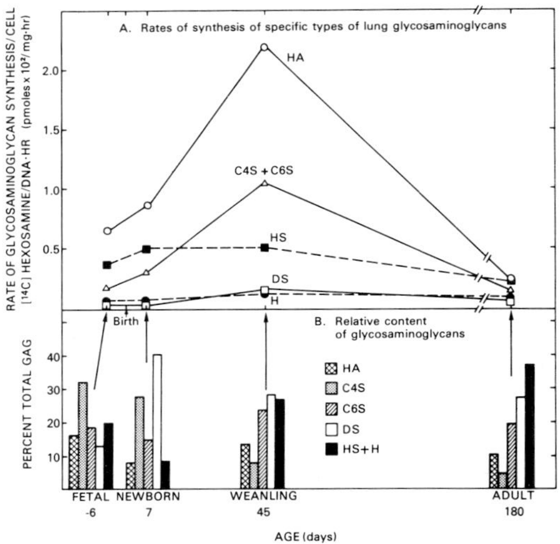

Fig. 10. Rates of synthesis and content of individual glycosaminoglycan types during development of the rabbit lung parenchyma (192). Rate of synthesis per cell of hyaluronic acid (HA) (o———o); chondroitin-4-sulfate (C4S) and chondroitin-6-sulfate (C6S), (△———△); heparan sulfate (HS), (■----■); dermatan sulfate (DS); (□———□), and heparin (H), (●----●). (B) Percentage of total proteoglycan accounted for by each glycosaminoglycan types at several ages. Abbreviations are as indicated in A. Although increases in rates of synthesis of some glycosaminoglycans precede accumulation of that glycosaminoglycan, the situation is complex, and other control mechanisms (e.g., degradation) are probably important in lung glycosaminoglycan accumulation; "−6" = 6 days before birth.

viously existing lung morphologic features disappear and no new clefts form in the rudimentary lung (218).

It is apparent that the control of lung connective tissue accumulation and the structure of lung itself are dependent on complex patterns of connective tissue synthesis and degradation. Extracellular factors, including the composition of connective tissue in the local milieu, seem to play important roles. As methods are developed to quantify the synthesis and degradation of each component of connective tissue, we will have powerful tools to investigate lung growth and development.

Connective Tissue and Lung Disease

General Principles

Two major groups of noninfectious disease of lung, the emphysematous and fibrotic disorders, are generally considered to involve aberrations of the normal connective tissue of lung. As we review the current knowledge of these disorders, several general principles should be kept in mind.

(1) The connective tissue of lung is complex and interdependent in anatomic arrangement and physical properties. Alterations in strong noncovalent interactions between proteoglycans and collagen, collagen and elastin, or elastin and microfibrillar components may be crucial.

(2) A significant proportion of lung connective tissue is in the large conductive and septal structures (16). If a disease is believed to be in the parenchyma, then parenchyma should be analyzed separately, because marked changes in parenchymal connective tissue may be required for average lung connective tissue to be affected.

(3) Even if parenchyma alone is analyzed, it should be remembered that it is composed of several distinct structures, each containing multiple connective tissue types. During the progression of parenchymal disease, the composition of each structure may change, possibly in opposite directions. Alterations in minor, yet physiologically crucial, substructures will not be detected until techniques are developed to quantify connective tissue on this level.

(4) Morphologically distinguishable subcategories of lung disease (e.g., panacinar versus centrilobular emphysema) should be analyzed separately. The biochemical abnormalities may be completely different.

(5) The marked insolubility and complexity of lung connective tissue severely limits the methodology that can be used to separate, purify, and quantify individual connective tissue components. Methods developed for other organs may not be specific for quantification of lung connective tissue components.

(6) Connective tissue composition represents a balance between synthesis and destruction. Accumulation could be due to a decrease in degradation; apparent destruction could be secondary to a decrease in synthesis.

(7) The response to injury could be ineffective repair, e.g., synthesis of normal quantities of connective tissue in abnormal locations. This anatomic "redistribution" of normal connective tissue will be extremely difficult to detect biochemically.

Emphysema

Although the primary focus in human emphysema has been on elastic tissue, there is some evidence implicating alterations of all 3 categories of connective tissue in this disease. Each will be considered separately.

Quantity of elastic fibers. Morphologically, destruction of elastic fibers is easily detected (182, 219, 220), but there is little evidence of biochemical derangement. All biochemical studies of elastic fibers in emphysema have been directed toward the elastin component. Examination of the whole lung has failed to reveal any difference in elastin content expressed as total lung elastin or per cent dry weight (208, 209, 221). Elastin content of the right middle lobe was somewhat decreased in patients with a_1-antitrypsin deficiency, but the differences were not significant (222, 223). Reports on elastin content of lung parenchyma in emphysema compared to normal have not been consistent, although the ratio of elastin to lung weight in peripheral emphysematous lung tissue has usually been found to be normal (212, 213, 224). In one study, the concentration of elastin in peripheral emphysematous lung was higher than normal, but the increase detected was small and not significant. In another, parenchyma from a small number of emphysematous lungs "subjacent to areas of bulla formation" was found to have a markedly decreased concentration of elastin (224). Unfortunately, histologic description of this lung tissue was not included; pathologic correlates could have given insight into how this tissue may have differed from "emphysematous parenchyma" analyzed in studies in which the quantity of elastin was normal.

Quality of elastic fibers. Amino acid analysis of elastin from emphysematous lung has also yielded conflicting results. In an early report, amino acid composition of elastin isolated by hot alkali methods from peripheral emphysematous lung showed no significant differences when compared to normal tissues (167). Other studies, using hot alkali or elastase methods of elastin isolation, have suggested that elastin from emphysematous lung has a higher ratio of polar to nonpolar amino acids than does elastin from normal lung (225–227). There are several explanations for these findings.

(*1*) As discussed previously, a high ratio of polar to nonpolar amino acids in elastin could be due to an artifact of analysis (i.e., the elastin was variably contaminated by microfibrils or other acidic structural proteins). This could be due to a relative loss of elastin during extraction, a stronger association between elastin and contaminating proteins, or a change in the composition of contaminating proteins in emphysematous lungs.

(*2*) Emphysema could result from selective degradation of nonpolar regions of elastin. If the polar groups of elastin were within an inner core surrounded by a shell of nonpolar regions, selective proteolysis of the nonpolar shell could result in altered "elastin" with a high ratio of polar to nonpolar amino acids (227).

(*3*) Less likely, emphysema could be a genetic disorder in which the primary sequence of tropoelastin is altered (e.g., higher polar amino acid content), thus leading to a faulty structure of elastin, predisposing to the development of emphysema (226).

Resolution of these possibilities will require studies using methods capable of separating elastin, microfibrils, and other insoluble nonelastin proteins.

Quantity of collagen. Studies of collagen content in emphysematous lung have revealed relatively few differences compared to age-matched, normal lung. Neither total collagen in the lung nor total collagen in the right middle lobe has been found to differ significantly from normal (208, 209, 221). Similarly, no differences in total right middle lobe collagen have been found in patients with emphysema associated with α_1-antitrypsin deficiency compared to normal subjects (222, 223). When parenchyma alone has been analyzed, collagen concentration from emphysematous lung has usually been reported as normal (213, 228). In a single study, collagen concentration in emphysematous tissue (expressed as hydroxyproline per wet weight of tissue) was 40 per cent higher than normal, and the difference was more pronounced in apical tissues, in which emphysematous changes are usually more prominent (212); however, lung weight and water content were both decreased, and the apparent increase in collagen concentration could, in part, reflect loss of noncollagen lung constituents.

Quality of collagen. Studies on collagen content of emphysematous lung preceded the recent discovery of the heterogeneity of lung collagen, and no information is available at present about the relative proportions of the types of collagen present in these lungs; however, the concentration of collagen in bronchial cartilage from patients with emphysema has been demonstrated not to change compared to that in bronchial cartilage from age-matched control subjects, suggesting that Type II collagen is unaffected (229). In another study, no significant differences in the amino acid composition of collagen extracted from normal and emphysematous lungs were found; however, the low proline, glycine, and alanine contents of the "collagen" that was analyzed strongly suggest contamination with noncollagen protein (213).

The solubility of collagen crudely reflects the degree of crosslinking or types of collagen present (Types III and IV are relatively insoluble). The data on the solubility of collagen of emphysematous lungs are skimpy; most studies showed no difference (213, 225, 228).

Morphologic studies suggest that there is considerable reorganization of collagen within the lung during development of emphysema. Within certain localized environments, such as alveolar basement membrane, there may be destruction of collagen, whereas in other areas, there may be local accumulation (182, 230). This type of reorganization of collagen is extremely difficult to detect biochemically. At this time, there is no biochemical evidence either for or against this concept; however, the finding of collagen antibodies in the serum of patients with emphysema (231) does suggest that collagen fragments are being "seen" by the immune system, possibly secondary to "reorganization."

Although these data suggest that change in lung collagen content or composition is not a prominent feature of emphysema, final conclusions must await the development of more sophisticated methods of analysis. Collagen content and composition must be examined not in whole lung and "parenchyma," but in individual subunits of structure. Potential changes in the interaction of collagen with other connective tissue elements must be explored, and possible changes in collagen metabolism, both synthesis and degradation, should be investigated before the role of collagen in the pathogenesis of emphysema can be resolved.

Proteoglycans. The role of proteoglycans in lung disease has received scant attention. The separation and quantification of proteoglycans is a formidable task because of their marked heterogeneity and relatively small contribution to lung connective tissue mass. Understanding of the potential importance of proteoglycans in fostering association between other connective tissue elements had led to speculation that these components are important determinants of normal lung structure and may play a central role in the pathogenesis of emphysema (232). Little data are available to support this concept. Hexosamine content and the ratio of galactosamine to glucosamine in emphysematous peripheral lung parenchyma are not different from normal (233); however, hexosamine determination is an extremely insensitive index of lung proteoglycan, because a large amount of hexosamine present in lung is found in nonproteoglycan lung protein and residual blood proteins.

When hexosamine content in lung proteoglycan was reinvestigated after prior separation of glycosaminoglycans from other glycoproteins, total parenchymal glycosaminoglycans (as judged by uronic acid content) were similar in normal and emphysematous peripheral lung tissue, but the relative content of galactosamine containing glycosaminoglycans (chondroitin-4-sulfate, chondroitin-6-sulfate, and dermatan sulfate) was significantly reduced (228). Specific glycosaminoglycan types were not isolated in this study, so the fractions(s) responsible for this change could not be determined. In another study, the ratio of galactosamine to glucosamine of bronchial cartilage from older patients with emphysema was significantly higher than that of bronchial cartilage from age-matched control subjects, but glycosaminoglycan content per se was not determined (229).

Changes in glycosaminoglycans in inflammatory disease of the lung appear to parallel changes in other inflamed tissue. The lungs of rats raised under nonaseptic conditions had more glycosaminoglycans, particularly hyaluronic acid and heparan sulfate, compared to germ-free rats (203). Thus, the inflammatory state of lung must also be considered when evaluating data from emphysematous lungs. Clearly, currently available data are too preliminary to reach any conclusion about the role of proteoglycans in emphysema.

Experimental protease-induced emphysema. Although other inducing agents have been used (234, 235), the exposure of lung to proteolytic enzymes has received the widest attention as an experimental model of emphysema. The morphologic and physiologic consequences of *in vivo* exposure of lung to these enzymes has been discussed in detail elsewhere; most investigators agree that inhalation of proteolytic enzymes leads to a state that closely resembles clinical emphysema, both morphologically and physiologically (236–247). We will concentrate primarily on the biochemical findings in protease-induced emphysema and what these findings imply.

General Characteristics of the Enzymes

Papain has been the enzyme used most extensively, although enzymes from a number of sources, including plants (bromelain, bromelin, and ficin) (245–248), alveolar macrophages (249), polymorphonuclear leukocytes (249–252), pancreas (elastase) (253), and bacteria (alcalase, maxatase, thermolysin, brinase, and pronase) (245, 254) are also capable of producing experimental emphysema. These enzymes all have generalized proteolytic activity; besides that, they have very little in common. They have different active sites, different optimal pH and ionic conditions, and are inactivated by different inhibitors (255). Because there are no common characteristics of the enzymes themselves, investigators have focused attention on the concept that the effectiveness of enzymes in producing emphysema is related to their ability to degrade a common substrate.

Specificity for Elastin

Light microscopic studies of lungs of animals exposed to these enzymes show elastic fiber destruction (242). Electron microscopic studies suggest that papain-induced emphysema is associated with early, selective destruction of the amorphous component of elastic fibers, leaving the microfibrillar component intact (247). Thus, it is not unreasonable to expect that the effectiveness of the enzymes in producing emphysema is related to their ability to degrade elastin. This is supported by studies demonstrating that purified preparations of human leukocyte elastase have elastolytic activity and will induce experimental emphysema, but rabbit leukocytes proteases have no elastolytic activity and will not produce emphysema (251, 252). The ability of intratracheally administered papain preparations and intravenously administered bacterial enzymes to produce emphysema correlates well with *in vitro* enzyme activity against elastin (179, 254); however, these enzymes have a wide spectrum of substrate specificity, and their relative potencies against other potential lung substrates, e.g., basement membrane and cellular elements, have not been investigated. In general, the bacterial enzymes capable of producing emphysema also have significant activity against denatured collagen (254).

Biochemical analyses of lungs from animals exposed to proteolytic enzymes do not directly show that there are decreased amounts of elastin (241, 256). These studies, however, are not definitive, and for now, the question must remain open. Amino acid analysis of "elastin" from lungs of rats given intravenous thermolysin revealed large increases in the ratio of polar to nonpolar amino acids (248). As discussed in the section on human emphysema, this finding may represent selective digestion of elastin leaving the microfibrils or could simply be an artifact of "elastin" isolation.

Specificity for Collagen or Proteoglycans

There is little direct evidence that enzyme-derived emphysema is secondary to collagen proteolysis. Total lung collagen content has been found not to change (241). Except for the dissolution of collagen fibrils seen early in papain-induced emphysema (241), morphologic studies have revealed no abnormalities in collagen (245–247). This is surprising, because the N- and C-terminal teleopeptides of tropocollagen are susceptible to many of the emphysema-producing enzymes. If these regions were cleaved, we would expect to find increased collagen solubility; this has not been studied.

When pure bacterial collagenase is used as an enzyme source, no morphologic or physiologic alterations characteristic of emphysema are seen (244, 257, 258). The lungs of these animals do show alterations in reticulin fibers, but not in collagen fibrils (244). The inability of collagenase to produce changes in the interstitium may be related to its inability to reach its substrate when administered intratracheally. In comparison, enzymes that do produce experimental emphysema are generally nonspecific proteases, and they may be better able to damage the alveolar epithelium and basement membrane, thus gaining access to the interstitium.

There is no information available on interstitial proteoglycans in enzyme-induced experimental emphysema, although the protein portions of the proteoglycans are probably susceptible to the enzymes.

Endogenous Factors

Although it is not yet clear which connective tissue component(s) are initially attacked, it is apparent that at least some of the initial destruction can be mediated by the enzymes themselves. The development of the histologic picture of emphysema begins very rapidly; in several models, damage to alveolar walls with enlargement of air spaces occurs within hours (242, 245, 253). In addition, emphysematous changes have been produced in excised lungs treated with enzymes *in vitro* (258). These data suggest that experimental emphysema is the result of enzymes ⟶ connective tissue damage ⟶ emphysema; however, the situation is not that simple, and there is ample evidence that the responses by lung tissues and extra-lung factors to the primary insult play a role. In studies in which lungs have been examined serially, the emphysematous lesion is seen to progress for periods varying from several weeks to several years after a single exposure to enzyme (242, 245, 253). This progression continued despite the fact that, at least in one study, enzymatic activity was almost completely inhibited within 2 hours of enzyme instillation, presumably by serum and tissue antiproteases (253).

A number of workers have suggested that the initial cellular and tissue damage produced by the enzymes secondarily recruits inflammatory and immunologic responses that perpetuate proteolysis of lung connective tissue. It has been demonstrated that collagen is chemotactic for polymorphonuclear leukocytes, particularly after it has been cleaved by animal collagenase (259). Enzyme-induced emphysema is accompanied by an accumulation of polymorphonuclear leukocytes, macrophages, and mononuclear cells, although this accumulation is not necessarily striking (242, 245, 253), each of which contains a wide variety of proteases with activity against elastic fibers, collagen, and proteoglycans (175, 176, 260–262). Many of these proteases are capable of producing emphysema themselves (251, 252). Thus, the introduction of proteolytic enzymes into lung parenchyma could upset the balance between proteolysis and inhibitors of proteolysis present in serum and lung tissue. This process may allow the continued destruction of parenchyma after the initial insult has been dissipated. Mechanical factors from normal respiration may also play a role in further disrupting alveolar connective tissue once it has been disturbed (263).

Repair Processes

Although proteolysis has been considered the keystone of the pathogenesis of emphysema for many years, changes in the synthesis of connective tissue elements could also play a role.

Early in the course of papain-induced emphysema, selective digestion of elastin results in the finding of isolated microfibrils. Later, only intact elastic fibers are found. This finding may be compatible with resynthesis of elastin elements, but the problem of morphologic quantification with electron microscopy leaves open the possibility that there was late proteolysis of microfibrils, leaving only normal elastic fibers that were never affected by the disease process (247).

Although synthesis of specific lung connective tissue elements in lung tissue exposed to proteolytic enzymes has not been studied, protein synthesis per unit mass of hampster lung tissue was almost twice normal in the 2 weeks after papain administration, whereas synthesis of lecithin (a component of lung surfactant) remained normal (241). When human fibroblasts were exposed to bacterial proteolytic enzymes capable of producing emphysema, collagen synthesis per cell was little affected, but total protein synthesis was markedly reduced, resulting in a marked increase in per cent collagen synthesis (264). These preliminary findings, coupled with the apparent proliferation of interstitial cells in lungs exposed to papain (241), raise the possibility that changes in the lung cell populations and changes in connective tissue synthesis by these cells may play roles in the pathogenesis of emphysema.

Summary

It is apparent that the enzyme models of emphysema have not completely resolved the issue of pathogenesis of emphysema *in vivo*; however, they have been extraordinarily useful and have led to some general principles. (*1*) The primary insult in emphysema is not known, but enzymatic attack, particularly of elastin, remains a strong possibility. It still must be shown that other events, such as alteration of basement membrane, proteolgycans, collagen-proteoglycan interactions, or microfibrillar component-elastin interactions are not important in the pathogenesis of emphysema. (*2*) After a primary enzymatic insult, there is progression of the lesion, possibly by lung and extra-lung factors mediating continued damage and possibly by reorganization of connective tissue. (*3*) There is still no direct biochemical evidence that in humans, even in Pi ZZ homozygous α_1-antitrypsin associated emphysema, that there is actually proteolysis of elastin *in vivo*.

Pulmonary Fibrosis

The fibrotic lung disorders are a subgroup of the so-called interstitial (16) or infiltrative diseases (265) of lung, of which there are more than 130 etiologic or morphologic categories. When the lung is injured by a variety of insults, there is often destruction of both cellular and noncellular elements of parenchyma. The remaining normal and injured cells are capable of reparative processes, and they attempt to restore normal parenchymal architecture and function (130). In many instances, however, the response is ineffective in restoring normality, and instead, the lung becomes "fibrotic," with destruction of architecture and loss of normal function.

There is little question that the fibrosis per se produces severe abnormalities in lung mechanics and gas exchange. Fulmer and associates (266) have, in preliminary studies, suggested that the maximal negative transthoracic pressure, the rate of decrease of the arterial P_{O_2} with increasing levels of exercise, and the rate of increase in the alveolar-arterial P_{O_2} difference with increasing levels of exercise correlate with the degree of parenchymal fibrosis, but not necessarily with the degree of parenchymal cellularity alone. Thus, it appears that parenchymal fibrosis is an important determinant of at least some of the abnormal functional parameters seen in this disease, including the development of arterial hypoxemia with exercise. It is reasonable, therefore, to direct our attention to the fibrosis itself as an important pathologic mechanism, the alleviation of which may lead to a lessening of abnormal lung function in this disease. It is also important to identify the primary insults or deficiencies that can initiate fibrosis, to understand how these insults make normal repair impossible, and to determine how the abnormal response (fibrosis) is mediated. Currently, 3 areas are under active investigation: collagen metabolism in human biopsy specimens; experimental animal models of pulmonary fibrosis; *in vitro* tissue culture models of the cellular elements involved in mediating the fibrotic response.

Biochemical measurements in human fibrotic disease. "Fibrosis" is a morphologic term that, translated into biochemical nomenclature, means "an increase in collagen." We would expect, therefore, that the lung of a patient with this disease would have increased amounts of collagen. Unfortunately, the problem is not that simple, and the application of biochemical methods to this disease has not yielded expected answers. As an example, the biopsy specimen shown in figure 11 is from a 60-year-old white woman with a 1-year history of breathlessness (16). Pulmonary function studies revealed a restrictive pattern, a moderately reduced diffusing capacity, a shift of the static volume-pressure curve downward and to the right, mild resting hypoxemia, and moderate hypoxemia with exercise; these findings are classic for the disorder. Although the biopsy specimen clearly shows "fibrosis," the amount of collagen per dry weight of lung was normal (patient, 21.7 ± 2.8 versus normal value, 26.1 ± 3.3 μg of hydroxyproline per mg dry weight), as was the rate of collagen synthesis per cell (patient, 0.328 versus normal value; 0.566 ± 0.092 nmole of [^{14}C]proline per mg of deoxyribonucleic acid (DNA) • hour). The percentage of total proteins synthesized that were collagen (patient, 1.8; normal value, 4.2 ± 0.8) was actually low (14, 16). These data do not state that, biochemically, the patient did not have fibrosis, but rather that there were abnormalities other than fibrosis, as yet only partially understood, that are inherent in the pathogenesis of the disorder. It must be realized that biochemical approaches to lung disease are limited by a severe handicap: to understand the disease, we must study it early in the course. To do this, the investigator is limited to the study of fresh biopsied material rather than whole lung. Thus, we cannot answer the question, Are there increases in the total amount of collagen in the lung and in the total amount of collagen synthesized by the entire lung? Rather, the data must be compared to parameters available in the biopsy specimen (e.g., the mass of the biopsy specimen or number of cells in the biopsy specimen). Re-examination of the biopsy specimen (figure 11) shows that it contains a great deal of "mass" that is abnormal and not collagen, and a vast number of cells that are not normal constituents of lung parenchyma, in particular, the nonlung mononuclear cells (lymphocytes, plasma cells, and macrophages). Thus, the amount of collagen may be vastly increased, but if other cellular and noncellular proteins are also increased to the same degree, the concentration of collagen will be normal. Likewise, because the number of cells per unit mass is increased (patient, 31.3 ± 2.5, versus normal value of 11.1 ± 3.4 mg of DNA per mg) (14, 16), and because a number of these cells (e.g., macrophages) do not make collagen (see section on collagen), the actual rate of collagen synthesis in the whole lung might be increased.

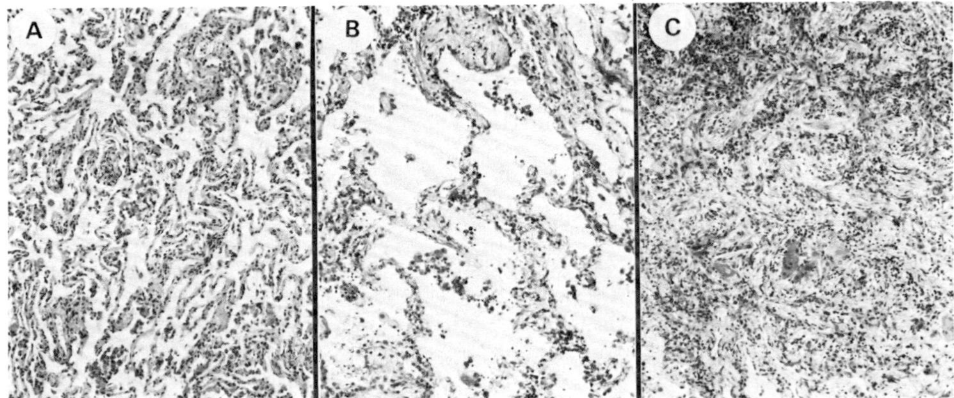

Fig. 11. Lung biopsy specimen from a 60-year-old woman with idiopathic fibrosis, 1 year after onset of symptoms. (A) Areas of minimally abnormal parenchyma are interspersed with (B) areas of active alveolitis and increased septal fibrosis and (C) areas of dense fibrosis and inflammation. It is apparent that the disease is very heterogeneous both in stage and distribution at any given site. In some stages, there are large increases in noncollagen parenchymal mass and in the number of noncollagen-producing cells (e.g., blood-derived cells) in addition to the fibrosis (hematoxylin and eosin stain; original magnification: $\times$ 130) (16).

Because it is obvious from biopsies of patients with these disorders that there is fibrosis present, why can we not demonstrate this abnormality on the biochemical level? From the above discussion, the answer is obvious, and it gives us clues to both pathogenesis and future studies. First, although fibrosis is part of the pathogenesis, there must be an increase in parenchymal components other than collagen (e.g., cells and other interstitial components). Second, studying a biopsy specimen may be too complex to unravel the molecular pathogenesis of this disorder. We may have to turn to models of fibrosis in experimental animals, or to even more simplified biochemical systems in which individual cell types can be studied alone and in response to external stimuli to understand events at the cellular level.

Experimental animal models of pulmonary fibrosis. A number of agents are used to initiate pulmonary fibrosis in animals, including physical agents, e.g., radiation (267, 268); O_2 (269); chemicals such as paraquat (270), N-nitroso-N-methylurethane (271, 272); drugs, e.g., bleomycin (273); viral infections (274); inhaled particles, such as silica (62, 275, 276), asbestos (277), and cadmium sulfate (278); toxic gases, e.g., ozone (279); immunologic mediators, such as bovine serum albumin immunization (280, 281), and antilung serum (282). Most of these models have been developed in attempts to parody the human disease in experimental animals, e.g., the effects of radiation and silicosis. Others, e.g., N-nitroso-N-methylurethane and the immunologic models, have been developed in attempts to mimic idiopathic pulmonary fibrosis (271, 278). Independent of their relevance to any human disease, all of the models are useful. As described in the previous section, pulmonary fibrosis is very complex; animal models are useful simply to develop new methodologies to study the human disease, just as the protease models have been useful in suggesting ways to study human emphysema. In this section, we will concentrate on the known connective tissue correlates of these animal models.

Although different radiation types, dosages, and animals result in somewhat different pathologic findings, serial observation has indicated that there are several general phases in the development of radiation fibrosis. The initial insult results in morphologic alterations in lung cells and interstitial edema. Both alveolar type II cells and endothelial cells appear to be relatively radiosensitive, and alterations in these cells and separation of the cells from the basement membrane are seen. Occasionally, immediate disruption of connective tissue fibrous elements is noted in this early stage. This is followed by a proliferative stage, characterized by accumulation of numerous cellular elements (macrophages, polymorphonuclear leukocytes, plasma cells, and mast cells), proliferation of interstitial cells and epithelial cells, and vascular destruction. Eventually, diffuse fibrosis, with marked distortion of normal architecture, results (283–295).

The marked alteration in lung cell populations that follows radiation, including changes in lung cells responsible for both connective synthesis and degradation, suggests that changes in cell populations can lead to imbalance in the rates of synthesis and proteolysis of connective tissue, resulting in connective tissue accumulation. Total lung collagen and concentration of lung collagen has been shown to increase after radiation (293–296), although the time course has been variable. In one report, elastin concentration transiently increased (296).

Rates of collagen synthesis have been found to increase after exposure to external cobalt-60 radiation, as well as after inhalation of several other nucleotides. This increase in collagen synthesis was delayed several weeks, occurred mostly during the period of cellular accumulation, and, although sustained for varying lengths of time, preceded evidence of increased collagen content (293–295). In addition, the period of increased synthesis was accompanied by an increase in the incorporation of proline into dialyzable hydroxyproline, indicating increased proteolysis of at least the newly synthesized collagen. In some cases, proteolysis of newly synthesized collagen was increased before the period of increased synthesis, although this was not reflected in a decrease in the total lung collagen content (295). The cellular events responsible for this increase in both collagen synthesis and degradation are uncertain. Increased numbers of collagen-synthesizing cells may be responsible, in part. A number of qualitative changes in cell function have been described after radiation, including altered macrophage function (297), fibroblast growth potential (298) and glycosaminoglycan synthesis by fibroblasts (299). Infiltration of macrophages and mast cells is found during the cellular phase and could influence the fibrotic response (292, 293). Connective tissue synthesis by individual lung cells has not been studied after radiation.

Experience with radiation-induced pulmonary fibrosis suggests that the balance between lung collagen synthesis and proteolysis can be modulated by external factors. Initiation and subsequent rapid withdrawal of steroids may activate subclinical lung radiation injury; reinitiation of steroids ameliorates this response (300).

Connective tissue elements themselves are relatively radioresistant, but there is *in vitro* evidence that radiation can cleave collagen and elastin, increase collagen crosslink formation, and depolymerize proteoglycans (268). Thus, it is conceivable that qualitative, as well as quantitative, changes in connective tissue could play a role in the pathogenesis of radiation-induced pulmonary fibrosis.

There is almost no information about proteoglycans in *in vivo* radiation exposure, although inhalation of plutonium by animals results in pulmonary fibrosis, together with an increase in total lung glycosaminoglycans, mostly chondroitin and dermatan sulfate (301).

As with the radiation model, fibrosis resulting from the intratracheal administration of silica to rats is accompanied by increases in lung collagen concentration and total lung collagen (275, 276). Treatment with steroids (275) or BAPN (276) has been shown to inhibit the silica-induced fibrotic response. Increased prolyl hydroxylase activity preceded morphologic evidence of collagen accumulation (62).

Other experimental models, e.g., exposure of rats to ozone (279), have promise in relation to the study of connective tissue homeostasis after lung injury. These models may have significant advantages, because the injury produced with toxic gases is much more diffuse than that with, for example, silicosis. A diffuse lesion greatly aids the biochemical investigator; localized reactions are more difficult to detect.

In vitro *tissue culture models of fibrosis*. It is obvious from the discussion of both human and experimental animal fibrosis that the pathogenesis of the disease is very complex. One way to approach this problem is to sidestep the complexity by reducing the number of variables involved. Tissue culture systems provide such simplicity; they invite the investigator to clarify pathogenic mechanisms by which both cell types and local milieu are controlled; however, these methods must be viewed simply as model systems that do not necessarily reflect what actually occurs *in vivo*. With that caveat, we will briefly describe the available data obtained using these

models. We will return to their consideration in the last section of this review.

An interesting use of these models has been their application to elucidating the role of the macrophage in silicosis. Direct exposure of fibroblasts to silica may produce cytopathic effects. Although there is no reported change in collagen accumulation (302–304), increased hyaluronic acid production has been found (305). Addition of an extract prepared from macrophages previously exposed to silica has been found to stimulate collagen production in fibroblasts, including lung fibroblasts (302–304), although negative results have also been reported (306). In addition, pretreatment of macrophages with polyvinylpyridine-*N*-oxide blunted their silica-induced fibrogenic activity (302). Similar experiments have also shown that intact alveolar macrophages by themselves are capable of stimulating collagen synthesis in fibroblasts (307). Extracts of alveolar macrophages obtained from silicotic animals have also been shown to increase collagen production in an *in vivo* system (308). In contrast to exposure to silica, exposure to asbestos directly stimulated collagen production by cells in culture, including rabbit lung fibroblasts (307).

There has been a great deal of interest in the possible role of immunologic mechanisms in promoting fibrotic disease. This interest comes from 3 sources: (*1*) in most cases, the pathologic findings in fibrotic lung disease accompanying the collagen-vascular disorders are identical to those seen in idiopathic pulmonary fibrosis (309, 310); (*2*) the pathologic findings in experimental immune injury to animal lung are similar to those of early idiopathic interstitial disease (311); (*3*) some investigators have noted abnormal serologic studies in patients with idiopathic fibrotic disease that are also seen in association with the collagen-vascular disorders, e.g., rheumatoid factor and antinuclear antibodies (312–315). The mechanisms by which the immunologic system might mediate the fibrotic process are being explored in *in vitro* model systems. Collaborative investigations in our laboratory with Kravis at the Scripps Institute and Ahmed at the Naval Medical Research Center have demonstrated that circulating lymphocytes in patients with pulmonary fibrosis secrete lymphokines when the lymphocytes are incubated with collagen, whereas those in normal subjects and patients with pneumonia or lung cancer do not. This information, in correlation with the knowledge that pulmonary alveolar macrophages (often the target for lymphocyte-produced lymphokines) have the potential to secrete collagenase and the potential to stimulate fibroblasts to secrete more collagen, suggests intriguing possibilities related to the pathogenesis of these disorders.

Relationship of Lung Connective Tissue to Lung Function

There is no question that connective tissue components strongly influence lung mechanical properties in health and that their alteration is important in producing impaired function in some disease states. The multiple types, distribution, and physical properties of lung connective tissue make it very difficult to define the contribution that each component makes to lung function; however, considerable effort has been spent trying to understand the remarkable mechanical behavior of lung tissue by correlating physiologic, morphologic, and biochemical data from normal and diseased human and experimental animal lungs. In this section, we will attempt to summarize this information by indicating some of the obstacles inherent in these correlative studies; by presenting several current models that attempt to explain the role of individual connective tissue components in determining mechanical properties; by reviewing the available experimental data, and by commenting on possible future approaches to this intriguing question.

Obstacles

(1) The interdependency of lung connective tissue makes it extremely difficult to establish the individual role of each connective tissue element; alteration of one component may drastically alter the contribution of another component to mechanical function.

(2) The heterogeneous substructures that form the lung are all interconnected through a so-called "fibrous continuum" (121). This generalized association of lung elements may be crucial for distributing pressure evenly throughout the lung. Destruction of the "fibrous continuum" at one level can affect structures at another level; e.g., in emphysema, alveolar destruction may reduce support of small airways.

(3) In tissues other than lung and in simplified model systems, it has been shown that specific types of glycosaminoglycans will associate with other connective tissue elements, influence the rate of synthesis of connective tissue compo-

nents, affect the hydration of connective tissue, and influence the rate of collagen fibril formation and subsequent stability of these fibrils (2, 192). Thus, it is not difficult to imagine that the quantity and quality of proteoglycans in the lung may significantly affect the mechanical properties of lung. Unfortunately, there is no specific information in this area, so that any studies on correlates of lung connective tissue with mechanical properties must be interpreted without knowledge of these factors.

(4) Lung elastic recoil depends on surface properties, tissue (fiber) mechanical properties, and the geometry of the alveolus. The contribution of surface properties can be minimized by using saline-filled lungs, but the relative contribution of fiber mechanical properties and alveolar geometry are very difficult to separate (e.g., the large alveoli found in emphysema could be due either to alterations in connective tissue components, resulting in loss of elastic recoil with expansion of individual alveoli, or to focal tissue destruction leaving larger "alveolar" spaces that have normal connective tissue (244).

Models

It is generally agreed that elastic fibers are an important determinant of lung elasticity in the physiologic pressure range, and that collagen is important in conferring tensile strength to lung. There is, however, no consensus as to how elastic fibers make this contribution to lung elasticity and whether collagen fibers are also an important determinant of elastic recoil at all lung volumes. Two general models have been proposed.

According to one model, at low lung volumes, collagen fibers are not under tension, and therefore, the collagen meshwork is able to expand easily (analogy has been made to the stretch of a nylon stocking). At high lung volumes, the collagen comes under stretch, and because of its high tensile strength, increasing pressure changes lung volume very little. Elastic fibers, however, would be under stretch at all lung volumes, and because of their elastic properties, a change in transpulmonary pressure would result in graded changes in lung volume. The sum of these effects would produce a pressure-volume curve similar to that seen in normal saline-filled lung (316, 317). According to this model, collagen would limit alveolar expansion and increase stability of the inflated lung by protecting elastic fibers from rupture, and prevent emptying of small alveoli into larger ones, a tendency resulting from the different surface properties of large and small alveoli (317). In emphysema, destruction of the elastic fibers could result in air spaces having elastic properties of collagen fibers only. Assuming that premature airway closure prevented interalveolar pressure from decreasing so low that collapse resulted from surface properties, these alveoli would remain inflated, but be capable of little further expansion (318).

Alternatively, it has been proposed that, rather than being a primary determinant of elasticity, elastic fibers could serve to orient properly the collagen fibrils in alveolar tissue (319). The constantly increasing slope of the normal pressure-volume curve could result from the "stiffness" of increasing number of collagen fibers being put under stretch as the lung volume increased (320). In emphysema, destruction of alveolar walls and disruption of elastin-collagen interaction could produce larger alveoli (increased resting length of tissue fibers) that could expand little with inspiration.

Experimental Evidence

Several experimental approaches have been used to study the role of individual connective tissue components in determining lung function in normal and diseased lungs: morphologic evaluation of the connective tissue; quantification of individual connective tissue components; investigation of the effects of increasing or decreasing crosslinks, and examination of the effects of proteolytic digestion of individual connective tissue elements. Each of these will be discussed individually. Although these data do not allow formulation of a single unifying model of the role of connective tissue in determining lung mechanical properties, certain generalizations will be made in a later section.

Morphologic studies. Within the normal parenchyma, the collagen and elastic fibers are arranged in a helical fashion as they encircle respiratory bronchioles and alveolar ducts (123). This remarkable orientation has led to the suggestion that lung elasticity is secondary to the coiling and uncoiling of this helix (analogous to a spring) rather than to significant extension of individual fibers (123). If lungs are fixed in inflation, collagen fibrils are straight, not wavy, as seen in completely deflated lung, suggesting that the intimately associated collagen-elastic fibers cannot undergo significant axial elongation *in vivo* because of the inelasticity of collagen (123).

Both clinical and protease-induced emphysema are characterized by morphologic abnormalities in elastic fibers and loss of lung elastic recoil. The association between these 2 phenomena was supported by examination of intact lung treated *in vitro* with proteolytic enzymes, in which enlargement of airspaces was found only in areas of lung with abnormal elastic fibers, and never in areas with intact elastic fibers (244). Because degradation of the elastin component of elastic fibers has been described as an early change in protease-induced emphysema, it is possible that some of the irreversible changes in lung function seen early in protease-induced emphysema, including loss of elastic recoil, are associated with loss of elastin.

Further support for a relationship between abnormalities in elastic fibers and loss of elastic recoil comes from studies using lungs from aged patients. By light microscopy, elastic fibers in alveoli and alveolar ducts are reduced in number, attenuated in diameter, frayed, and fragmented (182). Although age-related changes have been seen in other tissues by electron microscopy (321), no age-related abnormalities in elastic fibers have been so identified in lung (322). Functionally, aged patients have been noted to have (*1*) an increase in the ratio of functional residual capacity to total lung capacity (323, 324); (*2*) an increase in residual volume without change in total lung capacity (324, 325); (*3*) an increase in closing volume (325); (*4*) a decrease in uniformity of ventilation (326); (*5*) a shift of the compliance curve to the left (324, 325). Because most of these findings can be explained by a loss of lung elastic recoil with attendant early closure of airways, it appears that gross abnormalities in the quality of elastic fibers may be related to a loss of lung elastic recoil.

Quantity of connective tissue components. In most cases, alteration of normal physiologic function has not been accompanied by detectible change in the amount of connective tissue components. No consistent changes in parenchymal collagen or elastin content have been found to be associated with the alterations in pulmonary function found in clinical emphysema, protease-induced emphysema, lung aging, or idiopathic fibrosis. Except for a preliminary study (266), correlation between "fibrosis" and restrictive defects in pulmonary function have not been sought.

Effects of decreased crosslinks. Inhibition of elastin and collagen crosslink formation in experimental animals can be accomplished using a variety of agents, although the low turnover of adult lung connective tissue makes crosslink inhibition in lung less prominent than in tissues such as skin and bone.

Administration of DL-penicillamine to weanling rats for 7 to 9 weeks induced mild increases in compliance at low and mid lung volumes and reduced elastic recoil at all lung volumes (327), whereas morphologic assessment indicated enlargement of alveoli. Although penicillamine is capable of inhibiting crosslink formation of both collagen and elastin, study of the solubility and aldehyde content of lung collagen and elastin in animals treated with penicillamine suggested that only the formation of elastin crosslinks had been severely affected (328). Treatment of older rabbits for 2 weeks with penicillamine induced small increases in vital capacity and compliance without changing flows (329).

Growing rats fed BAPN showed increases in lung compliance, and analysis of lung aldehyde content indicated that the lungs had decreased crosslink content (330). In another study, growing rats treated with BAPN also showed increases in lung compliance and loss of lung tensile strength, despite the fact that morphologic alterations could not be demonstrated (331). In these studies, the alteration in crosslinks in individual fiber types was not determined, although BAPN does affect the solubility of lung collagen (12) and elastin (Franzblau, C.: Personal communication).

In marked contrast to penicillamine, semicarbazide enhanced the solubility of lung collagen, presumably by inhibiting crosslink formation, whereas the content of desmosine and isodesmosine was unchanged, suggesting no alteration in elastin crosslinking (332). Lungs showed no alteration in compliance, elastic recoil, or histopathologic features unless pressures greater than physiologic pressure were used, in which case evidence of reduced tensile strength was observed.

These studies have added considerable insight into the role of connective tissue in determining mechanical properties. They indicate that crosslink formation, and especially elastin crosslink formation, are very important determinants of lung elasticity, and that inhibition of elastin crosslinking results in distortion of parenchymal morphologic features and increased compliance. If collagen plays a role in lung elasticity at all lung volumes, as was suggested in the previous section, reduction of collagen crosslinks was not sufficient to alter this function acutely. Reduction in tensile strength by inhibition of collagen crosslinking could predispose the lung to rupture of terminal air spaces, as seen in overinflated, semicarbazide-treated lung, and thus play a role in pathogenesis of emphysema or age-related changes of pulmonary function (332).

Information on the effect of decreased elastin crosslinks is also available from the investigation of connective tissue from lungs of older patients. In one study, desmosine and isodesmosine contents decreased 30 to 40 per cent with age, although the content of the less stable lysinonorleucine crosslink increased 20 per cent (166). In another study, elastin crosslink content in aged lung tended to be reduced, although data were variable (225). These preliminary data are consistent with the concept that decreased elastin crosslink content may attend loss of elastic recoil.

Effects of increased crosslinks. Collagen from aged tissue (including lung) has been found to demonstrate a number of changes in physical properties, including decreased solubility, increased shrinking temperature, and resistance to proteolytic enzymes (206, 333–335). In tissues other than lung, these properties have been found to depend, in part, on the degrees of intra- and intermolecular crosslinking, which do increase with age (335).

There is some indirect evidence that increases in connective tissue crosslinking may have a role in altering lung function. Although crosslinks were not measured, studies of the elastic properties of isolated alveolar walls from aged and emphysematous lungs show increased resting length and decreased extensibility (336, 337).

Qualitatively similar changes can be induced by treating normal alveolar walls with formaldehyde (338). Such treatment is known to produce artificial methylene-derived crosslinks in both collagen and elastic fibers, although formaldehyde may exert other effects on lung alveolar walls. Exposing alveolar walls to formaldehyde and elastase produces abnormalities even closer to those seen in aged and emphysematous lung (338), suggesting that alterations in crosslinks are not the only determinant of decreased elastic recoil and that alterations in collagen-elastic fiber interactions are undoubtedly important.

It is not clear how these studies correlate with what is known about the crosslink composition of emphysematous and aged lung. Collagen crosslinks have never been quantified in emphysematous or aged lung, and elastin crosslinks may actually decrease with aging.

Enzymatic destruction of specific components. Isolated tracheal segments exposed to collagenase developed an increase in dead space, but distensibility was not affected in the physiologic pressure range. At high pressures, the airways were abnormally distensible. In contrast, trachea exposed to elastase became abnormally distensible only in the physiologic pressure range. Histologic studies confirmed relative specific disruption of elastic fibers by elastase and collagen by collagenase treatment (339). These studies suggest that collagen is important in determining tensile strength, but, at least in airways, elastin is the main determinant of elasticity.

After collagenase digestion, alveolar walls did not change resting length, but almost no force was required to stretch the walls, and they broke much sooner than normal alveolar walls. Exposure to elastase resulted in an increased resting length, but no change in the length at which alveolar walls broke (338). Digestion of alveolar walls with hyaluronidase did not alter mechanical properties. In a similar study, depletion of collagen from strips of lung parenchyma by collagenase digestion correlated well with the loss of lung tensile strength, whereas papain and elastase had no effect on tensile strength (319). These studies underscore the importance of collagen in providing tensile strength to the lung; in addition, the finding that alveolar walls digested with collagenase (in which elastic fibers were presumably intact) had little elasticity, even at resting length, strongly suggests an important role for collagen in fiber elastic recoil at all lung volumes.

Generalizations

It is apparent that these studies do not complete our understanding of the role of individual connective tissue elements in determining lung mechanical properties; however, certain generalizations are possible.

(1) Changes in the distribution, quality, or interaction of individual fiber components can produce dramatic alterations in lung function without accompanying changes in the quantity of the individual components.

(2) Likewise, biochemical alterations of lung connective tissue can produce significant functional changes without accompanying morphologic changes.

(3) Collagen is the principal determinant of lung tensile strength. The inelasticity and strength of collagen makes normal lung elasticity dependent on the proper orientation of collagen fibers.

(4) Elastic fibers are crucially important to lung mechanical properties in the normal physiologic pressure range. Morphologic evidence of disrupted elastic fibers is almost always accompanied by loss of lung elastic recoil. Whether the elastic fibers supply elasticity themselves, or serve to orient other connective tissue elements remains unknown.

(5) Inhibition of elastin crosslink formation results in loss of lung elastic recoil; inhibition of collagen crosslinking primarily affects lung tensile strength.

Future Approaches

It is obvious that the complex maze of lung connective tissue and the largely unexplored interactions between the elements leave the investigator of anatomic-biochemical-functional correlates in a technologic quandary; what methods can be used to unravel the specific contribution of each connective tissue type to the anatomic and functional integrity of the normal lung?

It is clear from the preceding section that correlative studies of pulmonary function, morphology, and biochemistry of clinical and experimental lung disease have given considerable information; these studies should continue to be useful in the future. Ideally, investigations should include knowledge of the mechanism of action by which the inciting agent or disease affects connective tissue, determination of the effect of this change on lung connective tissue, and assessment of the morphologic and physiologic consequences. If all of these parameters are investigated in a single study, it does not matter whether the enzymes used are nonspecific or the crosslink inhibitors affect more than one fibrous component; investigation of a wide variety of perturbations of connective tissue elements should eventually allow rational correlates of structure and function to be made.

One area that is particularly well suited to such correlative studies is the group of heritable connective tissue disorders. Recent biochemical advances should allow a detailed explanation at the molecular level of the abnormalities in many of these diseases. Although the heritable connective tissue disorders are usually considered diseases of skin and skeletal systems, it must be remembered that these are genetic disorders that, in many instances, result in a generalized defect in the quality or quantity of a connective tissue component. Thus, the lungs should be involved if the abnormal connective tissue component plays an important role in the maintenance of lung structure and function.

Detailed morphologic and physiologic evaluation of patients with these disorders, combined with a knowledge of the abnormality present in their lung connective tissue framework, could greatly aid assignment of the role of the abnormal connective tissue component in defining lung function. Currently, only preliminary information is available concerning alterations in pulmonary function and histopathologic features in patients with heritable connective tissue disorders, including several disorders in which the biochemical abnormalities already described suggest that major functional abnormalities in lung structure and function should exist. Some of the described connective tissue disorders, a brief description of the biochemical abnormality, and known alterations of pulmonary function are listed in table 4.

In contrast to the heritable disorders of connective tissue, our knowledge of the biochemical basis of the alterations in lung connective tissue resulting from aging and lung disease (both clinical and experimental) lags behind our knowledge of their morphologic and physiologic consequences. Approaches to improving our knowledge of the biochemical basis of lung disease are discussed in the next section in relation to therapy of lung disorders.

Approaches to the Understanding and Treatment of Lung Disorders Involving Connective Tissue

To appreciate the connective tissue abnormalities that are associated with lung disease, it is necessary first to understand the normal processes of lung connective tissue development, homeostasis, and aging. A tremendous amount of information concerning normal connective tissue synthetic and degradative mechanisms has been generated, but much of this information is from tissues other than lung. Although these mechanisms are, in general, similar from tissue to tissue, it is probable that there are local differences in which connective tissue elements are modified for specific structural requirements. The amounts, types, and quality of all lung connective components and the mechanisms controlling the synthesis and degradation of these components must be determined in each lung structure at each stage of development before we can fully

appreciate abnormalities associated with lung disease.

Formulating the pattern of pathogenesis of lung disease must include the identification of the primary stimulus to lung damage and the identification of the multitude of pulmonary and extrapulmonary factors that modulate the lung's response to the primary stimulus. For example, the association of a high incidence of early emphysema in patients with a_1-antitrypsin deficiency type Pi ZZ has given considerable insight into the pathogenesis of emphysema; however, a more complete understanding of the biochemical basis of this association would considerably enhance prospects for therapy. It must be remembered that the primary genetic defect responsible for type Pi ZZ a_1-antitrypsin has not been defined; the mechanisms and site at which a_1-antitrypsin normally operates, if, in fact, it is an important determinant in lung structure, are not known. The nature of the proteases (endogenous or exogenous to lung) that actually damage lung connective tissue *in vivo* has not been determined, and the lung's biochemical response to the primary insult is not known. As this information becomes available, possible therapeutic intervention, such as antiprotease replacement, inhibition of release of proteases, or control of connective tissue synthesis, will be easier to devise (355).

Similarly, there is also a paucity of information concerning the pathogenesis of the fibrotic disorders. Although a multitude of agents have been identified as being capable of inciting pulmonary "fibrosis," the nature of the primary lung damage remains unknown. A number of factors, including inflammatory and immune mechanisms, have been implicated in mediating the response that culminates in pulmonary fibrosis, but the mechanisms involved in the interactions of these systems with lung parenchyma are just begining to be understood. A more complete understanding of the biochemical basis of these disorders would help define sites for therapeutic intervention.

We have made frequent mention of the difficulty of studying these biochemical processes in intact lung. This difficulty arises from the large number of different cell types, and the heterogeneity, interactions, and insolubility of lung connective tissue. The anatomic maze of lung structure, with its multiple subcomponents, makes these complexities even more formidable. At this time, the most obvious solution is to "simplify" the lung by using *in vitro* models of

TABLE 4

USE OF THE HERITABLE DISORDERS OF CONNECTIVE TISSUE* TO UNDERSTAND THE CONTRIBUTION
OF CONNECTIVE TISSUE ELEMENTS TO LUNG FUNCTIONS

Disorder	Lung Abnormalities	Defect
Marfan's syndrome	Spontaneous pneumothorax, cystic disease, apical bullae, emphysema (340, p. 140; 342); controversial decrease in volumes, air trapping, increased airway resistance; decreased arterial saturation with exercise (343, 344).	Possible crosslink or maturation abnormality (340, p. 183; 345).
Homocystinuria	Unknown; patients probably will have loss of elastic recoil and high total lung capacity.	Deficiency in cystathionine synthetase → abnormal methionine metabolism → homocysteine ↑ → inhibition of normal connective tissue maturation (340, p. 224; 346).
Ehlers-Danlos (ED)	In general, spontaneous pneumothorax, mediastinal emphysema (340, p. 329). Two sisters with ED VI had obstructive defects (347). Functional abnormalities with ED IV should be profound.	ED IV = deficiency of synthesis of Type III tropocollagen (348); ED V = deficiency of lysyl oxidase (349); ED VI = deficiency of lysyl hydroxylase (347); ED VII = deficiency of procollagen peptidase (350).
Osteogenesis imperfecta	Congenital type, unknown (340, p. 390); tarda type, air-trapping, but may be secondary to kyphoscoliosis (351).	Congenital type, possible deficiency in snythesis of Type I collagen (352); tarda type, unknown.
Alkaptonuria	Severe hoarseness, fixed vocal cords, pigmentation of larynx and tracheal cartilage (340, p. 455; 353); other functional abnormalities, unknown.	Deficiency of homogentisic acid oxidase → homogentisic acid ↑ → possible abnormalities in lysyl oxidase or lysyl hydroxylase (353; Siegel, R.: Personal communication).
Pseudoxanthoma elasticum	Unknown; there should be significant abnormalities in elastic recoil.	Probably in the elastic fiber (340, p. 475).
The mucopolysaccharidoses	Hurler's: chest wall abnormalities, upper airway obstruction, no diffusion abnormality, although there is parenchymal disease (354); functional abnormalities in other disorders unknown.	Enzyme defects in glycosaminoglycan degradative pathways → glycosaminoglycan accumulation (340, p. 521; 187).

*The most extensive reviews of these disorders can be found in McKusick (340) and Stanbury and associates (341).

lung biochemical function. It should be kept in mind, however, that *in vitro* studies are only an aid to understanding *in vivo* processes and not an end in themselves. There are inherent artifacts in simplifying complex living systems; comparison to the *in vivo* situation must always be considered the true test of *in vitro* inferences.

Explant Culture Systems

Use of parenchyma, blood vessels, and tracheobronchial tree in explant culture has a number of advantages in studying lung connective tissue, primarily in reducing the number of variables that needs to be considered (1, 2, 215, 356). Small amounts of tissue can be used (100 mg of parenchyma from an open lung biopsy is often sufficient); tissue differentiation is maintained for at least 24 hours, and the rate of synthesis and degradation of many connective tissue types can be accurately quantified. Explant culture allows the control of tissue environment, the amounts of substrates available to lung cells, and the dose of pharmacologic agents being investigated. These methods should continue to yield useful information regarding the quantity and quality of connective tissue synthesis and degradation in lung structures from normal and diseased lung in humans and experimental animals. With lung explants, we should soon know whether there are abnormalities in the synthesis or degradation of each connective tissue component of parenchyma in human and experimental emphysema and fibrosis. It should also be possible to quantify the effect of therapeutic agents on these processes in parenchyma from patients and, thus, tailor, for each patient, a rational therapeutic regimen.

Dispersed Lung Cells and Tissue Culture Models

The complexity of lung structures makes it difficult to use explants to investigate connec-

TABLE 5

THERAPEUTIC AGENTS AND CONNECTIVE TISSUE SYNTHESIS AND DEGRADATION*

Effect	Agent	Comment
Crosslink inhibition	β-aminopropionitrile, penicillamine, semicarbazide (92, 160)	Decreases collagen accumulation in silicotic rats (276) and experimental granuloma (359).
Inhibit collagen secretion	Colchicine, vinblastine, vincristine (360)	May result in $\uparrow$ collagen proteolysis; preliminary studies suggest colchicine may be useful in human alcoholic cirrhosis (Rojkind, M.: Personal communication).
Decrease stability of tropocollagen	Proline analogs (58, 59, 359), iron chelators (15, 361)	Both prevent proline hydroxylation; no evidence so far that they are useful *in vivo* (361).
Inhibition of inflammatory and immune response to lung injury	Corticosteroids, azathioprine chlorambucil, superoxide desmutase	Our group currently has a double blind study with steroids and azathioprine in idiopathic fibrotic disease; superoxide desmutase may inhibit oxidative-induced collagen accumulation in fibroblasts *in vitro* (Bhatnagar, R. S., and Cross, C.: Personal communication).
Inhibit proteolytic enzymes	Elastase inhibitors (178)	May be useful in α_1-antitrypsin deficiency.
Enhance secretion of proteolytic enzymes	Oxyphenylbutazone, idomethacin (362)	Potential (but unproved) usefulness in the fibrotic disorders.
Enhance collagen accumulation	Ascorbic acid, vitamin A	Ascorbic acid may enhance collagen accumulation during periods of increased biosynthetic activity (363); vitamin A may prevent steroid inhibition of scar formation (364); vitamin A deficiency causes decreased lung tissue elasticity (365)
Decrease collagen accumulation	Reserpine, corticosteroids	Reserpine inhibits collagen accumulation in blood vessels of hypertensive rats (366); corticosteroids appear to decrease collagen synthesis (367), but they may also inhibit action of collagenase (368).

*An excellent review of this topic is available (359).

tive tissue synthesis and degradation by individual cell types. These complexities may be partially obviated by "dissecting" the explant system into individual cells, usually with the aid of enzymes. In the past few years, considerable advances have been made in the dispersion, isolation, and culture of individual lung cells. Cells representing more than 80 per cent of total lung cells (macrophages, alveolar epithelial, endothelial, and mesenchymal cells) can be isolated, purified, and maintained in culture for varying periods of time (17, 199, 357, 358; Hance, A. J., Bradley, K., and Crystal, R. G.: J Clin Invest, in press). Tissue culture models considerably simplify the investigation of the cells responsible for the synthesis and degradation of individual connective tissue types, the factors that influence cell turnover, mechanisms of cell-cell interactions, and the effects of environmental agents, antiproteases, immunologic mediators, and drugs on the synthesis and degradation of connective tissue.

In vitro models of emphysema might include investigation of the release of proteolytic enzymes from leukocytes, the effect of these enzymes on lung cells and their connective tissue products, and the protection afforded by serum and lung antiproteases on the processes. *In vitro* models of fibrosis might include the effect of lymphocytes, macrophages, fibrogenic agents (e.g., silica), and components of the immune system on the rate of synthesis and degradation of various types of connective tissue and the replication and differentiation of each type of parenchymal cell.

Several of the therapeutic agents currently under investigation with *in vitro* models are listed in table 5. Some are already being tested in clinical situations. Continued use of these models and the development of new methods to investigate connective tissue in intact lung should eventually allow the understanding and successful therapy of connective tissue abnormalities in lung disease.

Acknowledgment

The writers thank J. Fulmer, N. Elson, A. Horwitz, J. Karlinsky, R. Bienkowski, W. Wagner, K. Bradley, S. M. Breul, and, particularly, K. Cook for their help in preparing this manuscript.

References

1. Hance, A. J., and Crystal, R. G. : Collagen, in *The Biochemical Basis of Pulmonary Function,* R. G. Crystal, ed., Marcel Dekker, New York, in press.

2. Horwitz, A. L., Elson, N. A., and Crystal, R. G.: Proteoglycans and elastin, in *The Biochemical Basis of Pulmonary Function,* R. G. Crystal, ed., Marcel Dekker, New York, in press.

3. Piez, K. A., and Miller, A.: The structure of collagen fibrils, J Supramol Struct, 1974, *2,* 121.

4. Traub, W., and Piez, K. A.: The chemistry and structure of collagen, Adv Protein Chem, 1971, *25,* 243.

5. Gallop, P. M., Blumenfeld, O. O., and Seifter, S.: Structure and metabolism of connective tissue proteins, Annu Rev Biochem, 1972, *41,* 617.

6. Miller, E. J., and Matukas, V. J.: Biosynthesis of collagen: The biochemist's view, Fed Proc, 1974, *33,* 1197.

7. Reid, K. B. M., Lowe, D. M., and Porter, R. R.: Isolation and characterization of Clq, a subcomponent of the first component of complement, from human and rabbit sera, Biochem J, 1972, *130,* 749.

8. Bhattacharyya, S. N., Passero, M. A., DiAugustine, R. P., and Lynn, W. S.: Isolation and characterization of two hydroxyproline-containing glycoproteins from normal animal lung lavage and lamellar bodies, J Clin Invest, 1975, *55,* 914.

9. Bornstein, P., and Piez, K. A.: The nature of the intramolecular cross-links in collagen: The separation and characterization of peptides from the cross-link region of rat skin collagen, Biochemistry, 1966, *5,* 3460.

10. Miller, E. J.: A review of biochemical studies on the genetically distinct collagens of the skeletal system, Clin Orthop, 1973, *92,* 260.

11. Trelstad, R. L.: Human aorta collagens: Evidence for three distinct species, Biochem Biophys Res Commun, 1974, *57,* 717.

12. Bradley, K. H., McConnell, S. D., and Crystal, R. G.: Lung collagen composition and synthesis: Characterization and changes with age, J Biol Chem, 1974, *249,* 2674.

13. Bradley, K., McConnell-Breul, S., and Crystal, R. G.: Lung collagen heterogeneity, Proc Natl Acad Sci USA, 1974, *71,* 2828.

14. Bradley, K., McConnell-Breul, S., and Crystal, R. G.: Collagen in the human lung: Quantitation of rates of synthesis and partial characterization of composition, J Clin Invest, 1975, *55,* 543.

15. Grant, M. E., and Prockop, D. J.: The biosynthesis of collagen, N Engl J Med, 1972, *286,* 194, 242, 291.

16. Fulmer, J. D., and Crystal, R. G.: The biochemical basis of pulmonary function, in *The Biochemical Basis of Pulmonary Function,* R. G. Crystal, ed., Marcel Dekker, New York, in press.

17. Elson, N., Bradley, K., Hance, A., Kniazeff, A., Breul, S., Horwitz, A., and Crystal, R.: Synthe-

sis of collagen in cultured lung cells, Clin Res, 1975, *23*, 346A.

18. Hance, A. J., Horwitz, A. L., Cowan, M. J., Elson, N. A., Collins, J. F., Bienkowski, R. S., Bradley, K. H., McConnell-Breul, S., Wagner, W. M., and Crystal, R. G.: Biochemical approaches to the investigation of fibrotic lung disease, Chest, in press.

19. Green, H., and Goldberg, B.: Synthesis of collagen by mammalian cell lines of fibroblastic an nonfibroblastic origin, Proc Natl Acad Sci USA, 1965, *53*, 1360.

20. Ross, R., and Glomset, J. A.: Atherosclerosis and the arterial smooth muscle cell, Science, 1973, *180*, 1332.

21. Langness, U., and Udenfriend, S.: Collegan biosynthesis in nonfibroblastic cell lines, Proc Natl Acad Sci USA, 1974, *71*, 50.

22. Strawich, E., and Nimni, M. E.: Properties of a collagen molecule containing three identical components extracted from bovine articular cartilage, Biochemistry, 1971, *10*, 3905.

23. Miller, E. J.: Isolation and characterization of a collagen from chick cartilage containing three identical α chains, Biochemistry, 1971, *10*, 1652.

24. Mayne, R., Schiltz, J. R., and Holtzer, H.: Some overt and covert properties of chondrogenic cells, in *Biology of Fibroblast,* E. Kulonen and J. Pikkarainen, ed., Academic Press, New York, 1973, p. 61.

25. Chung, E., and Miller, E. J.: Collagen polymorphism: Characterization of molecules with the chain composition $[\alpha 1(III)]_3$ in human tissues, Science, 1974, *183*, 1200.

26. Epstein, E. H., Jr.: $[\alpha 1(III)]_3$ Human skin collagen: Release by pepsin digestion and preponderance in fetal life, J Biol Chem, 1974, *249*, 3225.

27. Epstein, E. H., Jr.: Isolation of $[\alpha 1(III)]_3$ collagen from pepsin digests of human skin, Clin Res, 1974, *22*, 327A.

28. Spiro, R. G.: Biochemistry of the renal glomerular basement membrane and its alterations in diabetes mellitus, N Engl J Med, 1972, *288*, 1337.

29. Kefalides, N. A., and Denduchis, B.: Structural components of epithelial and endothelial basement membranes, Biochemistry, 1969, *8*, 4613.

30. Hudson, B. G., and Spiro, R. G.: Fractionation of glycoprotein components of the reduced alkylated renal glomerular basement membrane, J Biol Chem, 1972, *247*, 4239.

31. Kefalides, N. A.: Structure and biosynthesis of basement membranes, Int Rev Connect Tissue Res, 1973, *6*, 63.

32. Fietzek, P. P., Rexrodt, F. W., Wendt, P., Stark, M., and Kühn, K.: The covalent structure of collagen amino-acid sequence of poptide $\alpha 1$-CB6-C2, Eur J Biochem, 1972, *30*, 163.

33. Grant, M. E., Kefalides, N. A., and Prockop, D. A.: The biosynthesis of basement membrane

collagen in embryonic chick lens. I. Delay between the synthesis of polypeptide chains and the secretion of collagen by matrix-free cells, J Biol Chem, 1972, *247*, 3539.

34. Burns, T. M., Spears, G. L., and Kerwar, S. S.: Further studies of the cell-free synthesis of procollagen-collagen by chick embryo polysomes, Arch Biochem Biophys, 1973, *159*, 880.

35. Diegelman, R. F., Bernstein, L., and Peterkofsky, B.: Cell-free collagen synthesis on membrane-bound polysomes of chich embryo connective tissue and localization of prolyl hydroxylase on the polysome-membrane complex, J Biol Chem, 1973, *248*, 6514.

36. Harwood, R., Grant, M. E., and Jackson, D. S.: The subcellular location of interchain disulfide bond formation during procollagen biosynthesis by embryonic chick tendon cells, Biochem Biophys Res Commun, 1973, *55*, 1188.

37. Collins, J. F., and Crystal, R. G.: Characterization of cell-free synthesis of collagen by lung polysomes in a heterologous system, J Biol Chem, 1975, *250*, 7332.

38. Siekevitz, P., and Palade, G. E.: A cytochemical study of the pancreas of the guinea pig, J Biophys Biochem Cytol, 1960, *7*, 619.

39. Boedtker, H., Crkvenjakov, R. B., Last, J. A., and Doty, P.: The identification of collagen messenger RNA, Proc Natl Acad Sci USA, 1974, *71*, 4208.

40. Lazarides, E., and Lukens, L. N.: Collagen synthesis on polysomes *in vivo* and *in vitro,* Nature [New Biol], 1971, *232*, 37.

41. Collins, J. F., and Crystal, R. G.: Protein synthesis, in *The Biochemical Basis of Pulmonary Function,* R. G. Crystal, ed., Marcel Dekker, New York, in press.

42. Bornstein, P.: The biosynthesis of collagen, Annu Rev Biochem, 1974, *43*, 567.

43. Vuust, J., and Piez, K. A.: Biosynthesis of the α chains of collagen studied by pulse-labeling in culture, J Biol Chem, 1970, *245*, 6201.

44. Sheer, C. J., Taubman, M. B., and Goldberg, B.: Isolation of a disulfide-stabilized three chain polypeptide fragment unique to the precursor of human collagen, J Biol Chem, 1973, *248*, 7035.

45. Tanzer, M. L., Church, R. L., Yaeger, J. A., Wampler, E., and Park, E.: Procollagen: Intermediate forms containing several types of peptide chains and non-collagen peptide extensions at NH_2 and COOH ends, Proc Natl Acad Sci USA, 1974, *71*, 3009.

46. Fessler, L. I., Morris, N. P., and Fessler, J. A.: Procollagen processing to collagen via a disulfide-linked triple stranded intermediate in chick calvaria. Fed Proc, 1975, *34*, 562A.

47. Davidson, J. M., and Bornstein, P.: Evidence for multiple steps in the limited conversion of procollagen to collagen, Fed Proc, 1975, *34*, 562A.

48. Goldberg, B., and Green, H.: Collagen synthesis on polyribosomes of cultured mammalian fibroblasts, J Mol Biol, 1967, *26*, 1.

49. Olsen, B. R., Berg, R. A., Kishida, Y., and Prockop, D. J.: Collagen synthesis: Localization of prolyl hydroxylase in tendon cells detected with ferritin-labeled antibodies, Science, 1973, *182*, 825.

50. Cutroneo, K. R., Guzman, N. A., and Sharawy, M. M.: Evidence for a subcellular vesicular site of collagen prolyl hydroxylation, J Biol Chem, *249*, 5989.

51. Hutton, J. J., Jr., Tappel, A. L., and Udenfriend, S.: Cofactor and substrate requirements of collagen proline hydroxylase, Arch Biochem Biophys, 1967, *118*, 231.

52. Rhoads, R. E., Udenfriend, S., and Bornstein, P.: *In vitro* enzymatic hydroxylation of prolyl residues in the α1-CB2 fragment of rat collagen, J Biol Chem, 1971, *246*, 4138.

53. Berg, R. A., and Prockop, D. J.: Affinity column purification of protocollagen proline hydroxylase from chick embryos and further characterization of the enzyme, J Biol Chem, 1973, *248*, 1175.

54. Miller, R. L., and Udenfriend, S.: Hydroxylation of proline residues in collagen nascent chains, Arch Biochem Biophys, 1970 *139*, 104.

55. Bornstein, P.: Comparative sequence studies of rat skin and tendon collagen. I. Evidence for incomplete hydroxylation of individual prolyl residues in the normal proteins, Biochemistry, 1967, *6*, 3082.

56. Margolis, R. L., and Lukens, L. N.: The role of hydroxylation in the secretion of collagen by mouse fibroblasts in culture, Arch Biochem Biophys, 1971, *147*, 612.

57. Barnes, M. J., and Kodicek, E.: Biological hydroxylations and ascorbic acid with special regard to collagen metabolism, Vitam Hor, 1972, *30*, 1.

58. Rosenbloom, J., and Prockop, D. J.: Incorporation of cis-hydroxyproline into protocollagen and collagen, J Biol Chem, 1971, *246*, 1549.

59. Lane, J. M., Dehm, P., and Prockop, D. J.: Effect of the proline analogue azetidine-2-carboxylic acid on collagen synthesis *in vivo*, Biochim Biophys Acta, 1971, *236*, 517.

60. Levene, C. I., and Bates, C. J.: Ascorbic acid and collagen synthesis, in *Biology of Fibroblast*, E. Kulonen and J. Pikkarainen, ed., Academic Press, New York, 1973, p. 397.

61. McGee, J. O'D, Langness, U., and Udenfriend, S.: Immunological evidence for an inactive precursor of collagen proline hydroxylase in cultured fibroblasts, Proc Natl Acad Sci USA, 1971, *68*, 1585.

62. Halme, J., Uitto, J., Kahanpää, K., Karhunen, P., and Lindy, S.: Protocollagen proline hydroxylase activity in experimental pulmonary fibrosis of rats, J Lab Clin Med, 1970, *75*, 535.

63. Popenoe, E. A., and Aronson, R. B.: Partial purification and properties of collagen lysine hydroxylase from chick embryos, Biochim Biophys Acta, 1972, *258*, 380.

64. Kivirikko, K. I., and Prockop, D. J.: Partial purification and characterization of protocollagen lysine hydroxylase from chick embryos, Biochim Biophys Acta, 1972, *258*, 366.

65. Kivirikko, K. I., Ryhänen, L., Anttinen, H., Bornstein, P., and Prockop, D. J.: Further hydroxylation of lysyl residues in collagen by protocollagen lysyl hydroxylase *in vitro*, Biochemistry, 1973, *12*, 4966.

66. Ryhänen, L., and Kivirikko, K. I.: Developmental changes in protocollagen lysyl hydroxylase activity in the chick embryo, Biochim Biophys Acta, 1974, *343*, 121.

67. Bailey, A. J., Robbins, S. P., and Belian, G.: Biological significance of the intermolecular crosslinks of collagen, Nature, 1974, *251*, 105.

68. Miller, E. J., Martin, G. R., Piez, K. A., and Powers, M. J.: Characterization of chick bone collagen and compositional changes associated with maturation, J Biol Chem, 1967, *242*, 5481.

69. Butler, W. T.: Partial hydroxylation of certain lysines in collagen, Science, 1968, *161*, 796.

70. Barnes, M. J., Constable, B. J., Morton, L. F., and Kodicek, E.: Hydroxylysine in the N-terminal teleopeptides of skin collagen from chick embryo and newborn rat, Biochem J, 1971, *125*, 925.

71. Spiro, R. G., and Spiro, M. J.: Studies on the biosynthesis of the hydroxylysine-linked disaccharide unit of basement membranes and collagens. I. Kidney glucosyltransferase, J Biol Chem, 1971, *246*, 4899.

72. Spiro, M. J., and Spiro, R. G.: Studies on the biosynthesis of the hydroxylysine-linked disaccharide unit of basement membranes and collagens. II. Kidney glycosyltransferase, J Biol Chem, 1971, *246*, 4910.

73. Brownell, A. G., and Veis, A.: The intracellular location of the glycosylation of hydroxylysine of collagen, Biochem Biophys Res Commun, 1975, *63*, 371.

74. Clark, C. C., Bhalla, A., and Kefalides, N. A.: The presence of mannose and glucosamine in newly synthesized tendon cell procollagen, Fed Proc, 1975, *34*, 696A.

75. Spiro, R. G., and Spiro, M. J.: Studies on the biosynthesis of the hydroxylysine-linked disaccharide unit of basement membranes and collagens. III. Tissue and subcellular distribution of glycosyltransferases and the effect of various conditions on the enzyme levels, J Biol Chem, 1971, *246*, 4919.

76. Eyre, D. R., and Glimcher, M. J.: Analysis of a crosslinked peptide from calf bone collagen: Evidence that hydroxylysyl glycoside participates

in the crosslink, Biochem Biophys Res Commun, 1973, *52*, 663.

77. Kang, A. H., Beachey, E. H., and Katzman, R. L.: Interaction of an active glycopeptide from chick skin collagen (α1-CB5) with human platelets, J Biol Chem, 1974, *249*, 1054.

78. Spiro, R. B.: Characterization and quantitative determination of the hydroxlysine-linked carbohydrate units of several collagens, J Biol Chem, 1969, *244*, 602.

79. Blumenkrantz, N., and Prockop, D. J.: Variations in the glycosylation of the collagen synthesized by chick embryo cartilage, Biochim Biophys, Acta, 1970, *208*, 461.

80. Dehm, P., Jimenez, S. A., Olsen, B. R., and Prockop, D. J.: A transport form of collagen from embryonic tendon: Electron microscopic demonstration of an NH_2-terminal extension and evidence suggesting the presence of cystine in the molecule, Proc Natl Acad Sci USA, 1972, *69*, 60.

81. Grant, M. E., Schofield, J. D., Kefalides, N. A., and Prockop, D. J.: The biosynthesis of basement membrane collagen in embryonic chick lens, J Biol Chem, 1973, *248*, 7432.

82. Schofield, J. D., Uitto, J., and Prockop, D. J.: Formation of interchain disulfide bonds and helical structure during biosynthesis of procollagen by embryonic tendon cells, Biochemistry, 1974, *13*, 1801.

83. Bellamy, G., and Bornstein, P.: Evidence for procollagen, a biosynthetic precursor of collagen, Proc Natl Acad Sci USA, 1971, *68*, 1138.

84. Lenaers, A., Ansay, M., Nusgens, B. V., and Lapiere, C. M.: Collagen made of extended α-chains, procollagen, in genetically-defective dermatosparaxic calves, Eur J Biochem, 1971, *23*, 533.

85. Veis, A., Anesey, J., Yuan, L., and Levy, S. J.: Evidence for an amino-terminal extension in high-molecular-weight collagens from mature bovine skin, Proc Natl Acad Sci USA, 1973, *70*, 1464.

86. Bailey, A. J., and Lapière, C. M.: Effect of an additional peptide extension of the N-terminus of collagen from dermatosparactic calves on the cross-linking of collagen fibers, Eur J Biochem, 1973, *34*, 91.

87. Goldberg, B., and Green, H.: An analysis of collagen secretion by established mouse fibroblast lines, J Cell Biol, 1964, *22*, 227.

88. Weinstock, M., and Leblond, C. P.: Formation of collagen, Fed Proc, 1974, *33*, 1205.

89. Kefalides, N. A., Tomichek, E., and Alper, R.: Peptides of basement membrane proteins after cyanogen bromide and potassium cyanide cleavage, in *Extracellular Matrix Influences on Gene Expression*, H. C. Slavkin and R. C. Greulich, ed., Academic Press, New York, 1975, pp. 129, 153.

90. Pinnell, S. R., and Martin, G. R.: The cross-linking of collagen and elastin: Enzymatic conversion of lysine in peptide linkage to α-amino-adipic-δ-semialdehyde (allysine) by an extract of bone, Proc Natl Acad Sci USA, 1968, *61*, 708.

91. Siegel, R. C.: Biosynthesis of collagen crosslinks: Increased activity of purified lysyl oxidase with reconstituted collagen fibrils, Proc Natl Acad Sci USA, 1974, *71*, 4826.

92. Barrow, M. V., Simpson, C. F., and Miller, E. J.: Lathyrism: A Review, Q Rev Biol, 1974, *49*, 101.

93. Brody, J. S., Kagan, H. M., Manalo, A. D., Hu, C. A., and Franzblau, C.: Lung lysyl oxidase and elastin synthesis during compensatory lung growth, Chest, in press.

94. Tanzer, M. L.: Cross-linking of collagen, Science, 1973, *180*, 561.

95. Miller, E. J., and Robertson, P. B.: The stability of collagen cross-links when derived from hydroxylysyl residues, Biochem Biophys Res Commun, 1973, *54*, 432.

96. Pickrell, J. A., and Shafer, J.: Lung connective tissue measurements. I. Amino acid analysis procedures for determination of canine lung connective tissue, Arch Intern Med, 1971, *127*, 891.

97. Seifter, S., and Harper, E.: Collagenases, in *Methods in Enzymology, Vol. XIX, Proteolytic Enzymes*, G. E. Perlmann and L. Lorand, ed., Academic Press, New York, 1970, p. 613.

98. Seifter, S., and Harper, E.: The collagenases, in *The Enzymes. III, Hydrolysis: Peptide bonds*, P. D. Boyer, ed., Academic Press, New York, 1971, p. 649.

99. Pérez-Tamayo, R.: Collagen degradation and resorption: Physiology and pathology, in *Molecular Pathology of Connective Tissues*, R. Pérez-Tamayo and M. Rojkind, ed., Marcel Dekker, New York, 1973, p. 229.

100. Davison, P. F.: Homeostasis in extracellular tissues: Insights from studies on collagen, CRC Crit Rev Biochem, 1973, *1*, 201.

101. Harris, E. D., and Krane, S. M.: Collagenases, N Engl J Med, 1974, *291*, 557, 605, 652.

102. Etherington, D. J.: The nature of the collagenolytic cathepsin of rat liver and its distribution in other rat tissues, Biochem, J, 1972, *127*, 685.

103. Burleigh, M., Barrett, A. J., and Lazarus, G. S.: Cathepsin B1: A lysosomal enzyme that degrades native collagen, Biochem J, 1974, *137*, 387.

104. Lazarus, G. S., Brown, R. S., Daniels, J. R., and Fullmer, H. M.: Human granulocyte collagenase, Science, 1968, *159*, 1483.

105. Robertson, P. B., Ryel, R. B., Taylor, R. E., Shyu, K. W., and Fullmer, H. M.: Collagenase: Localization in polymorphonuclear leukocyte granules in the rabbit, Science, 1972, *177*, 64.

106. Wahl, L. M., Wahl, S. M., Mergenhagen, S. E.,

and Martin, G. R.: Collagenase production by lymphokine-activated macrophages, Science, 1975, *187*, 261.

107. Harper, E., Bloch, K. J., and Gross, J.: The zymogen of tadpole collagenase, Biochemistry, 1971, *10*, 3035.

108. Harper, E., and Gross, J.: Collagenase, procollagenase and activator relationships in tadpole tissue cultures, Biochem Biophys Res Commun, 1972, *48*, 1147.

109. Oronsky, A. L., Perper, R. J., and Schroder, H. C.: Phagocytic release and activation of human leukocyte procollagenase, Nature, 1973, *246*, 417.

110. Gross, J., Harper, E., Harris, E. D., Jr., McCroskery, P. A., Highberger, J. H., Corbett, C., and Kang, A. H.: Animal collagenases: Specificity of action, and structures of the substrate cleavage site, Biochem Biophys Res Commun, 1974, *61*, 605.

111. Cohen, A. B.: Interrelationships between the human alveolar macrophage and alpha-1-antitrypsin, J Clin Invest, 1973, *52*, 2793.

112. Tuttle, W. C., and Jones, R. K.: Fluorescent antibody studies of alpha-1-antitrypsin in adult human lung, Am J Clin Pathol, in press.

113. Ohlsson, K., and Olsson, I.: The neutral proteases of human granulocytes: Isolation and partial characterization of two granulocyte collagenases, Eur J Biochem, 1973, *36*, 473.

114. Cowan, M. J., Breul, S. M., Hance, A., Bradley, K., Rowe, J., and Crystal, R. G.: Lung collagen accumulation: Synthesis versus proteolysis (abstract), Am Rev Respir Dis, 1975 *111*, 931.

115. Goldberg, A. L., and Dice, J. F.: Intracellular protein degradation in mammalian and bacterial cells, Annu Rev Biochem, 1974, *43*, 835.

116. Tencate, A. R.: Morphological studies of fibrocytes in connective tissue undergoing rapid remodelling, J Anat, 1972 *112*, 401.

117. Low, F. N.: Extracellular components of the pulmonary alveolar wall, Arch Intern Med, 1971, *127*, 847.

118. Luna, L. G.: Manual of Histologic Staining Methods of the Armed Forces Institute of Pathology, McGraw-Hill, New York, 1968.

119. Eastoe, J. E.: Composition of collagen and allied proteins, in *Treatise on Collagen*, G. N. Ramachandran, ed., Academic Press, New York, 1967, p. 1.

120. Pras, M., and Glynn, L. E.: Isolation of a noncollagenous reticulin component and its primary characterization, Br J Exp Pathol, 1973, *54*, 449.

121. Krahl, V. E.: Anatomy of the mammalian lung, in *Handbook of Physiology, Sec. 3, Respiration* vol. I, W. O. Fenn and H. Rahn, ed., American Physiological Society, Washington, D. C., 1964, p. 213.

122. Binet, J. P., Nezelof, C., and Fredet, J.: Five cases of lobar tension emphysema in infancy: Importance of bronchial malformation and value of postoperative steriod therapy, Dis Chest, 1962, *41*, 126.

123. Pierce, J. A., and Ebert, R. V.: Fibrous network of the lung and its change with age, Thorax, 1965, *20*, 469.

124. Brissie, R. M., Spicer, S. S., and Thompson, N. T.: The variable fine structure of elastin visualized with Verhoeff's iron hematoxylin, Anat Rec, 1975, *181*, 83.

125. Weibel, E. R.: Morphometrics of the lung, in *Handbook of Physiology, sec. 3, Respiration*, vol. I, American Physiological Society, Washington, D. C., 1964, p. 285.

126. Ryan, S. F.: The structure of the interalveolar septum of the mammalian lung, Anat Rec, 1969, *165*, 467.

127. Rosenquist, T. H., Bernick, S., Sobin, S. S., and Fung, Y. C.: The structure of the pulmonary interalveolar sheet, Microvasc Res, 1973, *5*, 199.

128. Weibel, E. R.: Morphological basis of alveolar-capillary gas exchange, Physiol Rev, 1973, *53*, 419.

129. Sobin, S. S., Bernick, S., Tremer, H. M., Rosenquist, T. H., Lindal, R., and Fung, Y. C.: The fibroprotein network of the pulmonary interalveolar sheet, Chest, 1974, *65*, 4S.

130. Bachofan, M., and Weibel, E. R.: Basic pattern of tissue repair in human lungs following unspecific injury, Chest, 1974, *65*, 14S.

131. Diverties, M. B., Cassan, S. M., and Brown, A. L., Jr.: Ultrastructural morphometry of the diffusion surface in a case of pulmonary asbestosis, Mayo Clin Proc, 1975, *50*, 193.

132. Legrand, M., Pariente, R., André, J., Chrétien, J., and Brouet, G.: Electron microscopic study of the human parietal pleura, Presse Med, 1971, *79*, 2515.

133. Roberts, W. C., and Ferrans, V. J.: Pure collagen plaques on the diaphragm and pleura, Chest, 1972, *61*, 357.

134. Dempsey, E. W., and Lansing, A. I.: Elastic tissue, Int Rev Cytol, 1954, *3*, 437.

135. Ross, R.: The elastic fiber: A review, J. Histochem Cytochem, 1973 *21*, 199.

136. Ross, R., and Bornstein, P.: Elastic fibers in the body, Sci Am, 1971, *224*, 44.

137. Ross, R., and Bornstein, P.: The elastic fiber. I. The separation and partial characterization of its macromolecular components, J Cell Biol, 1969, *40*, 366.

138. Robert, B., Szigieti, M., Derouette, J. C., Robert, L., Bouissou, H., and Fabre, M. T.: Studies on the nature of the "microfibrillar" component of elastic fibers, Eur J Biochem, 1971, *21*, 507.

139. Yu, S. Y., and Lai, S. E.: Structure of aortic elastic fiber: An electron microscopic study with special reference to staining by ruthenium red, J Electron Microsc (Tokyo), 1970, *19*, 362.

140. Franzblau, C.: Elastin, in *Comprehensive Biochemistry*, vol. 26, part C, M. Florkin and E. H. Stotz, ed., Elsevier, New York, 1970, p. 659.

141. Lansing, A. I., Rosenthal, T. B., Alex, M., and Dempsey, E. W.: The structure and chemical characterization of elastic fibers as revealed by elastase and by electron microscopy, Anat Rec, 1952, *114*, 555.

142. Weissman, N., Shields, G. S., and Carnes, W. H.: Cardiovascular studies on copper-deficient swine. IV. Content and solubility of the aortic elastin, collagen, and hexosamine, J Biol Chem, 1963, *238*, 3115.

143. Sandberg, L. B., Hackett, T. N., Jr., and Carnes, W. H.: The solubilization of an elastin-like protein from copper-deficient porcine aorta, Biochim Biophys Acta, 1969, *181*, 201.

144. Sandberg, L. B., Weissman, N., and Smith, D. W.: The purification and partial characterization of a soluble elastin-like protein from copper-deficient porcine aorta, Biochemistry, 1969, *8*, 2940.

145. Sandberg, L. B., Zeikus, R. D., and Coltrain, I. M.: Tropoelastin purification from copper-deficient swine: A simplified method, Biochim Biophys Acta, 1971, *236*, 542.

146. Grant, M. E., Steven, F. S., Jackson, D. S., and Sandberg, L. B.: Carbohydrate content of insoluble elastins prepared from adult bovine and calf ligamentum nuchae and tropoelastin isolated from copper-deficient porcine aorta, Biochem J, 1971, *121*, 197.

147. Sykes, B. C., and Partridge, S. M.: Isolation of a soluble elastin from lathyritic chicks, Biochem J, 1972, *130*, 1171.

148. Rucker, R. B., and Goettlich-Riemann, W.: Isolation and properties of soluble elastin from copper-deficient chicks, J Nut, 1972, *102*, 563.

149. Smith, D. W., Brown, D. M., and Carnes, W. H.: Preparation and properties of salt-soluble elastin, J Biol Chem, 1972, *247*, 2427.

150. Smith, D. W., and Carnes, W. H.: Biosynthesis of soluble elastin by pig aortic tissue *in vitro*, J Biol Chem, 1973, *248*, 8157.

151. Partridge, S. M.: Elastin structure and biosynthesis, in *Symposium on Fibrous Proteins*, W. G. Crewther, ed., Plenum Press, New York, 1967, p. 246.

152. Franzblau, C., and Lent, R. W.: Studies on the chemistry of elastin, Brookhaven Symp Biol, 1968, *21*, 358.

153. Siegel, R. C., Pinnell, S. R., and Martin, G. R.: Cross-linking of collagen and elastin: Properties of lysyl oxidase, Biochemistry, 1970, *9*, 4486.

154. Foster, J. A., Rubin, L., Kagan, H. M., Frazblau, C., Bruenger, E., and Sandberg, L. B.: Isolation and characterization of cross-linked peptides from elastin, J Biol Chem, 1974, *249*, 6191.

155. Gerber, G. E., and Anwar, R. A.: Structural studies in cross-linked regions of elastin, J Biol Chem, 1974, *249*, 5200.

156. Sandberg, L. B., Weissman, N., and Gray, W. R.: Structural features of tropoelastin related to the sites of cross-links in aortic elastin, Biochemistry, 1971, *10*, 52.

157. Ross, R., and Klebanoff, S. J.: The smooth muscle cell. I. *In vivo* synthesis of connective tissue proteins, J Cell Biol, 1971, *50*, 159.

158. Ross, R.: The smooth muscle cell. II. Growth of smooth culture and formation of elastic fibers, J Cell Biol, 1971, *50*, 172.

159. Foster, J. A., Bruenger, E., Gray, W. R., and Sandberg, L. B.: Isolation and amino acid sequence of tropoelastin peptides, J Biol Chem, 1973, *248*, 2876.

160. Levene, C. I.: Lathyrism, in *Molecular Pathology of Connective Tissue*, R. Pérez-Tamayo and M. Rojkind, ed., Marcel Dekker, New York, 1973, p. 175.

161. Rucker, R. B., Hussain, M. Z., Clifford, A., and Cross, C. E.: Isolation of a native soluble elastin from lung, Clin Res, 1974, *22*, 202A.

162. Naum, Y., and Morgan, T. E.: A microassay for elastin, Anal Biochem, 1973, *53*, 392.

163. Fitzpatrick, M., and Hospelhorn, V.D.: Studies of human pulmonary connective tissue. II. Amino acid composition of residues following collagenase digestion of lung connective tissue, Am Rev Respir Dis, 1965, *92*, 792.

164. Richmond, V.: Lung parenchymal elastin isolated by non-degradative means, Biochim Biophys Acta, 1974, *351*, 173.

165. Evans, H. E., Keller, S., and Mandl, I.: Lung tissue elastin composition in newborn infants with the respiratory syndrome and other diseases, J Clin Invest, 1974 *54*, 213.

166. John, R., and Thomas, J.: Chemical compositions of elastins isolated from aortas and pulmonary tissues of humans of different ages, Biochem J, 1972, *127*, 261.

167. Fitzpatrick, M., and Hospelhorn, V. D.: Studies of human pulmonary connective tissue. I. Amino acid composition of elastins isolated by alkaline digestion, J Lab Clin Med, 1962, *60*, 799.

168. Varadi, D. P.: Studies on the chemistry and fine structure of elastic fibers from normal adult skin, J Invest Dermatol, 1972, *59*, 238.

169. Hauschka, P. V., and Gallop, P. M.: Elastin biosynthesis in mouse lung, Fed Proc, 1974, *33*, 1536.

170. Slack, H. G. B.: Metabolism of elastin in the adult rat, Nature, 1954, *174*, 512.

171. Kao, K. Y. T., Hilker, D. M., and McGavack, T.: Connective tissue. V. Comparison of synthesis and turnover of collagen and elastin in tissues of rat at several ages, Proc Soc Exp Biol Med, 1961, *106*, 335.

172. Pierce, J. A., Resnick, H., and Henry P. H.: Collagen and elastin metabolism in the lungs, skin, and bones of adult rats, J Lab Clin Med, 1967, *69*, 485.

173. Robert, L., Moczar, M., and Robert, M.: Bio-

genesis maturation and aging of elastic tissue, Experientia, 1974, *30*, 211.

174. Hartley, B. S., and Shotton, D. M.: Pancreatic elastase, in *The Enzymes. III Hydrolysis: Peptide Bonds*, P. D. Boyer, ed., Academic Press, New York, 1971, p. 323.

175. Ohlsson, K., and Olsson, I.: The neutral proteases of human granulocytes: Isolation and partial characterization of granulocyte elastases, Eur J Biochem, 1974, *42*, 519.

176. Janoff, A.: Human granulocyte elastase, Am J Pathol, 1972, *68*, 579.

177. Blondin, J., Rosenberg, R., and Janoff, A.: An inhibitor in human lung macrophages active against human neutrophil elastase, Am Rev Respir Dis, 1972, *106*, 477.

178. Powers, J. C., and Tuhy, P. M.: Active-site specific inhibitors of elastase, Biochemistry, 1973, *12*, 4767.

179. Snider, G. L., Hayes, J. A., Franzblau, C., Kagan, H. M., Stone, P. S., and Korthy, A. L.: Relationship between elastolytic activity and experimental emphysema-inducing properties of papain preparations, Am Rev Respir Dis, 1974, *110*, 254.

180. Fischer, G.: Vergleichendanatomische untersuchungen über den bronchialbaum der Vögel, Zool (Stuttgart), 1905, *19*, 1.

181. Jones, A. W., and Barson, A. J.: Elastogenesis in the developing chick lung: A light and electron microscopical study, J Anat, 1971, *110*, 1.

182. Wright, R. R.: Elastic tissue of normal and emphysematous lungs: A tridimensional histologic study, Am J Pathol, 1961, *39*, 355.

183. Rhodin, J., and Dalhamn, T.: Electron microscopy of collagen and elastin in lamina propria of the tracheal mucosa of rat, Exp Cell Res, 1955 *9*, 371.

184. Karrer, H. E.: The fine structure of connective tissue in the tunica propria of bronchioles, J Ultrastruct Res, 1958, *2*, 96.

185. Low, F. N.: Microfibrils: Fine filamentous components of the tissue space, Anat Rec, 1962, *142*, 131.

186. Brody, J. S., Kagan, H. M., Manalo, A. D., Hu, C. A., and Franzblau, C.: Lung lysyl oxidase and elastin synthesis during compensatory lung growth, Clin Res, 1975, *23*, 427A.

187. Dorfman, A., and Matalon, R.: The mucopolysaccharidoses, in *The Metabolic Basis of Inherited Disease*, J. B. Stanbury, J. B. Wyngaarden, and D. S. Fredrickson, ed., McGraw-Hill, New York, 1972, p. 1218.

188. Schubert, M., and Hammerman, D.: *A Primer on Connective Tissue Biochemistry*, Lea and Febiger, Philadelphia, 1968.

189. Roden, L., Baker, J. R., Cifonelli, J. A., and Mathews, M. B.: Isolation and characterization of connective tissue polysaccharides, in *Methods in Enzymology*, vol. 28, S. P. Colowick and N.

O. Kaplan, ed., Academic Press, New York, 1972, p. 73.

190. Rodén, L.: Biosynthesis of acidic glycosaminoglycans, in *Metabolic Conjugation and Metabolic Hydrolysis*, vol. 2, W. H. Fishman, ed., Academic Press, New York, 1970, p. 345.

191. Rosenberg, L., Margolis, R., Wolfenstein-Todel, C., Pal, S., and Strider, W.: Organization of extracellular matrix in bovine articular cartilage, in *Extracellular Matrix Influences on Gene Expression*, H. C. Slavkin and R. C. Greulich, ed., Academic Press, New York, 1975, p. 415.

192. Horwitz, A. L., and Crystal, R. G.: Content and synthesis of glycosaminoglycans in the developing lung, J Clin Invest, 1975, in press.

193. Yeager, H.: Tracheobronchial secretions, Am J Med, 1971, *50*, 493.

194. Telser, A., Robinson, H. C., and Dorfman, A.: The biosynthesis of chondroitinsulfate protein complex, Proc Natl Acad Sci USA, 1965, *54*, 912.

195. Silbert, J. E.: Biosynthesis of mucopolysaccharides and protein-polysaccharides, in *Molecular Pathology of Connective Tissues*, R. Pérez-Tamayo and M. Rojkind, ed., Marcel Dekker, New York, 1973, p. 323.

196. Silbert, J. E.: Catabolism of mucopolysaccharides and protein-polysaccharides, in *Molecular Pathology of Connective Tissues*, R. Pérez-Tamayo and M. Rojkind, ed., Marcel Dekker, New York, 1973, p. 355.

197. Matalon, R., and Dorfman, A.: Sanfilippo A syndrome: Sulfamidase deficiency in cultured skin fibroblasts and liver, J Clin Invest, 1974, *54*, 907.

198. Buonassisi, V.: Sulfated mucopolysaccharide synthesis and secretion in endothelial cell cultures, Exp Cell Res, 1973, *76*, 363.

199. Sampson, P., Parshley, M. S., Mandl, I., and Turino, G. M.: Glycosaminoglycans produced in tissue culture by rat lung cells: Isolation from a mixed cell line and a deriv́ed endothelial clone, Connect Tissue Res, in press.

200. Trelstad, R. L., Hayashi, K., and Toole, B. P.: Epithelial collagens and glycosaminoglycans in the embryonic cornea: Macromolecular order and morphogenesis in the basement membrane, J Cell Biol, 1974, *62*, 815.

201. Groggins, J. F., Lazarus, G. S., and Fullmer, H. M.: Hyaluronidase activity of alveolar macrophages, J Histochem Cytochem, 1968, *16*, 688.

202. Wusteman, F. S.: Glycosaminoglycans of bovine lung parenchyma and pleura, Experientia, 1972, *28*, 887.

203. Wusteman, F. S., Johnson, D. B., and Dodgson, K. S.: The use of "normal" rats in studies on the acid mucopolysaccharides of lung, Life Sci, 1968, *7*, 1281.

204. Mason, R. M., and Wusteman, F. S.: The glycosaminoglycans of human tracheobronchial cartilage, Biochem J, 1970, *120*, 777.

205. Thurlbeck, W. M.: Postnatal growth and devel-

opment of the lung, Am Rev Respir Dis, 1975, *111*, 803.

206. Briscoe, A. M., Loring, W. E., and McClement, J. H.: Changes in human lung collagen and lipids with age, Proc Soc Exp Biol Med, 1959, *101*, 71.

207. Pierce, J. A., and Hocott, J. B.: Studies on the collagen and elastin content of the human lung, J Clin Invest, 1960, *39*, 8.

208. Wright, G. W., Kleinerman, J., and Zorn, E. M.: The elastin and collagen content of normal and emphysematous human lungs, Am Rev Respir Dis, 1960, *81*, 938.

209. Pierce, J. A., Hocott, J. B., and Ebert, R. V.: The collagen and elastin content of the lung in emphysema, Ann Intern Med, 1961, *55*, 210.

210. Boucek, R. J., Noble, N. L., and Marks, A.: Age and the fibrous proteins of the human lung, Gerontologia, 1961, *5*, 150.

211. Pierce, J. A.: Age related changes in the fibrous proteins of the lungs, Arch Environ Health, 1963, *6*, 56.

212. Pecora, L. J., Manne, W. R., Baum, G. L., Feldman, D. P., and Recauarren, S.: Biochemical study of ground substance in normal and emphysematous lungs, Am Rev Respir Dis, 1967, *95*, 623.

213. Johnson, R., and Andrews, F. A.: Lung scleroproteins in age and emphysema, Chest, 1970, *57*, 239.

214. Cowan, M. J., and Crystal, R. G.: Lung growth after unilateral pneumonectomy: Quantitation of collagen synthesis and content, Am Rev Respir Dis, 1975, *111*, 267.

215. Crystal, R., Bradley, K., McConnell-Breul, S., Collins, J., Hance, A., and Cowan, M.: Collagen in the lung: Development of a technology applicable to human lung disease, Chest, 1975, *67*, 30S.

216. Taderera, J. V. : Control of lung differentiations *in vitro*, Dev Biol, 1967, *16*, 489.

217. Loosli, C. G., and Potter, E. L.: The prenatal development of the human lung, Anat Rec, 1951, *109*, 320A.

218. Wessells, N. K., and Cohen, J. H.: Effects of collagenase on developing epithelia *in vitro*: Lung, ureteric bud, and pancreas, Dev Biol, 1968, *18*, 294.

219. Thurlbeck, W. M.: Pulmonary emphysema, Am J Med Sci, 1963, *246*, 332.

220. Lipets, V. Y.: Changes in the elastic fibers of the lungs in some conditions and their significance in the development of emphysema, Arkh Patol, 1965, *27*, 50.

221. Pierce, J. A., Hocott, J. B., and Ebert, R. V.: Studies of lung collagen and elastin, Am Rev Respir Dis, 1959, *80*, 45.

222. Adamson, J.: in *Pulmonary Emphysema and Proteolysis*, C. Mittman, ed., Academic Press, New York, 1972, p. 257.

223. Bruce, R. M., Adamson, J. S., and Pierce, J. A.: Collagen and elastin content of the lung in antitrypsin deficiency, Clin Res, 1970, *18*, 89A.

224. Briscoe, A. M., and Loring, W. E.: Elastin content of the human lung, Proc Soc Exp Biol Med, 1958, *99*, 162.

225. Fitzpatrick, M.: Studies of human pulmonary connective tissue. III. Chemical changes in structural proteins with emphysema, Am Rev Respir Dis, 1967, *96*, 254.

226. Fitzpatrick, M.: Studies of human pulmonary connective tissue. IV. Some differences in polypeptides derived from elastic protein, Am Rev Respir Dis, 1968, *97*, 248.

227. Keller, S., and Mandl, I.: Qualitative differences between normal and emphysematous human lung elastin, in *Pulmonary Emphysema and Proteolysis*, C. Mittman, ed., Academic Press, New York, 1972, p. 251.

228. Laros, C. D., Kuyper, C. M. A., and Janssen, H. M. J.: The chemical composition of fresh human lung parenchyma, Respiration, 1972, *29*, 458.

229. Saltzman, H. A., Sieker, H. O., and Green, J.: Hexosamine and hydroxyproline content in human bronchial cartilage from aged and diseased lungs, J Lab Clin Med, 1963, *62*, 78.

230. Martin, H. B., and Boatman, E. S.: Electron microscopy of human pulmonary emphysema, Am Rev Respir Dis, 1965, *91*, 206.

231. Michaeli, D., and Fudenberg, H. H.: Antibodies to collagen in patients with emphysema, Clin Immunol Immunopathol, 1974, *3*, 187.

232. Laros, C. D.: The pathogenesis of emphysema, Respiration, 1972, *29*, 442.

233. Saltzman, H. A., Schauble, M. K., and Sieker, M. K.: Hexosamine content of aged and chronically diseased lung, J Lab Clin Med, 1961, *58*, 115.

234. Freeman, G., and Haydon, G. B.: Emphysema after low level exposure to NO_2, Arch Environ Health, 1964, *8*, 125.

235. Snider, G. L., Hayes, J. A., Korthy, A. L., and Lewis, G. P.: Centrilobular emphysema experimentally induced by cadmium chloride aerosol, Am Rev Respir Dis, 1973, *108*, 40.

236. Gross, P. M., Babyak, M. A., Tolker, E., and Kaschak, M.: Enzymatically induced pulmonary emphysema, J Occup Med, 1964, *6*, 481.

237. Palecek, F., Palecekova, M., and Aviado, D. M.: Emphysema in immature rats: Condition produced by tracheal constriction and papain, Arch Environ Health, 1967, *15*, 332.

238. Goldring, I. P., Greenberg, L., and Ratner, I. M.: On the production of emphysema in Syrian hamsters by aerosol inhalation of papain, Arch Environ Health, 1968, *16*, 59.

239. Park, S. S., Goldring, I. P., Shim, C. S., and Williams, M. H, Jr.: Mechanical properties of the lung in experimental pulmonary emphysema,

J Appl Physiol, 1969, *26*, 738.

240. Pushpackom, R., Hogg, J. C., Woolcock, A. J., Angus, A. E., Macklem, P. T., and Thurlbeck, W. M.: Experimental papain-induced emphysema in dogs, Am Rev Respir Dis., 1970, *102*, 778.

241. Kilburn, K. H., Dowell, A. R., and Pratt, P. C.: Morphological and biochemical assessment of papain-induced emphysema, Arch Intern Med, 1971, *127*, 884.

242. Johanson, W. G., Jr., Pierce, A. K., and Reynolds, R. C.: The evolution of papain emphysema in the rat, J Lab Clin Med, 1971, *78*, 599.

243. Caldwell, E. J.: Physiologic and anatomic effects of papain on the rabbit lung, J Appl Physiol, 1971, *31*, 458.

244. Johanson, W. G., and Pierce, A. K.: Effects of elastase, collagenase and papain on structure and function of rat lungs, *in vitro*, J Clin Invest, 1972, *51*, 288.

245. Goldring, I. P., Park, S. S., Greenberg, L., and Ratner, I. M.: Sequential anatomic changes in lungs exposed to papain and other proteolytic enzymes, in *Pulmonary Emphysema and Proteolysis*, C. Mittman, ed., Academic Press, New York, 1972, p. 389.

246. Johanson, W. G., Jr., and Pierce, A. K.: Lung structure and function with age in normal rats and rats with papain emphysema, J Clin Invest, 1973, *52*, 2921.

247. Johanson, W. G., Jr., Reynolds, R. C., Scott, T. C., and Pierce, A. K.: Connective tissue in emphysema: An electron microscopic study of papain-induced emphysema in rats, Am Rev Respir Dis, 1973, *107*, 589.

248. Mandl, I., Keller, S., Hosannah, Y., and Blackwood, C. E.: Induction and prevention of experimental emphysema, in *Pulmonary Emphysema and Proteolysis*, C. Mittman, ed., Academic Press, New York, 1972, p. 439.

249. Mass, B., Ikeda, T., Marco, V., Meranze, D. R., Kimbel, P., and Weinbaum, G.: Experimental emphysema in dogs: Induction by leukocyte homogenates, Fed Proc, 1971, *30*, 293.

250. Marco, V., Mass, B., Meranze, D. R., Weinbaum, G., and Kimbel, P.: Induction of experimental emphysema in dogs using leukocyte homogenates, Am Rev Respir Dis, 1971, *104*, 595.

251. Kimbel, P., Mass, B., Ikeda, T., and Weinbaum, G.: Emphysema in dogs induced by leukocyte contents, in *Pulmonary Emphysema and Proteolysis*, C. Mittman, ed., Academic Press, New York, 1972, p. 411.

252. Mass, B., Ikeda, T., Meranze, D. R., Weinbaum, G., and Kimbel, P.: Induction of experimental emphysema: Cellular and species specificity, Am Rev Respir Dis, 1972, *106*, 384.

253. Kaplan, P. D., Kuhn, C., and Pierce, J. A.: The induction of emphysema with elastase. I. The evolution of the lesion and influence of serum,

J Lab Clin Med, 1973, *82*, 349.

254. Blackwood, C. E., Hosannah, Y., Perman, E., Keller, S., and Mandl, I.: Experimental emphysema in rats: Elastolytic titer of inducing enzyme as determinant of response, Proc Soc Exp Biol Med, 1973, *144*, 450.

255. The Enzymes. III. Hydrolysis: Peptide Bonds, P. D. Boyer, ed., Academic Press, New York, 1971.

256. Turino, G. M., and Lourenço, R. V.: The connective tissue basis of pulmonary mechanics, in *Pulmonary Emphysema and Proteolysis*, C. Mittman, ed., Academic Press, New York, 1972, p. 509.

257. Koo, K. W., Hayes, J. A., Kagen, H. M., Leith, D. E., Franzblau, C., and Snider, G. L.: Lung volumes and mechanics following elastase and collagenase in hamsters, Clin Res, 1974, *22*, 508A.

258. Karlinsky, J. B., Catanese, A., Honeychurch, C., Sherter, C. B., Hoppen, F., and Snider, G. L.: *In vitro* effects of elastase and collagenase on mechanical properties of hamster lungs, Chest, in press.

259. Chang, C., and Houck, J. C.: Demonstration of the chemotactic properties of collagen, Proc Soc Exp Biol Med, 1970, *134*, 22.

260. Senior, R. M., Bielefeld, D. R., and Jeffrey, J. J.: Collogenolytic activity in human macrophages, Clin Res, 1972, *20*, 88.

261. Harris, J. O., Olsen, G. N., Castle, J. R., and Maloney, A. S.: Comparison of proteolytic enzyme activity in pulmonary alveolar macrophages and blood leukocytes in smokers and non-smokers, Am Rev Respir Dis, 1975, *111*, 579.

262. Malemud, C. J., and Janoff, A.: Human neutrophil lysosomal elastase and chymotrypsin-like enzyme degrade rabbit articular cartilage proteoglycan, Fed Proc, 1975, *34*, 822.

263. Turino, G. M., Rodriguez, J. R., Greenbaum, L. M., and Mandl, I.: Mechanisms of pulmonary injury, Am J Med, 1974, *57*, 493.

264. Manner, G., Goldring, I. P., and Kuleba, M.: Effect of proteolytic enzymes on collagen and non-collagen protein synthesis in human lung fibroblasts, Connect Tissue Res, 1974, *2*, 283.

265. Murray, J. F.: Diffuse infiltrative diseases of the lung, in *Principles of Internal Medicine*, M. M. Wintrobe, ed., McGraw-Hill, New York, 1974, p. 1291.

266. Fulmer, J. D., Roberts, W. C., and Crystal, R. G.: Diffuse fibrotic lung disease: A correlative study, Chest, in press.

267. Van den Brenk, H. A. S.: Radiation effect on the pulmonary system, in *Pathology of Irradiation*, C. C. Berdjis, ed., Williams and Wilkins, Baltimore, 1971, p. 569.

268. Rantanen, J.: Radiation injury of connective tissue, Acta Radiol [Diag], 1973, *330* (Supplement, p. 1).

269. Välimäki, M., and Niinikoski, J.: Development and reversibility of pulmonary oxygen poisoning in the rat, Aerosp Med, 1973, *44*, 533.

270. Smith, P., Heath, D., and Kay, J. M.: The pathogenesis and structure of paraquatinduced pulmonary fibrosis in rats, J Pathol, 1974, *114*, 57.

271. Ryan, S. F.: Experimental fibrosing alveolitis, Am Rev Respir Dis, 1972, *105*, 776.

272. Herrold, K. McD.: Fibrosing alveolitis and atypical proliferative lesions of the lung, Am J Pathol, 1967, *50*, 639.

273. Aso, Y., Yoneda, K., and Kikkawa, Y.: Bleomycininduced pulmonary fibrosis: Morphologic and biochemical study, Am Rev Respir Dis, 1975, *111*, 904A.

274. Mellors, R. C., Aoki, T., and Huebner, R. J.: Further implication of murine leukemia-like virus in the disorders of NZB mice, J Exp Med, 1969, *129*, 1045.

275. Stacy, B. D., and King, E. J.: Silica and collagen in the lungs of silicotic rats treated with cortisone, Br J Ind Med, 1954, *11*, 192.

276. Levene, C. I., Bye, I., and Saffiotti, U.: The effect of β-aminopropionitrile on silicotic pulmonary fibrosis in the rat, Br J Exp Pathol, 1968, *49*, 152.

277. Davis, H. V., and Reeves, A. L.: Collagen biosynthesis in rat lungs during exposure to asbestos, Am Ind Hyg Assoc J, 1971, *32*, 599.

278. Carrington, C. B.: Organizing interstitial pneumonia: Definition of the lesion and attempts to devise an experimental model, Yale J Biol Med, 1968, *40*, 352.

279. Hussain, M. A., Mustafa, M. G., Chow, C. K., and Cross, C. E.: Ozone induced increase of lung proline hydroxylase activity and hydroxyproline content, Chest, in press.

280. Van Toorn, D. W.: Experimental interstitial pulmonary fibrosis, Pathol Eur, 1970, *5*, 97.

281. Brentjens, J. R., O'Connell, D. W. Pawlowski, I. B., Hsu, K. C., and Andres, G. A.: Experimental immune complex disease of the lung, J Exp Med, 1974, *140*, 105.

282. Read, J.: The pathological changes produced by anti-lung serum, J. Pathol, 1958, *76*, 403.

283. Jennings, T. L., and Arden, A.: Development of experimental radiation pneumonitis, Arch Pathol, 1961, *71*, 437.

284. De Villiers, A. J., and Gross, P.: Radiation pneumonitis: X-ray induced lesions in hamsters and rats, Arch Environ Health, 1967, *15*, 650.

285. Rubin, P., and Casarett, G. W.: Clinical Radiation Pathology, W. B. Saunders, Philadelphia, 1968.

286. Maisin, J.: The ultrastructure of the lung of mice to a supra-lethal dose of ionizing radiation to the thorax, Radiat Res, 1970, *44*, 545.

287. Adamson, I. Y. R., Bowden, D. H., and Wyatt, J. P.: A pathway to pulmonary fibrosis: An ultrastructural study of mouse and rat following radiation to the whole body and hemithorax, Am J Pathol, 1970, *58*, 481.

288. Sanders, C. L., Adee, R. R., and Jackson, T. A.: Fine structure of alveolar areas in the lung following inhalation of [^{239}PuO$_2$] particles, Arch Environ Health, 1971, *22*, 525.

289. Kurohara, S. S., and Casarett, G. W.: Effects of single thoracic x-ray exposure in rats, Radiat Res, 1972, *52*, 263.

290. Madrazo, A., Suzuki, Y., and Churg, J.: Radiation pneumonitis: Ultrastructural changes in pulmonary alveoli following high dose radiation, Arch Pathol, 1973, *96*, 262.

291. Faulkner, C. S., II, and Connolly, K. S.: The ultrastructure of Co-60 radiation pneumonitis in rats, Lab Invest, 1973, *28*, 545.

292. Watanabe, S., Watanabe, K., Ohishi, T., Aiba, M., and Kageyama, K.: Mast cells in the rat alveolar septa undergoing fibrosis after ionizing irradiation, Lab Invest, 1974, *31*, 555.

293. Pickrell, S. A., Harris, D. V., Hahn, F. F., Belasich, J. J., and Jones, R. K.: Biological alterations resulting from chronic lung irradiation. III. Effect of partial [^{60}Co] thoracic irradiation upon pulmonary collagen metabolism and fractionation in syrian hamsters, Radiat Res, 1975, *62*, 133.

294. Pickrell, J. A., Harris, D. V., Pfleger, R. C., Benjamin, S. A., Belasich, J. J., Jones, R. K., and McClellan, R. O.: Biological alterations resulting from chronic lung irradiation. II. Connective tissue alterations following inhalation of [^{144}Ce] fused clay aerosol in beagle dogs, Radiat Res, 1975, *63*, 299.

295. Pickrell, J. A., Harris, D. V., and Mauderly, J. L.: Altered collagen metabolism in radiation-induced interstitial pulmonary fibrosis, Chest, in press.

296. Trombropoulos, E. G., and Thomas, J. M.: Effect of 800R thoracic X-irradiation on lung tissue biochemistry, Radiat Res, 1970, *44*, 76.

297. Goldstein, E., and Lewis, J. P.: Patterns of pulmonary alveolar macrophage function following radiation injury, J Lab Clin Med, 1973, *82*, 276.

298. Lima, L., Malaise, E., and Macieira-Coelho, A.: Aging *in vitro*, Exp Cell Res, 1972, *73*, 345.

299. Yaron, M., Yaron, I., and Allalouf, D.: Effect of ionizing radiation on hyaluronic acid production by cultured human synovial fibroblasts, Isr J Med Sci, 1972, *8*, 1751.

300. Castellino, R. A., Glatstein, E., Turbow, M. M., Rosenberg, S., and Kaplan, H. S.: Latent radiation injury of lungs or heart activated by steroid withdrawal, Ann Intern Med, 1974, *80*, 593.

301. Tzeveleva, I. A.: Metabolism of glucosaminoglycans (acid mucopolysaccharides) in rabbit lungs after plutonium poisoning, Vopr Med Khim, 1970, *16*, 399.

302. Heppleston, A. G., and Styles, J. A.: Activity of a macrophage factor in collagen formation by

silica, Nature, 1967, *214*, 521.

303. Burrell, R., and Anderson, M.: The induction of fibrogenesis by silica-treated alveolar macrophages, Environ Res, 1973, *6*, 389.

304. Heppleston, A. G.: The biological response to silica, in *Biology of Fibroblast*, E. Kulonen and J. Pikkarainen, ed., Academic Press, New York, 1973, p. 529.

305. Richards, R. J., and Wusteman, F. S.: The effects of silica dust and alveolar macrophages on lung fibroblasts grown *in vitro*, Life Sci, 1974, *14*, 355.

306. Harington, J. S., Ritchie, M., King, P. C., and Miller, K.: The *in vitro* effects of silica-treated hamster macrophages on collagen production by hamster fibroblasts, J Pathol, 1973, *109*, 21.

307. Richards, R. J., Wusteman, F. S., and Dodgson, K. S.: The direct effects of dusts on lung fibroblasts grown *in vitro*, Life Sci, 1971, *10*, 1149.

308. Kilroe-Smith, T. A., Webster, I., van Drimmelen, M., and Marasas, L.: An insoluble fibrogenic factor in macrophages from guinea pigs exposed to silica, Environ Res, 1973, *6*, 298.

309. Spencer, H.: Interstitial pneumonia, Annu Rev Med, 1967, *18*, 423.

310. Spencer, H.: Pathology of the Lung, Pergamon Press, Oxford, 1968, p. 711.

311. Willoughby, W. F., Barbaras, J. E., and Wheelis, R. F.: Immunologic mechanisms in experimental interstitial pneumonitis, Chest, in press.

312. Tomasi, T. B., Fudenberg, H. H., and Finby, N.: Possible relationship between rheumatoid factors and pulmonary disease, Am J Med, 1962, *33*, 243.

313. Turner-Warwick, M., and Doniach, D.: Autoantibody studies in interstitial pulmonary fibrosis, Br Med J, 1965, *1*, 886.

314. Gohlich, A. J., Spieia, H., Tierstein, A. S., and Siltzbach, L. E.: Serological factors in idiopathic diffuse interstitial pulmonary fibrosis, Am J Med, 1965, *39*, 405.

315. Nagaya, H., Buckley, E., and Sieker, H. O.: Positive antinuclear factor in unexplained pulmonary fibrosis, Ann Intern Med, 1969, *70*, 1135.

316. Setnikar, I., Origine e significato della proprieta mechaniche del polmone, Arch Fisiol, 1955, *55*, 349.

317. Mead, J.: Mechanical properties of lungs, Physiol Rev, 1961, *41*, 281.

318. Hogg, J .C., Nepszy, S. F., Macklem, P. T., and Thurlbeck, W. M.: Elastic properties of the centrilobular space, J Clin Invest, 1969, *48*, 1306.

319. Senior, R. M., Bielefeld, D. R., and Abensohn, M. K.: The effects of proteolytic enzymes on the tensile strength of human lung, Am Rev Respir Dis, 1975, *111*, 184.

320. Mead, J.: Mechanical properties of the lung, in *The Lung*, A. A. Liebow and D. E. Smith, ed., Williams and Wilkins, Baltimore, 1968, p. 48.

321. Cox, R. C., and Little, K.: An electron microscopic study of elastic tissue, Proc R Soc Med, 1961, *155*, 232.

322. Adamson, J. S., Jr.: An electron microscopic comparison of the connective tissue from the lungs of young and elderly subjects, Am Rev Respir Dis, 1968, *98*, 399.

323. Permutt, S., and Martin, H. B.: Static pressure-volume characteristics of lungs in normal males, J Appl Physiol, 1960, *15*, 819.

324. Turner, J. M., Mead, J., and Wohl, M. E.: Elasticity of human lungs in relation to age, J Appl Physiol, 1968, *25*, 664.

325. Bates, D. V., Macklem, P. T., and Christie, R. V.: Respiratory Function in Disease, W. B. Saunders, Philadelphia, 1971, p. 96.

326. Edelman, N. H., Mittman, C., Norris, A. H., and Shock, N. W.: Effects of respiratory pattern on age differences in ventilation uniformity, J Appl Physiol, 1968, *24*, 49.

327. Hoffman, L., Mondshine, R. B., and Park, S. S.: Effect of penicillamine on elastic properties of rat lung, J Appl Physiol, 1971, *30*, 508.

328. Hoffman, L., Blumenfeld, O. O., Mondshine, R. B., and Park, S. S.: Effect of DL-pennicillamine on fibrous proteins of rat lung, J Appl Physiol, 1972, *33*, 42.

329. Caldwell, E. J., and Bland, J. H.: The effect of penicillamine on the rabbit lung, Am Rev Respir Dis, 1972, *105*, 75.

330. Boldstein, E. R., Haddad, R., and Hamosh, P.: Effect of β-aminopropionitrile on the elastic behavior of the rat lung, Clin Res, 1970, *18*, 89A.

331. Stanley, N. M., Cherniack, N. S., Altose, M. D., Saldana, M., and Fishman, A. P.: Effects of β-aminopropionitrile on the mechanical properties of rat lung, Am Rev Respir Dis, 1972, *105*, 999.

332. Stanley, N. N., Alper, R., Cunningham, E. L., Cherniack, N. S., and Kefalides, N. A.: Effects of a molecular change in collagen on lung structure and mechanical function, J Clin Invest, 1975, *55*, 1195.

333. Kohn, R. R., and Rollerson, E.: Aging of human collagen in relation to susceptibility to the action of collagenase, J Gerontol, 1960, *15*, 10.

334. Szemenyei, C., and Balint, A.: Studies on the aging process of the rat lung, Acta Sci Hung, 1973, *21*, 295.

335. Bornstein, P.: The cross-linking of collagen and elastin and its inhibition in osteolathyrism: Is there a relation to the aging process?, Am J Med, 1970, *49*, 429.

336. Sugihara, T. C., Martin, J., and Hildebrandt, J.: Length-tension properties of alveolar wall in man, J Appl Physiol, 1971, *30*, 874.

337. Sugihara, T., Hildebrandt, J., and Martin, C. J.: Viscoelastic properties of alveolar wall, J Appl Physiol, 1972, *33*, 93.

338. Sugihara, T., and Martin, C. J.: Simulation of lung tissue properties in age and irreversible obstructive syndromes using an aldehyde, J Clin

Invest, 1975, *56*, 23.

339. Turino, G. M., Lourenco, R. V., and McCracken, G. H.: Role of connective tissues in large pulmonary airways, J Appl Physiol, 1968, *25*, 645.

340. McKusick, V. A.: Heritable Disorders of Connective Tissue, C. V. Mosby, St. Louis, 1972.

341. The Metabolic Basis of Inherited Disease, J. B. Stanbury, J. B. Wyngaarden, and D. S. Fredrickson, ed., McGraw-Hill, New York, 1972.

342. Dwyer, E. M., and Troncale, F.: Spontaneous pneumothorax and pulmonary disease in the Marfan syndrome, Ann Intern Med, 1965, *62*, 1285.

343. Fuleihan, F. J. D., Suh, S. K., and Shepard, R. H.: Some aspects of pulmonary function in the Marfan syndrome, Bull Johns Hopkins Hosp, 1963, *113*, 320.

344. Chisholm, J. C., Cherniack, N. S., and Carton, R. W.: Results of pulmonary function testing in 5 persons with Marfan syndrome, J Lab Clin Med, 1968, *71*, 25.

345. Reye, R. D. K., and Bale, P. M.: Elastic tissue in pulmonary emphysema in Marfan syndrome, Arch Pathol, 1973, *96*, 427.

346. Gerritsen, T., and Waisman, H. A.: Homocystinuria, in *The Metabolic Basis of Inherited Disease*, J. B. Stanbury, ed., McGraw-Hill, New York, 1972, p. 404.

347. Pinnell, S. R., Krane, S. M., Kenzora, J. E., and Glimcher, M. J.: A heritable disorder of connective tissue: Hydroxylysine deficient collagen, N Engl J Med, 1972, *286*, 1013.

348. Pope, F. M., Martin, G. R., Lichtenstein, J. R., Penttinen, R., Gerson, B., Rowe, D. W., and McKusick, V. A.: Patients with Ehlers-Danlos syndrome type IV lack type III collagen, Proc Natl Acad Sci USA, 1975, *72*, 1314.

349. Di Ferrante, M., Leachman, R. D., Angelini, P., Donnelly, P. V., Francis G., and Almazan, A.: Lysyl oxidase deficiency in Ehlers-Danlos syndrome type V, Connect Tissue Res, 1975, *3*, 49.

350. Lichtenstein, J. R., Martin, G. R., Kohn, L. D., Byers, P. H., and McKusick, V. A.: Defect in conversion of procollagen to collagen in a form of Ehlers-Danlos syndrome, Science, 1973, *182*, 298.

351. Falvo, K. A., Klain, D. B., Krauss, A. N., Root, L., and Auld, P. A. M.: Pulmonary function studies in osteogenesis imperfecta, Am Rev Respir Dis, 1973, *108*, 1258.

352. Penttinen, R. P., Lichtenstein, J. R., Martin, G. R., and McKusick, V. A.: Abnormal collagen metabolism in cultured cells in osteogenesis imperfecta, Proc Natl Acad Sci USA, 1975, *72*, 586.

353. LaDu, B. N.: Alcaptonuria, in *The Metabolic Basis of Inherited Disease*, J. B. Stanbury, ed., McGraw-Hill, New York, 1972, p. 308.

354. Murray, J. F.: Pulmonary disability in the Hurler syndrome, N Engl J Med, 1959, *261*, 378.

355. Cohen, A. B.: Apha-1-antitrypsin: A systemic determinant of lung structure and function, in *The Biochemical Basis of Pulmonary Function*, R. G. Crystal, ed., Marcel Dekker, New York, in press.

356. Cowan, M. J., Collins, J. F., and Crystal, R. G.: Collagen and lung growth: A prototype of connective tissue differentiation, in *Eukaryotes at the Subcellular Level*, J. Last, ed., Marcel Dekker, New York, 1975, in press.

357. Kikkawa, Y., and Yoneda, K.: The type II epithelial cell of the lung. I. Method of isolation, Lab Invest, 1974, *30*, 76.

358. Douglas, W. H. J., and Kaighn, M. E.: Clonal isolation of differentiated rat lung cells, In Vitro, 1974, *10*, 230.

359. Chvapil, M.: Pharmacology of fibrosis and tissue injury, Environ Health Perspect, 1974, *9*, 283.

360. Ehrlich, H. P., and Bornstein, P.: Microtubules in transcellular movement of procollagen, Nature [New Biol], 1972, *238*, 257.

361. Chvapil, M., McCarthy, D., Madden, J. W., and Peacock, E. E.: Effect of 1,10-phenanthroline and desferrioxamine *in vivo* on prolyl hydroxylase and hydroxylation of collagen in various tissues of rats, Biochem Pharmacol, 1974, *23*, 2165.

362. Houck, J. C., and Sharma, V. K.: Induction of collagenolytic and proteolytic activities in rat and human fibroblasts by anti-inflammatory drugs, Science, 1968, *161*, 1361.

363. Rokosova, B., and Chvapil, M.: Relationship between the dose of ascorbic acid and its structural analogs and proline hydroxylation in various biological systems, Connect Tissue Res, 1974, *2*, 215.

364. Ehrlich, H. P., Tarver, H., and Hunt, T.: Effects of vitamin A and glucocorticoids upon inflammation and collagen synthesis, Ann Surg, 1973, *177*, 223.

365. Saksena, J. S., Mehta, J. A., and Naimark, A.: The effect of vitamin A deficiency in rabbits on the elastic properties of the lung and thoracic aorta, Can J Physiol Pharmacol, 1971, *49*, 127.

366. Ooshima, A., Fuller, G. C., Cardinale, G. J. Spector, S., and Udenfriend, S.: Increased collegan synthesis in blood vessels of hypertensive rats and its reversal by antihypertensive agents, Proc Natl Acad Sci USA, 1974, *71*, 3019.

367. Uitto, J., Teir, H., and Mustakallio, K. K.: Corticosteriod-induced inhibition of the biosynthesis of human skin collagen, Biochem Pharmacol, 1972, *21*, 2161.

368. Koob, T. J., Jeffrey, J. J., and Eisen, A. Z.: Regulation of human skin collagenase activity by hydrocortisone and dexamethasone in organ culture, Biochem Biophys Res Commun, 1974, *61*, 1083.

State of the Art

Cystic Fibrosis[1-3]

ROBERT E. WOOD,[4] THOMAS F. BOAT, and CARL F. DOERSHUK

Contents

[1] From the Department of Pediatrics, Rainbow Babies and Childrens Hospital, Case Western Reserve University School of Medicine, Cleveland, Ohio.

[2] Supported in part by Grants AM 08305, HL 13885, HL 06009, HL 17776, and HR 52957 from the U. S. Public Health Service, and by grants from the Cystic Fibrosis Foundation and the Health Fund of Greater Cleveland.

[3] Requests for reprints should be addressed to Carl F. Doershuk, M.D., 2103 Adelbert Road, Cleveland, Ohio 44106.

[4] Clinical Fellow, Cystic Fibrosis Foundation.

Introduction

Das Kind stirbt bald Wieder,
dessen Stirne beim Küssen salsig schmect. (1)

This saying from the German folklore, literally translated as "The child will soon die, whose brow tastes salty when kissed," is perhaps the earliest known reference to the condition now known as cystic fibrosis (Holsclaw, D. S.: Personal communication). Various early reports described the clinical manifestations, meconium ileus, and pathology of the pancreas (2–5). Fanconi and associates (6) related congenital cystic pancreatic fibrosis to bronchiectasis. Andersen (7) described it as a distinct entity, using the term cystic fibrosis of the pancreas. Subsequently, increasingly detailed descriptions of the pathophysiology, complications, and therapy have been published.

Cystic fibrosis is the most frequent lethal genetic syndrome among white children and is the cause of much of the chronic progressive pulmonary disease encountered in children. When initially recognized, it seemed invariably and rapidly fatal. However, increasing survival has resulted in more than 11,000 patients in the U.S. Cystic Fibrosis Data Registry (Warwick, W. R.: Unpublished data), with an estimated national total of 15,000 to 20,000 patients. An additional 800 to 1,000 new cases are diagnosed annually. Of the more than 110 centers established by the Cystic Fibrosis Foundation, 12 have more than 200 patients. The center program has encouraged clinical and basic research and has contributed to increasingly effective case detection and delivery of care. Of the 450 patients currently seen in our center, one-third are 15 years of age or older and the proportion is increasing. Our experience is similar to that at many other long-established centers, so that nationally there are some 2,000 known adults with cystic fibrosis.

The national 50 per cent survival rate is now 16 years (Warwick, W. R.: Unpublished data). Of the total patient group referred to our center for comprehensive care, 50 per cent survival now is being achieved beyond 26 years. In those cases in which diagnosis and treatment began while the pulmonary involvement was still reversible, survival of greater than 96 per cent is occurring beyond 18 years of treatment (8).

Although the age at diagnosis may be decreasing, the proportion of patients with active pulmonary disease at diagnosis remains high. This suggests that factors other than lessening severity of the disease are playing a role in the remarkable survival rate now being achieved by patients with cystic fibrosis. Some of the factors may include (1) recognition and correction of the vitamin deficiencies, together with availability and use of pancreatin therapy (9, 10); (2) increasingly effective antimicrobial drugs and improvement in their use and delivery; (3) more definite diagnosis using the pilocarpine iontophoresis sweat test and quantitative analysis (11); (4) recognition of cases with milder pulmonary and/or gastrointestinal involvement; (5) development of individual measures of pulmonary therapy, including mist (12) and postural drainage (13, 14); (6) development of a comprehensive care program (15) administered from the time of diagnosis for all patients (16); (7) increasing attention to psychosocial factors in the disease and its therapy; (8) development of a nationally linked network of diagnosis and care, teaching and research centers; (9) prompt recognition of complications with intervention by experienced physicians; (10) concentration of patients at centers based at major institutions, stimulating and facilitating research. In addition, there are probably other aspects not mentioned or still unrecognized.

Because of the increasing adolescent and adult population of patients with cystic fibrosis and their psychosocial, employment, and treatment needs, this review, whenever possible, will emphasize aspects pertinent to older patients.

Cystic fibrosis involves almost all organ systems, not just the respiratory tract. For this reason, we feel strongly that physicicians caring for patients with cystic fibrosis and researchers studying the disease need to be aware of all aspects and deal with them effectively.

Definition

No known biochemical or structural defect will account for all the pathophysiologic phenomena of cystic fibrosis. Thus, the definition of the disease rests on the clinical findings; cystic fibrosis is a syndrome, and not yet a disease.

There are 4 criteria for the diagnosis of cystic fibrosis. (*1*) A positive sweat test (sweat chloride > 60 mEq per liter) has been widely accepted as the *sine qua non*, if accompanied by at least one of the other diagnostic criteria. (*2*) Chronic obstructive pulmonary disease is found in almost all cases, with varying severity. (*3*) Exocrine pancreatic insufficiency is less universal, occurring in 80 to 90 per cent of patients. (*4*) Family history is not always present but is very helpful if confirmed cases are known. Most authorities require at least 2 of the criteria for a diagnosis, and the diagnosis is rarely made in the absence of a positive sweat test.

Incidence

Incidence figures for cystic fibrosis are necessarily minimal. The best diagnostic efforts currently available fail to detect all those who die at a young age or who have mild symptoms. The incidence is highest in white populations, ranging from 1:620 in South West African Afrikaners to 1:15,000 in Italy (table 1) and is generally highest in middle and western European countries and in locations with similar racial extractions. A figure of 1:2,000 has been proposed as a conservative and acceptable incidence in these countries.

The incidence of cystic fibrosis in nonwhite populations is clearly much lower, although not as thoroughly documented. The best survey of black populations in the United States estimated the incidence at 1:17,000 (18). A study in Hawaii demonstrated a 24-fold higher incidence of cystic fibrosis in Caucasian as compared with Oriental populations (17). Only occasional cases are reported in American Indian (39), African (40), American Oriental (41), Japanese (42), Malaysian (43), or Asian Indian (44) populations.

Genetics

Several pieces of evidence indicate that cystic fibrosis is transmitted as an autosomal recessive trait. (*1*) 24.3 per cent of children were affected in 232 sibships of index cases in Australia (32); (*2*) 0.55 per cent of first cousins of index cases in the same series were affected (32); and (*3*) the incidence of cystic fibrosis in children of mothers with cystic fibrosis is 1:46 (45).

It has been proposed that a single mutant allele is responsible for the manifestations of this syndrome (32, 35). More recently, patients with cystic fibrosis were categorized into 3 groups according to the metachromatic staining reaction of their skin fibroblasts (46). No distinct relation between severity of clinical manifestations and class of metachromasia was observed.

TABLE 1

ESTIMATED MINIMAL INCIDENCE OF CYSTIC FIBROSIS (LIVE BIRTHS)

Incidence	Year of Report	Location	Reference
1:90,000	1968	United States (Hawaii, Orientals)	17
1:17,000	1974	Washington, D.C. (blacks)	18
1:15,000	1970	Italy	19
1:10,000	1974	England (Pakistani immigrants)	20
1: 8,000	1962	Sweden	21
1:4,000–8,000	1971	European Soviet Union	22
1: 3,800	1968	United States (Hawaii, whites)	17
1: 3,700	1960	United States (Ohio)	23
1: 3,400	1966	United States (Middle and South Atlantic states)	24
1: 3,300	1963	Germany	25
1: 3,300	1972	Czechoslovakia	26
1: 3,200	1961	France	27
1: 3,000	1966	England	28
1: 2,900	1967	England	29
1: 2,600	1967	Czechoslovakia	30
1: 2,450	1966	United States (Buffalo, N.Y.)	31
1: 2,450	1965	Australia	32
1: 2,400	1968	England	33
1: 2,400	1962	United States (New England states)	34
1: 1,900	1962	United States (Indiana)	35
1: 1,860	1965	United States (Connecticut)	36
1: 1,000	1952	United States (Minnesota)	37
1: 620	1975	South West Africa (Dutch descent)	38

Later only 2 loci at which homozygosity produces cystic fibrosis were proposed, one resulting in metachromasia of cultured fibroblasts, and the other showing no metachromasia (47). The frequency of ametachromasia varied from 20 per cent in the United States (46) to 40 per cent in Denmark (48). Recent calculations based on affected first cousins of the proband are consistent with involvement of either 2 or 3 loci (49). Although it is tempting to support a hypothesis of multiple alleles for cystic fibrosis, especially in view of repeated difficulties with detection of a single pathogenetic mechanism, enthusiasm should be tempered by the recognition that fibroblast metachromasia is nonspecific (50) and not easily reproduced in cystic fibrosis cells by all investigators (51).

Cystic fibrosis in blacks also appears to be transmitted as an uncomplicated autosomal recessive trait (18). Although early reports suggested a similar course for cystic fibrosis in blacks and whites (52), our experience with 17 black patients suggests a more benign course for the pulmonary disease of black patients if they survive infancy. Once more the possibility of multiple loci is raised by these findings.

It can be calculated from incidence figures of 1:2,000 that approximately 5 per cent of most white populations are carriers of the cystic fibrosis gene. This makes cystic fibrosis the most frequent lethal genetic disease among whites (23). No detrimental effects of the carrier state are recognized (53–55). The high gene frequency in white populations probably cannot be maintained by spontaneous mutation alone (56). A heterozygote advantage, either increased survival to reproductive age or increased reproductive capacity, has been postulated (32, 47). Data from several sources (32, 57, 58) indicate that parents and grandparents of children with cystic fibrosis do produce more offspring. Although these studies do not prove a heterozygote reproductive advantage, such an advantage need only be 2 per cent to account for the high gene frequency (23, 32). This is a level that is difficult to detect.

Cystic fibrosis is not linked genetically with ABH blood group substances (59), MNS blood groups (60), or HL-A antigens (61). It has been diagnosed in patients with a number of other genetic diseases (table 2), but linkage with any of these diseases cannot be supported.

Pathophysiology

An autosomal recessive inheritance for cystic fibrosis suggests a discrete biochemical or structural defect. To date no single lesion has been proved to provide a unifying hypothesis for the pathophysiology of cystic fibrosis. If more than one allele is involved, definition of the basic defect will be more difficult. Distinguishing between primary and secondary defects has been an even greater practical problem. The effects of therapy must also be considered, because patients receive many medications. Many abnormalities have been described; yet, most of these appear to be one or several steps removed from the underlying defect. For example, malabsorption of fat-soluble vitamins is a secondary defect that in turn produces many metabolic and functional lesions.

Numerous studies have used parents of cystic

TABLE 2

OTHER GENETIC DISEASES IN PERSONS WITH CYSTIC FIBROSIS

Disease	No. of Cases	Reference
Downs syndrome	3	62
Cri-du-Chat syndrome	1	63
47, xxy double aneuploidy	1	64
Silver-Russell dwarfism	2	65, 66
Situs inversus (Kartagener's syndrome?)	2	67; Doershuk, C.F.: Unpublished observations
Rothmund-Thompson syndrome	1	68
Kallman's syndrome	1	69
Wiscott-Aldrich syndrome	1	70
Cleidocranial dysostosis	1	Stern, R. C.: Personal communication
Neurofibromatosis	1	Matthews, L. W.: Personal communication

fibrosis patients, reasoning that the basic defect should be demonstrable in obligate heterozygotes. However, because the mutation rate is unknown, and paternity is sometimes uncertain, such studies may be misleading. It is possible that one of the defects already described may be the actual basis of cystic fibrosis and that failure to demonstrate the defect in all patients or all parents has prevented its recognition as a basic defect.

Early studies of the pathophysiology of cystic fibrosis were comprehensively reviewed in 1967 (24). This review will concentrate on more recent developments.

Exocrine Gland Dysfunction

Obstruction of exocrine gland ducts or the passageways into which the exocrine secretions are discharged occurs in all (or very nearly all) patients with cystic fibrosis. Sites of obstruction include lung airways, paranasal sinuses, mucus-secreting salivary glands, small intestine, pancreas, biliary system, uterine cervix, and perhaps the male genital tract. Inspissation of secretions has been blamed for the obstructive events. Lack of water, alterations of electrolyte concentration, and abnormal organic constituents (especially mucous glycoproteins) have all been implicated in the pathogenesis of inspissated secretions. In addition, it has been suggested that autonomic control of the secretory process is disturbed in patients with cystic fibrosis. Evidence for and against the involvement of all 4 factors will be reviewed.

Water content. Cystic fibrosis secretions from several types of glands are relatively dehydrated (71–74) (table 3). Cervical mucus is generally dehydrated, but in addition the usual mid-cycle increase in water and sodium secretion is abolished, as evidenced by the absence of ferning (74). Total volumes of several cystic fibrosis secretions are diminished, including pancreatic juice, before and after pancreozymin or secretin stimulation (75, 76) and seminal fluid (77).

In general, the serous and hypotonic secretions (sweat, parotid saliva, tears) show only minor alterations of water content and have approximately the same flow rates and total volume as those of normal control subjects. In contrast, the protein or mucous glycoprotein-rich isotonic secretions (pancreatic juice, tracheobronchial or cervical mucus) have a reduced water content (78).

A paucity of water in mucous secretions may reflect decreased water secretion, increased secretion of solids without appropriately increased secretion of water, or increased reabsorption of water from the primary secretory fluid. There is little evidence to support any of these mechanisms. The hypothesis of "hyperpermeability" of mucus lining the exocrine gland duct systems (79) lacks direct experimental support. Evidence against ductal loss of water is available from studies of sweat duct perfusion with cystic fibrosis saliva containing inulin labeled with carbon-14 (80).

Electrolyte content. Representative values for electrolytes in cystic fibrosis and normal secretions are presented in table 4. Sodium and chloride concentrations in the sweat of cystic fibrosis patients are clearly elevated (89). Other serous fluids such as parotid saliva and tears contain little or no extra sodium and chloride (88, 90). Some mucous secretions of cystic fibrosis patients contain less than normal concentrations of sodium and chloride (e.g., tracheobronchial and cervical mucus). Increases of sodium and chloride concentrations in cystic fibrosis sweat probably arise from a decreased sodium reabsorption in the ducts. The isotonic primary secretions (91) in sweat glands normally become more hypotonic in the duct system as the result of sodium reabsorption in excess of water reabsorption. Cystic fibrosis secretions (saliva and sweat) when perfused through a rat parotid duct (92, 93) or a normal sweat gland duct have the capacity to block subsequent reabsorption of sodium by the duct. The marked lability of this

TABLE 3

PER CENT OF WATER CONTENT OF CYSTIC FIBROSIS
AND CONTROL SECRETIONS

	Cystic Fibrosis	Bronchiectatic	Normal	Reference
Sputum	89	95		71
	87	94		72
Meconium	55		77	73
Cervical mucus	60		90	74

TABLE 4

REPRESENTATIVE ELECTROLYTE VALUES (mM/LITER) FOR CYSTIC
FIBROSIS (CF) AND NORMAL (N) SECRETIONS*

		Na^+	K^+	Cl^-	HCO_3^-	Ca^{++}	Reference
Sweat	N	22	9	18	11	0.44	81
	CF	103	15	97	46	0.47	82
Parotid saliva	N	23.5	21.5	18.9	13.4	0.95	83
	CF	30.8	22.9	24.0	15.2	1.45	84
Submaxillary saliva	N	46.6	17.0	41.4	—	1.9	85
	CF	71.0	14.9	54.9	—	3.2	
Tears	N	140	26	134	—	2.5	86
	CF	137	23	133	—	4.8	87
Unstimulated pancreatic juice	N	107	11	94	—	—	88
	CF	125	10	90	—	—	
Tracheobronchial secretions	N	165	13.2	16.2	—	3.1	
	Br†	116	18.7	9.7	—	4.7	71
	CF	101	28.0	7.5	—	3.7	

*From reference 78.

†Br = sputum from subjects with bronchiectasis.

inhibitory activity (94) has greatly hampered attempts at purification or identification of a molecule that is responsible for this effect.

In the pancreas of all patients with cystic fibrosis, even those who produce digestive enzymes, secretion of water and electrolytes is severely impaired (75, 76). This is readily demonstrated by stimulation tests with secretin, which controls water and electrolyte release, and with pancreaozymin, which controls enzyme release (75). Bicarbonate secretion is particularly deficient in both nonstimulated and stimulated pancreatic secretions of all subjects with cystic fibrosis (75, 76). On the other hand, it is proton (H+) secretion, not bicarbonate, that is deficient in sweat of persons with cystic fibrosis (95). Bicarbonate concentrations in cystic fibrosis parotid saliva may be identical to those in control saliva (84). It is difficult to develop a unifying hypothesis for electrolyte abnormalities in cystic fibrosis when these abnormalities vary from one exocrine gland to another.

Much discussion has been generated concerning elevated calcium concentrations in cystic fibrosis secretions. Excess calcium in submaxillary saliva causes glycoprotein precipitation (96), but subsequent studies have shown that the glycoprotein is a low molecular weight, casein-like phosphoglycoprotein, not mucous glycoprotein (97). This calcium-phosphoglycoprotein complex and hydroxyapatite crystals (98) create the characteristic turbidity of cystic fibrosis submaxillary saliva. Calcium-phosphoglycoprotein complexes do not form in duodenal or tracheobronchial secretions and therefore play no major role in the generalized obstruction that characterizes cystic fibrosis (97). Calcium concentrations are not elevated in all cystic fibrosis secretions (table 4). The current concept of calcium secretion entails sequestration of this divalent cation in secretory organelles and release with exocrine macromolecules (99). The increased anionic character of mucous glycoproteins in some cystic fibrosis glands (see subsequent section) may promote increased sequestration and release of calcium. Studies of free (ionic) versus bound calcium show that about two-thirds is bound in both normal and cystic fibrosis saliva (100). Clearly, neither the reason for nor the consequence of increased calcium concentrations in cystic fibrosis secertions is fully recognized at this time. A more detailed compilation and discussion of electrolyte abnormalities in cystic fibrosis secretions is available in another review (78).

Content of organic substances. Exocrine secretions contain urea, monosaccharides, amino acids, fatty acids, and other organic acids, none of which have been implicated in the pathophysiology of cystic fibrosis (78). Of special interest are the polyamines (putrescine, spermidine, spermine), which are elevated in blood of cystic fibrosis subjects (101) and are present in smaller amounts in secretions (78). These polycations may affect glycoprotein synthesis (102), interact with macromolecules such as mucous glycoproteins (78), and alter transport mechanisms (103). Total protein concentrations are usually elevated in cystic fibrosis secretions (104). Examples of specific proteins present in increased concentrations in saliva include amylase, ribonuclease (105), and lysozyme (104). In contrast, arginine esterase activity may be decreased in cystic fibrosis saliva (106). Tracheobronchial mucous glycoproteins also are secreted in increased amounts (107) as the result of hyperplasia and hypertrophy of mucus-secreting elements. Intracellular gastric mucous stores appear normal ultrastructurally (108). Glycosyltransferases that synthesize and glycosidases that degrade mucous glycoproteins are not markedly altered in cystic fibrosis tissues, secretions, or sera (109, 110).

Mucous glycoproteins are able to form viscoelastic gels that contribute significantly to the behavior of secretions and that may play a major role in alterations of tracheobronchial secretions. Unfortunately, rheologic techniques that give consistent and meaningful data have not been used for most studies of cystic fibrosis secretions. In short, it is not certain that the physical properties of uninfected cystic fibrosis mucous secretions are altered (111, 112). Of course, purulent tracheobronchial secretions are more viscous than nonpurulent secretions (113), at least in part because of a high deoxyribonucleic acid content (114). These purulent secretions must

be treated with both reducing agent and deoxyribonuclease to achieve solubilization (Boat, T. F.: Unpublished observations).

The chemical determinants of the physical properties of mucous glycoproteins are not completely understood. The presence of intra- and intermolecular disulfide bonds seems to be required for gel formation (115). Sialic acid content also appears to influence viscosity; however, investigators have not agreed whether secretions containing sialic acid-rich mucous glycoprotein are more or less viscous (116, 117). Calcium interactions with intestinal mucous glycoprotein decrease viscosity (118).

A series of papers has dealt with the composition, certain structural features, and protein-protein interactions of tracheobronchial mucous glycoproteins from sputum of patients with bronchitis and cystic fibrosis (119–128). Sputum was separated routinely into soluble and gel (fibrillar) phases (119) and acidic (sulfate and sialic acid-containing) components isolated from the gel phase. Large amounts of acidic mucous glycoprotein were found consistently in cystic fibrosis sputum (126). Structural studies of acidic glycoproteins from the sputum of a cystic fibrosis donor have been reported (128).

We have isolated nasal and tracheobronchial mucous glycoproteins from control subjects and subjects with cystic fibrosis or other obstructive lung diseases (107, 129). The mucous glycoproteins were fractionated by ion-exchange chromatography into 2 major and 2 minor blood group–specific components. All 4 components are typical sulfated mucous glycoproteins, and all 4 are present in normal, bronchitic, and cystic fibrosis secretions. The 2 major components differ chiefly in sulfate content (2 per cent versus 6 to 7 per cent). Cystic fibrosis nasal and tracheobronchial secretions differ from normal in that they contain a predominance of the highly sulfated component. Bronchitic secretions, on the other hand, contain more of the sparsely sulfated component than normal. These and previous studies agree that the composite acidity of mucous glycoproteins is greater in cystic fibrosis than in normal or bronchitic secretions. Furthermore, increased mucous glycoprotein sulfation can be demonstrated by double isotope labeling of the secretory product of cultured cystic fibrosis respiratory epithelium (table 5). Therefore, excessive sulfation may be more than a response to respiratory tract inflammatory disease. These findings are supported by histochemical observations that, in contrast to normal, the number of

TABLE 5

$^{35}SO_4/^3H$ INCORPORATED* INTO MUCOUS GLYCOPROTEIN† RELEASED FROM RESPIRATORY EPITHELIAL EXPLANTS

Source of Epithelium	Ratio	Mean Ratio	SD
Cystic fibrosis			
Nose	0.47		
	0.26		
	0.43	0.41 ± 0.13	
	0.39		
Trachea	0.49	(P < 0.01)	
	0.43		
Not cystic fibrosis			
Nose	0.14		
	0.25	0.20 ± 0.05	
	0.21		
Trachea	0.23		
	0.16		
	0.16		
	0.23		

*Calculated as dpm/10^6 dpm of $^{35}SO_4^=$ and ^{3}H-6-D-glucosamine added to the culture medium.

†Purified from reduced and carboxymethylated total secretory product by BioGel A-5m chromatography.

sulfomucin-containing cells in the respiratory tract of children with cystic fibrosis remains high after birth (130).

Control of secretion. Various workers have postulated an involvement of the autonomic nervous system in the pathophysiology of cystic fibrosis. The most direct evidence demonstrates that the rate and magnitude of pupillary dilatation during dark adaptation by cystic fibrosis children are significantly impaired (131). This suggests inappropriate sympathetic autonomic response at a neural or neurohumoral level. Unfortunately, similar evidence for altered autonomic control of glandular secretion is lacking (24). We have demonstrated that explanted cystic fibrosis tracheal epithelium continues to hypersecrete *in vitro,* and that augmentation of secretion by addition of methacholine to culture medium parallels that of normal epithelial explants (132). This finding precludes an altered intrinsic responsiveness of cystic fibrosis tracheobronchial glands to cholinergic stimulation.

Animal models. Chronic administration of isoproterenol to rats in very large doses produces hypertrophy of parotid submaxillary glands (133). Flow rates of saliva are decreased but sodium concentrations are increased. Sera of these rats cause ciliary dyskinesia (133). Similar salivary gland changes are observed in rats fed pancreatin (134). Isoproterenol treatment also induces hypertrophy of bronchial submucosal glands and hyperplasia of goblet cells in the rat (135). Additional similarities of isoproterenol-treated rats to cystic fibrosis subjects have not been delineated.

More recently, histologic and histochemical similarities between submaxillary glands in reserpine-treated rats and subjects with cystic fibrosis have been noted (136, 137). Furthermore, secretory aberrations, which mimic in part those in cystic fibrosis subjects, and a ciliostatic effect of saliva from treated glands were demonstrated. The usefulness of this proposed model of cystic fibrosis in future investigations is at present uncertain.

Mucociliary Transport

Mucociliary transport, one of the major pulmonary defense mechanisms, physically removes natural debris and inhaled particulate matter including bacteria. Although a causal relation between failure of mucociliary transport and development of obstructive lung disease is difficult to prove, this assumption underlies many of the therapeutic modalities employed in cystic fibrosis and other chronic obstructive lung diseases. Clinical observers long ago presumed a failure of mucociliary transport, probably secondary to altered rheologic properties of the mucus. It was therefore surprising when mucociliary airway clearance in cystic fibrosis patients was reported to be at least as fast as in normal volunteers (138), when studied by measuring the retention of inhaled radioactive aerosol particles. We measured the rate of movement of discrete particles across the tracheal mucosa (139) and found it to be 5- to 10-fold lower than in normal volunteers of the same age. This observation is more consistent with logical expectations (140) and is similar to data obtained with the same method in adults with chronic bronchitis (141).

The mechanism by which mucociliary transport is impaired in cystic fibrosis is unknown. Many factors are necessary for effective mucociliary function. (*1*) The ciliated epithelium must be morphologically intact, although some transport may occur across islands of traumatized mucosa or squamous metaplasia (142). Little or no data is available on the ultrastructure of the bronchial mucosa in cystic fibrosis. With chronic infection some loss of cilia might occur. (*2*) The cilia must beat in a normal fashion, including rate, direction of beat, and coordination of beat. Mucociliary transport in bronchitic rats is impaired because the direction of the ciliary beat is altered (143). Beat frequency of cilia in excised nasal polyps was visually estimated to be normal (144). Ciliary beat pattern and frequency have not been studied systematically in cystic fibrosis, except for many *in vitro* studies of the effect of cystic fibrosis body fluids on nonhuman cilia. (*3*) Properties of the mucous layer are critical to effective mucociliary transport (145, 146). The mucous layer is presumed to consist of 2 layers: a superficial layer with high viscosity (gel) and a periciliary layer with low viscosity (sol). The nature of the sol layer is unknown, but theoretic considerations would require it to be relatively thin and of low viscosity (147, 148). Alterations of either the composition or depth of the sol or the gel layer could result in decreased effectiveness of ciliary propulsion. It has been calculated that a large amount of fluid must be absorbed from the bronchial mucous blanket as it moves toward the glottis (149). If water absorption were abnormally fast so that the sol layer was dehydrated, the net rate of transport could be reduced.

It is of great practical and theoretic importance to know if mucociliary transport is impaired in all patients with cystic fibrosis, or only in those with established pulmonary disease. Our studies have revealed several patients with very little pulmonary disease and yet with very slow mucociliary transport (139). Another study suggests that cystic fibrosis patients may be divided into several groups according to their clinical status and mucociliary clearance rates (150). The patients with little lung disease had relatively or completely normal rates of transport. The question remains, Are the alterations in mucociliary transport function the cause or the effect of the obstructive lung disease?

Immunology

Almost all patients with cystic fibrosis eventually develop chronic pulmonary infection, but extra-pulmonary infection is rare, except in infants. This implies a defect in local rather than systemic defense mechanisms. Local defenses in the lung include mucociliary transport, phagocytic cells, and immunoglobulin secretion. Mucociliary transport has been found to be impaired, as noted above, and this undoubtedly contributes to increased bacterial colonization of the lung.

Alveolar macrophage function has not been systematically studied. Although morphologically normal alveolar macrophages are found in lung washings, the majority of cells are polymorphonuclear leukocytes (PMN). In our experience, the ratio of PMN to macrophages ranges from 4:1 to 25:1, and many of the PMN appear to be dead or degenerating. There seems to be little correlation of the ratio of PMN to macrophages with the clinical state of the patient, suggesting a chronic inflammatory process even in those patients with clinically minimal disease.

Indirect studies of alveolar macrophage function have been performed using cystic fibrosis serum and rabbit alveolar macrophages. In 2 separate studies the phagocytosis and killing of *Pseudomonas aeruginosa* were impaired in the presence of serum from cystic fibrosis patients, but not from normal subjects. This has been attributed to defective opsonization (151) or to a heat-labile inhibitor (152). Until such studies are repeated with human alveolar macrophages, the significance of the observations remains unclear. Phagocytosis by peripheral leukocytes in cystic fibrosis is normal (151).

Immunoglobulin function in cystic fibrosis appears to be normal. Total circulating concentrations of IgG, IgA, and IgM are normal to ele-

vated (153), consistent with chronic infection. The responses to specific infecting agents, both viral and bacterial, appear normal. Secretory IgA function also seems normal (154). The majority of cystic fibrosis patients have high circulating titers to the bacterial flora in their lungs, which may account in part for the rarity of extrapulmonary infections (155–159). The question of complement abnormality has been raised (160, 161). No consistent alteration has been documented.

Although bacterial antibody titers are high in peripheral blood, relatively little antibody reaches the bronchial mucosa. For example, high titers were produced in response to immunization with a purified pseudomonas lipopolysaccharide antigen, but increases in titers in bronchial fluids and saliva were minimal (162). Both IgG and IgA secreting cells are found in the bronchial mucosa of cystic fibrosis patients and are increased in number in comparison to normal, whereas very small amounts of IgM are found in the respiratory tract (163, 164).

High local concentrations of antibody may assist in phagocytosis of infecting organisms but can also lead to deleterious effects. In allergic aspergillosis, for example, an Arthus-like reaction results in local tissue damage (165). A similar phenomenon has been noted with pseudomonas (166) and is postulated to occur in some cystic fibrosis patients (159).

Ciliary Factor(s)

The search for an identifiable gene product has played a major role in cystic fibrosis research. In 1967 a significant step was taken with the demonstration by Spock and associates (167) of a factor in the serum of cystic fibrosis patients and their parents that would disrupt the normal ciliary beat pattern of rabbit tracheal explants. Similar findings were soon reported with oyster gill cilia (168). Attempts to repeat these studies in a variety of ciliated systems, including chick embryo trachea (169), fresh water mussel gill (170, 171), human sperm, and ciliated protozoa (172) have produced varied results. Some workers were unable to demonstrate differences between normal and cystic fibrosis sera whereas others have reported success (173–176). Currently, the rabbit trachea and oyster gill are the only systems widely employed in research on "ciliary factors."

The molecular identity of the factor(s) is as yet unknown. The factor appears to be closely associated with immunoglobulins (167, 177–

180). Added IgG appears necessary for factor activity in the rabbit tracheal assay (180) but not in the oyster gill assay (178, 181). Factor activity is destroyed by heating or by proteolytic digestion (182). It is produced by fibroblasts and by long-term lymphoid cell cultures (174, 181, 183) and apparently can be labeled with radioactive amino acids (181). The molecular weight has been estimated at 7,000 to 10,000 by ultrafiltration studies (180, 184) and by separation of an active component from serum by gel filtration (185).

It has been postulated that the factor is a component of the complement system, C3a (186). C3a is normally inactivated by an enzyme (anaphylatoxin inactivator) with carboxypeptidase B-like activity, which removes the C-terminal arginine (187). A deficiency of this enzyme has been proposed to account for the activity of the ciliary factor in cystic fibrosis patients and heterozygotes (160). Other investigators have found carboxypeptidase B activity in cystic fibrosis serum to be increased (188). Kallikrein or a similar arginine esterase has variously been reported to be decreased (189) or normal (190). One of several enzymes of arginine esterase may be absent (191). The factor isolated from serum does not cross react with C3 or C3a by immunodiffusion (185). Factor activity in saliva has been reported to be closely associated with amylase (175).

The presence of a polypeptide factor in serum and fibroblasts of both homozygotes and presumptive heterozygotes strongly suggests a direct relation between the polypeptide and the cystic fibrosis gene. It is not yet known whether the factor is a normal product that accumulates because of a lack of normal degradation (160) or is an abnormal protein. "Factor" activity has been reported in normal sera after concentration (179) and in patients with a variety of other diseases (192). The relation of the ciliary factor to an apparently unique protein band found in some cystic fibrosis sera by isoelectric focusing (193, 194) is unknown.

As yet no pathophysiologic role has been defined for the presumed factor, and the mechanism by which the "factor" might alter ciliary activity is not known. Media from cystic fibrosis fibroblast cultures has been reported to inhibit red cell adenosine triphosphatase (ATPase) (195). In cilia from rabbit trachea and oyster gills, however, no alterations in ATPase activity or ATP consumption were found in the presence of cystic fibrosis serum (196). Cystic fibrosis serum and obligate heterozygote sera, but not normal sera, rapidly agglutinate suspensions of *Proteus vulgaris* (197). No relation has been established between the sodium transport inhibitory effect of cystic fibrosis saliva and the "ciliary factors."

A major problem in this important area of investigation is that all currently available methods for the detection of "factor" activity are bioassays. Changes in ciliary activity in these assays may be highly subjective and are often difficult to interpret. Furthermore, many variables affect the results, and the specificity of the assays is unknown. Until an objective, quantitative (preferably biochemical or immunologic) assay is developed, the detection of "factor" activity in biologic fluids or fibroblasts is far too unreliable to be used in diagnosis or genetic counseling (198, 199).

Transport Mechanisms

Alterations of transport mechanisms in cystic fibrosis are either primary or induced. Numerous studies have explored both these possibilities.

Membranes and their transport properties. Elevations of sweat sodium and chloride concentrations in the face of normal concentrations of these substances in precursor fluid (91) suggest that plasma membrane transport of electrolytes by duct epithelium is abnormal. Cystic fibrosis erythrocytes have been used as a simple model to delineate this abnormality but with inconclusive results. The sodium concentration in cystic fibrosis erythrocytes is normal (200). A reduction in both the ouabain-sensitive and ethacrinic acid-sensitive Na efflux of cystic fibrosis red cells has been claimed (201). However, a subsequent study has found a reduction only in the ethacrinic acid-sensitive portion of Na^+ efflux in red cells of homozygous men and older women, not in young female subjects and heterozygotes (202). More recently, normal total ouabain-sensitive and ouabain-insensitive Na transport were demonstrated (203). Transport of rubidium-86 and strontium-85 by cystic fibrosis red cells is normal (204). These ions are transported by the same mechanisms as Na^+ and Ca^{+2}, respectively.

Similarly, initial studies of cystic fibrosis red cell membrane ATPase showed diminution of the ouabain-sensitive activity (201), (Ca^{+2})-ATPase activity (205), and the ouabain-insensitive component of ATPase (200). Subsequent studies have demonstrated normal (Ca^{+2})-ATPase, normal (Mg^{+2})-ATPase, and ouabain-sensitive and -insensitive (Na$^+$-K$^+$)ATPase (206). In conclusion, there is little irrefutable evidence for abnormal intrinsic transport function in erythrocytes of patients with cystic fibrosis. Furthermore, (Na$^+$-K$^+$)ATPase activities are normal in cultured skin fibroblasts (207) and in sweat glands (208).

Transport of substances other than electrolytes by cystic fibrosis plasma membranes has received little attention. Uptake of leucine, glycine, deoxyglucose, and glucosamine by skin fibroblasts from patients with cystic fibrosis and control subjects was compared and no differences were found (209, 210).

Studies of membrane composition and specific membrane components have likewise turned up no promising leads. An initial report suggested membrane protein pattern differences (211); however, subsequent sodium dodecylsulfate (SDS)-polyacrylamide gel electrophoresis and lipid analyses of erythrocyte membrane proteins demonstrated no difference between cystic fibrosis and normal (206). Cyclic adenosine monophosphate–stimulated phosphorylation of red cell membranes was no different from that of control subjects (212). Similarly, the amount and spectrum of membrane components of skin fibroblasts from patients with cystic fibrosis showed no differences (210, 213). Synthetic rates of more than 30 protein species of the cystic fibrosis fibroblast membrane were found to be normal (214).

Induced alterations of membrane function. In 1967, Mangos and associates (92) described inhibition of rat parotid duct sodium reabsorption after retrograde perfusion of cystic fibrosis saliva. This effect has been linked, but only by indirect evidence, to the presence of a polycationic substance in saliva (94). In fact, cystic fibrosis saliva does not mimic poly-L-lysine effects on cultured fibroblasts (215). The sodium reabsorption inhibitory effect is present in saliva from mucus-secreting glands but not the serous secretion from the parotid gland (216). A similar effect is generated by perfusion of normal sweat gland ducts with cystic fibrosis sweat (83). These results may explain the elevated sodium and chloride concentrations in cystic fibrosis sweat and saliva.

However, studies of the transport of other substances by epithelia exposed to cystic fibrosis body fluids have been less conclusive. Plasma, saliva, and skin fibroblast culture media of patients with cystic fibrosis reportedly decrease ATPase activities in red cell membranes (195, 200, 217), but sodium influx and efflux are not altered by exposure to cystic fibrosis saliva (218). Rat jejunal uptake of arbutin, a glucose analogue, was reported to be inhibited after incubation with plasma (219) and transport of ^{14}C alanine was reduced by preincubation of rat jejunum with diluted cystic fibrosis saliva but not serum (220). In other studies, inhibition of mucosal-to-serosal flux of sodium or uptake of alanine in rat jejunum exposed to cystic fibrosis saliva could not be detected and uptake of 3-O-methyl-glucose by rat intestine was not inhibited (218). Sugar and amino acid transport by fibroblasts are not inhibited by cystic fibrosis saliva or dialyzed plasma (209). Sera from patients with cystic fibrosis decreased short circuit current and the short circuit current response to glucose in rat jejunum (221), suggesting interference with Na-dependent glucose transport in this system. It is also possible that transport inhibiting processes are not due to changes of membrane function but involve metabolic intracellular pathways (222). No investigator has been able to separate heterozygotes clearly from control populations on the basis of transport inhibition studies. Co-identity of Na transport inhibitory factors and ciliostatic factors is not likely. In summary: (*1*) the nature of a transport defect, if it exists, remains to be elucidated, and (*2*) a transport defect is probably secondary to another abnormality that is more fundamental to the genetic defect in cystic fibrosis.

Clinical and Pathologic Manifestations

The manifestations of cystic fibrosis involve many organ systems and the pattern of presentation is variable.

Respiratory

Pathology. Patients with cystic fibrosis presumably have morphologically normal lungs at birth, as seen in infants dying of meconium ileus. The earliest pulmonary lesions are dilation and hypertrophy of bronchial glands, and goblet cell metaplasia of the bronchiolar epithelium followed shortly by mucous plugging of peripheral airways (223–225). Infection soon follows, and bronchitis and bronchiolitis result. Unless the disease process can be arrested at this stage by effective treatment, a vicious cycle of obstruction, chronic infection, and more tissue damage develops. Bronchiolectasis, bronchiectasis, peribronchial fibrosis, and airway obstruction result in the progressive loss of pulmonary function and eventually in death. Pulmonary disease accounts for greater than 95 per cent of deaths of patients with cystic fibrosis other than those due to meconium ileus.

Areas of squamous metaplasia may be found in the bronchi of cystic fibrosis patients (223, 224). This is most likely due to infection, although vitamin A deficiency can also lead to this change. The apparent chronology of pulmonary lesions—obstruction preceding infection—suggests that squamous metaplasia is not a major contributing factor in mucociliary failure leading to the initial pathologic changes. Destruction of the ciliated epithelium may certainly contribute to the disease process in its later stages. Infection results in increased amounts of deoxyribonucleic acid and other cellular debris from bacteria and phagocytes, which increase the volume and viscosity of the bronchial secretions.

Emphysema has been noted in some patients but is less common than air trapping and dilation of the peripheral airways without destruction of alveolar septae (226, 227).

In many patients, bronchiectasis results in development of a rich vascular network of peribronchial granulation tissue (227, 228). This results in shunting of blood from the bronchial arteries to the pulmonary circulation, further compounding the problems of uneven distribution of ventilation/perfusion (227). In addition, minor trauma or increased infection may easily result in hemoptysis.

Pulmonary function. The earliest manifestation of pulmonary dysfunction in cystic fibrosis is an abnormality in the distribution of ventilation resulting in increased alveolar-arterial oxygen differences (229). This may occur before any detectable changes in flow rates or lung volumes. Tests of peripheral airway function such as frequency dependence of dynamic compliance (230) or flow rates at low lung volumes (231) may also show abnormalities in cystic fibrosis patients in whom more standard ventilatory measurements are still normal. The helium flow-volume technique may be an even more sensitive test for peripheral airway obstruction (232). These observations are consistent with the concept that the initial lesion is in the peripheral airways (228, 233). Closing volume is not a useful test for peripheral airway function in cystic fibrosis (232).

As pulmonary involvement progresses, large airway obstruction becomes manifest, with decreases in maximal mid-expiratory flow and

forced expiratory volume in 1 sec. Air trapping and loss of elastic recoil (234) result in elevation of residual volume and functional residual capacity. Thoracic gas volume at total lung capacity is usually normal to elevated even though vital capacity may be markedly decreased (235, 236).

Exercise tolerance is reduced in many patients and is limited by pulmonary mechanics (237). Exercise is not accompanied by a normal increase in the diffusing capacity for carbon monoxide (238). Although there is little reactive bronchoconstriction after exercise, there is more bronchodilation than normal during exercise, suggesting a significant degree of bronchomotor tone (239, 240). However, most patients do not have large increases in expiratory flow rates after isoproterenol and some may even decrease their flow rate (239, 240a; see also 389), probably because of a decrease in bronchial wall rigidity (241). Patients with advanced disease have abnormal collapse of large airways during forced expiration (242, 243).

Radiology. The radiographic manifestations of pulmonary disease in cystic fibrosis (244–246) are often seemingly out of proportion to the clinical status of the patient. Bronchial thickening and irregular areas of hyperinflation are the earliest radiologic signs of disease. Patches of atelectasis and infiltration, hilar adenopathy, and more hyperinflation with depression of the diaphragms and increased anterioposterior diameter are common with moderate to advanced disease. Radiographic changes may be more pronounced in the apices, especially on the right, but usually become diffuse. In advanced disease, segmental or lobar atelectasis, cyst formation, extensive bronchiectasis, retained secretions, and extensive infiltrates are seen. Pneumothorax or pneumomediastinum, which sometimes are clinically inapparent, may be found. It is not unusual for older, relatively asymptomatic patients to be referred for treatment of presumed tuberculosis after having had a screening roentgenogram. Bronchograms are not usually helpful except for evaluation of the occasional patient with localized disease who is considered for lobectomy.

Microbiology. Impairment of pulmonary clearance renders the lung susceptible to infection; patients with cystic fibrosis are no exception. They may be infected with any organism, but the flora usually seen are greatly influenced by therapy. In the 1940s and 1950s the predominant pathogen was *Staphylococcus aureus* (247,

248). It has been postulated that *S. aureus* was responsible for the majority of the early permanent damage to the lung (249).

A significant decrease in the frequency of isolation of *S. aureus* has been noted during the past 10 to 15 years (250), with a concomitant increase in *P. aeruginosa* (158, 250). At present, pseudomonas appears to be the most common pathogen isolated from cystic fibrosis patients (250–252). Pseudomonas is the initial pathogen in some patients but more often appears during the course of therapy. Once established, it is extremely difficult to eradicate, whereas the *S. aureus* can often be successfully treated.

A peculiar feature of pseudomonas in cystic fibrosis is the very high frequency of mucoid strains (158, 252, 253), which are rarely isolated from other human sources. Mucoid pseudomonas is associated with a high incidence of serum precipitating antibodies and is believed by some to be much more pathogenic than nonmucoid strains (156, 158, 159, 254, 255). These investigators have noted a very high incidence of the mucoid strain in cystic fibrosis patients at death and a lower incidence in older patients, suggesting that those with mucoid pseudomonas died earlier. It has been suggested that the large number of precipitating antibodies usually found in association with mucoid strains may lead to a Type III hypersensitivity reaction in the lung with increased tissue damage (159).

Another organism found with significant frequency in cystic fibrosis is *Haemophilus influenzae*. In some series the incidence of serum precipitating antibodies to *H. influenzae* has been as high as 80 per cent (156).

Other bacteria including streptococci, klebsiella, *Escherichia coli*, and proteus are also found with some frequency. Fungi such as candida and aspergillus are seen but rarely implicated in clincal symptomatology. Viral respiratory infections may exacerbate bacterial infection. Influenza and measles cause particularly severe pulmonary involvement. Mycobacteria are rarely encountered.

Clinical. The most prominent and constant symptom of pulmonary involvement is cough (246, 256). At first the cough may be dry and hacking, but with progression of the disease it becomes productive and is often increased at night. Decreasing exercise tolerance and increased respiratory rate are common signs of increasing severity of disease. Physical findings vary with the extent of pulmonary damage. Initially, the chest may be clear to auscultation, with rales and rhonchi appearing only during acute exacerbations. Progressive airway obstruction leads to air trapping with increased anteroposterior diameter of the chest and hyperresonance. Wheezing may be heard with acute infections. Rales and rhonchi may become permanent features, and the increased work of breathing leads to retractions and costal flaring. Digital clubbing is often an early manifestation.

The course of the pulmonary disease is highly variable and greatly influenced by therapy but tends to be progressive. Some patients remain essentially asymptomatic or have only a cough, clubbing, or increased anteroposterior diameter of the chest for long periods of time. Some infants have severe obstructive disease presenting as wheezing (257). Those who survive infancy become less symptomatic as they grow older, possibly because of growth of the lung and consequently less severe airway obstruction. Exacerbations resulting from viral or bacterial infection are common and often lead to pneumonia. Once bronchiectasis has developed, the course tends to accelerate, with more frequent exacerbations and eventually respiratory failure, cor pulmonale, and death.

Pulmonary disease in cystic fibrosis is usually diffuse but frequently more pronounced in the apices, especially the right. Recurrent right upper lobe pneumonia should be considered to be due to cystic fibrosis until proved otherwise. An occasional patient may develop severe bronchiectasis in a single lobe and benefit from lobectomy.

Common pulmonary complications include atelectasis, hemoptysis, pneumothorax, mucoid impaction of the bronchi, and cor pulmonale, as discussed in a later section.

The upper airway is often involved in cystic fibrosis. Chronic pansinusitis occurs in almost all patients. Nasal polyps are present in 10 to 15 per cent (258, 259). Some of the cough (especially at night) may be due to sinus drainage and sometimes responds to appropriate therapy. Mouth breathing is common and may interfere with normal humidification of inspired air.

The combination of pulmonary and gastrointestinal involvement frequently results in poor weight gain, short stature, delayed maturation, delayed menarche, and primary or secondary amenorrhea.

Gastrointestinal

The diagnosis of cystic fibrosis is frequently suggested by gastrointestinal manifestations of the disease. As is the case with pulmonary dysfunction, the gastrointestinal problems vary from mild to severe.

Obstruction. The earliest possible problem is meconium ileus, which occurs in 7 per cent (260) to 25 per cent (261) of newborns with cystic fibrosis. This obstructive lesion is usually suspected between 24 and 48 hours of age because of abdominal distention, emesis, and failure to pass meconium. Abdominal roentgenograms show dilated loops of bowel and a collection of granular ("ground glass") material in the lower central abdomen but usually no air-fluid levels. Introduction of barium through the rectum outlines an unexpanded colon (262, 263). Occasionally, a sterile peritonitis occurring *in utero* can be detected in the newborn by roentgenographic demonstration of peritoneal (262) or scrotal (264) calcifications. Meconium ileus also may be accompanied by secondary volvulus and intestinal stenosis or atresia (262, 263). The long-term prognosis for infants surviving surgery approaches that of the entire patient population (263, 265).

A similar obstructive lesion, meconium ileus equivalent, may occur occasionally in older children and adults (266–268) and should be suspected in any patient with pain and obstipation. In our experience, intestinal obstruction beyond the newborn period occurs more often in persons who have had previous abdominal surgery. This condition must be differentiated from intussusception, which has an increased frequency in cystic fibrosis (269), and other less frequent causes of obstruction. Intussusception may occur without pain or evidence of obstruction, and retention of fecal material in the cecum may be accompanied by a nontender, mobile, right lower quadrant mass (270).

Maldigestion. After the newborn period, manifestations of pancreatic insufficiency occur in 80 to 90 per cent of patients (271, 272). These manifestations include frequent, bulky, loose, greasy stools and failure to gain weight despite a ravenous appetite. A protuberant abdomen and decreased muscle mass are often seen. Poor growth and delayed maturation may result from poor nutrition. Excessive flatus is a common complaint. Whereas cystic fibrosis is often included in the differential diagnosis of diarrhea, frequent watery stools are not characteristic. More characteristic is the passage of orange oil droplets with the fecal material. The extent of steatorrhea can vary from minimal to 70 per cent of ingested fat but bears little relation to intestinal symptoms or state of nutrition (273). Malabsorption, in addition to maldigestion, may play a variable but minor role in the production of intestinal symptoms (274–279). In general, the intestinal manifestations of cystic fibrosis should be considered the result of maldigestion rather than malabsorption.

Several additional manifestations of maldigestion may appear, sometimes as the presenting complaint (table 6).

Biliary disease. Fatty change, the most common hepatic lesion in cystic fibrosis, occurs in about 30 per cent of patients (291, 292) despite pancreatic enzyme replacement, adequate diet, and vitamin supplementation. A second process, unique to cystic fibrosis (293) and perhaps more important clinically, is focal biliary cirrhosis with eosinophilic concretions in the intrahepatic ducts. This lesion, although responsible for occasional cases of prolonged neonatal jaundice (294, 295), is rarely apparent in infants and young children (293). It is found at postmortem examination in 20 to 25 per cent of patients (291). Older patients presumably have experienced more focal insults and have an increased chance for diffuse cirrhotic changes. Accordingly, elevations of hepatic alkaline phosphatase, α-glutamyl transpeptidase, and transaminases (296, 297) in serum increase with age; however, cirrhosis may be present without any elevation of liver enzymes (298). Hepatic congestion sec-

TABLE 6

**LESS FREQUENT GASTROINTESTINAL
MANIFESTATIONS OF CYSTIC FIBROSIS**

1. Hypoproteinemia, anasarca (280, 281)
2. Fat-soluble vitamin deficiences: vitamin K (282)
                                      vitamin A (283)
                                      vitamin E (284, 285)
3. Rectal prolapse (286)
4. Duodenal irritation and ulceration (287, 288)
5. Pseudotumor cerebri due to catch-up growth after malnutrition (289)
6. Appendiceal mass (290)

ondary to cor pulmonale and drug hepatotoxicity also elevates liver enzymes in serum (296).

Severe complications of liver disease, including liver failure and portal hypertension with bleeding esophageal varices or hypersplenism occur in only 2 to 3 per cent of patients (293). As life expectancy improves, the cumulative effects of focal biliary cirrhosis may be expected to increase the frequency of these life-threatening complications. Unexplained cirrhosis in a child or adult warrants a sweat chloride analysis.

Gallstones and biliary colic occasionally occur in older adolescent and adult patients (299). Roentgenographic examination may show a small or nonfunctioning gallbladder (300). Postmortem observations often reveal a hypoplastic gallbladder, filled with mucoid material and displaying extensive mucous metaplasia of the epithelium (301).

Pancreatic disease. Despite extensive pathologic changes, inflammatory disease of the pancreas is rarely seen in cystic fibrosis. Pancreatic calcifications are observed infrequently and have no correlation with symptoms or signs referrable to the pancreas. Recurrent acute pancreatitis occasionally occurs in adolescents and young adults who have residual exocrine function (302). Glucose intolerance due to disruption of islets by extensive fibrosis will be discussed (see Complications and Their Treatment).

Salivary gland disease. Enlargement of the submandibular salivary glands can be detected in more than 90 per cent of patients with cystic fibrosis (303). Eosinophilic plugging and dilatation of ducts (303, 304) are seen in all mucus-secreting salivary glands (sublingual, submandibular, submucosal). The parotid duct system is usually normal when examined by sialography (305). No clinically important alterations of salivary gland function are recognized.

Genitourinary Manifestations

Men. Sterility in men with cystic fibrosis was reported initially in 1966 (306) and confirmed in 1968· (307, 308). Documentation of a normal semen analysis in 3 and paternity in 2 patients (309, 310) has led to an estimate of only 2 to 3 per cent fertility in postpubertal men. Bilateral absence or atrophy of the body of the epididymis, vas deferens, and seminal vesicles provides an anatomic basis for sterility (310). Early developmental failure of wolffian duct structures has been proposed (311, 312). Although wolffian duct derivatives are affected as early as the first week of life (311), an intrauterine obstructive process and secondary obliteration of the genital tract cannot be excluded as a pathogenetic mechanism (313, 314). Decreased semen volume and absence of semen coagulation are concomitants of aspermia in men with cystic fibrosis (83). Their semen is low in fructose content, high in citrate and acid phosphatase content, and has a low pH (83). These findings reflect an absence of the seminal vesicles and the presence of an intact, functional prostate gland. The incidence of inguinal hernia (15 per cent), hydrocele (4.0 per cent), and undescended testicle (3.4 per cent) is also increased (315) and may be increased in male siblings (316). The relation of these 3 conditions to anatomic changes of the wolffian duct structures is unknown.

Women. In contrast to men, women with cystic fibrosis display no major reproductive abnormalities. Delayed menarche is the rule, but the average delay is only 2 years (8). Severe nutritional and/or pulmonary disease is usually evident in cases of more prolonged delay of menarche. Secondary amenorrhea may also occur and, likewise, often appears to result from exacerbations of pulmonary disease.

Examination of the uterine cervix in the newborn period or later in childhood frequently shows mucous cell hyperplasia, distention of cervical glands with mucous secretions, and copious mucus in the cervical canal (317). No inflammatory response is noted at early ages. Polypoid cervicitis may occur in women with cystic fibrosis who are taking oral contraceptives (318). Cervical mucus in postpubertal women is less voluminous, contains more protein and 3- to 4-fold more total solids than cervical mucus from normal women, and forms a sticky plug that tenaciously resists removal. It does not pull into a thread (spinbarkeit) or fern at mid-cycle. The latter is due to the fact that cyclic increases of volume (water) and sodium concentration do not occur (319).

Despite the rather severe changes in cervical mucous composition, pregnancy does occur. The actual incidence of fertility is unknown but probably is rather low. A survey in early 1975 revealed the occurrence of more than 100 pregnancies in 70 women with cystic fibrosis in the United States (45). From 70 pregnancies with a known outcome, 46 viable infants were produced (45), only one of whom had cystic fibrosis.

Sweat Gland

Although abnormal electrolyte concentrations

in sweat are the most constant clinical finding in cystic fibrosis, no abnormality of sweat gland morphology has been described. Micropuncture studies have revealed normal composition of the sweat in the secretory coil (91), leading to the presumption that reabsorption of salt or water or both (24, 78) may be impaired. The physiology of the sweat gland in cystic fibrosis has been reviewed (320).

Clinical manifestations of the sweat gland abnormality are related to the high rate of salt loss. Excessive losses of salt and fluid may lead to heat prostration (321, 322), especially in hot weather, a clinical observation that led di Sant'Agnese and associates (323) to the discovery of the sweat defect.

Sweat salt loss must be considered in the care of hospitalized patients receiving intravenous fluids and diuretics. Hyponatremia and hyperkalemic alkalosis have been described (324). Adults with cystic fibrosis have lower mean systolic and diastolic blood pressures, presumably owing to chronic salt loss in their sweat (325).

Diagnosis

Sweat Testing

The cornerstone of the diagnosis of cystic fibrosis is a positive sweat test (table 7). It cannot be overemphasized that this rather simple test is subject to many potential errors; about half the patients referred to our center from another hospital with a positive sweat test yield normal results in our laboratory. Because of the prognostic implication of a positive test result, it has been recommended that sweat testing be performed only where the test is done frequently and where very careful control of the technique is maintained (326).

Both sample collection and analysis are important. Qualitative methods, such as palm prints, are mentioned only in condemnation. The most reliable method is the pilocarpine iontophoresis method of Gibson and Cooke (11), coupled with chemical analysis of ionic composition. Details of procedure and analysis are available (327). It is of great importance that sufficient sweat (at least 100 mg) be collected for accurate determination, and sweat volumes should be reported along with the electrolyte concentration to assist in interpretation of results. Thermal stimulation or collection of unstimulated sweat are less reliable for clinical diagnosis than iontophoresis.

Electrolyte composition should be measured by well-established, quantitative methods. Sodium is usually determined by flame photometry, and chloride by a titrimetric technique. Electrical conductivity methods are widely used but are much less reliable. Direct-reading skin electrodes are useful only for screening. Both of these methods give false positive and false negative results (326).

Sweat test results must be interpreted with care. Ideally, both chloride and sodium content should be measured, but in practice often only a chloride analysis is performed because it is more reliable and discriminates better between normal and cystic fibrosis populations. The most generally accepted upper limit of normal is 60 mEq per liter for chloride, although some laboratories accept up to 70 mEq per liter, especially in older children and adolescents. Values above 50 mEq per liter are suspicious and should be repeated. Normal adults may have slightly higher values; it is easier to rule out cystic fibrosis with a low value than to diagnose it in an adult with a sweat chloride of 60 to 80 mEq per liter (328, 329). A positive report must always be verified before a final diagnosis is made.

TABLE 7

INDICATIONS FOR SWEAT TESTING

Pulmonary	Gastrointestinal	Other
Chronic cough	Meconium ileus, steatorrhea, malabsorption	Family history of cystic fibrosis
Recurrent or chronic pneumonia		Failure to thrive
Staphylococcal pneumonia	Rectal prolapse	Salty sweat, salty taste when kissed, salt frosting of skin
Recurrent bronchiolitis	Childhood cirrhosis (portal hypertension or bleeding esophageal varices)	
Atelectasis		Nasal polyps
Hemoptysis	Hypoprothrombinemia beyond newborn period	Heat prostration, hyponatremia, and hypochloremia, especially in infants
Mucoid pseudomonas infection		
		Pansinusitis
		Aspermia

The most common cause of a false positive test is laboratory error (326). In addition, elevated sweat chloride concentration has been associated with several conditions other than cystic fibrosis (table 8). Most conditions associated with false positive results should be readily distinguishable from cystic fibrosis. Edema may give false negative results (340, 341).

Cystic fibrosis may not be diagnosed by a positive sweat test in the absence of other criteria. At least one of the other 3 criteria must be present: documented family history of cystic fibrosis, chronic pulmonary disease, or pancreatic insufficiency (342).

Pancreatic Function

Pancreatic dysfunction may be documented by duodenal intubation and measurement of bicarbonate and enzyme content of the duodenal fluid. This is best done after stimulation by secretin and pancreozymin (75). In the 10 to 20 per cent of patients without clinical evidence of pancreatic insufficiency, stimulation tests may reveal normal to increased enzyme concentration, but markedly diminished water and electrolyte (especially bicarbonate) secretion; however, such testing is rarely performed in practice. The most common laboratory procedure used to document pancreatic insufficiency indirectly is the measurement of stool trypsin and/or chymotrypsin (343), a test subject to many errors and unreliable in patients older than approximately 2 years (342). Tests for fat absorption may be helpful but are nonspecific. In the majority of patients, serum pancreatic isoamylase is either absent or markedly diminished in comparison to serum salivary isoamylase (344). This test may be valuable in screening for pancreatic function.

Screening

There are at least 3 possible approaches to screening for cystic fibrosis: (1) sweat testing, (2) evaluation of pancreatic function, or (3) detection of some product of the defective gene. The latter is not yet feasible. Sweat testing is unacceptable for screening of normal populations because of the high cost and relative unreliability of the sweat test during the immediate newborn period (326, 345). In high risk groups, however, sweat testing is justified, and if carefully performed can give accurate results after the first week of life. Mass screening has been attempted with a direct reading chloride sensitive electrode, but this method has not proved satisfactory (326).

Infants with pancreatic insufficiency due to cystic fibrosis have an increased albumin in their meconium (346, 347). This has been screened by several methods, most recently the Boehringer Mannheim test strip. This test was reported feasible for screening because it detected 60 cases of cystic fibrosis in 69,000 infants screened (348). Experience in other centers has been less rewarding: the color changes on the test strip may be ambiguous, infants without pancreatic insufficiency may have false negative tests, and normal infants with melena or intestinal atresia may have false positive tests. Some premature infants may also give false positive reactions. The future of this particular test is unclear. A national cooperative study by the Cystic Fibrosis Foundation should be completed in 1976 and should provide the necessary answers.

Prenatal Diagnosis and Heterozygote Testing

In the absence of a definitive test for the defective gene products, prenatal diagnosis and heterozygote screening are unavailable. Early enthusiasm for the use of various bioassays for

---

TABLE 8

CONDITIONS OTHER THAN CYSTIC FIBROSIS REPORTED TO BE ASSOCIATED
WITH ELEVATED CONCENTRATIONS OF SWEAT ELECTROLYTES

Condition	Reference
Adrenal insufficiency, untreated	330
Ectodermal dysplasia	331, 332
Hereditary nephrogenic diabetes insipidus	333
Glucose-6-phosphatase deficiency	334
Pupillatonia, hyporeflexia, and segmental hypohydrosis with autonomic dysfunction	335
Hypothyroidism	336
Mucopolysaccharidoses	337
Malnutrition	320, 338
Fucosidosis	339

the "ciliary factor" has been tempered with time, and it is now generally agreed that these "tests" should not be used for genetic counseling (199).

Diagnosis in Adults

In the past decade the average age of cystic fibrosis patients has increased significantly. This is due not only to improved therapy but also to greater awareness of the possibility of diagnosis in adolescents and young adults. Unfortunately, for many physicians the mental image of cystic fibrosis remains that of chronically ill infants and death in the first decade. Thus, a relatively healthy adolescent or adult with chronic bronchitis may escape suspicion for cystic fibrosis.

The diagnosis of cystic fibrosis in adults may be more difficult than in children (349). Adult patients with severe malabsorption by laboratory criteria may verbally deny gastrointestinal symptoms and even report "normal" stools and stool patterns. They may be much less symptomatic than children, even with fecal fat losses as high as 70 per cent (273). A review of 66 adults with cystic fibrosis (350) revealed that those in whom gastrointestinal symptoms were absent or greatly delayed were diagnosed at a much later age (20 years). Some of the indications for sweat testing are listed (table 7).

Diagnostic Problems

What about the patient with respiratory symptoms and a borderline sweat test? The most obvious approaches are to repeat the sweat test and evaluate pancreatic function. Careful attention should be given to the technique of the sweat test and to the metabolic state of the patient at the time the test is performed, because edema, dehydration, electrolyte imbalance, and perhaps other factors can influence the sweat test. Pretreatment with mineralocorticoids (9α-fluorohydrocortisone) has been advocated to help identify normal persons with borderline elevated sweat tests (351); however, because cystic fibrosis patients also respond to mineralocorticoids, this cannot be used as a diagnostic test (352). Many patients with borderline sweat tests have clinically normal pancreatic function, and sophisticated tests (pancreozymin-secretin stimulation) may be required to demonstrate pancreatic involvement. Isolation of mucoid pseudomonas from the respiratory tract is a very helpful sign and strongly suggests the diagnosis of cystic fibrosis.

Although "factor assays" and other research tools are not helpful for diagnosis in our present state of knowledge (353), hopefully a specific test for the gene product will become available.

Treatment

Because of the multiple system involvement, the poor prognosis encountered in the past, progression in most patients, and rapid progression encountered in some, a comprehensive and intensive plan of therapy for cystic fibrosis is mandatory. The pulmonary involvement leads to most of the morbidity and mortality; thus, considerable attention and expertise are required in this area.

Comprehensive care includes parent education and, as soon as practicable, continuing patient education and encouragement. A chronic, serious condition like cystic fibrosis, chronic asthma, or bronchitis requires regularly scheduled follow-up visits at frequent intervals (in our practice, every 6 to 8 weeks). An experienced and available physician should supervise the patient's over-all program to detect changes or progression as early as possible and to recommend and evaluate the use of appropriate therapeutic measures.

Because no one person can be knowledgeable about or deal with all the aspects of cystic fibrosis, it is mandatory to create a team approach, using other health professionals including laboratory, respiratory and physical therapy, nursing, dietary, and counseling personnel, who develop increasingly specific knowledge of cystic fibrosis and its problems. Another advantage of the center concept is the accessibility of specialty consultants experienced with cystic fibrosis.

Symptoms such as increasing cough, wheezing, hemoptysis, chest pain, or intestinal obstruction must be dealt with early and correctly before significant changes occur. Experience, team work, and ready access of the patient to such care each serve to improve the chance of success in long-term survival.

Prevention

If preventive health care plays a role anywhere in medicine, it would seem to have a place in the care of cystic fibrosis. Rubeola immunization and especially annual influenza vaccination represent minimal preventive measures. We have emphasized the latter immunization since 1961 and have been progressively impressed with its effectiveness and infrequent rate of reaction.

Other important aspects include protection of young infants from unnecessary exposure to infection, discouragement of smoking by the parents or patient, maintenance of good nutrition, and encouragement of a reasonable level of activity. Psychosocial factors are extremely important and should include encouragement of a positive attitude and development of reasonable long-term goals. If these things are to be achieved, a close personal relationship between center personnel and patients must be developed and maintained.

Although the pulmonary involvement cannot be prevented in most cases, the delay of significant involvement until lung and airway maturity are reached is a reasonable and achievable goal and well worth the effort.

Pulmonary Therapy

Pulmonary disease accounts for much of the morbidity and almost all the mortality in cystic fibrosis patients. Programs for pulmonary therapy along with other aspects of care were begun by several groups in the 1950s and developed by Matthews and co-workers (15) into a concept of comprehensive care. Survival of cystic fibrosis patients has improved greatly so that in many centers 50 per cent survival is obtained well beyond 18 years. The reasons for the improved survival have not been adequately explored.

Because the basic defect remains unknown, treatment is essentially empirical and symptomatic. Although some aspects of therapy are controversial, the effect of the over-all program including close supervision, continuity of care, aggressive intervention, and an optimistic outlook is more important than minor variations in use of individual measures. Individual measures should not be evaluated with the anticipation that each measure should be effective for all patients. Therapy trials must be made with carefully selected patients and well-defined goals because there are many variables.

Antimicrobial therapy. Improved patient survival may be attributed in large part to improvements in antimicrobial therapy, routes of delivery, and increased therapeutic aggressiveness (354, 355). Because the predominant flora in most cystic fibrosis patients are usually staphylococcus or pseudomonas, some have tended to rely on empirical drug regimens, but in our experience specific therapy based on cultures has been more rewarding, especially in younger patients. Antimicrobial sensitivities, especially of gram-negative organisms, cannot be predicted; we rely on *in vitro* sensitivity results to guide our choice of drugs (356). Full therapeutic dosage (table 9) and relatively long treatment periods (at least 2 to 3 weeks) should be used (342, 357). Response to therapy should be monitored clinically and changes made empirically if necessary. Enhanced renal clearance of some antimicrobial drugs has been noted in cystic fibrosis patients (358) and may warrant administration at more frequent intervals than usually recommended.

TABLE 9

SYSTEMIC ANTIMICROBIAL THERAPY*

Antimicrobial Agent	Oral Dose per Day (mg/kg)	Parenteral Dose per Day (mg/kg)	Maximum Dose (mg/day)
Oxacillin	100–200		
Cloxacillin	50–100		
Dicloxacillin	30–50		
Penicillin	30–50		
Ampicillin	100–200		
Amoxicillin	50–100		
Cephalexin	50–100		
Chloramphenicol	50–100		
Tetracycline	50–100		
Methacycline	10–15		
Sulfonamides	150–200		
Novobiocin	30–50		
Erythromycin	50–100		
Gentamicin		7	210–250
Tobramycin		7	210–250
Colistin		7	210–250
Carbenicillin		300–1,000	
Oxacillin		150–200	
Nafcillin		150–200	

*Adapted from reference 342.

Continuous bacterial colonization of the lower respiratory tract is extremely common. Even young, apparently healthy patients frequently produce purulent secretions during cough stimulated by a deep pharyngeal swab. We believe such patients should have specific antimicrobial therapy for their organisms intermittently during the year. Increased cough and sputum production, night cough, decreased appetite, and weight loss or failure to gain weight with or without fever are indicators of increasing bacterial infection. Such patients require more intensive, specific antimicrobial therapy. When the patient reports that symptoms increase promptly each time therapy is stopped, this is a strong indication for continuous antimicrobial therapy.

Isolation of several pathogens on culture may require therapy with multiple agents. Oral therapy may result in the eradication of gram-positive organisms but rarely eliminates pseudomonas; however, suppression of this significant pathogen is probably beneficial (359). Tetracycline, sulfisoxazole, and/or chloramphenicol are often used for this purpose. Further comments on outpatient use of antimicrobial drugs are available (342, 357).

If the response to oral therapy is not satisfactory, the patient should be admitted without delay to the hospital for intravenous therapy (table 9). A decade ago, intravenous therapy implied an arm board, continuous infusion, confinement to bed or room, and impairment in carrying out physical activity or postural drainage. With the heparin lock, discontinuous therapy is possible via a relatively inconspicuous intravenous site (354), and full mobility allows exercise, full postural drainage, and leave from the hospital for school or employment. In some cases intravenous therapy can be maintained at home (360).

As for outpatient management, we rely on *in vitro* sensitivity testing to determine our choice of drugs and often use multiple drugs. Opinion varies on the effectiveness of intravenous therapy (361–367). Because it is difficult to achieve adequate concentrations of drug in the bronchi, adjustment of dosage to the highest safe level is desirable. This may be facilitated by measurement of serum antimicrobial concentrations. Aerosolization of drugs may be useful to increase further the delivery of medication to the site(s) of infection in the airways. In selected cases direct instillation of drug into the tracheobronchial tree via a tracheostomy or endotracheal tube may be efficacious (368). This form of treatment should be considered whenever a route for administration exists. Alternatively, a transtracheal catheter may be placed for repeated administration.

Patients receiving intensive and intravenous therapy often have significant remission of symptoms within 3 to 5 days; however, early relapse is common unless therapy is continued beyond this point. In our experience this usually means 10 to 14 days of in-hospital therapy for each episode.

Mist tent therapy. Mist tent therapy was defined and initiated in the 1950s (12). Various factors in achieving optimal mist therapy and the potential detrimental effects have been reviewed (369–371). Early studies of therapeutic response to mist tents in patients with pulmonary involvement as measured by pulmonary function testing were encouraging (369, 371). Later studies (372, 373) have not shown this beneficial response in many patients.

A common approach to evaluation of mist therapy has been the attempted quantification of water deposition in the lung and study of its distribution by using radioactive aerosols. In studies with nebulized water containing technetium-99 Na pertechnitate and measurement of its deposition in the lungs of subjects by slow rectilinear scanning, very little radioactivity was detected in the lungs. This was interpreted to mean that very little of the water had reached the lungs (374, 375). However, Na pertechnitate is rapidly absorbed from the lungs (half-times of 7 to 13 min) (376), so that significant deposition and distribution may be masked by absorption and/or mucociliary clearance. Greater deposition has been found with the use of an ultrasonic nebulizer than with a jet nebulizer (374) and in cystic fibrosis patients compared with control subjects (375). Another study observed that many counts remained in the nebulizer (377), and in all studies the concentration of radioactivity in the mist reaching the patient was unknown, thus making estimates of fluid deposition uncertain. We have observed, through a fiberoptic bronchoscope, apparently large amounts of mist particles reaching at least the subsegmental bronchi even during nasal breathing.

The interpretation of these studies is difficult, because the behavior of water particles in the respiratory tract is complex and poorly understood. Surprisingly, even inhaled radioactive water vapor ($H_2^{15}O$) is detected almost exclusively in the upper (378) rather than in the lower airways. Inhaled water droplets may well change size by evaporation or condensation in their passage through the nose and trachea (379), and the influence of the addition of solutes such as NaCl or propylene glycol is unclear. Because each particle generated by the nebulizer would contain a constant amount of radioactivity (ignoring the effects of coalescence) regardless of water loss or gain, the amount of radioactivity deposited in the lungs may correlate poorly with the mass water deposition in the lung at a given site. Extrapolation from studies of solid particles to water droplets can also be misleading.

A more basic question is what effect the deposition of water will actually have on the secretions and/or their removal from the lung. In normal dogs, mist had no effect on mucociliary transport (380) but did increase cough transport (381). These data are not directly applicable to the patient with cystic fibrosis, in whom mucociliary transport may be severely impaired (139). In the presence of airway obstruction, peripheral deposition may be decreased, possibly limiting effectiveness (382). The relation of mucous viscosity to mucociliary transport is not well understood (146), but viscosity and elastic recoil have been related to mucociliary transport (383). The viscoelastic properties of sputum *in vitro* may be altered by exposure of the sputum to mist (384, 385). *In vivo* exposure to mist did not alter the rheologic properties of sputum (386). All such studies are technically difficult and their interpretation is still open to question.

Mist therapy and the behavior of liquid droplets in airways remain subjects for discussion and investigation. Mist therapy should not serve as the standard of care for all cystic fibrosis patients, but rather as only one component in a many-faceted, over-all therapeutic program (15). Current pulmonary function tests may be too insensitive to demonstrate efficacy, especially because patients who might benefit most could be those with relatively little airway disease. Further study of mist and other therapy should include long-term, carefully controlled clinical trials using measures of morbidity, clinical status, and more sensitive pulmonary function tests. Such studies should evaluate patients with established lung disease separately from those with little lung disease. Attention should be given to the effect of patient hydration on mucociliary transport and to alternative methods to stimulate pulmonary clearance of secretions (139). Mist therapy is expensive, may be time-consuming and

uncomfortable, and has potential dangers such as inhalation of a contaminated solution. Currently available data suggest that further studies on the physiology of the airways and on mist therapy are needed (387).

Over and above the question regarding deposition of bulk water by mist therapy, simple humidification of inspired air may be of importance in cystic fibrosis patients. Normally, 25 per cent of the humidification of inspired air occurs in the larynx, trachea, and major bronchi, and with mouth breathing this requirement may increase to 75 per cent (370).

Intermittent aerosol therapy. Intermittent aerosol therapy is used to deliver medication rather than bulk liquid to the bronchial mucosa. Because most agents used are potent, the actual volume of liquid delivered need not be great. One significant problem is that airway obstruction by abnormal secretions leads to failure of the aerosol to deposit in precisely those areas most in need of the medication. In patients with minimal airway disease, aerosols are distributed evenly throughout the lung (377). Because intermittent positive pressure breathing therapy is more expensive, has not been shown to add additional benefit, and may be detrimental, we use it rarely in treating cystic fibrosis.

Agents commonly used for aerosol therapy include phenylephrine and bronchodilators such as isoproterenol. Phenylephrine is used to reduce mucosal edema by local vasoconstriction (15), although there is little data demonstrating objective effects. Improvement has occurred in airway resistance and thoracic gas volume in infants with cystic fibrosis after institution of aerosol therapy with orciprenaline in propylene glycol and glycerin (388).

Not all cystic fibrosis patients respond with increased flow rates after isoproterenol. Some decrease their flow rates, probably by a reduction in bronchial wall rigidity (389). Cystic fibrosis patients tend not to demonstrate bronchospasm after inhaling an aerosol as do some asthmatics (390), and the routine use of a bronchodilator has been condemned (389). However, it has recently been demonstrated that mucociliary transport can be increased in cystic fibrosis patients by the subcutaneous administration of terbutaline, a β_2-adrenergic stimulator (139). It is possible that routine administration of β-adrenergic agents may be beneficial.

Mucolytic agents (most commonly, *N*-acetylcysteine) have also been delivered to the airways as aerosols, but opinions vary regarding the value of this approach. *N*-acetylcysteine induces cough, possibly owing to a change in the physical characteristics of the bronchial secretions or simply to mucosal irritation. Decreasing the viscosity of bronchial secretions might improve cough transport but may also result in complete failure of mucociliary transport and pooling of secretions (391).

Intermittent antimicrobial aerosols have been used to supplement systemic administration of drugs (392). These are often given after postural drainage to improve the distribution of the drug.

Postural drainage, breathing exercises, and exercise therapy. Segmental postural drainage, assisted by chest clapping and vibration, and followed by vigorous coughing, has gained widespread acceptance for the treatment of airways obstruction (393), especially in cystic fibrosis. Use of a tilt board or drainage table (357) can facilitate therapy and positioning and minimize discomfort. Self therapy is frequently encouraged in older patients to increase their independence.

Anecdotal evidence for improvement is provided by many patients, although beneficial effects are not perceived by all. Available data indicate that these maneuvers increase sputum expectoration 2-fold over coughing alone during a 20-min period (394) and may increase vital capacity and expiratory flow rates in selected patients (395, 396). In light of the large time and energy demands this therapy places on both the patient and parents, spouse, or friends, the following questions need to be addressed. (*1*) Which patients will benefit from postural drainage? (*2*) Can acute beneficial effects be translated into long-term improvement or arrest of progression? (*3*) Can the onset of significant obstructive lung disease be delayed by routine administration of postural drainage? (*4*) Can mechanical percussors be used as effectively as manual percussion? (*5*) Can adolescent and adult patients effectively administer their own postural drainage?

Breathing exercises aimed at improving lung mechanics are not widely used but are advocated by some physicians. There is little evidence that children or adults carry exercise breathing patterns over into routine living patterns or are able to use these learned breathing techniques to improve ventilation when shortness of breath appears (397).

Persons with chronic obstructive lung disease frequently complain that they must stop strenuous activity to cough and expectorate sputum. The volume of mucus expectorated during strenuous activity may be greater than that produced during a comparable period of inactivity. The benefits from this forced expectoration can only be presumed. The most active patients with cystic fibrosis seem to be those whose lungs are most free of disease; however, it is not clear which is cause and which effect. Additional beneficial effects of exercise may include maintenance of adequate muscle mass and consequently maximal ventilatory efforts and vigorous cough. Those physical activities (if any) that are most helpful for mucous clearance remain undefined. The possibility that regular strenuous activity can be substituted at least in part for the more laborious postural drainage deserves attention.

Endoscopy and lavage. Treatment of obstructive airway disease may sometimes include tracheobronchial suctioning or lavage. The flexible fiberoptic bronchoscope (398) has made endoscopy simpler and better tolerated but has limitations in smaller patients. Bronchoscopy is indicated for treatment of atelectasis and mucoid impaction and for investigation of hemoptysis.

Bronchopulmonary lavage has been performed by a variety of techniques (399–401), ranging from the instillation of a few milliliters of saline or mucolytic agent through a bronchoscope to the use of many liters through a double-lumen endotracheal tube. Indications for such procedures have not been clearly defined, and definitive physiologic evidence for efficacy is lacking.

Expectorants. Although accumulation of secretions in the tracheobronchial tract is a major cause of lung dysfunction in patients with cystic fibrosis, drugs that clearly assist with the physical removal of these secretions and can be used routinely are not available. Reducing agents that depolymerize the mucous glycoproteins (*N*-acetylcysteine) do reduce the viscosity of sputum *in vitro* (402, 403) and apparently assist with removal of secretions if directly instilled into the tracheobronchial tract in sufficient volumes (404). Delivery of this agent by aerosol suffers from the theoretic disadvantage that deposition is largely limited to the airways that are unobstructed and well ventilated (405). Use of *N*-acetyl-L-cysteine in concentrations greater than 5 per cent may cause inflammation of the mucosa (406), and chronic use of nebulized *N*-acetyl-L-cysteine at any concentration may result in tracheitis. Addition of isoproterenol to the aerosol decreases the incidence of *N*-acetyl-L-cysteine–induced bronchospasm (404). Nucleases (Dornase®) and proteases used as liquifying agents for purulent secretions display similar *in vitro* effectiveness and many of the problems with delivery and side effects seen with *N*-acetylcysteine (407).

Iodides and glycerol guaicolate in safe systemic doses do not increase water secretion into the tracheobronchial lumen (408), clearly change the rheologic properties of the secretions, or effect clinical improvement (409–410a). The former agent has the added disadvantage of distressing side effects such as iodism and goiter formation. Other systemic or nebulized "expectorants" have no more impressive clinical effectiveness.

Patient hydration under certain circumstances may improve mucous clearance. Aerosolization of water in a solution physiologic for tracheobronchial secretions should not be irritating, may reduce sputum viscosity (411), and appears at present to be one of the few safe approaches to sputum liquefaction.

Pulmonary surgery. In general, patients with cystic fibrosis tolerate thoracic surgery surprisingly well, provided aggressive preoperative and postoperative antimicrobial and pulmonary therapies are carried out (412, 413). Lung disease due to cystic fibrosis tends to be generalized and severe focal disease usually is not encountered (414). Occasional patients develop symptomatic lobar bronchiectasis, accompanied by persistent fever, anorexia, or weight loss. Lobectomy may delay the development of similar problems in other areas of the lung. The other frequent indication for surgery is pneumothorax (see Complications and Their Treatment).

Gastrointestinal Therapy

Pancreatic enzyme replacement. **Preparations** of animal pancreas given with ingested food tend to reduce but not fully correct stool fat and nitrogen losses (10, 273, 415, 416). Adjustment of enzyme dosage and product should be individualized for each patient. There is a theoretic basis for the addition of bile salts in some patients otherwise not well controlled (277, 417). Reduction of gastric acidity before meals may increase effectiveness of the pancreatin in some cases; sodium bicarbonate may be especially effective (418, 419). However, the use of L-arginine and sodium bicarbonate have no significant effect on fat or nitrogen balance (420).

The available products have been reviewed (421). Enzyme dosage is empirical and requirements vary. Dosage should be adjusted to reduce overt steatorrhea and maintain nutrition. Reduction of fat intake is frequently necessary in infants and children, but less so in older patients. We usually recommend taking one-half the enzyme dose partway through the meal and the remainder at the end. Some (422) have recommended extremely large amounts of enzymes to increase the absorption of fatty acids (423). However, the cost, recent shortage, and patient resistance preclude this approach in most patients. Some patients develop constipation with too great a dosage whereas others may have frequent loose green stools or abdominal pain. Intolerance to hog pancreatic extracts can be a problem with some patients and some family members who develop episodes of rhinitis, watery eyes, or bronchospasm (Type I hypersensitivity reaction) (424–426). Papase®, a non-animal extract of papaya fruit, can provide a reasonable alternate for proteolytic digestion in such situations.

For those patients with considerable flatus, the use of 50 mg of simethicone 1 to 4 times daily has been quite beneficial.

Vitamin supplementation. Because pancreatic insufficiency results in malabsorption of fat-soluble vitamins (A, D, E, and K) a multi-vitamin supplement is usually recommended. Vitamin E deficiency is usually corrected when daily doses of up to 1 mg per kg of water-miscible vitamins are given orally (427). Although ceroid pigment in the smooth muscle of the intestine is found in cystic fibrosis, clinical manifestations are not apparent (428), so vitamin E supplementation has not been uniformly recommended. Vitamin K may be necessary in the newborn period, during times of stress, and during periods of hemoptysis, intense antimicrobial therapy, or surgery. The usual dose is 5 mg orally given daily or every other day. Most patients do not require vitamin K regularly.

Patients with chelosis may benefit from extra riboflavin (5 to 10 mg daily) or additional B vitamins. The chelosis may also respond to local steroid-antifungal applications.

Vitamin B_{12} deficiency has been reported (429) and is corrected by use of pancreatic extract (430). Although supplementation usually is not necessary (429), it is suggested that in older patients the vitamin B_{12} deficiency may become more obvious (431).

Nutritional supplementation. Medium chain triglyceride oils can be more readily absorbed without digestion, reduce fecal fats without much change in circulatory fats (432), and provide a useful source of calories; however, many patients find them unpalatable. The same is true of many of the high-calorie nutritional supplements now available. Total replacement of calories with an artificial replacement/supplement diet including medium chain triglyceride, a glucose polymer, and beef serum hydrolysate has been reported (433, 434). Significant improvement in weight and clinical status has occurred in some patients used as their own controls. Mildly affected patients showed the most improvement in growth and well-being when the diet represented the major part of their nutritional intake; however, it is difficult to keep many children on the diet (435). The use of artificial replacement diets must still be considered experimental and may result in deficiency states (436, 437). Because adequate nutrition seems difficult to achieve in many patients, continued study of the gastrointestinal involvement and controlled study of nutritional therapy are needed. Androgenic steroids have been used to increase weight gain and muscle mass and may be useful in selected patients (438, 439).

Complications and Their Treatment

Pulmonary

Atelectasis. Airway obstruction is the hallmark of the pulmonary involvement. This begins in the peripheral airways and may cause relatively few symptoms, with focal areas of atelectasis and over-inflation apparent radiographically. Segmental or lobar atelectasis is common in infants and older patients with more advanced disease. Occasionally, obstruction of subsegmental airways produces a radiographic picture of "mucoid impaction" (440) that may lead quickly to extensive bronchiectasis and should be treated vigorously.

Treatment of atelectasis is similar to that in other diseases. Postural drainage and inhalation therapy are intensified and appropriate antimicrobial drugs are given. Bronchoscopy may result in quick resolution.

Pneumothorax. This complication is increasingly frequent in adolescent and adult patients with cystic fibrosis. It occurs with equal frequency in men and women, and on the left and right sides. The occurrence of respiratory distress due to intrapleural tension is relatively frequent and has led to a rapid death in several instances (441). Prompt diagnosis and appropriate treatment are essential when this emergency arises.

A significant number of pneumothoraces in patients with cystic fibrosis are small (< 10 to 15 per cent), asymptomatic (441), and detected only by chest roentgenograms. Observation, initially in the hospital and then at home, constitutes appropriate therapy. Larger or symptomatic pneumothoraces must be treated by evacuation of intrapleural air. This has usually been achieved by inserting a large intercostal catheter into the pleural space and attaching the catheter to water-seal drainage or suction (441, 442). Disadvantages of this therapy for patients with cystic fibrosis include a high incidence of persistent air leakage despite expansion of the lung (443) and a high recurrence rate (441, 442). Both problems usually are circumvented by one of two approaches. Pleural inflammation produced by repeated intrapleural instillations of quinacrine hydrochloride or silver nitrate (412, 443) during a 3-day period has resulted uniformly in cessation of air leakage within 24 to 48 hours and has apparently been effective in reducing the incidence of recurrence (412). Alternatively, thoracotomy with closure of the air leak, obliteration of blebs, apical pleural stripping, and dry sponge abrasion of the remaining pleural surface promotes early resolution and rehabilitation and decreases the incidence of recurrence (412). Neither procedure has been attended by increased morbidity or mortality or by significant loss of pulmonary function in comparison with standard tube thoracotomy (412).

Hemoptysis. Hemoptysis is relatively common and ranges from mere streaking to massive blood loss. Although small amounts of bleeding may be associated with little or no morbidity, infection should be suspected and the patient treated accordingly. Massive blood loss (requiring transfusion) is a bad prognostic sign (444) and signals the need for vigorous intervention.

Hospitalization is usually advised for hemoptysis of more than 15 to 30 ml, especially if recurrent. In some patients, *S. aureus* may play a role despite nonrecovery on cultures. The addition or intensification of appropriate antimicrobial therapy can bring cessation of bleeding. Postural drainage with clapping and forced cough may be stopped temporarily. Measurement of prothrombin time and oral or parenteral administration of vitamin K as indicated may be helpful. Bleeding may also be associated with drug therapy such as aspirin and carbenicillin.

Localization of the site(s) of bleeding is often difficult but may be improved with fiberoptic bronchoscopy (445). Endoscopy is more successful in localizing the bleeding site if performed during active bleeding. Bleeding may then be stopped by lavage with iced saline, topical application of epinephrine, or by tamponade with a balloon-tipped catheter (446). Bronchial arteriography is of limited value in the evaluation of hemoptysis in cystic fibrosis (447).

Respiratory failure. Increasing dyspnea, cyanosis, and sputum production, accompanied by retention of CO_2, herald the onset of respiratory failure. Some patients develop respiratory failure rather quickly with an acute infection, whereas others do so much more slowly. In the latter case, signs of right heart failure eventually appear, and the patient usually responds if therapy is directed toward cor pulmonale as well. The primary goal of therapy is the relief of hypoxemia and airway obstruction. With judicious use of O_2, intensive intravenous antimicrobial therapy, and bronchial hygiene, most patients survive at least the first episode of respiratory failure.

The mode of death is very frequently major airway obstruction with massive quantities of thick secretions. Direct endotracheal suctioning may be useful; however, in debilitated and fatigued patients with an ineffective cough, improvement is transient. Mechanical ventilation is seldom helpful for more than a few days and may impact secretions in the smaller airways (although the endotracheal tube provides a route for frequent suctioning). Many feel that intubation and mechanical ventilation are contraindicated in cystic fibrosis patients with advanced pulmonary disease in resipratory failure although this may be as much a philsophical stance as a medical one. Short-term ventilatory support may be helpful when acute respiratory failure is superimposed on only moderately severe respiratory disease.

Because of the critical role of cough in bronchial hygiene, the attitude and cooperation of the patient are most important to the success of therapy for respiratory failure. Active emotional support is essential. A patient with advanced disease can die in a matter of hours to days after deciding to "give up" despite the fact that his or her condition was relatively good at the time.

Cor pulmonale. The majority of patients with cystic fibrosis die as a result of the pulmonary involvement and its complications. With progressive loss of pulmonary function and hypoxemia, pulmonary hypertension develops and results in cor pulmonale. Cardiac failure may occur at any age, depending on the severity of the pulmonary involvement, and may be acute, especially if severe hypoxemia and acidosis develop. Because pulmonary hypertension may be reversible with relief of hypoxemia, aggressive therapy is recommended (448).

The physical signs of cardiac failure in cystic fibrosis may be partially masked by the manifestations of tthe pulmonary involvement. Hyperinflation often results in apparent hepatomegaly, may make the heart shadow on a chest roentgenogram appear small or normal, and makes recognition of the accentuated pulmonic component of the second heart sound difficult. Classical signs may, of course, be present, including distended neck veins, gallop rhythm, hepatomegaly, and edema. The localization and occurrence of edema are variable. In some patients right upper quadrant abdominal pain may be the presenting symptom of cardiac failure. Some patients may have associated left ventricular failure due, presumably, to low oxygen saturation.

Laboratory confirmation of cor pulmonale is difficult. The scalar electrocardiogram may be normal (449–451) although the vectorcardiogram can be more helpful (451, 452). Vectorcardiographic changes (terminal rightward forces) have been correlated with pulmonary function test results and in some cases are reversible (451). The electrocardiographic pattern of right ventricular hypertrophy is affected by overdistention of the lung (453). Right axis deviation greater than 90° may be a useful indicator of cor pulmonale (450, 454).

Pulmonary artery pressures correlate best with arterial O_2 tension (Pa_{O_2}). Almost all patients with pulmonary hypertension have a $Pa_{O_2} < 45$ mm Hg (table 10) (450). Hypoalbuminemia is

TABLE 10

INDICATIONS OF CHRONIC COR PULMONALE IN
CYSTIC FIBROSIS (450)

Right ventricular hypertrophy by standard electrocardiogram or orthogonal vectorcardiogram.

Arterial oxygen tension < 50 mm Hg, especially if the carbon dioxide is > 45 mm Hg.

A vital capacity of less than 60 per cent of predicted.

Clinical signs of congestive heart failure.

Roentgenographic evidence of enlarged pulmonary artery or cardiac size.

often seen with heart failure and may be evident before clinically apparent cardiac involvement (455, 456).

Treatment of cor pulmonale is directed toward relief of hypoxemia and airway obstruction and to specific support of cardiac function. Low-flow O_2 with frequent blood gas determinations to keep the Pa_{O_2} above 50 mm Hg without producing increasing CO_2 retention is very helpful. Diuresis and restriction of salt and fluid intake reduce venous pressure (457). Electrolyte imbalances (hypokalemia, hypochloremia) may occur with diuretic therapy and should be corrected. Digitalization may be useful for acute management (342). Some investigators recommend continuation of digitalis in those who have had an episode of failure or initiation in those in whom impending failure is suspected.

Tolazoline reduces pulmonary artery pressure at high altitude (458) and at sea level (459), especially when combined with O_2, but it has not been possible to predict which patients respond favorably even with cardiac catheterization (459). Antihistamines prevent hypoxic pulmonary vasoconstriction in dogs (460), but 5 of our patients with cystic fibrosis studied at cardiac catheterization showed no beneficial effect.

In the past, cardiac failure usually meant death within a month or two. In recent years, however, the prognosis has been improving, and a number of older patients have survived for 2 years or more after cardiac failure. These patients have been maintained on a vigorous, comprehensive pulmonary care program, including digoxin and diuretics. Only one of our patients has required continuous low-flow O_2 therapy at home.

Allergic aspergillosis. Approximately one third of patients with cystic fibrosis have precipitins for *Aspergillus fumigatus* in their serum (461), usually indicating colonization of the sputum with this organism. Occasionally, a patient develops allergic aspergillosis, including increased cough, wheezing, dyspnea, new lung infiltrates, fever, eosinophilia, and/or expectoration of red-brown sputum plugs or casts. Multiple serum precipitins and skin hypersensitivity to extracts of *A. fumigatus* are present (462). We have seen 4 typical episodes of this syndrome in a population of more than 700 patients. Treatment with systemic steroids eliminated the acute symptoms in each case, but resolution of infiltrates required therapy for several months. Concomitant use of aerosolized amphotericin B has been advocated (463), but its efficacy is un-

proved. Parenteral administration of amphotericin B, because of severe toxicity, is usually not recommended. Because bronchiectasis may result from an Arthus reaction attending allergic bronchopulmonary aspergillosis (462–464), prompt recognition and treatment seem important.

Tuberculosis. Tuberculosis is encountered infrequently in cystic fibrosis. We have found fewer than 10 purified protein derivative converters and only 2 active cases in an 18-year period involving more than 700 patients. *Mycobacterium tuberculosis* infections should be appropriately evaluated and treated as in any other patient. Occasionally, an undiagnosed patient may be referred for treatment of tuberculosis when the correct diagnosis is cystic fibrosis.

Atypical mycobacteria (*M. fortuitum*) have been recovered from the sputum of 3 of our patients. The differentiation between colonization, innocuous infection, and serious disease is difficult. One patient with very resistant *M. fortuitum* died but we were unable to demonstrate conclusively significant active infection with this organism.

Hypertrophic osteoarthropathy. Clubbing of fingers and toes is an almost universal phenomenon in patients with cystic fibrosis, but periostitis and arthritis with pain, edema, and decreased activity are uncommonly observed. Only 6 instances of this complication have been recorded in any detail (465–467). This complication may occur during prepubertal years, but in our experience has appeared most often in adolescent or adult patients. No specific therapy is available. Vigorous treatment and subsequent improved control of the lung disease may ameliorate related symptoms (466).

Other Complications

Meconium ileus, meconium ileus equivalent, intussusception. Traditionally, meconium ileus has been treated surgically (263); however, good results have been obtained recently in selective cases using gastrograffin enemas (468).

Cramping abdominal pain is not uncommon in patients with cystic fibrosis and is probably usually due to the large amounts of fecal material associated with maldigestion. Often a change in pancreatin dosage will relieve symptoms. In some patients cramping pain may be the sign of a more serious complication, such as intussusception (269), meconium ileus equivalent (268), volvulus, or appendicitis.

Meconium ileus equivalent or intussusception

may require surgical intervention for relief of obstruction; however, either may respond to one or more high enemas with hygroscopic radiographic contrast material (342, 469). Enemas containing *N*-acetylcysteine, pancreatin, and/ or mineral oil may be used to complete the cleansing of the bowel after relief of obstruction. Large volumes (up to 4 liters) may be required to reach the ileocecal area. If obstruction is not promptly relieved or if definite evidence of vascular compromise is present, surgery should be performed without delay.

Recurrent cramping abdominal pain may be a sign of impending obstruction, with or without a palpable mass. Some patients have responded to the regular oral administration of mineral oil or of *N*-acetylcysteine (470), although both are rather unpalatable.

We have seen several patients who received drugs for other purposes (opiates, atropine) that resulted in decreased gastrointestinal motility for a period of several days and produced the clinical picture of meconium ileus equivalent. Such drugs should be given with great caution to patients with cystic fibrosis.

Rectal prolapse. Prolapse of the rectum may occur in up to 20 per cent of untreated infants with cystic fibrosis and should alert one to the diagnosis of cystic fibrosis (286). It occurs occasionally in older children and adults and appears related to pancreatic enzyme deficiency, bulky stools, poor nutrition, and/or poor perineal muscle tone. In addition to manual reduction with each occurrence, adequate pancreatin replacement and decreased fat and roughage in the diet generally result in improvement. We have used surgical placement of a silastic perianal sling in one 5-year-old child with relief of chronic recurrences.

Biliary disease. The incidence of focal biliary cirrhosis probably exceeds 25 per cent of patients with cystic fibrosis who reach late adolescence or adulthood (see gastrointestinal manifestations). On the other hand, clinical signs of hepatic involvement occur in only 2 to 4 per cent of patients (291, 293, 471). These clinical signs nearly always reflect portal hypertension and include splenomegaly and hypersplenism, significant bleeding from esophageal varices, and ascites. Frank hepatic failure is a rare event.

The major therapeutic question concerns the risks and efficacy of a shunting procedure to ameliorate portal hypertension. Twenty-three portal systemic shunt procedures have been reported (471–473). Seventeen of these patients

had experienced variceal bleeding; 7 of 12 patients died within the first 4 postoperative months (472, 473). In a more recent report of 5 patients, no deaths were reported in the first postoperative year (471). Rebleeding occurred in only 2 of 10 patients who survived 1 to 10 years after surgery. Repeat bleeding was caused by a nonfunctioning shunt. Intellectual performance, educational achievement, and work records have been excellent in shunted patients (471). Hepatic complications after portal-systemic shunting are minimal. As experience is gained with major surgery for patients with cystic fibrosis, it is apparent that the immediate risks of surgery can be minimized by careful pre-, intra-, and postoperative pulmonary care (413). We recommend that variceal bleeding in cystic fibrosis patients be treated by portal-systemic shunting (471).

Pancreatitis. Some patients who do not have clinical pancreatic insufficiency may have recurrent attacks of acute pancreatitis (302), usually precipitated by fatty meals, alcohol ingestion, or tetracycline therapy. Pancreatitis may be the presenting symptom of cystic fibrosis. Avoidance of the precipitating agent usually precludes recurrences. Prolonged elevation of serum amylase and lipase suggests constant inflammation of the pancreas (302). Treatment is similar to that for other patients with pancreatitis (474) and should include antacids, low fat diet, and pancreatin supplement (302).

Diabetes. The incidence of symptomatic glucose intolerance in cystic fibrosis is estimated to be at least 1 per cent, 2 to 3 times higher than the incidence in the general population under 25 years of age (475). Onset can be at any age (476). The occurrence is not related to the severity of the disease (477), and the incidence will probably increase with increasing length of survival. The incidence of glucosuria or an abnormal glucose tolerance test ranges from 25 per cent to 75 per cent of cystic fibrosis subjects, depending on the criteria and type of test (478). Glucose intolerance due to anatomic disorganization of the islets of Langerhans produced by fibrosis of the pancreas and not due to diabetes mellitus as such is discussed (479, 480). The capacity for insulin release is decreased even when nutrition is good (478, 479, 481–483). There may be increased peripheral tissue sensitivity to insulin to compensate partly for the insulin deficiency (478).

Ketoacidosis is rarely encountered. Thorough education and continued follow-up are important, and management must be individualized

(476). Most patients are treated with a mixture of regular and neutral protein Hagedorn insulin. In our experience, oral hypoglycemic agents have not been useful. The period of follow-up has generally been too brief to permit observation for complications associated with diabetes mellitus; however, retinal vascular changes (477) and glomerular lesions (483a) have been reported.

The development of diabetes is not clearly associated with subsequent increased pulmonary symptoms but may precipitate psychologic problems, such as depression. The diabetes is usually not life threatening and is more of a nuisance than a factor in prognosis.

Psychosocial Aspects

The psychosocial aspects of cystic fibrosis in children have been discussed in a number of articles (484–493). These articles deal both with patients' coping responses and with the effects on family members of a child with a chronic, potentially fatal illness. On the basis of this information and our own experience, we believe that extensive education and counseling of the child and the parents at the time of initial diagnosis and frequent monitoring of patient and family functioning at the time of routine examinations can markedly increase the chances for both to approach normality in living.

A new set of psychosocial considerations has emerged as physicians and other medical personnel care for increasingly large numbers of teenagers and adults with cystic fibrosis (494, 495). The transition to independent living may be difficult for the adolescent who has been forced into a dependent relationship with his or her parents because of daily medical care needs. Responsibility for performance of therapy should be shifted gradually during grade school years and completed sometime during adolescence. This approach will, we hope, eliminate some of the self-destructive adolescent noncompliance with therapy that is linked to control by and dependence on parents.

Early vocational planning is important and may require professional assistance. Persons with cystic fibrosis need skills that are in demand and that are utilized in environments acceptable for those with chronic lung disease (8). College education or its equivalent is often desirable and frequently completed. Medical therapies on campus are handled comfortably by those patients who have developed good self-care routines. Financial assistance for college, trade school, or apprenticeship training often can be obtained from local vocational rehabilitation services.

Financing medical care at and beyond 21 years of age can be a major hurdle. The cost of medications alone may exceed $100 to $200 a month. Medical insurance for adults usually is available only through group policies. Several states have implemented medical programs for adults with cystic fibrosis that continue the support provided by Crippled Children's Services. Stable employment usually allows adults with cystic fibrosis to be financially independent. It is our experience that these adults generally have excellent work records (8).

Increasing numbers of young adults are married. Adequate premarital counseling of patient and potential spouse concerning health, need for prescribed therapies, infertility, risks of pregnancy, effects of chronic lung disease on sexual function, and genetic implications is very important and should be undertaken, at least in part, by a physician who is knowledgeable about these facets of cystic fibrosis. Birth control is often desired but should be considered carefully because of potential harmful effects of medications such as oral contraceptives (45). Continued contact with patient and spouse is necessary to identify and deal with new or ongoing problems.

Most older patients with cystic fibrosis cope

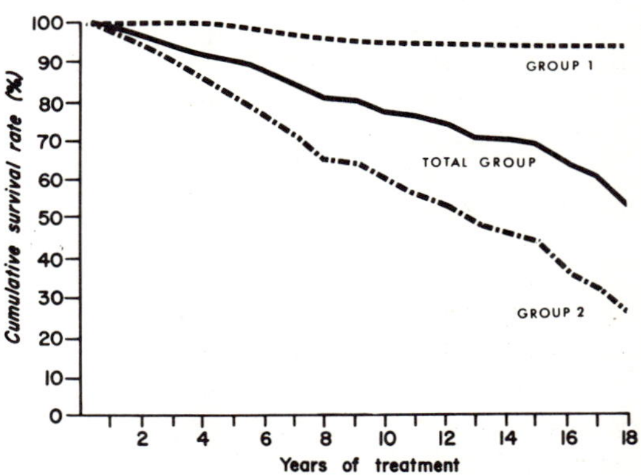

Fig. 1. Life table analysis of 535 patients with cystic fibrosis covering 18 years of treatment and 4,720 patient years of follow-up from 1957 to 1975 (solid line). The results for Group 1 ($\geq$ 19 points) are represented by the dashed line and includes 280 patients and 2,666 patient follow-up years. The dotted line represents 255 Group 2 (< 19 points) patients with 2,054 patient follow-up years. The abscissa is years of treatment, not years of age.

admirably with their situation. As with any group having a severe chronic illness, psychological disturbances do arise. Anticipation of prolonged illness and death, concerns about body image and infertility, and insecurity in social encounters may lead to manifestations of anxiety or depression. Early recognition and appropriate referral for psychological counseling are important in dealing with these manifestations. Group meetings with skilled leadership may assist young adults with the management of daily difficulties (495); however, increased anxiety may result from dealing with more disabled persons or experiencing the death of a fellow patient. The goal of any counseling effort for adults with cystic fibrosis should be the development of independent attitudes and life-styles.

Evaluation and Prognosis

The development of a clinical scoring system (497), modified for infants and young children (498), has proved useful for evaluating and following patients. A more complex system includes prognostic factors and pulmonary function results for those patients old enough to cooperate (499).

Shwachman (500) and others (501; Warwick, W. R.: Unpublished data) have noted an improving prognosis. This has been our experience (16). We have used the chest roentgenogram alone to define patient groups and to predict survival (16). The chest roentgenogram is scored independently by a radiologist, with a perfect score being 25 points. Our patients have been divided into 2 groups according to highest roentgenogram score achieved during the first year of treatment. Patients whose degree of pulmonary involvement was sufficiently reversible to return to near normal as evidenced by a score of 19 or more points during the first year of treatment were placed in Group 1. Group 2 patients did not improve during the first year of treatment and never achieved a score over 18 points. Both groups were continued on comprehensive treatment. Patients in Group 1, who constitute 53 per cent of the total population, have had a decidedly different survival outcome, with only 13 deaths during an 18-year period compared with 106 deaths in Group 2. When the follow-up experience was subjected to life table analysis (502), the difference in survival was readily apparent (figure 1). Despite the presence of pulmonary involvement by chest roentgenogram at initiation of therapy, the reversibility shown during the first year of treatment resulted in a 93 per cent rate of survival after 18 years of treatment (Group 1).

National life table data suggest that males have better survival rates than females, based on age in years (Warwick, W. R.: Unpublished data); however, cumulative survival for both males and females remains the same in our group of 535 patients (74 per cent rate of survival) to 18 years of age. Subsequently, the male survival is slightly better, so that at 26 years of age the male survival rate is 51 per cent and the female rate is 47 per cent, but the differences are not significant.

There are few reports of long-term pulmonary function testing in cystic fibrosis (16, 503). In a subpopulation of 59 patients treated for 13 to 18 years, we observed progressive loss of pulmonary function for both males and females in Group 2. Many females in Group 1 also showed loss of function during the 13- to 18-year period of treatment. In contrast, the mean test values remained normal or near normal for the 24 males in Group 1 (table 11). Forty-two per cent of the Group 1 males had appreciable pulmonary involvement at the time of diagnosis (mean score 15.6 points $\pm$ 6.0 SD; n = 26) but were still able to respond to therapy in the first treatment

TABLE 11

SELECTED PULMONARY FUNCTION RESULTS FOR 59 PATIENTS WITH
CYSTIC FIBROSIS AFTER 13 TO 18 YEARS OF TREATMENT

		No. of Patients	Age (years)	Vital Capacity (% pred.)	Residual Volume* (% pred.)	RV/TLC*	FEV$_1$/FVC
Group 1	male	26	18 ± 3	96 ± 24	180 ± 53	0.35 ± 0.12	0.68 ± 0.13
	female	15	19 ± 3	83 ± 22	223 ± 60	0.42 ± 0.11	0.68 ± 0.13
Group 2	male	10	24 ± 5	62 ± 13	304 ± 132	0.57 ± 0.11	0.58 ± 0.10
	female	8	22 ± 3	67 ± 18	284 ± 61	0.55 ± 0.12	0.62 ± 0.10

*Residual volume to total lung capacity ratio.
†Forced expiratory volume in 1 sec to forced vital capacity ratio.

year and had better mean values than females for vital capacity, residual volume, and ratio of residual volume to total lung capacity at the end of the treatment period. Diagnosis and treatment before the development of significant pulmonary involvement improves the chances of achieving normal or near-normal function in adolescence, especially in males.

Acknowledgment

The authors are indebted to Dr. Frank P. Primiano, Jr., and Dr. Jay G. Horowitz for the life table data; Dr. Pierre A. Vauthy, Marvin D. Lough, and the pulmonary function laboratory technicians for the pulmonary function data; Dr. LeRoy W. Matthews and Dr. Robert C. Stern for their contributions to the Cystic Fibrosis Center program; Judith Wood for the bibliography; and Kathleen Hollosy, Marjorie Bruch, Joyce Protiva, and Ruth Fagan for assistance with the manuscript.

References

1. Rochholz, E. L.: Kinderlied und Kinderspiel aus der Schweiz, Weber, Leipzig, 1857, p. 280.
2. Landsteiner, K.: Darmverschluss durch eingedicktes meconium Pancreatitis, Allg Pathol, 1905, *16*, 903.
3. Garrod, A. E., and Hurtley, W. H.: Congenital family steatorrhoea, Q J Med, 1913, *6*, 242.
4. Blackfan, K. D., and Wolbach, S. B.: Vitamin A deficiency in infants: A clinical and pathological study, J Pediatr, 1933, *3*, 679.
5. Blackfan, K. D., and May, C. D.: Inspissation of secretion, dilatation of the ducts and acini, atrophy and fibrosis of the pancreas in infants: A clinical note, J Pediatr, 1938, *13*, 627.
6. Fanconi, G., Uehlinger, E., and Knauer, C.: Das Coeliakiesyndrom bei angeborener zystischer Pankreasfibromatose und Bronkiektasien, Wien Med Wochenschr, 1936, *86*, 753.
7. Andersen, D. H.: Cystic fibrosis of the pancreas and its relation to celiac disease: A clinical and pathologic study, Am J Dis Child, 1938, *56*, 344.
8. Stern, R. C., Boat, T. F., Doershuk, C. F., Tucker, A. S., Primiano, F. P., and Matthews, L. W.: Course of ninety-five patients with cystic fibrosis, J Pediatr, in press.
9. Andersen, D. H.: Celiac syndrome. III. Dietary therapy for congenital pancreatic deficiency, Am J Dis Child, 1945, *70*, 100.
10. Harris, R., Norman, A. P., and Payne, W. W.: The effect of pancreatin therapy on fat absorption and nitrogen retention in children with fibrocystic disease of the pancreas, Arch Dis Child, 1955, *30*, 424.
11. Gibson, L. E., and Cooke, R. E.: A test for concentration of electrolytes in sweat in cystic fibrosis of the pancreas utilizing pilocarpine iontophoresis, Pediatrics, 1959, *23*, 545.
12. Denton, R., and Smith, R. M.: Portable humidifying unit. II. Large capacity metal nebulizer, Am J Dis Child, 1951, *82*, 433.
13. Doyle, B.: Physical therapy in the treatment of cystic fibrosis, Phys Ther Rev, 1959, *39*, 24.
14. Thacker, E. W.: Postural drainage and respiratory control, Lloyd-Luke Ltd., London, 1959.
15. Matthews, L. W., Doershuk, C. F., Wise, M., Eddy, G., Nudelman, H., and Spector, S.: A therapeutic regimen for patients with cystic fibrosis, J Pediatr, 1964, *65*, 558.
16. Doershuk, C. F., Matthews, L. W., Tucker, A. S., and Spector, S.: Evaluation of a prophylactic and therapeutic program for patients with cystic fibrosis, Pediatrics, 1965, *36*, 675.
17. Wright, S. W., and Morton, N. E.: Genetic studies on cystic fibrosis in Hawaii, Am J Hum Genet, 1968, *20*, 157.
18. Kulczycki, L. L., and Schauf, V.: Cystic fibrosis in blacks in Washington, D.C., Am J Dis Child, 1974, *127*, 64.
19. Antonelli, M., and Donfrancesco, A.: Indagine clinico-statistica sulla epidemiologia della fibrosi cistica (F.C.) in Italia nel quadrienno 1966-1969, Fracastoro, 1970, *63*, 207.
20. Goodchild, M. C., Insley, J., Rushton, D. I., and Gaze, H.: Cystic fibrosis in 3 Pakistani children, Arch Dis Child, 1974, *49*, 739.
21. Selander, P.: The frequency of cystic fibrosis of the pancreas in Sweden, Acta Paediatr, 1962, *51*, 65.
22. Reiderman, M. I.: Studies on the incidence of mucoviscidosis based on urban clinical data in European USSR, Sov Genet, 1973, *7*, 111.
23. Steinberg, A. G., and Brown, D. C.: On the incidence of cystic fibrosis of the pancreas, Am J Hum Genet, 1960, *12*, 416.
24. di Sant'Agnese, P. A., and Talamo, R. C.: Pathogenesis and pathophysiology of cystic fibrosis of the pancreas, N Engl J Med, 1967, *277*, 1287, 1344, 1399.
25. Vivell, O., Jacobi, H., and Münchbach, K.: Zur mukoviscidosis in Kindesalter, Monatsschr Kinderheilkd, 1963, *111*, 62.
26. Brunecky, Z.: The incidence and genetics of cystic fibrosis, J Med Genet, 1972, *9*, 33.
27. Bernheim, M., Monnet, P., Jeune, M., Robert, J. M., and Comby, J.: La maladie fibrokystique des parenchymes glandulaires, Pediatrie, 1961, *16*, 17.
28. Carter, C. O.: Genetical aspects of cystic fibrosis of the pancreas, Mod Probl Pediatr, 1967, *10*, 372.
29. Pugh, R. J., and Pickup, J. D.: Cystic fibrosis in the Leeds region, Arch Dis Child, 1967, *42*, 544.
30. Houstek, J., and Vavrova, V.: Notre experience a propos de la mucoviscidose, Rev Med Liege, 1967, *22*, 421.
31. Sultz, H. A., Schlesinger, E. R., and Mosker,

W. E.: The Erie County survey of long-term childhood illness, Am J Public Health, 1966, *56*, 1461.

32. Danks, D. M., Allan, J., and Anderson, C. M.: A genetic study of fibrocystic disease of the pancreas, Ann Hum Genet, 1965, *28*, 323.

33. Hall, B. D., and Simkiss, M. J.: Incidence of fibrocystic disease in Wessex, J Med Genet, 1968, *5*, 262.

34. Kramm, E. R., Crane, M. M., Sirken, M. G., and Brown, M. L.: Cystic fibrosis pilot survey in three New England states, Am J Public Health, 1962, *52*, 2041.

35. Merritt, A. D., Hanna, B. L., Todd, C. W., Jr., and Meyers, T. L.: Incidence of mode of inheritance of cystic fibrosis, J Lab Clin Med, 1962, *60*, 998.

36. Honeyman, M. S., and Siker, E.: Cystic fibrosis of the pancreas: An estimate of the incidence, Am J Hum Genet, 1965, *17*, 461.

37. Goodman, H. O., and Reed, S. C.: Heredity of fibrosis of the pancreas: Possible mutation rate of the gene, Am J Hum Genet, 1952, *4*, 59.

38. Super, M.: Cystic fibrosis in the South West African Afrikaner, S Afr Med J, 1975, *49*, 818.

39. Harris, R. L., and Riley, H. D., Jr.: Cystic fibrosis in the American Indian, Pediatrics, 1968, *41*, 733.

40. Macdougall, L. G.: Fibrocystic disease of the pancreas in African children, Lancet, 1962, 2, 409.

41. Wang, C-I, Sumi, W. T., Stanton, R., Kwok, S., and Yamazaki, J. N.: Cystic fibrosis in an Oriental child, N Engl J Med, 1968, *279*, 1216.

42. Ikai, K., Sugie, I., Sugino, I., Nitta, H., Iida, T., Ogava, J., and Suecki, T.: Cystic fibrosis found by re-examination of histology of the pancreas and postmortem protocol in Japanese children and sweat test on siblings, Acta Paediatr Jap, 1965, *7*, 23.

43. Kandar, H. R.: Cystic fibrosis of the pancreas with respiratory allergy in children, Antiseptic, 1961, *58*, 863.

44. Reddy, C. R., Devi, C. S., Anees, A. M., Murthy, D. P., and Reddy, G. E.: Cystic fibrosis of the pancreas in India, J Pediatr, 1969, *75*, 522.

45. Cohen, L. F.: Problems in reproductive physiology and anatomy in young adults with cystic fibrosis, in *GAP Conference Report*, T. F. Boat and I. Harwood, ed., Cystic Fibrosis Foundation, Atlanta, Ga., 1975, p. 6.

46. Danes, B. S., and Bearn, A. G.: Cystic fibrosis of the pancreas. A study in cell culture, J Exp Med, 1969, *129*, 775.

47. Bearn, A. G.: The relevance of biological markers to the pathogenesis of inherited disease, in *Fundamental Problems of Cystic Fibrosis and Related Diseases*, J. A. Mangos and R. C. Talamo, ed., Intercontinental Medical Book Corp., New York, 1973, p. 21.

48. Danes, B. S., and Flensborg, E. W.: Cystic fibrosis: Cell culture studies on a Danish population, Am J Hum Genet, 1971, *23*, 297.

49. Conneally, P. M., Merritt, A. D., and Yu, P-L.: Cystic fibrosis: Population genetics, Tex Rep Biol Med, 1973, *31*, 639.

50. Taysi, K., Kistenmacher, M. L., Punnett, H. H., and Mellman, W. J.: Limitations of metachromasia as a diagnostic aid in pediatrics, N Engl J Med, 1969, *281*, 1108.

51. Reed, G. B., Bain, A. D., McCrae, W. M., and Scott, F. M.: Cellular metachromasia in cystic fibrosis, J Pathol, 1970, *101*, 251.

52. Kulczycki, L. L., Guin, G. H., and Mann, N.: Cystic fibrosis in Negro children, Clin Pediatr (Phila), 1964, *3*, 692.

52a. Stern, R. C., Doershuk, C. F., Boat, T. F., Tucker, A. S., Primiano, F. P., Jr., and Matthews, L. W.: Course of cystic fibrosis in 17 black patients, J Pediatr, in press.

53. Batten, J., Muir, D., Simon, G., and Carter, C.: Prevalence of respiratory disease in heterozygotes for the gene for fibrocystic disease of pancreas, Lancet, 1963, *1*, 1348.

54. Orzalesi, M. M., Kohner, C. D., Cook, C. D., and Shwachman, H.: Anamnesis, sweat electrolyte and pulmonary function studies in parents of patients with cystic fibrosis of pancreas, Acta Paediatr, 1963, *52*, 267.

55. Hallett, W. Y., Knudson, A. G., Jr., and Massey, F. J.: Absence of detrimental effect of the carrier state for the cystic fibrosis gene, Am Rev Respir Dis, 1965, *92*, 714.

56. Bearn, A. G.: Genetics of cystic fibrosis, Clin Gastroenterol, 1973, *2*, 515.

57. Baumann, T.: Die Mucoviscidosis als rezessives und irregulär dominantes Erbleiden: eine klinische und genetische Studie, Helv Paediatr Acta, 1958, *13* (Supplement 8, p. 1.)

58. Knudson, A. G., Jr., Wayne, L., and Hallett, W. Y.: On the selective advantage of cystic fibrosis heterozygotes, Am J Hum Genet, 1967, *19*, 388.

59. Virtanen, S.: Salivary secretion of ABH blood group substances in cystic fibrosis of the pancreas, J Pediatr, 1966, *68*, 139.

60. Steinberg, A. G., and Morton, N. E.: Sequential test for linkage between cystic fibrosis of the pancreas and the MNS locus, Am J Hum Genet, 1956, *8*, 177.

61. Götz, M., Ludwig, H., and Polymenidis, Z.: HLA antigens in cystic fibrosis, Z. Kinderheilkd, 1974, *117*, 183.

62. Milunsky, A.: Cystic fibrosis and Down's syndrome, Pediatrics, 1968, *42*, 501.

63. Smith, D. W., Docter, J. M., Ferrier, P. E., Frias, J. L., and Spock, A.: Possible localization of the gene for cystic fibrosis of the pancreas to the short arm of chromosome 5, Lancet, 1968, 2, 309.

64. Lindenbaum, R. H., Blackwell, N. L., and de

Sa', D. J.: A case of double aneuploidy, 47, XXY, 14-, t (13q14q) +, also probably homozygous for the cystic fibrosis gene, J Med Genet, 1972, *9*, 232.

65. Taussig, L. M., Braunstein, G. D., White, B. J., and Christiansen, R. L.: Silver-Russell dwarfism and cystic fibrosis in a twin, Am J Dis Child, 1973, *125*, 495.

66. Fluge, G., and Aarskog, D.: Silver-Russell dwarfism and cystic fibrosis (letter to the editor), Am J Dis Child, 1974, *127*, 760.

67. Burnell, R. H., and Robertson, E. F.: Cystic fibrosis in a patient with Kartagener syndrome, Am J Dis Child, 1974, *127*, 746.

68. Lewis, M. B.: Rothmund-Thompson syndrome and fibrocystic disease, Australas J Dermatol, 1972, *13*, 105.

69. Lox, C. D., Davis, J. R., Christian, C. D., and Heine, M. W.: Anosomic hypogonadotropic hypogonadism: Kallman's syndrome, a case history complicated by cystic fibrosis, Ariz Med, 1974, *31*, 508.

70. Bitar, J., and Lightwood, R.: The Wiskott-Aldrich syndrome associated with mucoviscidosis in the same patient, J Pediatr, 1967, *71*, 123.

71. Matthews, L. W., Spector, S., Lemm, J., and Potter, J. L.: Studies on pulmonary secretions. I. The over-all chemical composition of pulmonary secretions from patients with cystic fibrosis, bronchiectasis, and laryngectomy, Am Rev Respir Dis, 1963, *88*, 199.

72. Chernick, W. S., and Barbero, G. J.: Composition of tracheobronchial secretions in cystic fibrosis of the pancreas and bronchiectasis, Pediatrics, 1959, *24*, 739.

73. Kopito, L., and Shwachman, H.: Mineral composition of meconium, J Pediatr, 1966, *68*, 313.

74. Kopito, L. E., Kosasky, H. J., Sturgis, S. H., Lieberman, B. L., and Shwachman, H.: Water and electrolytes in human cervical mucus, Fertil Steril, 1973, *24*, 499.

75. Hadorn, B., Zoppi, G., Shmerling, D. H., Prader, A., McIntyre, I., and Anderson, C. M.: Quantitative assessment of exocrin pancreatic function in infants and children, J Pediatr, 1968, *73*, 39.

76. Zoppi, G., Shmerling, D. H., Gaburro, D., and Prader, A.: The electrolyte and protein contents and outputs in duodenal juice after pancreozymin and secretin stimulation in normal children and in patients with cystic fibrosis, Acta Paediatr Scand, 1970, *59*, 692.

77. Rule, A. H., Kopito, L., and Shwachman, H.: Chemical analysis of ejaculates from patients with cystic fibrosis, Fertil Steril, 1970, *21*, 515.

78. Dearborn, D. G.: Water and electrolytes of exocrine secretions, in *Cystic Fibrosis: Projections into the Future*, J. A. Mangos and R. C. Talamo, ed., Intercontinental Medical Book Corp., New York, 1976, p. 179.

79. Gibson, L. E., Matthews, W. J., Minihan, P. T., and Patti, J. A.: Relating mucus, calcium and sweat in a new concept of cystic fibrosis, Pediatrics, 1971, *48*, 695.

80. Mangos, J. A.: Microperfusion study of the sweat gland abnormality in cystic fibrosis, Tex Rep Biol Med, 1973, *31*, 651.

81. di Sant'Agnese, P. A., and Powell, G. F.: The eccrine sweat defect in cystic fibrosis of the pancreas, Ann NY Acad Sci, 1962, *93*, 555.

82. Paunier, L., Girardin, E., Sizonenko, P. L., Wyss, M., and Megevand, A.: Calcium and magnesium concentrations in sweat of normal children and patients with cystic fibrosis, Pediatrics, 1973, *52*, 446.

83. Kaiser, D., Drack, E., and Rossi, E.: Inhibition of net sodium transport in single sweat glands of patients with cystic fibrosis of the pancreas, Pediatr Res, 1971, *5*, 167.

84. Chauncey, H. H., Levine, D. M., Kass, G., Shwachman, H., Henriques, B. L., and Kulczycki, L. L.: Composition of human saliva, Arch Oral Biol, 1962, *7*, 707.

85. Chernick, W. S., Barbero, G. J., and Parkins, F. M.: Studies on submaxillary saliva in cystic fibrosis, J Pediatr, 1961, *59*, 890.

86. Shwachman, H., and Antonowicz, I.: The sweat test in cystic fibrosis, Ann NY Acad Sci, 1962, *93*, 600.

87. Botelho, S. Y., Goldstein, A. M., and Rosenlund, M. L.: Tear sodium, potassium, chloride and calcium at various flow rates: Children with cystic fibrosis and unaffected siblings with and without corneal staining, J Pediatr, 1973, *83*, 601.

88. di Sant'Agnese, P. A., Grossman, A., Darling, R. C., and Denning, C. R.: Saliva, tears, and duodenal contents in cystic fibrosis of the pancreas, Pediatrics, 1958, *22*, 507.

89. di Sant'Agnese, P. A., and Powell, G. F.: The eccrine sweat defect in cystic fibrosis of the pancreas, Ann NY Acad Sci, 1962, *93*, 555.

90. Mandel, I. D., Thompson, R. H., Wotman, S., Taubman, M., Kutscher, A. H., Zegarelli, E., Denning, C. R., Botwick, J. T., and Fahn, B. S.: Parotid saliva in cystic fibrosis. II. Electrolytes and protein bound carbohydrates, Am J Dis Child, 1965, *110*, 646.

91. Schultz, I. J.: Micropuncture studies of the sweat formation in cystic fibrosis patients, J Clin Invest, 1969, *48*, 1470.

92. Mangos, J. A., McSherry, N. R., and Benke, P. J.: A sodium transport inhibitory factor in the saliva of patients with cystic fibrosis of the pancreas, Pediatr Res, 1967, *1*, 436.

93. Mangos, J. A., and McSherry, N. R.: Sodium transport: Inhibitory factor in sweat of patients with cystic fibrosis, Science, 1967, *158*, 135.

94. Mangos, J. A., and McSherry, N. R.: Studies on the mechanism of inhibition of sodium transport in cystic fibrosis of the pancreas, Pediatr

Res, 1968, *2*, 378.

95. Kaiser, D.: Excretion of proteins, bicarbonate and cations by the single sweat gland of patients with cystic fibrosis, in *Fundamental Problems of Cystic Fibrosis and Related Diseases*, J. A. Mangos and R. C. Talamo, ed., Intercontinental Medical Book Corp, New York, 1973, p. 247.

96. Gugler, E., Pallavicini, J. C., Swerdlow, H., and di Sant'Agnese, P. A.: The role of calcium in submaxillary saliva of patients with cystic fibrosis, J Pediatr, 1967, *71*, 585.

97. Boat, T. F., Wiesman, U. N., and Pallavicini, J. C.: Purification and properties of the calcium-precipitable protein in submaxillary saliva of normal and cystic fibrosis subjects, Pediatr Res, 1974, *8*, 531.

98. Warton, K. L., and Blomfeld, J.: Hydroxyapatite in the pathogenesis of cystic fibrosis, Br Med J, 1971, *3*, 570.

99. Satir, B., Schooley, C., and Satir, P.: Membrane fusion in a model system: Mucocyst secretion in Tetrahymena, J Cell Biol, 1973, *56*, 153.

100. Braddock, L. I., Nagelberg, I., Margallo, E., and Barbero, G. J.: Calcium binding in submaxillary saliva in cystic fibrosis, in *Cystic Fibrosis Club Abstracts*, Cystic Fibrosis Foundation, Atlanta, 1969, p. 17.

101. Lundgren, D. W., Farrell, P. M., and di Sant'Agnese, P. A.: Polyamine alterations in blood of male homozygotes and heterozygotes for cystic fibrosis, Clin Chim Acta, 1975, *62*, 357.

102. Baker, A. P., and Hillegass, L. M.: Enhancement of UDP-Galactose: Mucin galactosyltransferase activity by spermine, Arch Biochem Biophys, 1974, *165*, 597.

103. Munro, G. F., Hercules, K., Morgan, J., and Sauerbier, W.: Dependence of the putrescine content of E. coli on the osmotic strength of the medium, J Biol Chem, 1972, *247*, 1272.

104. Mandel, I. D., Kutscher, A., Denning, C. R., Thompson, R. H., and Zegarelli, E. V.: Salivary studies in cystic fibrosis, Am J Dis Child, 1967, *113*, 431.

105. Chernick, W. S., Eichel, H. J., and Barbero, G. J.: Submaxillary salivary enzymes as a measure of glandular activity in cystic fibrosis, J Pediatr, 1964, *65*, 694.

106. Rao, G. J. S., and Nadler, H. L.: Deficiency of trypsin-like activity in saliva of patients with cystic fibrosis, J Pediatr, 1972, *80*, 573.

107. Boat, T. F., and Cheng, P. W.: Mucous glycoproteins, in *Cystic Fibrosis: Projections into the Future*, J. A. Mangos and R. C. Talamo, ed., Intercontinental Medical Book Corp., New York, 1976, p. 165.

108. Lillibridge, C. B., Brown, M. R., and Hall, J. G.: The electron microscopic appearance of presecreted gastric mucus in cystic fibrosis, Pediatrics, 1974, *53*, 913.

109. Butterworth, J.: Properties of microsomal glycoprotein galactosyltransferase of cultured human fibroblasts in relation to cystic fibrosis, Clin Chim Acta, 1974, *56*, 159.

110. Butterworth, J., Scott, F., McCrae, W. M., and Brain, A. D.: Lysosomal enzymes of cultured fibroblasts of cystic fibrosis patients, Clin Chim Acta, 1972, *40*, 139.

111. Lorin, M. I., Denning, C. R., and Mandel, I. D.: Viscosity of exocrine secretions in cystic fibrosis: Sweat, duodenal fluid, and submaxillary saliva, Biorheology, 1972, *9*, 27.

112. Bettelheim, F. A., Epstein, S., and Gorvoy, J. D.: Rheology of submaxillary secretions of cystic fibrosis patients and normal individuals, Biorheology, 1971, *8*, 129.

113. Sturgess, J. M., Palfry, A. J., and Reid, L.: The viscosity of bronchial secretion, Clin Sci, 1970, *38*, 145.

114. Potter, J. L., Spector, S., Matthews, L. W., and Lemm, J.: Studies on pulmonary secretions. III. The nucleic acids in whole pulmonary secretions from patients with cystic fibrosis, bronchiectasis, and laryngectomy, Am Rev Respir Dis, 1969, *99*, 909.

115. Snary, D., Allen, A., and Pain, P. H.: Structural studies on gastric mucoproteins: Lowering of molecular weight after reduction with 2-mercaptoethanol, Biochem Biophys Res Commun, 1970, *40*, 844.

116. Deman, J., Mareel, M., and Bruyneel, E.: Effects of calcium and bound sialic acid on the viscosity of mucin, Biochim Biophys Acta, 1973, *297*, 486.

117. Friberg, S., Morein, B., and Rydhag, L.: Bovine respiratory secretion as a two phase system, Am Rev Respir Dis, 1973, *108*, 1010.

118. Forstner, J. F., and Forstner, G. G.: Effects of calcium on intestinal mucin, Pediatr Res, in press.

119. Biserte, G., Havez, R., and Cuvelier, R.: Les glycoprotéides des sécrétions bronchiques, Expos Annu Biochim Med, 1963, *24*, 85.

120. Havez, R., Roussel, P., Degand, P., and Biserte, G.: Étude des structures fibrillaires de la sécrétion bronchique humaine, Clin Chim Acta, 1967, *17*, 281.

121. Havez, R., Deminatti, M., Roussel, P., Degand, P., Randoux, A., and Biserte, G.: Étude des glycoprotéines carboxyliques et sulfatées de la sécrétion bronchique humaine, Clin Chim Acta, 1967, *17*, 463.

122. Havez, R., Roussel, P., Degand, P., Randoux, A., and Biserte, G.: Biochemical exploration of bronchial hypersecretions, in *Protides of the Biological Fluids*, vol. 16, H. Peeters, ed., Pergamon, New York, 1968, p. 343.

123. Degand, P., Roussel, P., Randoux, A., Moschetto, Y., and Havez, R.: Étude des glycopeptides du mucus fibrillaire de la sécrétion bronchique, in *Protides of the Biological Fluids*, vol. 16, H. Peeters, ed., New York, Pergamon, 1968, p. 361.

124. Havez, R., Roussel, P., Degand, P., Delmas-Marsalet, Y., and Biserte, B.: Étude de substances de groupe sanguin A isolées du mucus bronchique, Bull Soc Chim Biol, 1969, *51*, 245.

125. Roussel, P., Lamblin, G., Degand, P., and Havez, R: Isolement des mucines bronchiques sécrétées au cours de la mucoviscidose, Clin Chim Acta, 1972, *36*, 315.

126. Lamblin, G., Degand, P., Roussel, P., Havez, R., Hartemann, E., and Fillat, M.: Les glycopeptides du mucus bronchique fibrillaire dans la mucoviscidose, Clin Chim Acta, 1972, *36*, 329.

127. Degand, P., Roussel, P., Lamblin, G., Durand, G., and Havez, R.: Definition biochimique des mucines dans l'expectoration, Bull Physiopathol Respir (Nancy), 1973, *9*, 199.

128. Roussel, P., Lamblin, G., Degand, P., Walker-Nasir, E., and Jeanloz, R. W.: Heterogeneity of the carbohydrate chains of sulfated bronchial glycoproteins isolated from a patient suffering from cystic fibrosis, J Biol Chem, 1975, *250*, 2114.

129. Boat, T. F., Kleinerman, J. I., Carlson, D. M., Maloney, W. H., and Matthews, L. W.: Human respiratory tract secretions. I. Mucous glycoproteins secreted by cultured nasal polyp epithelium from subjects with allergic rhinitis and with cystic fibrosis, Am Rev Respir Dis, 1974, *110*, 428.

130. Lamb, D., and Reid, L.: The tracheobronchial submucosal glands in cystic fibrosis: A qualitative histochemical study, Br J Dis Chest, 1972, *66*, 239.

131. Rubin, L. S., Barbero, G. J., Chernick, W. S., and Sibinga, M. S.: Pupillary reactivity as a measure of anatomic balance in cystic fibrosis, J Pediatr, 1963, *63*, 1120.

132. Boat, T. F., and Kleinerman, J. I.: Human respiratory secretions. 2. Effect of cholinergic and adrenergic agents on *in vitro* release of protein and mucous glycoprotein, Chest, 1975, *67*, 32S.

133. Mangos, J. A., McSherry, N. R., Benke, P. J., and Spock, A.: Studies on the pathogenesis of cystic fibrosis: The isoproterenol treated rat as an experimental model, in *Proceedings of the 5th International Cystic Fibrosis Conference*, D. Lawson, ed., Cystic Fibrosis Trust, London, 1969, p. 25.

134. Mangos, J. A., Benke, P. J., and McSherry, N.: Salivary gland enlargement and functional changes during feeding of pancreatin to rats, Pediatr Res, 1969, *3*, 562.

135. Sturgess, J., and Reid, L.: The effect of isoprenaline and pilocarpine on (a) bronchial mucus-secreting tissue, and (b) pancreas, salivary glands, heart, thymus, liver, and spleen, Br J Exp Pathol, 1973, *54*, 388.

136. Martinez, J. R., Adelstein, E., Quissel, D., and Barbero, G. J.: The chronically reserpinized rat as a possible model for cystic fibrosis. I. Submaxillary gland morphology and ultrastructure, Pediatr Res, 1975, *9*, 463.

137. Martinez, J. R., Adshead, P. C., Quissel, D. O., and Barbero, G. J.: The chronically reserpinized rat as a possible model for cystic fibrosis. II. Composition and cilioinhibitory effects of submaxillary saliva, Pediatr Res, 1975, *9*, 470.

138. Sanchis, J., Dolovich, M., Rossman, C., Wilson, W., and Newhouse, M.: Pulmonary mucociliary clearance in cystic fibrosis, N Engl J Med, 1973, *288*, 651.

139. Wood, R. E., Wanner, A., Hirsch, J., and Farrell, P. M.: Tracheal mucociliary transport in patients with cystic fibrosis and its stimulation by terbutaline, Am Rev Respir Dis, 1975, *111*, 733.

140. Waring, W. W.: Cilia and cystic fibrosis, N Engl J Med, 1973, *288*, 681.

141. Santa Cruz, R., Landa, J., Hirsch, J., and Sackner, M. A.: Tracheal mucous velocity in normal man and patients with obstructive lung disease: Effects of terbutaline, Am Rev Respir Dis, 1974, *109*, 458.

142. Hilding, A. C.: Ciliary streaming in the lower respiratory tract, Am J Physiol, 1957, *191*, 404.

143. VanAs, A., and Webster, I.: The organization of ciliary activity and mucus transport in pulmonary airways, S Afr Med J, 1972, *46*, 347.

144. Magid, S. L., Smith, C. C., and Dolowitz, D. A.: Nasal mucosa in pancreatic cystic fibrosis, Arch Otolaryngol, 1967, *86*, 212.

145. Sadé, J., Eliezer, N., Silberberg, A., and Nevo, A. C.: The role of mucus in transport by cilia, Am Rev Respir Dis, 1970, *102*, 48.

146. King, M., Gilboa, A., Meyer, F. A., and Silberberg, A.: On the transport of mucus and its rheologic simulates in ciliated systems, Am Rev Respir Dis, 1974, *110*, 740.

147. Lucas, A. M., and Douglas, L. C.: Principles underlying ciliary activity in the respiratory tract. II. A comparison of nasal clearance in man, monkey, and other mammals, Arch Otolaryngol, 1934, *20*, 518.

148. Blake, J.: On the movement of mucus in the lung, J Biomech, 1975, *8*, 179.

149. Asmundsson, T., and Kilburn, K. H.: Mucociliary clearance rates at various levels in dog lungs, Am Rev Respir Dis, 1970, *102*, 388.

150. Yeates, D. B., Sturgess, J. M., Crozier, D., Levison, H., and Aspin, N.: Mucociliary transport in the trachea of patients with cystic fibrosis, Arch Dis Child, 1976, *51*, 28.

151. Biggar, W. D., Holmes, B., and Good, R. A.: Opsonic defect in patients with cystic fibrosis of the pancreas, Proc Natl Acad Sci USA, 1971, *68*, 1716.

152. Boxerbaum, B., Kagumba, M., and Matthews, L. W.: Selective inhibition of phagocytic activ-

ity of rabbit alveolar macrophages by cystic fibrosis serum, Am Rev Respir Dis, 1973, *108*, 777.

153. Schwartz, R. H.: Serum immunoglobulin levels in cystic fibrosis, Am J Dis Child, 1966, *111*, 408.

154. South, M. A., Warwick, W. J., Wollheim, F. A., and Good, R. A.: The IgA system. III. IgA levels in the serum and saliva of pediatric patients—Evidence for a local immunological system, J Pediatr, 1967, *71*, 645.

155. Halbert, S. P., di Sant'Agnese, P. A., and Kotek, F. R.: Staphylococcal antibodies in cystic fibrosis of the pancreas, Pediatrics, 1960, *26*, 792.

156. Burns, M. W., and May, J. R.: Bacterial precipitins in serum of patients with cystic fibrosis, Lancet, 1968, *1*, 270.

157. Habboushe, C., Iacocca, V., Braddock, L., and Barbero, G.: Pseudomonas agglutinins in patients with cystic fibrosis, Pediatrics, 1971, *48*, 973.

158. May, J. R., Herrick, N. C., and Thompson, D.: Bacterial infection in cystic fibrosis, Arch Dis Child, 1972, *47*, 908.

159. Hoiby, N., and Wiik, A.: Antibacterial precipitins and autoantibodies in serum of patients with cystic fibrosis, Scand J Respir Dis, 1975, *56*, 38.

160. Conover, J. H., Conod, E. J., and Hirschhorn, K.: Complement components in cystic fibrosis, Lancet, 1973, *2*, 1501.

161. Polley, M. J., and Bearn, A. G.: Cystic fibrosis: Current concepts, J Med Genet, 1974, *11*, 249.

162. Pennington, J. E., Reynolds, H. Y., Wood, R. E., Robinson, R. A., and Levine, A. S.: Use of a *Pseudomonas aeruginosa* vaccine in patients with acute leukemia and cystic fibrosis, Am J Med, 1975, *58*, 629.

163. Martinez-tello, F. J., Braun, D. G., and Blanc, W. A.: Immunoglobulin production in bronchial mucosa and bronchial lymph nodes, particularly in cystic fibrosis of the pancreas, J Immunol, 1968, *101*, 989.

164. Falk, G. A., Okinaka, A. J., and Siskind, G. W.: Immunoglobulins in the bronchial washings of patients with chronic obstructive pulmonary disease, Am Rev Respir Dis, 1972, *105*, 14.

165. Turner-Warwick, M., and Pepys, J.: Some aspects of immunopathology and lung disease, Br J Dis Chest, 1967, *61*, 113.

166. Gordon, D. S., Hunter, R. G., O'Reilly, R. J., and Conway, B. P.: *Pseudomonas aeruginosa* allergy and humoral antibody mediated hypersensitivity pneumonia, Am Rev Respir Dis, 1973, *108*, 127.

167. Spock, A., Hieck, H. M. C., Cress, H., and Logan, W. S.: Abnormal serum factor in patients with cystic fibrosis of the pancreas, Pediatr Res, 1967, *1*, 173.

168. Bowman, B. H., Lockhart, L. H., and McCombs, M. L.: Oyster ciliary inhibition by cystic fibrosis factor, Science, 1969, *164*, 325.

169. Cherry, J. D., Roden, V. J., Rejent, A. J., and Dorner, R. W.: The inhibition of ciliary activity in tracheal organ cultures by sera from children with cystic fibrosis and control subjects, J Pediatr, 1971, *79*, 937.

170. Besley, G. T. N., Patrick, A. D., and Norman, A. P.: Inhibition of the motility of gill cilia of *Dreissensia* by plasma of cystic fibrosis patients and their parents, J Med Genet, 1969, *6*, 278.

171. Posselt, H.-G., and Bender, S.: Heterozygote testing in cystic fibrosis: Experimental studies with cilia of the mussel Dreissena Polymorpha, Z. Kinderheilkd, 1971, *110*, 93.

172. McCombs, M. L., and Bowman, B. H.: Rivanol treatment of cystic fibrosis serum: Effect of supernatant upon ciliary action, Clin Genet, 1970, *1*, 171.

173. Conover, J. H., Bonforte, R. J., Hathaway, P., Paciuc, S., Conod, E. J., Hirschhorn, K., and Kopel, F. B.: Studies on ciliary dyskinesia factor in cystic fibrosis. I. Bioassay and heterozygote detection in serum, Pediatr Res, 1973, 7, 220.

174. Danes, B. S., and Bearn, A. G.: Oyster ciliary inhibition by cystic fibrosis culture medium, J Exp Med, 1972, *136*, 1313.

175. Doggett, R. G., and Harrison, G. M.: Cystic fibrosis: *in vitro* reversal of the ciliostatic character of serum and salivary secretions by heparin, Nature [New Biol], 1973, *243*, 251.

176. Iacocca, V. F., Braddock, L. I., and Barbero, G. J.: Confirmation of the inhibitory effect of cystic fibrosis sera on oyster cilia, J Pediatr, 1971, *79*, 508.

177. Bowman, B. H., McCombs, M. L., and Lockhart, L. H.: Cystic fibrosis: Characterization of the inhibitor to ciliary action in oyster gills, Science, 1970, *167*, 871.

178. Danes, B. S., Litwin, S. D., Hutteroth, T. H., Cleve, H., and Bearn, A. G.: Characterization of cystic fibrosis factor and its interaction with human immunoglobulin, J Exp Med, 1973, *137*, 1538.

179. Schmoyer, I. R., Brooks, S. P., and Fischer, J. F.: Isolation and characterization of a ciliary dyskinetic factor from cystic fibrosis heterozygous serum, Life Sci, 1972, *11*, Part 2, 1037.

180. Beratis, N. G., Conover, J. H., Conod, E. J., Bonforte, R. J., and Hirschhorn, K.: Studies on ciliary dyskinesia factor in cystic fibrosis. III. Skin fibroblasts and cultured amniotic fluid cells, Pediatr Res, 1973, 7, 958.

181. Bowman, B. H., Barnett, D. R., Matalon, R., Danes, B. S., and Bearn, A. G.: Cystic fibrosis: Fractionation of fibroblast media demonstrating ciliary inhibition, Proc Natl Acad Sci USA, 1973, *70*, 548.

182. Barnett, D. R., Kurosky, A., Bowman, B. H., and Barranco, S. C.: Loss of the ciliary inhibi-

tory effect of the cystic fibrosis factor following proteolytic digestion and heat denaturation, Tex Rep Biol Med, 1973, *31*, 697.

183. Conover, J. H., Beratis, N. G., Conod, E. J., Ainbender, E., and Hirschhorn, K.: Studies on ciliary dyskinesia factor in cystic fibrosis. II. Short term leukocyte cultures and long term lymphoid lines, Pediatr Res, 1973, 7, 224.

184. Barnett, D. R., Kurosky, A., Bowman, B. H., Hutchison, H. T., Schmoyer, I., and Carson, S. D.: Cystic fibrosis: Molecular weight estimation of the ciliary inhibitor, Tex Rep Biol Med, 1973, *31*, 703.

185. Bowman, B. H., Lankford, B. J., Fuller, G. M., Carson, S. D., Kurosky, A., and Barnett, D. R.: Cystic fibrosis: The ciliary inhibitor is a small polypeptide associated with immunoglobulin G, Biochem, Biophys Res Commun, 1975, *64*, 1310.

186. Conover, J. H., Conod, E. J., and Hirschhorn, K.: Studies on ciliary dyskinesia factor in cystic fibrosis. IV. Its possible identification as anaphylatoxin (C3a)-IgG complex, Life Sci, 1974, *14*, 253.

187. Bokisch, V. A., and Muller-Eberhard, H. J.: Anaphylatoxin inactivator of human plasma: It isolation and characterization as a carboxypeptidase, J Clin Invest, 1970, *49*, 2427.

188. Lieberman, J.: Carboxypeptidase-B-like activity and C3 in cystic fibrosis, Am Rev Respir Dis, 1975, *111*, 100.

189. Rao, G. J. S., Posner, L. A., and Nadler, H. L.: Deficiency of kallikrein activity in plasma of patients with cystic fibrosis, Science, 1972, *177*, 610.

190. Lieberman, J.: Plasma arginine esterase activity in cystic fibrosis, Am Rev Respir Dis, 1974, *109*, 399.

191. Rao, G. J. S., and Nadler, H. L.: Arginine esterase in cystic fibrosis of the pancreas, Pediatr Res, 1974, *8*, 684.

192. Conover, J. H., Conod, E. J., and Hirschhorn, K.: Ciliary dyskinesia factor in immunological and pulmonary disease, Lancet, 1973, *1*, 1194.

193. Wilson, G. B., and Fudenberg, H. H.: Studies on cystic fibrosis using isoelectric focusing. I. An assay for detection of cystic fibrosis homozygotes and heterozygote carriers from serum, Pediatr Res, 1975, *9*, 635.

194. Altland, K., Schmidt, S. R., Kaiser, G., and Knoche, W.: Demonstration of a factor in the serum of homozygotes and heterozygotes for cystic fibrosis by a non-biological technique, Humangenetik, 1975, *28*, 207.

195. Schmoyer, I. R., and Baglia, F. A.: Cystic fibrosis: Effect of media from cultured cystic fibrosis fibroblasts on ATPase activity, Biochem Biophys Res Commun, 1974, *58*, 1066.

196. Farrell, P. M., Fox, G. N., and Spicer, S. S.: Determination and characterization of ciliary ATPase in the presence of serum from cystic fibrosis patients, Pediatr Res, 1976, *10*, 127.

197. Cohen, F. L., and Daniel, W. L.: Effects of cystic fibrosis sera on *Proteus vulgaris* motility, J Med Genet, 1974, *11*, 253.

198. Wood, R. E., and di Sant'Agnese, P. A.: Bioassay of cystic fibrosis factor, Lancet, 1973, *2*, 1452.

199. Ciliary Inhibitory Factor of Cystic Fibrosis: GAP Conference Report, Cystic Fibrosis Foundation, Atlanta, Ga., 1973.

200. Cole, C. H., and Dirks, J. H.: Changes in erythrocyte membrane ATPase in patients with cystic fibrosis of the pancreas, Pediatr Res, 1972, *6*, 616.

201. Balfe, J. W., Cole, C., and Welt, L. G.: Red-cell transport defect in patients with cystic fibrosis and in their parents, Science, 1968, *162*, 689.

202. Lapey, A., and Gardner, J. D.: Abnormal erythrocyte sodium transport in cystic fibrosis (CF), Pediatr Res, 1970, *4*, 478.

203. Feig, S. A., Segel, G. B., Kern, K. A., Osher, A. B., and Schwartz, R. H.: Erythrocyte transport function in cystic fibrosis, Pediatr Res, 1974, *8*, 594.

204. Hadden, J. W., Hansen, L. G., Shapiro, B. L., and Warwick, W. J.: Erythrocyte enigmas in cystic fibrosis, Proc Soc Exp Biol Med, 1973, *142*, 577.

205. Horton, C. R., Cole, W. Q., and Bader, H.: Depressed (Ca++)-transport ATPase in cystic fibrosis erythrocytes, Biochem Biophys Res Commun, 1970, *40*, 505.

206. McEvoy, F. A., Davies, R. J., Goodchild, M. C., and Anderson, C. M.: Erythrocyte membrane properties in cystic fibrosis, Clin Chim Acta, 1974, *54*, 195.

207. Quissell, D. O., and Pitot, H. C.: Number of ouabain binding sites in fibroblasts from normal subjects and patients with cystic fibrosis, Nature, 1974, *247*, 115.

208. Gibbs, G. E., Griffin, G., and Reimer, K.: Quantitative microdetermination of enzymes in sweat gland. V. Ouabain-sensitive sodium-potassium of activated adenosinetriphosphatase, Pediatr Res, 1967, *1*, 24.

209. Benke, P. J., Erbstoeszer, M., and Pitot, H. C.: Transport of labeled compounds in control and cystic fibrosis cells *in vitro*, Lancet, 1972, *1*, 182.

210. Fletcher, D. S., and Lin, T-Y.: Incorporation of L-leucine and D-glucosamine into skin fibroblasts derived from cystic fibrosis and normal individuals, Clin Chim Acta, 1973, *44*, 5.

211. Fitzpatrick, D. F., Landon, E. J., and James, V.: Serum binding of calcium and the red cell membrane in cystic fibrosis, Nature [New Biol], 1972, *235*, 173.

212. Duffy, M. J., and Schwartz, V.: Cyclic AMP stimulated phosphorylation of erythrocyte membranes from cystic fibrosis and control subjects, Clin Chim Acta, 1973, *49*, 397.

213. Baig, M. M., Cetorelli, J. J., and Roberts, R. M.: Plasma membrane components of skin fibro-

blasts from normal individuals and patients with cystic fibrosis, J Pediatr, 1975, *86*, 72.

214. Changus, J. E., Quissell, D. O., Sukup, M. R., and Pitot, H. C.: Studies on the synthesis of plasma membrane proteins of fibroblasts from patients with cystic fibrosis, Am J Pathol, 1975, *80*, 317.

215. Benke, P. J., Herrick, N., and Pitot, H. C.: Studies on basic charged molecules and cell membranes in cystic fibrosis, Proc Soc Exp Biol Med, 1971, *137*, 1283.

216. Taylor, A., Mayo, J. W., Boat, T. F., and Matthews, L. W.: Standardized assay for the sodium reabsorption inhibitory effect and studies of its salivary gland distribution in patients with cystic fibrosis, Pediatr Res, 1974, *8*, 861.

217. Cole, C. H., and Sella, G.: Inhibition of ouabain-sensitive ATPase by the saliva of patients with cystic fibrosis of the pancreas, Pediatr Res, 1975, *9*, 763.

218. Taussig, L. M., and Gardner, J. D.: Effects of saliva and plasma from cystic fibrosis patients on membrane transports, Lancet, 1972, *1*, 1367.

219. Brown, G. A., Oshin, A., Goodchild, M. C., and Anderson, C. M.: Inhibition of sugar transport by plasma from cystic fibrosis patients, Lancet, 1971, *2*, 639.

220. Morin, C. L., Desjeux, J. F., and Authier, L.: Effect of saliva and serum from patients with cystic fibrosis on intestinal uptake of amino acids in rat, Biomedicine, 1973, *19*, 133.

221. Araki, H., Field, M., and Shwachman, H.: A new assay for cystic fibrosis factor: Effects of sera from patients with cystic fibrosis on the *in vitro* electrical properties of rat jujunum, Pediatr Res, 1975, *9*, 932.

222. Shapiro, B. L., Lee, S. M., and Warwick, W. J: The pentose phosphate pathway in cystic fibrosis erythrocytes, Biochem Biophys Res Commun, 1970, *39*, 816.

223. Zuelzer, W. W., and Newton, W. A.: The pathogenesis of fibrocystic disease of the pancreas. A study of 36 cases with special reference to the pulmonary lesions, Pediatrics, 1949, *4*, 53.

224. Esterly, J. R., and Oppenheimer, E. H.: Observations in cystic fibrosis of the pancreas. III. Pulmonary lesions, Johns Hopkins Med J, 1968, *122*, 94.

225. Reid, L., and De Haller, R.: The bronchial mucous glands, their hypertrophy and change in intracellular mucus, Bibl Paediatr, 1967, *86*, 195.

226. Esterly, J. R., and Oppenheimer, E. H.: Cystic fibrosis of the pancreas: Structural changes in the peripheral airways, Thorax, 1968, *23*, 670.

227. Bowden, D. H., Fischer, V. W., and Wyatt, J. P.: Cor pulmonale in cystic fibrosis: A morphometric analysis, Am J Med, 1965, *38*, 226.

228. Wentworth, P., Gough, J., and Wentworth, J. E.: Pulmonary changes and cor pulmonale in mucoviscidosis, Thorax, 1968, *23*, 582.

229. Lamarre, A., Reilly, B. J., Bryan, A. C., and Levison, H.: Early detection of pulmonary function abnormalities in cystic fibrosis, Pediatrics, 1972, *50*, 291.

230. Landau, L. I., and Phelan, P. D.: The spectrum of cystic fibrosis. A study of pulmonary mechanics in 46 patients, Am Rev Respir Dis, 1973, *108*, 593.

231. Zapletal, A., Motoyama, E. K., Gibson, L. E., and Bouhuys, A.: Pulmonary mechanics in asthma and cystic fibrosis, Pediatrics, 1971, *48*, 64.

232. Fox, W. W., Bureau, M. A., Taussig, L. M., Martin, R. R., and Beaudry, P. H.: Helium flow-curves in the detection of early small airway disease, Pediatrics, 1974, *54*, 293.

233. Mellins, R. B.: The site of airway obstruction in cystic fibrosis, Pediatrics, 1969, *44*, 315.

234. Mansell, A., Dubrawsky, C., Levison, H., Bryan, A. C., and Crozier, D. N.: Lung elastic recoil in cystic fibrosis, Am Rev Respir Dis, 1974, *109*, 190.

235. Beier, F. R., Renzetti, A. D., Mitchell, M., and Watanabe, S.: Pulmonary pathophysiology in cystic fibrosis, Am Rev Respir Dis, 1966, *94*, 430.

236. Cook, C. D., Helliesen, P. J., Kulczycki, L., Barrie, H., Freidlander, L., Agathan, S., Harris, G. B. C., and Schwachman, H.: Studies of respiratory physiology in children. II. Lung volumes and mechanics of respiration in 64 patients with cystic fibrosis of the pancreas, Pediatrics, 1959, *24*, 181.

237. Godfrey, S., and Mearns, M.: Pulmonary function and response to exercise in cystic fibrosis, Arch Dis Child, 1971, *46*, 144.

238. Zelkowitz, P. S., and Giammona, S. T.: Effects of gravity and exercise on the pulmonary diffusing capacity in children with cystic fibrosis, J Pediatr, 1969, *74*, 393.

239. Day, G., and Mearns, M. B.: Bronchial lability in cystic fibrosis, Arch Dis Child, 1973, *48*, 355.

240. Levison, H., and Godfrey, S.: Pulmonary aspects of cystic fibrosis, in *Cystic Fibrosis: Projections into the Future*, J. A. Mangos and R. C. Talamo, ed., Intercontinental Medical Book Corp., New York, 1976, p. 3.

240a. Lifschitz, M. I., and Denning, C. R.: Asessment of bronchospasm in patients with cystic fibrosis, Am Rev Respir Dis, 1969, *99*, 399.

241. Bouhuys, A., and Van deWoestijne, K. P.: Mechanical consequences of airway smooth muscle relaxation, J Appl Physiol, 1971, *30*, 670.

242. Mellins, R. B., Levine, R., Ingram, R. H., and Fishman, A. P.: Obstructive disease of the airways in cystic fibrosis, Pediatrics, 1968, *41*, 560.

243. Landau, L. I., Taussig, L. M., Macklem, P. T., and Beaudry, P. H.: Contribution of inhomogeneity of lung units to the maximal expiratory flow-volume curve in children with asthma

and cystic fibrosis, Am Rev Respir Dis, 1975, *111*, 725.

244. Hodson, C. J., and France, N. E.: Pulmonary changes in cystic fibrosis of the pancreas, a radio-pathological study, Clin Radiol, 1962, *13*, 54.

245. Schwartz, E. E., and Holsclaw, D. S.: Pulmonary involvement in adults with cystic fibrosis, Am J Roentgenol Radium Ther Nucl Med, 1974, *122*, 708.

246. di Sant'Agnese, P. A.: The pulmonary manifestations of fibrocystic disease of the pancreas, Dis Chest, 1955, *27*, 654.

247. Huang, N. N., VanLoon, E. L., and Sheng, K. T.: The flora of the respiratory tract of patients with cystic fibrosis of the pancreas, J Pediatr, 1961, *59*, 512.

248. Iacocca, V. F., Sibinga, M. S., and Barbero, G. J.: Respiratory tract bacteriology in cystic fibrosis, Am J Dis Child, 1963, *106*, 315.

249. Lawson, D.: Bacteriology of the respiratory tract in cystic fibrosis—a hypothesis, in *The Control of Chemotherapy*, P. J. Watt, ed., E. & S. Livingstone, Ltd., Edinburgh, 1970, p. 69.

250. Mearns, M. B., Hunt, G. H., and Rushworth, R.: Bacterial flora of respiratory tract in patients with cystic fibrosis 1950-1971, Arch Dis Child, 1972, *47*, 902.

251. Hoiby, N.: Epidemiological investigations of the respiratory tract bacteriology in patients with cystic fibrosis, Acta Pathol Microbiol Scand, 1974, *82B*, 541.

252. Reynolds, H. Y., Levine, A. S., Wood, R. E., Zierdt, C. H., Dale, D. C., and Pennington, J. E.: *Pseudomonas aeruginosa* infections: Persisting problems and current research to find new therapies, Ann Intern Med, 1975, *82*, 819.

253. Doggett, R. G., Harrison, G. M., Stillwell, R. N., and Wallis, E. S.: An atypical *Pseudomonas aeruginosa* associated with cystic fibrosis of the pancreas, J Pediatr, 1966, *68*, 215.

254. Doggett, R. G., and Harrison, G. M.: *Pseudomonas aeruginosa*: Immune status in patients with cystic fibrosis, Infect Immun, 1972, *6*, 628.

255. Hoiby, N.: *Pseudomonas aeruginosa* infection in cystic fibrosis. Relationship between mucoid strains of *P. aeruginosa* and the humoral immune response, Acta Pathol Microbiol Scand [B], 1974, *82*, 551.

256. Holsclaw, D. S.: Common pulmonary complications of cystic fibrosis, Clin Pediatr (Phila), 1970, *9*, 346.

257. Lloyd-Still, J. D., Khaw, K.-T., and Shwachman, H.: Severe respiratory disease in infants with cystic fibrosis, Pediatrics, 1974, *53*, 678.

258. Shwachman, H., Kulczycki, L. L., Mueller, H. L., and Flake, C. G.: Nasal polyposis in patients with cystic fibrosis, Pediatrics, 1962, *30*, 389.

259. Rulon, J. T., Brown, H. A., and Logan, G. B.: Nasal polyps and cystic fibrosis of the pancreas, Arch Otolaryngol, 1963, *78*, 192.

260. Harris, G. B. C., Neuhauser, E. B. D., and Shwachman, H.: Roentgenographic spectrum of cystic fibrosis, Postgrad Med, 1963, *34*, 251.

261. Oppenheimer, E. H., and Esterly, J. R.: Observations in cystic fibrosis of the pancreas. II. Neonatal intestinal obstruction, Bull Hopkins Hosp, 1962, *111*, 1.

262. Holsclaw, D. S., Eckstein, H. B., and Nixon, H. H.: Meconium ileus: A 20-year review of 109 cases, Am J Dis Child, 1965, *109*, 101.

263. Donnison, A. B., Shwachman, H., and Gross, R. E.: A review of 164 children with meconium ileus seen at the Children's Hospital Medical Center, Boston, Pediatrics, 1966, *37*, 833.

264. Berdon, W. E., Baker, D. H., Becker, J., and DeSanctis, P.: Scrotal masses in healed meconium peritonitis, N Engl J Med, 1967, *277*, 585.

265. McPartlin, J. F., Dickson, J. A. S., and Swain, V. A. J.: Meconium ileus: Immediate and long-term survival, Arch Dis Child, 1972, *47*, 207.

266. Fisher, O. D.: Intestinal obstruction as a late complication of fibrocystic disease of the pancreas, Arch Dis Child, 1954, *29*, 262.

267. Cordonnier, J. K., and Izant, R. J.: Meconium ileus equivalent, Surgery, 1963, *54*, 667.

268. Hunton, D. B., Long, W. K., and Tsumagari, H. Y.: Meconium ileus equivalent: An adult complication of fibrocystic disease, Gastroenterology, 1966, *50*, 99.

269. Holsclaw, D. S., Rocmans, C., and Shwachman, H.: Intussusception in patients with cystic fibrosis, Pediatrics, 1971, *48*, 51.

270. di Sant'Agnese, P. A., and Lepore, M. J.: Involvement of abdominal organs in cystic fibrosis of the pancreas, Gastroenterology, 1961, *40*, 64.

271. Kopel, F. B.: Gastrointestinal manifestations of cystic fibrosis, Gastroenterology, 1972, *62*, 483.

272. Hadorn, B., Johansen, P. G., and Anderson, C. M.: Pancreozymin secretin test of exocrine pancreatic function in cystic fibrosis and the significance of the result for the pathogenesis of the disease, Can Med Assoc J, 1968, *98*, 377.

273. Lapey, A., Kattwinkel, J., di Sant'Agnese, P. A., and Laster, L.: Steatorrhea and azotorrhea and their relation to growth and nutrition in adolescents and young adults with cystic fibrosis, J Pediatr, 1974, *84*, 328.

274. Reemstma, K., di Sant'Agnese, P. A., and Malm, J. R.: Cystic fibrosis of the pancreas: Intestinal absorption of fat and fatty acid labeled ^{131}I, Pediatrics, 1958, *22*, 525.

275. Gryboski, J. D., Thayer, W. R., Gabrielson, I. W., and Spiro, H. M.: Disacchariduria in gastrointestinal disease, Gastroenterology, 1963, *45*, 633.

276. Antonowicz, I., Reddy, V., Khau, K. T., and Shwachman, H.: Lactase deficiency in patients with cystic fibrosis, Pediatrics, 1968, *42*, 492.

277. Weber, A. M., Roy, C. C., Morin, C. L., and LaSalle, R.: Malabsorption of bile acids in chil-

dren with cystic fibrosis, N Engl J Med, 1973, *289*, 1001.

278. Heizer, W. D., Smith, T. W., and Goldfinger, S. E.: Absorption of digoxin in patients with malabsorption syndromes, N Engl J Med, 1971, *285*, 257.

279. Moss, A. J., Finkelstein, S., Cradine, C., Young, G. A., Dooley, R. R., and Osher, A. B.: Absorption of digoxin in cystic fibrosis, J Pediatr, 1975, *86*, 295.

280. Lee, P. A., Roloff, D. W., and Howatt, W. F.: Hypoproteinemia and anemia in infants with cystic fibrosis, JAMA, 1974, *228*, 585.

281. Dolan, T. F., Jr., Rowe, D. S., and Gibson, L. E.: Edema and hypoproteinemia in infants with cystic fibrosis, Clin Pediatr (Phila), 1970, *9*, 295.

282. Torstenson, O. L., Humphrey, G. B., Edson, J. R., and Warwick, W. J.: Cystic fibrosis presenting with severe hemorrhage due to vitamin K malabsorption: A report of 3 cases, Pediatrics, 1970, *45*, 857.

283. Petersen, R. A., Petersen, V. S., and Robb, R. M.: Vitamin A deficiency with xerophthalmia and night blindness in cystic fibrosis, Am J Dis Child, 1968, *116*, 662.

284. Underwood, B. A., and Denning, C. R.: Blood and liver concentrations of vitamins A and E in children with cystic fibrosis of the pancreas, Pediatr Res, 1972, *6*, 26.

285. Blanc, W. A., Reid, J. D., and Andersen, D. H.: Avitaminosis E in cystic fibrosis of the pancreas, Pediatrics, 1958, *22*, 494.

286. Kulczycki, L. L., and Shwachman, H: Studies in cystic fibrosis of the pancreas: Occurrence of rectal prolapse, N Engl J Med, 1958, *259*, 409.

287. Taussig, L. M., Saldino, R. M., and di Sant'Agnese, P. A.: Radiographic abnormalities of the duodenum and small bowel in the cystic fibrosis of the pancreas (mucoviscidosis), Radiology, 1973, *106*, 369.

288. Alterman, K.: Duodenal ulceration and fibrocystic pancreas disease, Am J Dis Child, 1961, *101*, 210.

289. Bray, P. F., and Herbst, J. J.: Pseudotumor cerebri as a sign of "catchup" growth in cystic fibrosis, Am J Dis Child, 1973, *126*, 78.

290. Dolan, T. F., Jr., and Meyers, A.: Mild cystic fibrosis presenting as an asymptomatic distended appendiceal mass, Clin Pediatr (Phila), 1975, *14*, 862.

291. Craig, J. M., Haddad, H., and Shwachman, H.: The pathologic changes in the liver in cystic fibrosis of the pancreas, Am J Dis Child, 1957, *93*, 357.

292. Sharp, H. L., and Warwick, W. J.: Hepatic function and structure in cystic fibrosis, in *Cystic Fibrosis Club Abstracts,* Cystic Fibrosis Foundation, Atlanta, Ga., 1968, p. 4.

293. di Sant'Agnese, P. A., and Blanc, W. A.: A distinctive type of biliary cirrhosis of the liver associated with cystic fibrosis of the pancreas, Pediatrics, 1956, *18*, 387.

294. Valman, H. B., France, N. E., and Wallis, P. G.: Prolonged neonatal jaundice in cystic fibrosis, Arch Dis Child, 1971, *46*, 805.

295. Cooper, H. S., and Oppenheimer, E. H.: Cystic fibrosis manifested as focal biliary cirrhosis in a newborn infant with congenital heart disease, Johns Hopkins Med J, 1974, *135*, 268.

296. Boat, T. F., Doershuk, C. F., Stern, R. C., and Matthews, L. W.: Serum alkaline phosphatase in cystic fibrosis, Clin Pediatr (Phila), 1974, *13*, 505.

297. Kattwinkel, J., Taussig, L. M., Statland, B. E., and Verter, J. I.: The effects of age on alkaline phosphatase and other serologic liver function tests in normal subjects and patients with cystic fibrosis, J Pediatr, 1973, *82*, 234.

298. Webster, R., and Williams, H.: Hepatic cirrhosis associated with fibrocystic disease of the pancreas, Arch Dis Child, 1953, *28*, 343.

299. Rovsing, H., and Sloth, K.: Micro-gallbladder and biliary calculi in mucoviscidosis, Acta Radiol [Diagn], (Stockh), 1973, *14*, 588.

300. Feigelson, J., Pecau, Y., and Sauvegrain, J.: Liver function studies and biliary tract investigations in mucoviscidosis, Acta Paediatr Scand, 1970, *59*, 539.

301. Esterly, J. R., and Oppenheimer, E. H.: Observations in cystic fibrosis of the pancreas. I. The gallbladder, Bull Johns Hopkins Hosp, 1962, *110*, 247.

302. Shwachman, H., Lebenthal, E., and Khaw, K.-T.: Recurrent acute pancreatitis in patients with cystic fibrosis with normal pancreatic enzymes, Pediatrics, 1975, *55*, 86.

303. Barbero, G. J., and Sibinga, M. S.: Enlargement of the submaxillary salivary glands in cystic fibrosis, Pediatrics, 1962, *29*, 788.

304. Warwick, W. J., Bernard, B., and Meskin, L. H.: The involvement of the labial mucous salivary gland in patients with cystic fibrosis, Pediatrics, 1964, *34*, 621.

305. Leake, D., Khaw, K.-T., and Shwachman, H.: Parotid gland sialograms in cystic fizrosis, J Pediatr, 1970, *76*, 301.

306. Denning, C. R., and Vande Wiele, R. L.: Sterility studies in the male patients with cystic fibrosis, in *Cystic Fibrosis Club Abstracts,* Cystic Fibrosis Foundation, Atlanta, Ga., 1966, p. 18.

307. Denning, C. R., Sommers, S. C., and Quigley, H. J., Jr.: Infertility in male patients with cystic fibrosis, Pediatrics, 1968, *41*, 7.

308. Kaplan, E., Shwachman, H., Perlmutter, A. D., Rule, A., Khaw, K.-T., and Holsclaw, D. S.: Reproductive failure in males with cystic fibrosis, N Engl J Med, 1968, *279*, 65.

309. Feigelson, J., Pecau, Y., and Shwachman, H.: À-propos d'une paternité chez un malade atteint de mucoviscidose: Études des fonctions

génitales et de la filiation, Arch Fr Pediatr, 1969, *26*, 937.

310. Taussig, L. M., Lobeck, C. C., di Sant'Agnese, P. A., Ackerman, D. R., and Kattwinkel, J.: Fertility in males with cystic fibrosis, N Engl J Med, 1972, *287*, 586.

311. Valman, H. B., and France, N. E.: The vas deferens in cystic fibrosis, Lancet, 1969, *2*, 566.

312. Holsclaw, D. S., Perlmutter, A. D., Jockin, H., and Shwachman, H.: Genital abnormalities in male patients with cystic fibrosis, J Urol, 1971, *106*, 568.

313. Landing, B. H., Wells, T. R., and Wang, C.-I.: Abnormality of the epididymis and vas deferens in cystic fibrosis, Arch Pathol, 1969, *88*, 569.

314. Oppenheimer, E. H., and Esterly, J. R.: Observations on cystic fibrosis of the pancreas. V. Developmental changes in the male genital system, J Pediatr, 1969, *75*, 806.

315. Holsclaw, D. S., and Shwachman, H.: Increased incidence of inguinal hernia, hydrocele and undescended testicle in males with cystic fibrosis, Pediatrics, 1971, *48*, 442.

316. Wang, C.-I., Kwok, S., and Edelbrock, H.: Inguinal hernia, hydrocele, and other genitourinary abnormalities, Am J Dis Child, 1970, *119*, 236.

317. Oppenheimer, E. H., and Esterly, J. R.: Observations on cystic fibrosis of the pancreas. VI. The uterine cervix, J Pediatr, 1970, *77*, 991.

318. Dooley, R. R., Braunstein, H., and Osher, A. B.: Polypoid cervicitis in cystic fibrosis patients receiving oral contraceptives, Am J Obstet Gynecol, 1974, *118*, 971.

319. Kopito, L., Kosasky, H. J., and Shwachman, H.: Water and electrolytes in cervical mucus from patients with cystic fibrosis, Fertil Steril, 1973, *24*, 512.

320. Lobeck, C. C.: Cystic fibrosis, in *The Metabolic Basis of Inherited Disease*, ed. 3, J. B. Stanbury, J. B. Wyngaarden, and D. S. Fredrickson, ed., McGraw Hill, New York, 1972, p. 1605.

321. Kessler, W. R., and Andersen, D. H.: Heat prostration in fibrocystic disease of pancreas and other conditions, Pediatrics, 1951, *8*, 648.

322. di Sant'Agnese, P. A.: Salt depletion in cold weather in infants with cystic fibrosis of the pancreas, JAMA, 1960, *172*, 2014.

323. di Sant'Agnese, P. A., Darling, R. C., Perera, G. A., and Shea, E.: Abnormal electrolyte composition of sweat in cystic fibrosis of the pancreas, Pediatrics, 1953, *12*, 549.

324. Gottleib, R. P.: Metabolic alkalosis in cystic fibrosis, J Pediatr, 1971, *79*, 930.

325. Liberman, J., and Rodbard, S.: Low blood pressure in young adults with cystic fibrosis. An effect of chronic salt loss in sweat?, Ann Intern Med, 1975, *82*, 806.

326. Problems in Sweat Testing: GAP Conference Report. Cystic Fibrosis Foundation, Atlanta, Ga., 1975.

327. Gibson, L. E., di Sant'Agnese, P. A., and Shwachman, H.: Procedure for the Quantitative Iontophoretic Sweat Test for Cystic Fibrosis, Cystic Fibrosis Foundation, Atlanta, Ga,. 1975.

328. Jones, J. D., Steige, H., and Logan, G. B.: Variations of sweat sodium values in children and adults with cystic fibrosis and other diseases, Mayo Clin Proc, 1970, *45*, 768.

329. Coltman, C. A., and Atwell, R. J.: The electrolyte composition of normal adult sweat, Am Rev Respir Dis, 1966, *93*, 62.

330. Conn, J. W.: Electrolyte composition of sweat: Clinical implication as an index of adrenal function, Arch Intern Med, 1949, *83*, 416.

331. Robinson, G. C., Miller, J. R., and Bensimon, J. R.: Familial ectodermal dysplasia with sensori neural deafness and other anomalies, Pediatrics, 1962, *30*, 797.

332. Morse, W. I., Cochrane, W. A., and Landrigan, P. L.: Familial hypoparathyroidism with pernicious anemia, steatorrhea and adrenocortical insufficiency: A variant of mucoviscidosis, N Engl J Med, 1961, *264*, 1021.

333. Lobeck, C. C., Barta, R. A., and Mangos, J. A.: Study of sweat in pitressin-resistant diabetes insipidis, J Pediatr, 1963, *62*, 868.

334. Harris, R. C., and Cohen, H. I.: Sweat electrolytes in glycogen storage disease, type 1, Pediatrics, 1963, *31*, 1044.

335. Esterly, N. B., Cantolino, S. J., Alter, B. P., and Brusilow, S. W.: Pupillatonia, hyporeflexia, and segmental hypohydrosis: Autonomic dysfunction in a child, J Pediatr, 1968, *73*, 852.

336. Strickland, A. L.: Sweat electrolytes in thyroid disorders, J Pediatr, 1973, *82*, 284.

337. Durand, P., Borrone, C., Della Cella, G., and Liotta, A.: Le mucopolisaccaridosi, Recent Prog Med (Roma), 1968, *44*, 279.

338. Mace, J. W., and Scharberger, J. E.: Elevated sweat chloride in a child with malnutrition, Clin Pediatr (Phila), 1971, *10*, 285.

339. Durand, P., Borrone, C., and Della Cella, G.: Fucosidosis, J Pediatr, 1969, *75*, 665.

340. MacLean, W. C., Jr., and Tripp, R. W.: Cystic fibrosis with edema and falsely negative sweat test, J Pediatr, 1973, *83*, 86.

341. Vlachos, P., and Liakakos, D.: Cystic fibrosis with edema and falsely negative sweat test (letter to the editor), J Pediatr, 1974, *84*, 926.

342. Guide to Diagnosis and Management of Cystic Fibrosis, Cystic Fibrosis Foundation, Atlanta, Ga., 1971.

343. Barbero, G. J., Sibinga, M. S., Marino, J. M., and Seibel, R.: Stool trypsin and chymotrypsin, Am J Dis Child, 1966, *112*, 536.

344. Taussig, L. M., Wolf, R. O., Wood, R. E., and Deckelbaum, R. J.: Use of serum amylase iso-

enzymes in evaluation of pancreatic function, Pediatrics, 1974, *54*, 229.

345. Hardy, J. D., Davis, S. H. H., Higgins, M. U., and Polycarpou, P. N.: Sweat tests in the newborn period, Arch Dis Child, 1973, *48*, 316.

346. Green, M. N., and Shwachman, H.: Presumptive tests for cystic fibrosis based on serum protein in meconium, Pediatrics, 1968, *41*, 989.

347. Kollberg, H., and Hellsing, K.: Screening for cystic fibrosis by analysis of albumin in meconium, Acta Paediatr Scand, 1975, *64*, 477.

348. Stephan, U., Busch, E. W., Kollberg, H., and Hellsing, K.: Cystic fibrosis detection by means of a test-strip, Pediatrics, 1975, *55*, 35.

349. Tomashefski, J. F., Christoforidis, A. J., and Abdullah, A. K.: Cystic fibrosis in young adults: An overlooked diagnosis, with emphasis on pulmonary function and radiological patterns, Chest, 1970, *57*, 28.

350. Lober, C., Wood, R. E., di Sant'Agnese, P. A., Rourk, M. H., and Spock, A.: Patterns of presentation of cystic fibrosis of the pancreas seen in patients over age 20, Chest, 1974, *66*, 332.

351. Lobeck, C. C., and McSherry, N. R.: Response of sweat electrolyte concentrations for 9-alpha-fluoro-hydrocortisone in patients with cystic fibrosis and their families, J Pediatr, 1963, *62*, 393.

352. Grand, R. J., di Sant'Agnese, P. A., Talamo, R. C., and Pallavicini, J. C.: The effects of exogenous aldosterone or sweat electrolytes. II. Patients with cystic fibrosis of the pancreas, J Pediatr, 1967, *70*, 357.

353. Rennert, O. M.: Evaluation of laboratory tests proposed as aids for the diagnosis of cystic fibrosis, Ann Clin Lab Sci, 1973, *3*, 1.

354. Stern, R. C., Pittman, S., Doershuk, C. F., and Matthews, L. W.: Use of a "Heparin Lock" in the intermittent administration of intravenous drugs, Clin Pediatr (Phila), 1972, *11*, 521.

355. Mearns, M. B.: Treatment and prevention of pulmonary complications of cystic fibrosis in infancy and early childhood, Arch Dis Child, 1972, *47*, 5.

356. Saggers, B. A., and Lawson, D.: In vivo penetration of antibiotics into sputum in cystic fibrosis, Arch Dis Child, 1968, *43*, 404.

357. Doershuk, C. F., and Matthews, L. W.: Cystic fibrosis and obstructive pulmonary disease, in *Ambulatory Pediatrics*, M. Green and R. J. Haggerty, ed., W. B. Saunders, Philadelphia, 1968, p. 707.

358. Jusko, W. J., Mosovich, L. L., Gerbracht, L. M., Mattar, M. E., and Yaffe, S. J.: Enhanced renal excretion of dicloxacillin in patients with cystic fibrosis, Pediatrics, 1975, *56*, 1038.

359. Basic and Clinical Research on Pseudomonas; GAP Conference Report, Cystic Fibrosis Foundation, Atlanta, Ga., in press.

360. Rucker, R. W., and Harrison, G. M.: Outpatient intravenous medications in the management of cystic fibrosis, Pediatrics, 1974, *54*, 358.

361. Phair, J. P., Tan, J. S., Watanakunakorn, C., Schwab, L., and Sanders, L. W.: Carbenicillin treatment of Pseudomonas pulmonary infection. Use in children with cystic fibrosis, Am J Dis Child, 1970, *120*, 22.

362. Marks, M. I., Prentice, R., Swarson, R., Cotton, E. K., and Eickhoff, T. C.: Carbenicillin and gentamicin: Pharmacologic studies in patients with cystic fibrosis and pseudomonas pulmonary infections, J Pediatr, 1971, *79*, 822.

363. Huang, N. N., Hiller, E. J., Macri, C. M., Capitanio, M., and Cundy, K. R.: Carbenicillin in patients with cystic fibrosis: Clinical pharmacology and therapeutic evaluation, J Pediatr, 1971, *78*, 338.

364. Boxerbaum, B., Doershuk, C. F., and Matthews, L. W.: Use of carbenicillin in cystic fibrosis, J Infect Dis, 1970, *122* (Suppl., p. 59).

365. Boxerbaum, B., Pittman, S., Doershuk, C. F., Stern, R. C., and Matthews, L. W.: Use of gentamicin in children with cystic fibrosis, J Infect Dis, 1971, *124* (Suppl., p. 293).

366. Kluge, R. M., Standiford, H. C., Tatem, B., Young, V. M., Schimpff, S. C., Greene, W. H., Calia, F. M., and Hornick, R. B.: The carbenicillin-gentamicin combination against *Pseudomonas aeruginosa;* correlation of effect with gentamicin sensitivity, Arch Intern Med, 1974, *81*, 584.

367. Hawley, H. B., Lewis, R. M., Swartz, D. R., and Gump, D. W.: Tobramycin therapy of pulmonary infections in patients with cystic fibrosis, Curr Ther Res, 1974, *16*, 414.

368. Klastersky, J., Geuning, C., Monawad, E., Daneau, D.: Endotracheal gentamicin in bronchial infections in patients with tracheostomy, Chest, 1972, *61*, 117.

369. Doershuk, C. F., Matthews, L. W., Gillespie, C. T., Lough, M. D., and Spector, S.: Evaluation of jet-type and ultrasonic nebulizers in mist tent therapy for cystic fibrosis, Pediatrics, 1968, *41*, 723.

370. Parks, C. R.: Mist therapy : Rationale and practice, J Pediatr, 1970, *76*, 305.

371. Matthews, L. W., Doershuk, C. F., and Spector, S.: Mist tent therapy of the obstructive pulmonary lesion of cystic fibrosis, Pediatrics, 1967, *39*, 176.

372. Motoyama, E. K., Gibson, L. E., and Zigas, C. J.: Evaluation of mist tent therapy in cystic fibrosis using maximum expiratory flow volume curve, Pediatrics, 1972, *50*, 299.

373. Chang, N., Levison, H., Cunningham, K., Crozier, D. N., and Grosett, O.: An evaluation of nightly mist tent therapy for patients with cystic fibrosis, Am Rev Respir Dis, 1973, *107*, 672.

374. Wolfsdorf, J., Swift, D. L., and Avery, M. E.:

Mist therapy reconsidered: An evaluation of the respiratory deposition of labelled water aerosols produced by jet and ultrasonic nebulizers, Pediatrics, 1969, *43*, 799.

375. Bau, S. K., Aspin, N., Wood, D. E., and Levison, H.: The measurement of fluid deposition in humans following mist tent therapy, Pediatrics, 1971, *48*, 605.

376. Yeates, D. B., Aspin, N., Bryan, A. C., and Levison, H.: Regional clearance of ions from the airways of the lung, Am Rev Respir Dis, 1973, *107*, 602.

377. Alderson, P. O., Secker-Walker, R. H., Strominger, D. B., Markham, J., and Hill, R. L.: Pulmonary deposition of aerosols in children with cystic fibrosis, J Pediatr, 1974, *84*, 479.

378. West, J. B., and Dollery, C. T.: Absorption of inhaled radioactive water vapour, Nature, 1961, *189*, 588.

379. Morrow, P. E.: Aerosol characterization and deposition, Am Rev Respir Dis, 1974, *110* (Supplement, p. 88).

380. Parks, C. R., Woodrum, D. E., Graham, C. B., Cheney, F. W., and Hodson, W. A.: Effect of water nebulization on normal canine pulmonary mucociliary clearance, Am Rev Respir Dis, 1971, *104*, 99.

381. Parks, C. R., Alden, E. R., Standaert, T. A., Woodrum, D. E., Graham, C. B., and Hodson, W. A.: The effect of water nebulization on cough transport of pulmonary mucus in the mouth-breathing dog, Am Rev Respir Dis, 1973, *108*, 513.

382. Goldberg, I. S., and Lourenço, R. V.: Deposition of aerosol in pulmonary disease, Arch Intern Med, 1973, *131*, 88.

383. Dulfano, M. J., and Adler, K. B.: Physical properties of sputum. VII. Rheologic properties and mucociliary transport, Am Rev Respir Dis, 1975, *112*, 341.

384. Lifschitz, M. I., and Denning, C. F.: Quantitative interaction of water and cystic fibrosis sputum, Am Rev Respir Dis, 1970, *102*, 456.

385. Dulfano, M. J., Adler, K., and Wooten, O.: Physical properties of sputum. IV. Effects of 100 per cent humidity and water mist, Am Rev Respir Dis, 1973, *107*, 130.

386. Rosenbluth, M., and Chernick, V.: Influence of mist tent therapy on sputum viscosity and water content in cystic fibrosis, Arch Dis Child, 1974, *49*, 606.

387. Aerosol therapy, Am Rev Respir Dis, 1974, *110* (Supplement, p. 7).

388. Phelan, P. D., Gracey, M., Williams, H. E., and Anderson, C. M.: Ventilatory function in infants with cystic fibrosis: Physiological assessment of inhalation therapy, Arch Dis Child, 1969, *44*, 393.

389. Landau, L. I., and Phelan, P. D.: The variable effect of a bronchodilating agent on pulmonary function in cystic fibrosis, J Pediatr, 1973, *82*, 863.

390. Barker, R., and Levison, H.: Effects of ultrasonically nebulized distilled water of airway dynamics in children with cystic fibrosis and asthma, J Pediatr, 1972, *80*, 396.

391. Carson, S., Goldhamer, R., and Carpenter, R.: Mucus transport in the respiratory tract, Am Rev Respir Dis, 1966, *93* (Supplement, p. 86).

392. Lake, K. B., Van Dyke, J. J., and Rumsfeld, J. A.: Combined topical pulmonary and systematic gentamicin: The question of safety, Chest, 1975, *68*, 62.

393. Mellins, R. B.: Pulmonary physiotherapy in the pediatric age group, Am Rev Respir Dis, 1974, *110* (Supplement, p. 137).

394. Lorin, M. I., and Denning, C. R.: Evaluation of postural drainage by measurement of sputum volume consistency, Am J Phys Med, 1971, *50*, 215.

395. Motoyama, E. K.: Assessment of lower airway obstruction in cystic fibrosis, in *Fundamental Problems of Cystic Fibrosis and Related Diseases*, J. A. Mangos, and R. C. Talamo, ed., Intercontinental Medical Book Corp, New York, 1973, p. 335.

396. Tecklin, J. S., and Holsclaw, D. S.: Evaluation of bronchial drainage in patients with cystic fibrosis, Phys Ther, 1975, *55*, 1081.

397. Sharp, J. T., Danon, J., Druz, W. S., Goldberg, N. B., Fishman, H., and Machnach, W.: Respiratory muscle function in patients with chronic obstructive pulmonary disease: Its relationship to disability and to respiratory therapy, Am Rev Respir Dis, 1974, *110*, (Supplement, p. 154).

398. Sackner, M. A.: Bronchofiberscopy, Am Rev Respir Dis, 1975, *111*, 62.

399. Cezeaux, G., Jr., Telford, J., Harrison, G., and Keats, A. S.: Bronchial lavage in cystic fibrosis. A comparison of agents, JAMA, 1967, *199*, 15.

400. Kylstra, J. A., Rausch, D. C., Hall, K. D., and Spock, A.: Volume-controlled lung lavage in the treatment of asthma, bronchiectasis, and mucoviscidosis, Am Rev Respir Dis, 1971, *103*, 651.

401. Altman, P., Kulczycki, L. L., Randolph, J. G., and McClenathan, J. E.: Bronchoscopy and bronchial lavage in children with cystic fibrosis, J Pediatr Surg, 1973, *8*, 809.

402. Sheffner, A. L., Medler, E. M., Jacobs, L. W., and Sarett, H. P.: The in vitro reduction in viscosity of human tracheobronchial secretions by acetylcysteine, Am Rev Respir Dis, 1964, *90*, 721.

403. Hirsch, S. R., Zastrow, J. E., and Kory, R. C.: Sputum liquifying agents: A comparative *in vitro* evaluation, J Lab Clin Med, 1969, *74*, 346.

404. Lieberman, J.: The appropriate use of mucolytic agents, Am J Med, 1970, *49*, 1.

405. Lourenço, R. V., Loddenkemper, R., and Car-

ton, R. W.: Patterns of distribution and clearance of aerosols in patients with bronchiectasis, Am Rev Respir Dis, 1972, *106*, 857.

406. Shaw, A.: Safety of *N*-acetylcysteine in treatment of meconium obstruction of the newborn, J Pediatr Surg, 1969, *4*, 119.

407. Lieberman, J.: Measurement of sputum viscosity in a cone-plate viscometer. I. Characteristics of sputum viscosity, Am Rev Respir Dis, 1968, *97*, 654.

408. Boyd, E. M.: Expectorants and respiratory tract fluid, Pharmacol Rev, 1954, *6*, 521.

409. Forbes, J., and Wise, L.: Expectorants and sputum viscosity, Lancet, 1957, *2*, 767.

410. Hirsch, S. R., Viernes, P. F., and Kory, R. C.: The expectorant effect of glycerol guaiacolate in patients with chronic bronchitis, Chest, 1973, *63*, 9.

410a. Dolan, T. F., and Gibson, L. E.: Complications of iodide therapy in patients with cystic fibrosis, J Pediatr, 1971, *79*, 684.

411. Palmer, K. N. V.: Reduction of sputum viscosity by a water aerosol in chronic bronchitis, Lancet, 1960, *1*, 91.

412. Stowe, S. M., Boat, T. F., Mendelsohn, H., Stern, R. C., Tucker, A. S., Doershuk, C. F., and Matthews, L. W: Open thoracotomy for pneumothorax in cystic fibrosis, Am Rev Respir Dis, 1975, *111*, 611.

413. Doershuk, C. F., Reyes, A. L., Regan, A. G., and Matthews, L. W.: Anesthesia and surgery in cystic fibrosis, Anesth Analg (Cleve), 1972, *51*, 413.

414. Kulczycki, L. L., Craig, J. M., and Shwachman, H.: Resection of pulmonary lesions associated with cystic fibrosis of the pancreas, N Engl J Med, 1957, *257*, 203.

415. Steigmann, F., Snyder, D., and Fernandez, A.: Pancreatic enzyme replacement therapy in malabsorption of pancreatic, hepatic, and gastric origin, Am J Dig Dis, 1962, *7*, 464.

416. Goodchild, M. C., Sagaro, E., Brown, G. A., Cruchley, P. M., Jukes, H. R., and Anderson, C. M.: Comparative trial of pancrex V forte and nutrizym in treatment of malabsorption in cystic fibrosis, Br Med J, 1974, *3*, 712.

417. Bile acid malabsorption in cystic fibrosis, Nutr Rev, 1974, *32*, 232.

418. Veeger, W., Abels, J., Hellemans, N., and Nieweg, H. O.: Effect of sodium bicarbonate and pancreatin on the absorption of vitamin B_{12} and fat in pancreatic insufficiency, N Engl J Med, 1962, *267*, 1341.

419. Haro, E. N., and Faloon, W. W.: The effect of bicarbonate on pancreatic enzyme activity, Clin Res, 1964, *12*, 207.

420. Kattwinkel, J., Agus, S. G., Taussig, L. M., di Sant'Agnese, P. A., and Laster, L.: The use of L-arginine and sodium bicarbonate in the treatment of malabsorption due to cystic fibrosis, Pediatrics, 1972, *50*, 133.

421. Littman, A., and Hanscom, D. H.: Current concepts: Pancreatic extracts, N Engl J Med, 1969, *281*, 201.

422. Crozier, D. N.: Cystic fibrosis: A not-so-fatal disease, Pediatr Clin North Am, 1974, *21*, 935.

423. Rosenlund, M. L., Kim, H. K., and Kritchevsky, D.: Essential fatty acids in cystic fibrosis, Nature, 1974, *251*, 719.

424. Bergner, A., and Bergner, R. K.: Pulmonary hypersensitivity associated with pancreatin powder exposure, Pediatrics, 1975, *55*, 814.

425. Dolan, T. F., Jr., and Meyers, A.: Bronchial asthma and allergic rhinitis associated with inhalation of pancreatic extracts, Am Rev Respir Dis, 1974, *110*, 812.

426. Pilat, L., and Teculescu, D.: Bronchial asthma and allergic rhintis associated with inhalation of pancreatic extracts, Am Rev Respir Dis, 1975, *112*, 275.

427. Harries, J. T, and Muller, D. P.: Absorption of different doses of fat soluble and water miscible preparations of vitamin E in children with cystic fibrosis, Arch Dis Child, 1971, *46*, 341.

428. Farrell, P. M., Fratantoni, J. C., Bieri, J. T., and di Sant'Agnese, P. A.: Effects of vitamin E deficiency in man, Acta Paediatr Scand, 1975, *64*, 150.

429. Deren, J. J., Arora, B., Toskes, P. P., Hansell, J., and Sibinga, M.: Malabsorption of crystalline vitamin B_{12} in cystic fibrosis, N Engl J Med, 1973, *288*, 949.

430. Toskes, P. P., Deren, J. J., Fruiterman, J., and Conrad, M. E.: Specificity of the correction of vitamin B_{12} malabsorption by pancreatic extract and its clinical significance, Gastroenterology, 1973, *65*, 199.

431. Barness, L. A.: Vitamin B_{12} absorption in cystic fibrosis, N Engl J Med, 1973, *289*, 45.

432. Huang, N. N.: Medium chain triglycerides in cystic fibrosis, in *Medium Chain Triglycerides*, J. R. Senior, ed., University of Pennsylvania Press, Philadelphia, 1968, p. 207.

433. Allan, J. D., Mason, A., and Moss, A. D.: Nutritional supplementation in treatment of cystic fibrosis of the pancreas, Am J Dis Child, 1973, *126*, 22.

434. Berry, H. K., Kellogg, F. W., Hunt, M. N., Ingberg, R. L., Richter, L., and Gutjahr, C.: Dietary supplement and nutrition in children with cystic fibrosis, Am J Dis Child, 1975, *129*, 165.

435. Barclay, R. P., and Shannon, R. S.: Trial of artificial diet in treatment of cystic fibrosis of pancreas, Arch Dis Child, 1975, *50*, 490.

436. Dodge, J. A., Salter, D. G., and Yassa, J. G.: Essential fatty acid deficiency due to artificial diet in cystic fibrosis (letter to the editor), Br Med J, 1975, *2*, 192.

437. Sherman, J. O., Hamly, C. A., and Khachadurian, A. K.: Use of an oral elemental diet in

infants with severe intractable diarrhea, J Pediatr, 1975, *86*, 518.

438. Dooley, R. R., Moss, A. J., Wright, P. M., and Hassakis, P. C.: Norethandrolone in cystic fibrosis of pancreas, J Pediatr, 1969, *74*, 95.

439. Good, T. A., and Bessman, S. P.: Anabolic steroids in cystic fibrosis of the pancreas, Am J Dis Child, 1966, *111*, 272.

440. Waring, W. W., Brunt, C. H., and Hilman, B. C.: Mucoid impaction of the bronchi in cystic fibrosis, Pediatrics, 1967, *39*, 166.

441. Boat, T. F., di Sant'Agnese, P. A., Warwick, W. J., and Handwerger, S. A.: Pneumothorax in cystic fibrosis, JAMA, 1969, *209*, 1498.

442. Lifschitz, M. I., Bowman, F. O., Denning, C. R., and Wylie, R. H.: Pneumothorax as a complication of cystic fibrosis, Am J Dis Child, 1968, *116*, 633.

443. Kattwinkel, J., Taussig, L. M., McIntosh, C. L., di Sant'Agnese, P. A., Boat, T. F., and Wood, R. E.: Intrapleural instillation of quinacrine for recurrent pneumothorax: Use in a patient with cystic fibrosis, JAMA, 1973, *226*, 557.

444. Holsclaw, D. S., Grand, R. J., and Shwachman, H.: Massive hemoptysis in cystic fibrosis, J Pediatr, 1970, *76*, 829.

445. Smiddy, J. F., and Elliott, R. C.: The evaluation of hemoptysis with fiberoptic bronchoscopy, Chest, 1973, *64*, 158.

446. Gottlieb, L. S., and Hillberg, R.: Endobronchial tamponade therapy for intractable hemoptysis, Chest, 1975, *67*, 482.

447. Fellows, K. E., Stigol, L., Shuster, S., Khaw, K.-T., and Shwachman, H.: Selective bronchial arteriography in patients with cystic fibrosis and massive hemoptysis, Radiology, 1975, *114*, 551.

448. Goldring, R. M., Fishman, A. P., Turino, G. M., Cohen, H. I., Denning, C. R., and Andersen, D. H.: Pulmonary hypertension and cor pulmonale in cystic fibrosis of the pancreas, J Pediatr, 1964, *65*, 501.

449. Liebman, J., Doershuk, C. F., Rapp, C., and Matthews, L.: The vector-cardiogram in cystic fibrosis, Circulation, 1967, *35*, 552.

450. Siassi, B., Moss, A. J., and Dooley, R. R.: Clinical recognition of cor pulmonale in cystic fibrosis, J Pediatr, 1971, *78*, 794.

451. Liebman, J., Krause, D. A., Doershuk, C. F., Downs, T. D., and Matthews, L. W.: Orthogonal vectorcardiogram in cystic fibrosis. Diagnostic significance and correlation with pulmonary function tests; a four year follow-up, Chest, 1973, *63*, 218.

452. Moss, A. J., Harper, W. H., Dooley, R. R., Murray, J. F., and Mack, J. F.: Cor pulmonale in cystic fibrosis of the pancreas, J Pediatr, 1965, *67*, 797.

453. Flaherty, J. T., Blumenschein, S. D., Spock, A., Canent, R. V., Gallie, T. M., Boineau, J. P., and Spach, M. S.: Cardiac potentials in pulmonary disease. Overdistension of the lung versus cor pulmonale (right ventricular hypertrophy), Am J Cardiol, 1967, *20*, 29.

454. Millerd, F. J. C.: The electrocardiogram in chronic lung disease, Br Heart J, 1967, *29*, 43.

455. Strober, W., Peter, G., and Schwartz, R. H.: Albumin metabolism in cystic fibrosis, Pediatrics, 1969, *43*, 416.

456. Pittman, F. E., Denning, C. R., and Baker, H. G.: Albumin metabolism in cystic fibrosis, Am J Dis Child, 1964, *108*, 360.

457. Whitman, V., Stern, R. C., Bellet, P., Doershuk, C. F., Liebman, J., Boat, T. F., Borkat, G., and Matthews, L. W.: Studies on cor pulmonale in cystic fibrosis. I. Effects of diuresis, Pediatrics, 1975, *55*, 83.

458. Kelminson, L. L., Cotton, E. K., and Vogel, J. H. K.: The reversibility for pulmonary hypertension in patients with cystic fibrosis, Pediatrics, 1967, *39*, 24.

459. Liebman, J., Lucas, R. V., Moss, A., and Rosenthal, A.: Cor pulmonale and related cardiovascular effects of cystic fibrosis, in *Cystic Fibrosis: Projections into the Future,* J. A. Mangos and R. C. Talamo, ed., Intercontinental Medical Book Corp, New York, 1976, p. 41.

460. Susmano, A., and Carleton, R. A.: Prevention of hypoxic pulmonary hypertension by chlorpheniramie, J Appl Physiol, 1971, *31*, 531.

461. Schwartz, R. H., Johnstone, D. E., Holsclaw, D. S., and Dooley, R. R.: Serum precipitins to *Aspergillus fumigatus* in cystic fibrosis, Am J Dis Child, 1970, *120*, 432.

462. Pepys, J., Riddell, R. W., Citron, K. M., Clayton, Y. M., and Short, E. I.: Clinical and immunologic significance of *Aspergillus fumigatus* in sputum, Am Rev Respir Dis, 1959, *80*, 167.

463. Slavin, R. G., Stanczyk, D. J., Lonigro, A. J., and Broun, G. O.: Allergic bronchopulmonary aspergillosis: A North American rarity, Am J Med, 1969, *47*, 306.

464. Henderson, A. H.: Allergic aspergillosis: Review of 32 cases, Thorax, 1968, *23*, 501.

465. Grossman, H., Denning, C. R., and Baker, D. H.: Hypertrophic osteoarthropathy in cystic fibrosis, Am J Dis Child, 1964, *107*, 1.

466. Athreya, B. H., Borns, P., and Rosenlund, M. L.: Cystic fibrosis and hypertrophic osteoarthropathy in children, Report of three cases, Am J Dis Child, 1975, *129*, 634.

467. Van Leersum, H. G.: Hypertrophisce osteo arthropathie bij een kind, lijdend aan mucoviscidosis, J Belge Radiol, 1966, *49*, 65.

468. Wagget, J., Johnson, D. G., Borns, P., and Bishop, H. C.: The nonoperative treatment of meconium ileus by Gastrografin enema, J Pediatr, 1970, *77*, 407.

469. McPartlin, J. F., Dickson, J. A. S., and Swain, V. A. J.: The use of Gastrografin in the relief

of residual and late bowel obstruction in cystic fibrosis, Br J Surg, 1973, *60*, 707.

470. Lillibridge, C. B., Docter, J. M., and Eidelman, S.: Oral administration of *N*-acetyl cysteine in the prophylaxis of "meconium ileus equivalent," J Pediatr, 1967, *71*, 887.

471. Stern, R. C., Stevens, D. P., Boat, T. F., Doershuk, C. F., Izant, R. J., and Matthews, L. W.: Symptomatic hepatic disease in cystic fibrosis: Incidence, course, and outcome of portal systemic shunting, Gastroenterology, in press.

472. Danielson, G. K., Kyle, G. C., and Denton, R.: Portal hypertension in cystic fibrosis, JAMA, 1966, *195*, 217.

473. Tyson, K. R. T., Schuster, S. R., and Shwachman, H.: Portal hypertension in cystic fibrosis, J Pediatr Surg, 1968, *3*, 271.

474. Banks, P. A.: Acute pancreatitis, Gastroenterology, 1971, *61*, 382.

475. Joslin's Diabetes Mellitus, ed. 11, A. Marble, P. White, R. F. Bradley, and L. P. Krall, ed., Lea and Febiger, Philadelphia, 1971, p. 12.

476. Rosan, R. C., Shwachman, H., and Kulczycki, L. L.: Diabetes mellitus and cystic fibrosis of the pancreas, Am J Dis Child, 1962, *104*, 625.

477. Chazan, B. I., Balodimos, M. C., Holsclaw, D. S., and Shwachman, H.: Microcirculation in young adults with cystic fibrosis: Retinal and conjunctival vascular changes in relation to diabetes, J Pediatr, 1970, *77*, 86.

478. Wilmshurst, E. G., Soeldner, J. S., Holsclaw, D. S., Kaufmann, R. L., Shwachman, H., Aoki, T. T., and Gleason, R. E.: Endogenous and exogenous insulin responses in patients with cystic fibrosis, Pediatrics, 1975, *55*, 75.

479. Handwerger, S., Roth, J., Gorden, P., di Sant'-Agnese, P., Carpenter, D. F., and Peter, G.: Glucose intolerance in cystic fibrosis, N Engl J Med, 1969, *281*, 451.

480. Clodi, H. P., and Pfeiffer, E. F.: Mechanism of glucose intolerance in cystic fibrosis, N Engl J Med, 1970, *282*, 455.

481. Milner, A. D.: Blood glucose and serum insulin levels in children with cystic fibrosis, Arch Dis Child, 1969, *44*, 351.

482. Milunsky, A., Bray, G. A., Londono, J., and Loridan, L.: Insulin, glucose, growth hormone and free fatty acids: Determinations in patients with cystic fibrosis, Am J Dis Child, 1971, *121*, 15.

483. Kjellman, N.-I. M., and Larsson, Y.: Insulin release in cystic fibrosis, Arch Dis Child, 1975, *50*, 205.

483a. Oppenheimer, E. H.: Glomerular lesions in cystic fibrosis: Possible relation to diabetes mellitus, acquired cyanotic heart disease and cirrhosis of the liver, Johns Hopkins Med J, 1972, *131*, 351.

484. Turk, J.: Impact of cystic fibrosis on family functioning, Pediatrics, 1964, *34*, 67.

485. Meyerowitz, J. H., and Kaplan, H. B.: Familial responses to stress: The case of cystic fibrosis, Soc Sci Med, 1967, *1*, 249.

486. Tropauer, A, Franz, N. M., and Dilgard, V. W.: Psychological aspects of care of children with cystic fibrosis, Am J Dis Child, 1970, *119*, 424.

487. McCollum, A. T., and Gibson, L. E.: Family adaptation to the child with cystic fibrosis, J Pediatr, 1970, *77*, 571.

488. McCollum, A. T.: Cystic fibrosis: Economic impact upon the family, Am J Public Health, 1971, *61*, 1335.

489. Psychosocial Aspects of Cystic Fibrosis: A Model for Chronic Lung Disease, P. R. Patterson, C. R. Denning, and A. H. Kutscher, ed., Columbia University Press, New York, 1973.

490. Gayton, W. F., and Friedman, S. B.: Psychosocial aspects of cystic fibrosis: A review of the literature, Am J Dis Child, 1973, *126*, 856.

491. Galdstone, R.: Growing up with cystic fibrosis, in *Fundamental Problems of Cystic Fibrosis and Related Diseases*, J. A. Mangos and R. C. Talamo, ed., Intercontinental Medical Book Corp, New York, 1973, p. 377.

492. Meyers, A., Dolan, T. F., and Mueller, D.: Compliance and self-medication in cystic fibrosis, Am J Dis Child, 1975, *129*, 1011.

493. Allan, J. L., Townley, R. R. W., and Phelan, P. D.: Family response to cystic fibrosis, Aust Paediatr J, 1974, *10*, 136.

494. Boyle, I. R., Sack, S., Millican, F., and di Sant'-Agnese, P. A.: Emotional adjustment in adolescents and young adults with cystic fibrosis, in *Fundamental Problems of Cystic Fibrosis and Related Diseases*, J. A. Mangos and R. C. Talamo, ed., Intercontinental Medical Book Corp, New York, 1973, p. 385.

495. Rosenlund, M. L., and Lustig, H. S.: Young adults with cystic fibrosis: The problems of a new generation, Ann Intern Med, 1973, *78*, 959.

496. Problems in reproductive physiology and anatomy in young adults with cystic fibrosis, GAP Conference Report, Cystic Fibrosis Foundation, Atlanta, Ga. 1975.

497. Shwachman, H., and Kulczycki, L. L.: Long-term study of 105 patients with cystic fibrosis: Studies made over 5 to 14 year period, Am J Dis Child, 1958, *96*, 6.

498. Doershuk, C. F., Matthews, L. W., Tucker, A. S., Nudelman, H., Eddy, G., Wise, M., and Spector, S.: A five year clinical evaluation of a therapeutic program for patients with cystic fibrosis, J Pediatr, 1964, *65*, 677.

499. Taussig, L. M., Kattwinkel, J., Friedewald, W. T., and di Sant'Agnese, P. A.: A new prognostic score and clinical evaluation system for cystic fibrosis, J Pediatr, 1973, *82*, 380.

500. Shwachman, H., Kulczycki, L. L., and Khaw, K.-T.: Studies in cystic fibrosis: A report on

sixty-five patients over 17 years of age, Pediatrics, 1965, *36*, 689.

501. Huang, N. N., Macri, C. N., Girone, J., and Sproul, A.: Survival of patients with cystic fibrosis, Am J Dis Child, 1970, *120*, 289.

502. Cutler, S. J., and Ederer, F.: Evaluation and prognosis: Maximal utilization of the life-table method in evaluating survival. J Chronic Dis, 1958, *8*, 699.

503. Mearns, M. B., and Simon, G.: Patterns of lung and heart growth as determined from serial radiographs of 76 children with cystic fibrosis, Thorax, 1973, *28*, 537.

Bronchial Asthma: The Possible Role of the Chemical Mediators of Immediate Hypersensitivity in the Pathogenesis of Subacute Chronic Disease[1,2]

K. FRANK AUSTEN and ROBERT P. ORANGE

Contents

Introduction

Chemical Mediators of Immediate Hypersensitivity
    Histamine (β-imidazolylethylamine)
    Eosinophil Chemotactic Factor of Anaphylaxis
      (ECF-A)
    Slow-Reacting Substance of Anaphylaxis (SRS-
      A)
    Platelet Activating Factor (PAF)
    Other Potential Mediators

Biochemical Characteristics of Target Cell Activa-
    tion, Mediator Generation, and Release
    Activation
    Generation of Unstored Mediators
    Secretion of Preformed and Newly Formed Me-
      diators

Potential Interrelationships of the Chemical Me-
    diators

Introduction

After years of *in vitro* studies on the mechanisms of release, physicochemical characteristics,
and pathobiologic effects of the chemical mediators, it is pertinent to re-examine these findings
as they might apply to the pathophysiology of
bronchial asthma. It is, of course, easier to re-

late this knowledge to anaphylaxis because of
the acute nature of the *in vitro* model. Nonetheless, sufficient information now exists to
allow speculation on the events that may trans-
cribe an acute reaction into a subacute or even
a chronic state in the presence of repeated
stimuli or inadequate control mechanisms or
both. This review will deal briefly with the
studies of the cellular origin of the chemical
mediators, the biochemical characteristics of
their generation and release, and the current
knowledge of their structure and function before focusing on an evolving integrated view of
their primary and sequential effects as they
might pertain to the expression of bronchial
asthma. Division of the pathobiologic events in-

____

[1] From the Departments of Medicine, Harvard
Medical School and Robert B. Brigham Hospital,
Boston, Mass., and the Department of Immunology,
The Hospital for Sick Children, University of Toron-
to, Toronto, Ontario, Canada.

[2] Supported by grants AI-07722, AI-10356, and
HL-17382 from the National Institutes of Health,
and MT-4605 from the Medical Research Council
of Canada.

volved in bronchial asthma into *pathopharmacologic phases* and *inflammatory phases* not only provides insight into the sequence of events in a given patient and the heterogeneity of responses within patient groups but also is entirely consistent with our evolving knowledge of mast cell-dependent phenomena.

Chemical Mediators of Immediate Hypersensitivity

Human lung (1, 2) and nasal polyp (3) fragments obtained from allergic subjects release histamine, slow-reacting substance of anaphylaxis (SRS-A), and eosinophil chemotactic factor of anaphylaxis (ECF-A) after being challenged with specific allergen; the same chemical mediators as well as platelet activating factor (PAF) (4) are obtained from normal respiratory tissue (5, 6) after it has been passively sensitized with IgE antibody and challenged with specific antigen. Similarly, there is evolving evidence that basophil-rich leukocyte suspensions release the same 4 primary mediators (7–10). In contrast, chemical mediators such as the prostaglandins, which are readily formed as altered membranes make available substrate (11), or bradykinin, which is derived by a sequential plasma protein reaction sequence after activation or Hageman factor by altered basement membrane of collagen (12), are considered secondary rather than primary mediators of the acute allergic reaction in lung tissue (table 1). In addition to the direct effects on the target tissues, the prostaglandins (13) and bradykinin (14) may have a profound influence on the concentration of cyclic nucleotides in lung fragments, and thus they may serve as modulators of the release and/or action of the primary mediators. The primary mediators differ not only in structure and function but also because histamine, an amine, and ECF-A, an acidic peptide, are stored preformed, whereas SRS-A, an acidic sulfate ester, and PAF are generated immediately before release.

Histamine (β-imidazolylethylamine)

Mast cells, which are located prominently in the perivascular connective tissue, contain histamine in association with the granules. Regardless of whether histamine is contained in mast cells, in circulating elements such as basophils and platelets, or in the parietal region of the

TABLE 1

CHEMICAL MEDIATORS OF IMMEDIATE HYPERSENSITIVITY

Mediators	Physicochemical Characteristics	State in Tissues	Biologic Activities
Primary			
Histamine	β-imidazolylethylamine	Preformed	Stimulates irritant receptors, constricts bronchial smooth muscle, increases venular permeability
Slow-reacting substance of anaphylaxis	Acidic sulfate ester, mol wt < 500	Precursor	Constricts bronchial smooth muscle, increases venular permeability
Eosinophil chemotactic factor of anaphylaxis	Acidic peptide(s), mol wt 500 to 600	Preformed	Selectively attracts and deactivates eosinophils
Platelet-activating factor	Phospholipids, mol wt 300 to 500		Aggregation and degranulation of platelets
Basophil kallikrein of anaphylaxis	Unknown	Unknown	Formation of bradykinin
Neutrophil chemotactic factor of anaphylaxis	Mol wt > 10,000	Preformed	Chemotaxis of neutrophils
Secondary			
Prostaglandins	C_{20} Hydroxy acids	Precursor	Regulate bronchomotor tone and pulmonary vascular resistance
Bradykinin	Nonapeptide	Precursor	Stimulates irritant receptors, constricts bronchial smooth muscle, increases venular permeability

stomach, it is formed from L-histidine and degraded by either oxidative deamination or by methylation and oxidative deamination (15). The *in vivo* pathobiologic effects of histamine include the production of leaking venules, attributed to partial disconnection of the endothelium, and elicitation of a profound increase in respiratory airway resistance with concomitant reduction in compliance (16). The actions of histamine on pulmonary mechanics, conductance, and compliance are significantly ameliorated by pretreatment of the experimental animal with atropine, and to this extent they are attributed to vagal reflexes initiated by airway irritant receptors (16) rather than to a direct effect on smooth muscle (17).

Eosinophil Chemotactic Factor of Anaphylaxis (ECF-A)

ECF-A is a preformed mediator that has been specifically associated with the rat mast cell (18) and the human leukemic basophil (10) by its extraction from essentially pure populations of these cell types; in the rat mast cell, its association with the granules has also been demonstrated by subcellular fractionation (18). ECF-A extracted or released immunologically from human or guinea pig lung fragments, rat mast cells, and leukemic human basophils exhibits a molecular weight of 500 to 600 by gel filtration on Sephadex G-25 (10, 18) and is susceptible to inactivation by digestion with subtilisin or pronase, but not with chymotrypsin or trypsin (19). High voltage electrophoresis on paper at neutral pH after gel filtration has resolved ECF-A from human lung into 2 discrete peaks of eosinophilotactic activity that migrate anodally, indicating that at least 2 acidic peptides have the functional attributes of ECF-A (20). ECF-A is the most active eosinophilotactic factor for purified human eosinophils when compared to complement-derived C3a, C5a, or active site (kallikrein, plasminogen activator) principles at concentrations exhibiting similar neutrophil chemotactic activity (20). Eosinophils demonstrate diminished chemotactic responsiveness, termed deactivation, after interaction with ECF-A (21). Deactivation is rapid and selective, in that ECF-A deactivates human eosinophils more markedly than neutrophils or mononuclear leukocytes. It may be that deactivation represents a mechanism by which specifically attracted eosinophils are held at a site for the purpose of exerting some regulatory function, such as the inactivation of SRS-A (22, 23).

Slow-Reacting Substance of Anaphylaxis (SRS-A)

SRS-A is an acidic, sulfur-containing (24) chemical mediator of approximately 500 molecular weight (25), which is inactivated by limpet (24) and human eosinophil (22) arylsulfatases. In contrast to the preformed mediators, histamine and ECF-A, SRS-A appears in tissues or cells only after immunologic activation and immediately before its release (26, 27). The mast cell has been presumed to be the cell source because the generation of SRS-A follows IgE-dependent reactions in human lung (5) and nasal polyp (3) fragments and in human lung (26) and peripheral leukocyte (9) cell suspensions; the generation of a material with the functional and physicochemical characteristics of SRS-A from human leukemic basophils activated with the calcium ionophore (10) supports this view. SRS-A generation continues *in vitro* at a time when the tissue or cellular lung content has reached a plateau and the release of preformed mediators is complete (26), a phenomenon explicable by the involvement of an additional cell type or by the interaction of antigen with IgE at sites not required for the release of preformed mediators. That more than one cell type and more than one immunoglobulin class can participate in SRS-A generation is illustrated in the rat by the release of SRS-A into the peritoneal cavity by either an IgE-mast cell dependent (28) or an IgGa-complement-neutrophil dependent (29) mechanism. SRS-A increases vascular permeability upon intracutaneous injection (30), and decreases pulmonary compliance independent of cholinergic mechanisms when injected intravenously into guinea pigs (17, 31).

Platelet Activating Factor (PAF)

PAF, assessed by its ability to release histamine or radiolabeled serotonin from rabbit and human platelets, has been released from rabbit (32, 33) and human (34) cell suspensions and from human lung fragments (4) by IgE-dependent mechanisms. That the source of this chemical mediator is basophils or mast cells is further indicated by the release of a platelet-activating principle from suspensions of leukemic human basophils upon interaction with the calcium ionophore (10). Whether this activity represents a single factor remains to be determined, but it seems unlikely in that PAF was extractable from human leukocyte suspensions (34) and lung fragments (4) before immunologic activation, whereas the material derived from the leukemic basophils was not present until after the introduction of the calcium ionophore (10). Material extracted from rabbit peripheral leukocytes, deproteinated with 80 per cent ethanol, and subjected to Sephadex LH-20 gel filtration exhibited a molecular weight of approximately 1,100 (34). In contrast, PAF generated in the peritoneal cavity of rats prepared with hyperimmune antiserum and challenged with specific antigen deproteinated with 80 per cent ethanol, separated from water soluble mediators by adsorption on Amberlite XAD-2 and elution with 80 per cent ethanol, and subjected to silicic acid chromatography reveals an apparent molecular weight of 300 to 500 on Sephadex LH-20 (35). PAF, which chromatographed with SRS-A on silicic acid and Sephadex LH-20, could be distinguished functionally from SRS-A because it was stable to treatment with human eosinophil arylsulfatase but was inactivated by phospholipase D of both the cabbage (35) and the human eosinophil. It differed from the prostaglandins in its elution characteristics on silicic acid and its failure to contract the gerbil colon. The generation of a mediator capable of activating a cell type with the potentiality of the platelet adds a significant further dimension to possible consequences of immediate type hypersensitivity reactions.

Other Potential Mediators

Recent evidence indicates that antigen challenge of IgE-sensitized human lung fragments (36) and peripheral leukocytes (37) results in the release of activities capable of hydrolyzing synthetic substrates such as tosyl-L-arginine methyl ester (TAMe). Supernatants from antigen-challenged human leukocyte suspensions also appear to contain kallikrein activity in that they cleave bradykinin from its natural substrate, kininogen. Whether the TAMe esterase activity and the kallikrein activity represent the same or different enzymes in the supernatants has not been established. The antigen dose response relationships and the kinetics of release of the leukocyte-derived kallikrein generally paralleled those of histamine release, and the release of this enzyme is similarly modulated by agents influencing cellular concentrations of cyclic adenosine 3', 5'-monophosphate (cyclic AMP) (38). Such a cellular kallikrein may implicate the kinins as primary mediators of immediate hypersensitivity in addition to their possible secondary function via the Hageman factor–dependent activation of plasma prekallikrein (12).

In addition to the mediators mentioned above, antigen challenge of sensitized human lung fragments results in the release of prostaglandins E_1, E_2, and F_{2_α} (39), whereas no rabbit aorta-constricting substance is detectable. It has also been demonstrated that prostaglandins are released upon anaphylactic contraction of sensitized guinea pig trachea (40). The observation that eicosatrienoic acid inhibits prostaglandin formation but does not affect SRS-A (41) release whereas disodium cromoglycate inhibits the release of SRS-A and prostaglandins supports the view that the prostaglandins are not formed by a pathway common to the primary mediators and may be best considered secondary mediators.

A second chemotactic factor, predominantly a neutrophil chemotactic factor of anaphylaxis, has recently been recognized. Extracts of human leukemic basophils (10) and of human lung fragments (18) contain a chemotactic activity preferential for neutrophils relative to eosinophils that separates from ECF-A by filtering in the exclusion volume on Sephadex G-25; the same activity appears to be released by an IgE-dependent activation of human lung fragments or purified rat mast cells. Although this mediator is only now being characterized, it is of particular interest because its release might account for the accumulation of neutrophils at the site of allergic tissue injury, which through the release of lysosomal enzymes would aggravate the tissue injury process.

Biochemical Characteristics of Target Cell Activation, Mediator Generation, and Release

The composite events that follow antigen bridging of membrane-bound IgE antibody include the biochemical concomitants of the membrane interaction, designated activation, the generation of unstored mediators, and the selective secretion of newly formed and preformed mediators of diverse structure and function (figure 1).

Activation

Although there is no definitive analysis of the biochemical events of cell activation that follow immediately upon antigen bridging of membrane-bound IgE molecules, studies of the reaction sequence in the human lung link calcium ion influx and activation of a proesterase to the initial membrane perturbation. Antigen challenge of sensitized tissue in the presence of diisopropyl fluorophosphate (DFP) yields no mediator release, whereas removal of DFP before antigen introduction permits full release; thus, activation of a serine proesterase is essential for mediator release (42). Antigen challenge in the presence of DFP, followed by washing and transfer of tissue to normal buffer, permits histamine release in inverse relation to the duration of the initial incubation in the presence of DFP; the irreversible nature of serine esterase inactivation by DFP implies that the release of histamine upon transfer of lung fragments to normal buffer reflects the continued activation of residual proesterase during a finite period after initial antigen challenge (43). Omission of calcium ions from the DFP-containing buffer at the time of antigen challenge protects the esterase from inactivation by DFP because full histamine release is observed when the challenged tissue is transferred to normal buffer (43). Apparently, antigen challenge does not activate the proesterase to the DFP-susceptible state in the absence of calcium ions, but such an activation does occur without new antigen when the buffer conditions are normalized. Both the omission of calcium ions and the presence of DFP are required to maintain the proesterase state in the face of antigen because selective calcium absence permits mediator release, whereas the introduction of DFP alone prevents release through inhibition of the activated esterase. The action of calcium ions could be either on the rate of initial activation or on autocatalytic feedback activation of the initial esterase formed. It is tempting to speculate that IgE fixed to a binding subunit of membrane-located proesterase is re-

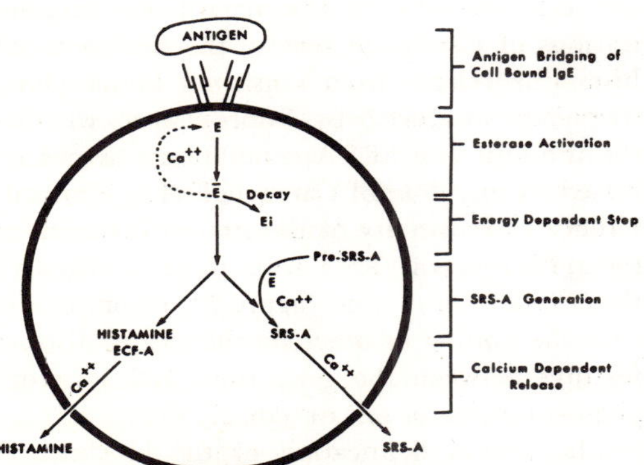

Fig. 1. Biochemical characteristics of target cell activation, and mediator generation and release. Proesterase (E) is converted to an active chymotrypsin-like esterase (Ē), which then decays (Ei). SRS-A = slow-reacting substance of anaphylaxis; ECF-A = eosinophil chemotactic factor of anaphylaxis.

sponsible for local activation in the presence of antigen and calcium ions. Depending upon the location of the proesterase in relation to other membrane structures, the calcium ions would act at the surface or require transport to control the rate of activation (figure 1).

Generation of Unstored Mediators

Only SRS-A has been studied in sufficient detail to permit consideration of its formation. The capacity to extract SRS-A from the lung fragments or cells after their immunologic activation, together with the measurement of SRS-A in both the extract and the surrounding fluid, permits the study of total SRS-A generation (26, 27). That the material extracted was SRS-A was established by differential bioassay, physicochemical characteristics during purification steps, and inactivation of purified SRS-A by arylsulfatase. Intracellular accumulation of SRS-A occurred within one-half min of IgE-dependent activation and reached a plateau by 2 min, whereas release was often not apparent until 2 to 5 min and continued through 15 to 30 min, indicating that SRS-A is generated well beyond the plateau in the cellular level of SRS-A and beyond the release of preformed mediators (26). With limited IgE-dependent direct or reversed anaphylactic activation, intracellular SRS-A accumulation occurred without the release of any mediators, indicating that cellular formation of SRS-A may be a highly sensitive marker of an immediate hypersensitivity reaction. The quantity of total SRS-A generated was augmented by the introduction of 8-bromo-cyclic 3',5'-guanosine monophosphate (8-bromo-cyclic GMP) and inhibited by dibutyryl cyclic AMP, revealing a site of cyclic nucleotide modulation in addition to that of mediator secretion (26). The capacity of certain conditions, such as the introduction and removal of DFP before antigen challenge (43) or challenge in the presence of certain ratios of isoproterenol to carbamylcholine (44) or in the presence of cytochalasins A or B (27), to suppress SRS-A release while permitting or even augmenting histamine release may well be explicable by an action on the formation of SRS-A distinct from secretion of newly formed and preformed mediators. Further, these findings reveal biochemical requirements for SRS-A formation distinct or qualitatively different from those for release. The immunologic release of histamine and SRS-A from human lung tissue can be divided broadly into an antigen-dependent activation phase and a calcium ion–dependent release phase by using ethylenediamine tetraacetic acid (EDTA) (45), as has been previously described for human leukocytes (46). No SRS-A is detectable either in the diffusates or in the tissues during the activation phase (47); however, when calcium is added to the activated tissues, histamine is released and SRS-A is both formed and released, indicating that SRS-A generation may be a late step in the reaction (figure 1). These findings (47), taken together with the kinetic data (26), suggest that initial immunologic activation of the tissues may involve a common enzymatic sequence that leads to the release of histamine and ECF-A and initiation of the independent steps involved in the generation of SRS-A.

Secretion of Preformed and Newly Formed Mediators

Although antigen challenge of IgE-sensitized human tissues results in the release of numerous physicochemically distinct chemical mediators, there may be a striking variation in both the quality and quantity of the mediators released from differing tissues and from the same tissues of various persons. For example, antigen challenge of sensitized nasal polyps appears to result in the release of more histamine than SRS-A as compared to lung tissue (3), and there appears to be no correlation between the absolute amounts of histamine and SRS-A released from differing human lung specimens challenged with specific antigen or anti-IgE (47). Human leukemic basophils challenged with calcium ionophore yield a much higher percentage of their ECF-A than histamine (10), and in rat mast cells, the enhancement of histamine release by phosphatidylserine is not associated with augmentation of ECF-A release (D. J. Stechschulte and S. I. Wasserman: Unpublished observation). In addition, human ECF-A activity has been recovered from an undifferentiated bronchogenic carcinoma that did not contain detectable amounts of histamine (19). These qualitative and quantitative variations in mediator release may account for the differences in the pathobiology of local hypersensitivity reactions in differing tissues and in the responses of various patients to comparable antigen challenge.

It is now well established in human lung that agents capable of stimulating adenylate cyclase, such as β-adrenergic agonists (5) and prostaglandins (13), increase tissue concentrations of cyclic AMP and inhibit mediator generation and/or release. Phosphodiesterase inhibitors such as aminophylline also block mediator release and demonstrate synergistic effects with β-adrenergic agents; conversely, imidazole stimulates phosphodiesterase activity with lowering of tissue concentrations of cyclic AMP and enhancement of the release of both histamine and SRS-A (44). Alpha-adrenergic agonists and low concentrations of prostaglandins, especially of the $PGF_{2\alpha}$ class, also decrease tissue concentrations of cyclic AMP and enhance the release of chemical mediators (5, 13, 48). Thus, there appears to be an inverse relationship between tissue concentrations of cyclic AMP and the degree of mediator release observed. Implicit in these observations is the presence of β- and α-adrenergic prototype receptors and receptors for certain of the prostaglandins on the target cells in human lung (figure 2A).

Cholinergic stimulation of sensitized lung fragments with acetylcholine or carbamylcholine chloride (Carbachol ®) results in enhancement of the IgE-dependent release of chemical mediators. The enhancement is not associated with a decrease in cyclic AMP concentrations (48) and is blocked by the addition of atropine, indicating that the cholinergic receptors on the target cells in human lung tissue are of the muscarinic prototype. Cholinergic stimulation results in an increase in tissue concentrations of cyclic GMP (49, 50), and the addition of 8-bromo-cyclic GMP to human lung fragments effects a dose-dependent enhancement of histamine release and SRS-A generation (26, 48). The opposing effects of cyclic AMP and cyclic GMP on modulating IgE-dependent mediator generation and release (48) have also been observed in other tissues and cells (51–54). In this regard, low concentrations of Carbachol reverse the inhibition of histamine release from sensitized human lung fragments produced by isoproterenol whereas the inhibition of SRS-A generation was not reversed by any dose of Carbachol (44). This difference in sensitivity of the step (s) involved in the generation of SRS-A from those involved in the release of histamine (figure 2A) is compatible with the finding of other biochemically distinct features between the generation and secretory phases of mediator release (26, 27, 43).

The partial delineation of the biochemical steps involved in the immunologic release of chemical mediators from human lung tissue permits the development of a theoretic model for mechanisms of pharmacologic modulation (figures 2A, B). The interaction of specific antigen with tissue-fixed IgE antibody results in membrane perturbation with a finite duration of effects at 37° C even in the absence of calcium ions (27). The membrane effects result in the transport of extra-cellular calcium ions to the site of a proesterase (E), which is converted to an active chymotrypsin-like serine esterase (Ē); the esterase engages in further autocatalytic activation and acts upon its substrate, perhaps removing an inhibitory protein. The influx of calcium ions may be critical to either initial activation or autocatalytic activation of the proesterase to the esterase, which then decays (Ei). The subsequent energy-dependent step is inhibitable by 2-deoxyglucose (43) (figure 2B). Whether the energy requirement is related to the function of a "contractile protein" has not been established, but dense bands of microfilaments have been observed around mast cell granules, particularly during degranulation (55). A striking dissociation of the immunologic release of histamine and SRS-A from human lung fragments is observed upon challenge in the presence of the fungal metabolites, cytochalasin A and cytochalasin B. These compounds enhance the release of histamine while inhibiting the concomitant formation of SRS-A and appear to act before the calcium ion-dependent release phase of the reaction (56) (figure 2B). The mechanism involved in the enhancement of histamine release may be analogous to the mechanisms involved in the facilitated exocytosis of

lysosomal enzymes (57–59), the dispersion of melanin granules (60), and the glucose-induced secretion of insulin from pancreatic islet cells (61); these latter effects are attributed to action on a subcortical web of microfilaments, which may represent a cytochalasin-sensitive barrier to the exocytosis of granules (62). Indeed, it has been observed that cytochalasin B may disorganize and/or disrupt oriented bundles of 40 to 50 A° subplasmalemmal microfilaments in cultivated mouse macrophages (63).

The ability of the cytochalasins to inhibit the formation and release of SRS-A in a dose-dependent fashion suggests either a contrasting role for microfilament function in activating the pathway leading to SRS-A generation or an effect of the cytochalasins on a membrane transport system (64) required for SRS-A generation. A further distinction between histamine secretion and SRS-A generation is observed with cysteine pretreatment of human lung fragments, which produces a selective and marked enhancement of the formation of SRS-A (65) (figure 2B). Whether cysteine is contributing a reactive sulfide for SRS-A formation or is involved in the stabilization or activation of an antigen-induced enzyme has not been elucidated.

Previous studies (66, 67) have indicated a role for microtubules in the release of histamine from rat mast cells stimulated with compound 48/80 and from human peripheral leukocytes chal-

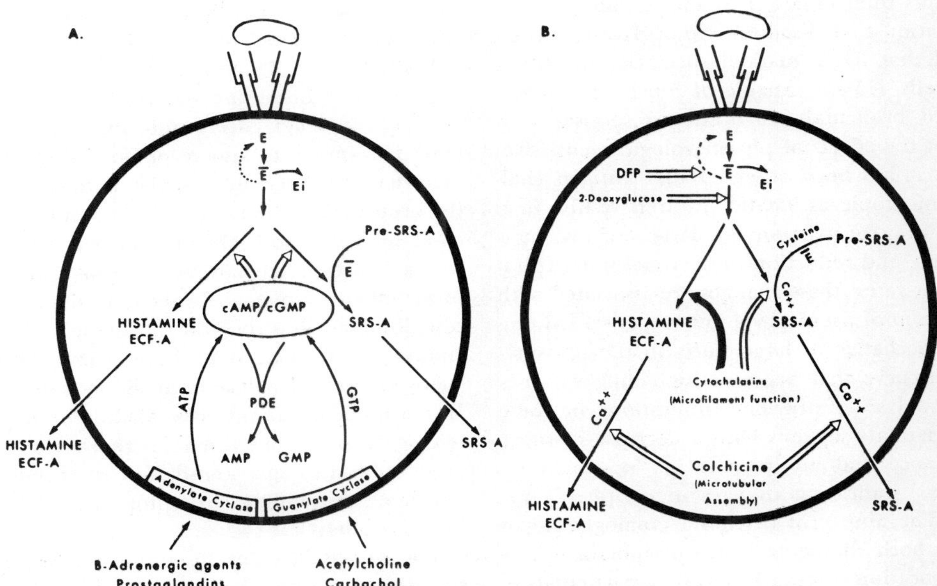

Fig. 2. Theoretic sites of pharmacologic modulation of the immunologic release of chemical mediators. See text for details and explanations of abbreviations.

lenged with specific antigen. Colchicine, an agent that binds to the microtubular subunit protein to prevent microtubule assembly and function (68), inhibits the release of histamine and appears to be acting in the calcium ion-dependent release phase of the reaction in leukocytes (67) (figure 2B). The findings that agents that chelate calcium ions, alter cyclic nucleotide concentrations, or inhibit microtubule assembly (43, 67) all act in the later phases of the release reaction are compatible with the evidence that there may be an integral relationship between calcium ion flux, the relative concentrations of cyclic nucleotides, and microtubular assembly and function (69). A calcium binding regulator protein may control adenylate cyclase, guanylate cyclase, and phosphodiesterase activities (70). The intracellular ratio of cyclic AMP/cyclic GMP may affect the degree of phosphorylation or dephosphorylation (71) of the proteins (ATPases) associated with assembled microtubules (72) that control the movement of intracellular organelles.

Potential Interrelationships of the Chemical Mediators

The observation that bronchial provocation reactions demonstrate a high degree of antigen specificity leads to the conclusion that allergic bronchospasm may result from the antigen-induced release of chemical mediators from the IgE-sensitized target cells in these tissues (73, 74). This interpretation is substantiated by the observation that disodium cromoglycate, a compound that has a marked specificity for tissue mast cells (75), is capable of blocking antigen-induced bronchial provocation responses (76) but not the effects of pharmacologic agents. Recently, it has been observed that antigen challenge of atopic asthmatic children results in a significant constriction of large airways, gas trapping, and reduction in maximal mid-expiratory flow rates; these changes are associated with a spectrum of pressure-volume responses varying from no change to large shifts in the pressure-volume curve that begin at high lung volumes (77). Analysis of the flow limitations in these latter patients suggests both a decrease in static compliance and an increase in "upstream resistance," indicating changes in peripheral airways. The ability of disodium cromoglycate to inhibit both the central and peripheral effects of provocation reactions suggests a participation of chemical mediators in the initiation of responses that ultimately result in both flow re-

duction and gas trapping. However, the similar time courses of the bronchial provocation response *in vivo* and of the immunologic release of chemical mediators *in vitro* are more analogous to an acute anaphylactic reaction than to the subacute or chronic abnormalities observed in the asthmatic patient. Furthermore, neither the *in vivo* nor the *in vitro* model satisfactorily accounts for the nonspecific hyperreactivity of the asthmatic airway (78) or for certain of the characteristic pathologic features (79, 80). On the other hand, recent advances in the understanding of the diversity of primary chemical mediators and their interactions with primary and secondary effector cells (figure 3) may permit development of an integrated concept of the mechanisms involved in the evolution of the sustained asthmatic abnormalities.

It has been appreciated for more than 15 years that allergen provocation induces an exquisite hyperreactivity of the asthmatic airways to nonspecific irritants, including histamine and mecholyl (81). This observation suggests that the antigen-induced release of chemical mediators in lung tissue results in a functional change in reactivity that may be expressed as a lowered response threshold of irritant receptors. Inflammation in peripheral airways also may lower the threshold for stimulation of irritant receptors (82, 83). Nonspecific stimulation of irritant receptors results in vagally mediated bronchoconstriction, which is blocked by atropine (83–87). The fact that only part of the bronchoconstrictor effect of histamine injected directly into the bronchial artery of dogs is present after vagotomy suggests that histamine has both direct effects and indirect reflex effects on bronchomotor tone (88). Histamine is also a potent permeability factor; it may increase vascular permeability in the bronchial capillary bed, which results in mucosal edema in both central and peripheral airways (figure 3). Histamine-induced changes in bronchomotor tone and mucosal edema could contribute to lowering the threshold of the irritant receptors to nonspecific stimuli but it seems unlikely that histamine alone is sufficient. In addition, histamine may modulate mediator release from primary and perhaps secondary target cells through stimulation of membrane-associated histamine-2 receptor sites (89, 90) linked to adenylate cyclase.

The direct effect of histamine on bronchial smooth muscle may be potentiated by the concomitant release of SRS-A. Exposure of atropinized isolated smooth muscle strips to SRS-A

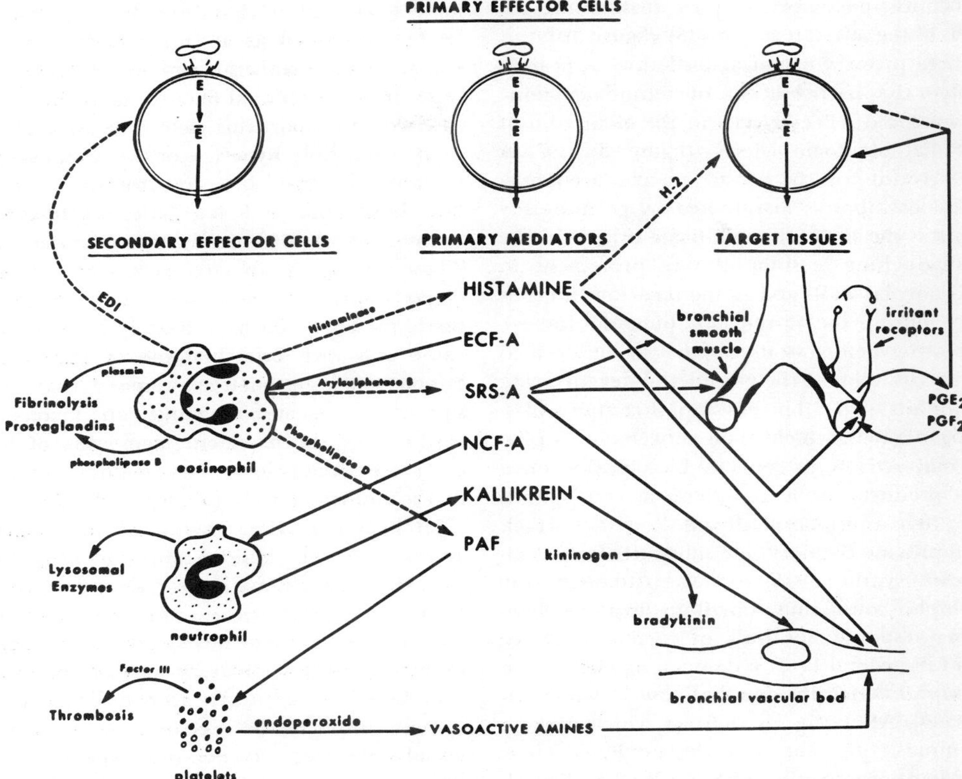

Fig. 3. Diversity of primary chemical mediators and their interactions with primary and secondary effector cells and with target tissues.

results in subsequent potentiation of the histamine responses (91), and a similar synergism may exist for vascular responses. SRS-A appears to be a potent constrictor of human bronchial smooth muscle (91–93) *in vitro,* and partially purified preparations of SRS-A increase vascular permeability in the skin of rats (94), guinea pigs, and monkeys (30). The intravenous administration of SRS-A to unanesthetized guinea pigs results in decreases in pulmonary compliance with minimal decreases in conductance, whereas histamine and bradykinin have comparable effects on compliance and conductance, and PGF_{2_α} has an early preferential effect on conductance (31) followed by a late equal effect on both parameters. The effects observed with SRS-A on compliance are not blocked by atropine (17).

The effects of both histamine and SRS-A on the smooth muscle of the target tissues in lung may result in the secondary elaboration of prostaglandins, which in turn may have profound effects on bronchomotor tone, the pulmonary vasculature, and the primary effector cells (figure 3). Both PGE_1 and PGE_2 appear to cause dilatation of bronchial smooth muscle *in vivo* and *in vitro,* whereas PGF_{2_α} causes bronchoconstriction (95–97). The exquisite sensitivity of the asthmatic airway to aerosolized PGF_{2_α} (98) suggests an action on irritant receptors that would appreciably amplify the bronchoconstrictor effects of histamine and SRS-A. Both histamine and PGF_{2_α} increase pulmonary vascular resistance (99) in isolated guinea pig lungs and contract the circular smooth muscle of the pulmonary artery. Prostaglandins are highly active as potentiators of the vascular permeability changes induced by histamine and bradykinin, and the intradermal injection of low doses of PGE_1 enhances passive cutaneous anaphylactic, reversed passive Arthus, and delayed hypersensitivity reactions in the skin of guinea pigs (100). Besides potentiating the effects of the primary mediators on smooth muscle, the prostaglandins may have direct effects on the primary target cells. Low concentrations of PGE_1 and especially PGF_{2_α} are capable of decreasing cellular levels of cyclic AMP and enhancing the antigen-induced release of chemical mediators, thereby augmenting the effects of the initial reaction (13) (figure 3).

Three primary chemical mediators appear to involve the participation of secondary, non–IgE-sensitized, effector cells in the elicitation of their pathobiologic effects (figure 3). ECF-A may account for the attraction and accumulation of eosinophils marginated by permeability factors at the site of allergic tissue injury. In the asthmatic lung, eosinophils are prominent in the bronchial walls and in the tenacious mucous plugs filling the bronchial lumens. Indeed, Charcot-Leyden crystals appear to be formed from crystalloids of the granules of degenerating eosinophils (101). The eosinophil contains plasminogen (102), which upon conversion to plasmin may activate or generate biologically active split products from complement components (103, 104) and phospholipase B (105), which could provide the fatty acid substrates for prostaglandin synthesis (figure 3). Although the eosinophil could thus contribute to the inflammatory response, the bulk of current evidence would in general favor a dampening effect: The eosinophil is rich in phospholipase D, which inactivates PAF (106), histaminase, which destroys histamine (107), and arylsulfatase B, which is capable of inactivating SRS-A (22, 23). The elaboration of prostaglandins possibly attributable to the action of eosinophil phospholipase B may result in effective inhibition of primary target cell degranulation (108) (figure 3).

PAF may also contribute to both the acute and chronic changes observed in the asthmatic lung, because this low molecular weight mediator appears to cause the local aggregation and degranulation of platelets. The elaboration of vasoactive amines and perhaps platelet factor III may result in contraction of bronchopulmonary smooth muscle and in fibrin deposition. Finally, either ECF-A and/or neutrophil chemotactic factor of anaphylaxis may account for the presence of neutrophils in the cellular infiltrates associated with bronchial asthma; such secondary effector cells would provide kallikrein, acid hydrolases, and cathepsin (109, 110). Thus, the immunologic release of the primary mediators of immediate hypersensitivity may recruit diverse effector cells (eosinophils, neutrophils, and platelets) and multiple plasma protein effector systems (fibrinolytic, clotting, and kinin-generating) in a sustained inflammatory reaction sufficient to alter the response threshold of the irritant receptors.

Both the anatomic and the immunopharmacologic data suggest that bronchial asthma may be best regarded as an inflammatory state of central and peripheral airways; evolving concepts of the functional derangements in this disease would support this view. The asthmatic patient is not only hyperresponsive to nonspecific irritants but may also demonstrate significant flow limitations and ventilation/perfusion abnormalities while clinically asymptomatic (111). These findings are in agreement with the results of postmortem examination of lungs from asthmatic patients who have died from some other cause and with bronchial biopsy material obtained from symptom-free asthmatics that reveals significant mucous plugging, an increase in thickness of the basement membrane of bronchial smooth muscle, and eosinophilic infiltrates in the bronchial wall (79, 80, 112). The bronchial hyperreactivity, functional abnormalities, and pathologic findings in the apparently asymptomatic asthmatic may all reflect the inflammatory phase of the response to specific allergen. The chemical mediators, in addition to initiating the inflammatory state of the disease, may directly or indirectly alter cyclic nucleotide concentrations in the effector cells but more especially the target tissues. Such changes in the ratio of the cyclic nucleotides could underlie the hyperirritability of the irritant receptors in the *pathopharmacologic stage* of the disease as well as in the *inflammatory phase*. The inflammatory phase may then reinforce the reactivity of the irritant receptors by additional mechanisms, biochemical or anatomic. It thus appears appropriate to consider therapy in this disease not only in terms of the acute and highly reversible pathopharmacologic phase but also for the chronic inflammatory stage that may be more subtle to diagnoses but yet more persistent in its effects.

References

1. Schild, H. O., Hawkins, D. F., Mongar, J. L., and Herxheimer, H.: Reactions of isolated human asthmatic lung and bronchial tissue to a specific antigen, Lancet, 1951, *2*, 376.
2. Brocklehurst, W. E.: The release of histamine and formation of a slow reacting substance (SRS-A) during anaphylactic shock, J Physiol, 1960, *151*, 416.
3. Kaliner, M., Wasserman, S. I., and Austen, K. F.: Immunologic release of chemical mediators from human nasal polyps, N Engl J Med, 1973, *289*, 277.
4. Bogart, D. B., and Stechschulte, D. J.: Release

of platelet activating factor from human lung, Clin Res, 1974, *22*, 652A.

5. Orange, R. P., Austen, W. G., and Austen, K. F.: Immunological release of histamine and slow reacting substance of anaphylaxis from human lung. I. Modulation by agents influencing cellular levels of cyclic 3',5'-adenosine monophosphate, J Exp Med, 1971, *134*, 136s.

6. Kay, A. B., and Austen, K. F.: The IgE-mediated release of an eosinophil leukocyte chemotactic factor from human lung, J Immunol, 1971, *107*, 899.

7. Katz, G., and Cohen, S.: Experimental evidence of histamine release in allergy, JAMA, 1941, *117*, 1782.

8. Parish, W. E.: Reaginic and nonreaginic antibody reactions on anaphylactic participating cells, in *Mechanisms in Allergy: Reagin Mediated Hypersensitivity*, L. Goodfriend, A. H. Sehon, and R. P. Orange, ed., Marcel Dekker, New York, 1973, p. 197.

9. Grant, J. A., and Lichtenstein, L. M.: Release of slow reacting substance of anaphylaxis from human leukocytes, J Immunol, 1974, *112*, 897.

10. Lewis, R. A., Goetzel, E. J., Wasserman, S. I., Valone, F. H., Rubin, R. H., and Austen, K. F.: The release of four mediators of immediate hypersensitivity from human leukemic basophils, J Immunol, 1975, *114*, 87.

11. Weeks, J. R.: Prostaglandins, Ann Rev Pharmacol, 1972, *12*, 317.

12. Cochrane, C. G., Revak, S. D., Aikin, B. S., and Wuepper, K. D.: The structural characteristics and activation of Hageman factor, in *Inflammation: Mechanisms and Control*, I. H. Lepow and P. A. Ward, ed., Academic Press, New York, 1972, p. 119.

13. Tauber, A. I., Kaliner, M., Stechschulte, D. J., and Austen, K. F.: Immunological release of histamine and slow reacting substance of anaphylaxis from human lung. V. Effects of prostaglandins on release of histamine, J Immunol, 1973, *111*, 27.

14. Stoner, J., Manganiello, V. C., and Vaughn, M.: Effects of bradykinin and indomethacin on cyclic GMP and cyclic AMP in lung slices, Proc Natl Acad Sci USA, 1973, *70*, 3830.

15. Schayer, R. W.: Histamine and circulatory homeostasis, Fed Proc, 1965, *24*, 1295.

16. Nadel, J. A.: Neurophysiologic aspects of asthma, in *Asthma: Physiology, Immunopharmacology and Treatment*, K. F. Austen and L. Lichtenstein, ed., Academic Press, New York, 1973, p. 29.

17. Drazen, J. M., and Austen, K. F.: Atropine modification of the pulmonary effects of chemical mediators in the guinea pig, J Appl Physiol, 1975, *38*, 834.

18. Wasserman, S. I., Goetzl, E. J., and Austen, K. F.: Preformed eosinophil chemotactic factor of anaphylaxis (ECF-A), J Immunol, 1974, *290*, 420.

19. Wasserman, S. I., Goetzl, E. J., Ellman, L., and Austen, K. F.: Tumor-associated eosinophilotactic factor, N Engl J Med, 1974, *290*, 420.

20. Goetzl, E. J., Wasserman, S. I., and Austen, K. F.: Modulation of the eosinophil chemotactic response in immediate hypersensitivity, in *Progress in Immunology II*, vol. 4, L. Brent and J. Holborow, ed., North Holland Publishing Co., Amsterdam, 1974, p. 41.

21. Wasserman, S. I., Whitmer, D., Goetzl, E. J., and Austen, K. F.: Chemotactic deactivation of human eosinophils by the eosinophil chemotactic factor of anaphylaxis, Proc Soc Exp Biol Med, 1975, *148*, 301.

22. Wasserman, S. I., Goetzl, E. J., and Austen, K. F.: Inactivation of slow reacting substance of anaphylaxis by human eosinophil arylsulfatase, J Immunol, 1975, *114*, 645.

23. Wasserman, S. I., Goetzl, E. J., and Austen, K. F.: Inactivation of human SRS-A by intact human eosinophils and by eosinophil arylsulfatase (abstract), J Allergy Clin Immunol, 1975, *55*, 72.

24. Orange, R. P., Murphy, R. C., and Austen, K. F.: Inactivation of slow reacting substance of anaphylaxis (SRS-A) by arylsulfatases, J Immunol, 1974, *113*, 316.

25. Orange, R. P., Murphy, R. C., Karnovsky, M. L., and Austen, K. F.: The physicochemical characteristics and purification of slow reacting substance of anaphylaxis, J Immunol, 1973, *110*, 760.

26. Lewis, R. A., Wasserman, S. I., Goetzl, E. J., and Austen, K. F.: Formation of SRS-A in human lung tissue and cells before release, J Exp Med, 1974, *140*, 1133.

27. Orange, R. P.: The formation and release of slow reacting substance of anaphylaxis in human lung tissues, in *Progress in Immunology II*, vol. 4, L. Brent and J. Holborow, ed., North Holland Publishing Co., Amsterdam, 1974, p. 29.

28. Orange, R. P., Stechschulte, D. J., and Austen, K. F.: Immunochemical and biologic properties of rat IgE. II. Capacity to mediate the immunologic release of histamine and slow reacting substance of anaphylaxis (SRS-A), J Immunol, 1970, *105*, 1087.

29. Morse, H. C., III, Bloch, K. J., and Austen, K. F.: Biologic properties of rat antibodies. II. Time-course of appearance of antibodies involved in antigen-induced release of slow reacting substance of anaphylaxis (SRS-Arat); association of this activity with rat IgGa, J Immunol, 1968, *101*, 658.

30. Orange, R. P., Stechschulte, D. J., and Austen, K. F.: Cellular mechanisms involved in the release of slow reacting substance of anaphylaxis,

Fed Proc, 1969, *28*, 1710.

31. Drazen, J. M., and Austen, K. F.: Effects of intravenous administration of slow reacting substance of anaphylaxis, histamine, bradykinin and prostaglandin $F_{2\alpha}$ on pulmonary mechanics in the guinea pig, J Clin Invest, 1974, *53*, 1679.

32. Henson, P. M.: Release of vasoactive amines from rabbit platelets induced by sensitized mononuclear leukocytes and antigen, J Exp Med, 1970, *131*, 287.

33. Siraganian, R. P., and Osler, A. G.: Destruction of rabbit-platelets in the allergic response of sensitized leukocytes. II. Evidence of basophil involvement, J Immunol, 1971, *106*, 1252.

34. Benveniste, J.: Platelet-activating factor, a new mediator of anaphylaxis and immune complex deposition from rabbit and human basophils, Nature, 1974, *249*, 581.

35. Kater, L. A., Austen, K. F., and Goetzl, E. J.: Identification and partial purification of a platelet activating factor (PAF) from rat (abstract), Fed Proc, 1975, *34*, 4340.

36. Webster, M. E., Horakova, Z., Beaven, M. A., Takahaski, H., and Newball, H. H.: Release of arginine esterase and histamine from human lung passively sensitized with ragweed antibody, Fed Proc, 1974, *33*, 761.

37. Newball, H. H., Lichtenstein, L. M., and Talamo, R. C.: Leukocyte arginine esterase—a potential new mediator of allergic reactions, J Allergy, 1975, *55*, 72.

38. Newball, H. H., Lichtenstein, L. M., and Talamo, R. C.: Basophil kallikrein of anaphylaxis (BK-A), Fed Proc, 1975, *34*, 1045.

39. Piper, P., and Walker, J. L.: The release of spasmogenic substance from human chopped lung tissue and its inhibition, Br J Pharmacol, 1973, *47*, 291.

40. Orehek, J., Douglas, J. S., Lewis, A. J., and Bouhuys, A.: Prostaglandin regulation of airway smooth muscle tone, Nature, 1973, *245*, 84.

41. Dawson, W., and Tomlinson, R.: Effect of cromoglycate and eicosatraynoic acid on the release of prostaglandins and SRS-A from immunologically challenged guinea pig lungs, Br J Pharmacol, 1974, *52*, 107P.

42. Orange, R. P., Kaliner, M. A., and Austen, K. F.: The immunological release of histamine and slow reacting substance of anaphylaxis from human lung. III. Biochemical control mechanisms involved in the immunologic release of the chemical mediators, in *Second International Symposium on the Biochemistry of Acute Allergic Reactions*, K. F. Austen and E. L. Becker, ed., Blackwell, Oxford, 1971, p. 189.

43. Kaliner, M., and Austen, K. F.: A sequence of biochemical events in the antigen-induced release of chemical mediators from sensitized human lung tissue, J Exp Med, 1973, *138*, 1077.

44. Kaliner, M., and Austen, K. F.: Hormonal control of the immunologic release of histamine and slow reacting substance of anaphylaxis from human lung, in *Cyclic AMP, Cell Growth and the Immune Response*, W. Braun, W. Lichtenstein, and C. W. Parker, ed., Springer-Verlag, New York, 1974, p. 163.

45. Orange, R. P., and Austen, K. F.: Immunologic and pharmacologic receptor control of the release of chemical mediators from human lung, in *The Biologic Role of the Immunoglobulin E System*, K. Ishizaka and D. H. Dayton, ed., U.S. Dept. of Health, Education and Welfare, Bethesda, Md., 1973, p. 151.

46. Lichtenstein, L. M., and DeBernardo, R.: The immediate allergic response: In vitro action of cyclic AMP-active and other drugs on the two stages of histamine release, J Immunol, 1971, *107*, 1131.

47. Orange, R. P., and Langer, H: Bronchial asthma: Hyperreactivity of airways and target cells, in *Allergology*, Excerpta Medica, Amsterdam, 1974, p. 325.

48. Kaliner, M., Orange, R. P., and Austen, K. F.: Immunologic release of histamine and slow reacting substance of anaphylaxis from human lung. IV. Enhancement by cholinergic and alpha adrenergic stimulation, J Exp Med, 1972, *136*, 556.

49. Kuo, J., Lee, T., Reyes, P. L., Watson, K. D., Donnelly, Jr., T. E., and Greengard, P.: Cyclic nucleotide-dependent protein kinases. X. An assay method for the measurement of guanosine 3′,5′-monophosphate in various biological materials and a study of agents regulating its levels in heart and brain, J Biol Chem, 1972, *247*, 16.

50. Lee, T. P., Kuo, J. F., and Greengard, P.: Regulation of myocardial cyclic AMP by isoproterenol, glucagon and acetylcholine, Biochem Biophys Res Commun, 1971, *45*, 991.

51. Triner, L., Vulliemoz, Y., Verosky, M., and Nahas, G. G.: Acetylcholine and the cyclic AMP system in smooth muscle, Biochem Biophys Res Commun, 1972, *46*, 1966.

52. George, W. J., Polson, J. D., O'Toole, A. G., and Goldberg, H. D.: Elevation of guanosine 3′,5′-cyclic phosphate in rat heart after perfusion with acetylcholine, Proc Natl Acad Sci USA, 1970, *66*, 398.

53. Schultz, G., Hardman, J. G., and Sutherland, E. .W: Cyclic nucleotides and smooth muscle function, in *Asthma: Physiology, Immunopharmacology and Treatment*, K. F. Austen and L. M. Lichtenstein, ed., Academic Press, New York, 1973, p. 123.

54. Hadden, J. W., Hadden, E., and Goldberg, N. D.: Cyclic GMP and cyclic AMP in lymphocyte metabolism and proliferation, in *Cyclic AMP, Cell Growth and the Immune Response*, W. Braun, L. M. Lichtenstein, and C. W. Parker, ed., Springer-Verlag, New York, 1974, p. 237.

55. Trotter, C. M., and Orr, T. S. C.: A fine structure study of some cellular components in allergic reactions. I. Degranulation of human mast cells in allergic asthma and perennial rhinitis, Clin Allergy, 1973, *3*, 411.

56. Orange, R. P.: Dissociation of the immunologic release of histamine and slow reacting substance of anaphylaxis from human lung using cytochalasins A and B, J Immunol, 1975, *114*, 182.

57. Henson, P. M., and Oades, Z.: Enhancement of immunologically induced granule exocytosis from neutrophils by cytochalasin B, J Immunol, 1973, *110*, 290.

58. Zurier, R. B., Hoffstein, S., and Weissmann, G.: Cytochalasin B: Effect on lysosomal enzyme release from human leukocytes, Proc Natl Acad Sci USA, 1973, *71*, 844.

59. Hawkins, D.: Neutrophilic leukocytes in immunologic reactions in vitro: Effect of cytochalasin B, J Immunol, 1973, *110*, 294.

60. McGuire, J., and Moellmann, G.: Cytochalasin B: Effects on microfilaments and movement of melanin granules within melanocytes, Science, 1972, *175*, 642.

61. Orci, L., Gabbay, K. H., and Malaisse, W. J.: Pancreatic beta-cell web: Its possible role in insulin secretion, Science, 1972, *175*, 1128.

62. Colten, H. R., and Gabbay, K. H.: Histamine release from human leukocytes: Modulation by a cytochalasin B-sensitive barrier, J Clin Invest, 1972, *51*, 1972.

63. Axline, S. G., and Reaven, E. P.: Inhibition of phagocytosis and plasma membrane mobility of the cultivated macrophage by cytochalasin B: Role of subplasmalemmal microfilaments, J Cell Biol, 1974, *62*, 647.

64. Estensen, R. D., and Plagemann, P. G. W.: Cytochalasin B: Inhibition of glucose and glucosamine transport, Proc Natl Acad Sci USA, 1972, *69*, 1430.

65. Orange, R. P.: Selective enhancement of the immunologic release of a slow reacting substance of anaphylaxis (SRS-A) by cysteine, Fed Proc, 1975, *34*, 1046.

66. Gillespie, E., Levine, R. J., and Malawista, S. E.: Histamine release from rat peritoneal mast cells: Inhibition by colchicine and potentiation by deuterium oxide, J Pharmacol Exp Ther, 1968, *164*, 158.

67. Gillespie, E., and Lichtenstein, L. M.: Histamine release from human leukocytes: Studies with deuterium oxide, colchicine, and cytochalasin B, J Clin Invest, 1972, *51*, 2941.

68. Gillespie, E.: Cyclic AMP and microtubules, in *Cyclic AMP, Cell Growth, and the Immune Response*, W. Braun, L. M. Lichtenstein, and C. W. Parker, ed., Springer-Verlag, New York, 1974, p. 317.

69. Cyclic AMP, Cell Growth and the Immune Response, W. Braun, L. M. Lichtenstein, and C. W. Parker, ed., Springer-Verlag, New York, 1974.

70. Brostrom, C. O., Huang, Y., Breckenridge, B. M., and Wolff, D. J.: Identification of a calcium-binding protein as a calcium-dependent regulator of brain adenylate cyclase, Proc Natl Acad Sci USA, 1975, *72*, 64.

71. Smith, R. J., and Ignarro, L. J.: Bioregulation of lysosomal enzyme secretion from human neutrophils: Roles of guanosine 3',5'-monophosphate and calcium in stimulus-secretion coupling, Proc Natl Acad Sci USA, 1975, *72*, 108.

72. Sloboda, R. D., Rudolph, S. A., Rosenbaum, J. L., and Greengard, P.: Cyclic AMP-dependent endogenous phosphorylation of a microtubule-associated protein, Proc Natl Acad Sci USA, 1975, *72*, 177.

73. Peipers, A.: A study of provocation tests on patients with bronchial asthma, Acta Allergol, (Kbh), 1971, *5*, 143.

74. Aas, K.: Bronchial provocation tests in asthma, Arch Dis Child, 1970, *45*, 221.

75. Cox, J. S. G., Beach, J. E., Blair, A. M. J. N., Clarke, A. J., King, J., Lee, T. B., Loveday, D. E. E., Moss, G. E., Orr, T. S. C., Ritchie, J. T., and Sheard, P.: Disodium cromoglycate (Intal), in *Advances in Drug Research*, vol. 5. M. J. Harper and A. B. Simmonds, ed., Academic Press, New York, 1970, p. 115.

76. Altounyan, R. E. C.: Inhibition of experimental asthma by a new compound—disodium cromoglycate, "Intal," Acta Allergol (Kbh), 1967, *22*, 487.

77. Mansell, A., Dubrawsky, C., Levison, H., Bryan, A. C., Langer, H., Collins-Williams, C., and Orange, R. P.: Lung mechanics in antigen-induced stress, J Appl Physiol, 1974, *37*, 297.

78. Curry, J. J.: Action of histamine on respiratory tract in normal and asthmatic subjects, J Clin Invest, 1946, *25*, 785.

79. Bohrod, M. J.: Pathological manifestations of allergies and related mechanisms in diseases of the lungs, Int Arch Allergy, 1958, *13*, 39.

80. Dunhill, M. S.: The pathology of asthma with special reference to changes in the bronchial mucosa, J Clin Pathol, 1960, *13*, 27.

81. Tiffeneau, R.: Recherches quantitatives sur les mediateurs bronchoconstrictifs produits par inhalation continue d'allergenes, Pathol Biol, 1959, *7*, 2293.

82. Parker, C. D., Bilbo, R. E., and Reed, C. E.: Methacholine aerosol as a test for bronchial asthma, Arch Intern Med, 1965, *115*, 452.

83. Simonsson, B. G., Jacobs, F. M., and Nadel, J. A.: Role of autonomic nervous system and the cough reflex in the increased responsiveness of airways in patients with obstructive airway disease, J Clin Invest, 1967, *46*, 1812.

84. DuBois, A. B., and Dautrebande, L.: Acute effect of breathing inert dust particles and of carbachol aerosol on the mechanical character-

istics of the lungs in man. Changes in response after inhaling sympathomimetic aerosols, J Clin Invest, 1958, *37*, 1746.

85. Herxheimer, H.: Atropine cigarettes in asthma and emphysema, Br Med J, 1959, *2*, 167.

86. Bouhuys, A., Jonsson, R., Lichtneckerts, S., Lindell, S. E., Lundgren, C., Lundin, G., and Pingquist T. F.: Effects of histamine on pulmonary ventilation in man, Clin Sci, 1960, *19*, 79.

87. Nadel, J. A.: Structure-function relationships in the airways: Bronchoconstriction mediated via vagus nerves or bronchial arteries; peripheral lung constriction mediated via pulmonary arteries, Med Thorac, 1965, *22*, 231.

88. DeKock, M. A., Nadel, J. A., Zwi, S., Colebatch, H. J. H., and Olsen, C. R.: New method for perfusing bronchial arteries: Histamine bronchoconstriction and apnea, J Appl Physiol, 1966, *21*, 185.

89. Lichtenstein, L., and Henney, C. S.: Adenylate cyclase-linked hormone receptors: An important mechanism for the immunoregulation of leucocytes, in *Progress in Immunology II,* vol. 2, L. Brent and J. Holborow, ed., North-Holland Publishing Co., Amsterdam, 1974, p. 73.

90. Zurier, R. B., Weissmann, G., Hoffstein, S., Kammerman, S., and Tai, H. H.: Mechanisms of lysosomal enzyme release from human leukocytes. II. Effects of cAMP and cGMP, autonomic agonists, and agents which affect microtubule function, J Clin Invest, 1974, *53*, 297.

91. Brocklehurst, W. E.: Slow reacting substance and related compounds, Prog Allergy, 1962, *6*, 539.

92. Schild, H. O., Hawkins, D. F., Mongar, J. L., and Herxheimer, H.: Reactions of isolated human asthmatic lung and bronchial tissue to a specific allergen, Lancet, 1951, *2*, 376.

93. Orange, R. P., and Austen, K. F.: Slow reacting substance of anaphylaxis, Adv Immunol, 1969, *10*, 106.

94. Brocklehurst, W. E.: Chemical mediators of anaphylaxis, in *Clinical Aspects of Immunology* P. F. H. Gell and R. R. A. Coombs, ed., ed. 2, Blackwell, Oxford, 1968, p. 611.

95. Main, I. H. M.: The inhibitory actions of prostaglandins on respiratory smooth muscle, Br J Pharmacol Chemother, 1964, *22*, 511.

96. Sweatman, W. J., and Collier, H. O.: Effects of prostaglandins on human bronchial smooth muscle, Nature, 1968, *217*, 69.

97. Collier, H. O. J., and James, G. E. L.: Humoral factors affecting pulmonary inflation during acute anaphylaxis in the guinea pig in vivo, Br J Pharmacol Chemother, 1967, *30*, 238.

98. Mathé, A. A., and Hedqvist, P.: Effect of prostaglandins $F_{2\alpha}$ and E_2 on airway conductance in healthy subjects and asthmatic patients, Am Rev Respir Dis, 1975, *111*, 313.

99. Okpako, D. T.: The actions of histamine and prostaglandins $F_{2\alpha}$ and E_2 on pulmonary vascular resistance of the lung of the guinea pig, J Pharm Pharmacol, 1972, *24*, 40.

100. Williams, T. J., and Morley, J.: Prostaglandins as potentiators of increased vascular permeability in inflammation, Nature, 1973, *246*, 215.

101. Welsh, R. A.: The genesis of Charcot-Leyden crystals in the eosinophil leucocyte in man, Am J Pathol, 1959, *35*, 1091.

102. Barnhart, M. I., and Riddle, J. M.: Cellular localization of profibrinolysin (plasminogen), Blood, 1963, *21*, 306.

103. Ratnoff, O. D., and Naff, G. B.: The conversion of Cl to Cl esterase by plasmin and trypsin, J Exp Med, 1967, *125*, 337.

104. Ward, P.: A plasmin-split fragment of C3 as a new chemotactic factor, J Exp Med, 1967, *126*, 189.

105. Ottolenghi, A.: The relationship between eosinophil leukocytes and phospholipase B activity in some rat tissues, Lipids, 1970, *5*, 531.

106. Kater, L. A., Austen, K. F., and Goetzl, E. J.: Inactivation of platelet-activating factor (PAF) by eosinophil phospholipase D (abstract), Arthritis Rheum, in press.

107. Zeiger, R. S., and Colten, H. R.: Histamine metabolism in cells of the allergic response, Pediatr Res, 1974, *8*, 147.

108. Hubscher, T.: Role of the eosinophil in the allergic reactions. I. EDI—An eosinophil-derived inhibitor of histamine release, J Immunol, 1975, *114*, 1379.

109. Movat, H. A., Steinberg, S. G., Habal, F. M., and Ranadive, N. S.: Demonstration of a kinin-generating enzyme in the lysosomes of human polymorphonuclear leukocytes, Lab Invest, 1973, *29*, 669.

110. Cochrane, C. G., and Aikin, B. S.: Polymorphonuclear leukocytes in immunologic reactions: The destruction of vascular basement membrane in vivo and in vitro, J Exp Med, *124*, 733.

111. Levison, H., Collins-Williams, C., Reilly, B. J., and Orange, R. P.: Asthma: Current concepts, Pediatr Clin North Am, 1974, *21*, 951.

112. Glynn, A. A., and Michaels, L.: Bronchial biopsy in chronic bronchitis and asthma, Thorax, 1960, *15*, 142.

Bronchial Provocation Tests in Etiologic Diagnosis and Analysis of Asthma[1]

J. PEPYS AND B. J. HUTCHCROFT[2]

Contents

[1] From the Department of Clinical Immunology, Cardiothoracic Institute, Brompton, London SW3, and the Department of Medicine, Charing Cross Hospital, Fulham Palace Road, London W6, England.

[2] Dr. Hutchcroft is supported by a Medical Research Council scholarship.

When investigating the allergy of asthma, defined as "airways obstruction reversible spontaneously or by treatment," bronchial provocation testing can be of value and may even be indispensable for accurate etiologic diagnosis. In addition to the extensive literature on its use, mainly for the investigation of immediate type asthmatic reactions (1–8), others (9, 10) have also reported nonimmediate, or late, reactions, which could be blocked by corticosteroid drugs. In this review, emphasis will be placed on the clinical use of bronchial provocation tests for etiologic diagnostic purposes and for assessment of the effects of therapeutic agents on the reactions elicited. We have used a pragmatic approach to determine whether the relevant suspected agents are capable of eliciting asthmatic reactions in the patient. These reactions, in turn, have thrown light, with reciprocal interplay, on a range of at least 5 patterns of asthmatic reaction, on possible immunopathologic mechanisms, and on their responses to some of the main therapeutic agents. Accumulated experience under clinical conditions, which, to a large extent, preclude experimental studies, is a major source of basic information on this test procedure, and may be a guide to previously unrecognized patterns of clinical asthma that may be discerned, or should be sought, in the patient's history.

The desirability of bronchial provocation tests is often discussed on ethical grounds, which must clearly be an important consideration in tests designed to provoke the clinical manifestations under investigation, and that might provoke undue allergic reactions. In practice, one of the primary obligations of the clinician in asthma, as in any other disease, is to make a precise etiologic diagnosis. This is particularly relevant to allergic disorders, in which avoidance of the causal agent may terminate or reduce the disorder. The provisos that make bronchial provocation tests acceptable for this purpose are that they should be safe and reproducible, and that they should be made under controlled conditions. The test exposure should be less, preferably far less, than that likely to be encountered clinically. Bronchial provocation tests are time-consuming and require much patience; in contrast, quite simple measurements of ventilatory function have provided the basis for the findings discussed here. When these requirements can be met, failure to do the tests could be regarded as an act of omission. Testing also has obvious clinical limitations, and it is within this framework

that the results elicited and their interpretation must be assessed.

Some of our own experience in bronchial provocation tests made for etiologic diagnostic purposes in patients at the Brompton Hospital will be described under the following headings: (1) asthmatic reactions to tests with familiar, common allergens; (2) asthmatic reactions to less familiar, uncommon causes, such as chemical dusts, fumes, and gases; (3) effects of sodium cromoglycate, corticosteroids, and inhaled bronchodilators in relation to each group of tests used; (4) patterns of reactions to tests using a variety of very different agents.

Patients Tested

With few exceptions, the tests were done on inpatients as part of their clinical investigation. Volunteer, healthy control subjects were also tested when possible. Other control data were derived from tests in which the subjects were exposed to a number of agents, each of which was expected to affect some, but not all, subjects.

It was considered unacceptable to expose patients to agents that were not relevant to their potential clinical exposure. The limits this imposed on control information were balanced against the high degree of sensitivity in affected subjects and the often very limited effective test exposures, in contrast to the far heavier and more prolonged exposures tolerated by most apparently unaffected co-workers.

With few exceptions, patients were tested when their ventilatory function was considered satisfactory (tables 1, 2, 6, 7, and 9) and when there was little variation on control days. Whenever possible, the patients were unaware of the nature of the materials to which they were exposed in the course of the tests.

Test Materials

Common allergens were tested as extracts in Coca's fluid, either obtained commercially or prepared in our own laboratories. Chemical dusts, vapors, and gases were produced and tested in the forms in which they were met at work to provide a simulated "occupational" exposure.

Test Concentrations

The object of the etiologic diagnostic test is to establish the smallest exposure capable of eliciting a definite, reproducible reaction. The factors that determine initial test concentrations include assessment of the degree of sensitivity from the clinical history and from skin tests when appropriate, and the known potency of the test agent. Care is needed when unfamiliar materials are tested, and it is our practice to take precautions, particularly with regard to possible toxic or irritant effects of chemical agents, and to initiate the tests with quantities much smaller than those likely to be met at work.

Prick tests were made with extracts of common allergens, and bronchial provocation tests were initiated with the concentration that produces a wheal no larger in diameter than 3 mm. If the initial challenge gave a negative reaction, subsequent tests were made by increasing the period of exposure and/or testing with 10-fold higher concentrations up to 10 mg of freeze-dried extracts per ml or 2.5 to 5 per cent (weight/vol) concentrations of commercial extracts.

Inhalation Procedure

A volume of 5 ml of the extract solution was placed in a Wright nebulizer, and an aerosol was produced by passing O_2 or air through at a flow of 8 liter per min. The same nebulizer was used throughout for each patient, because nebulizers vary in the particle size and volume delivered. The aerosol was passed into a 500-ml rebreathing bag that was linked to a BLB oronasal mask from which the patient inhaled in a natural, unforced way. The effects of differences in procedure have been measured (Woolfe, R., Killian, D., Hargreave, F. E., and Newbase, M. N.: Unpublished data); different doses of inhaled material reach the lungs and are distributed differently, according to whether the subject uses tidal breathing or slow or fast vital capacity efforts, and these can influence the clinical response. Aerosols are also produced by a variety of other methods by other workers; some use closed spirometric systems (3, 9), whereas others administer calculated amounts of aerosol given during a period or a series of repeated, single doses, although these techniques provide little evidence of the amounts reaching the sites of reaction in the bronchi. The dosage in our method, as estimated in terms of the test concentration and duration of exposure, serves to give closely reproducible reactions on repetition of the tests.

Duration of Exposure

The duration of exposure was carefully controlled to prevent unduly severe immediate reactions in particular, and also troublesome late reactions. The inhalation started with a brief period of 30 to 60 sec, followed by a 10-min interval during which the 1-sec forced expiratory volume (FEV_1) and forced vital capacity (FVC) were measured. When there was no clinical reaction or decrease in FEV_1 or FVC, another 1- to 2-min exposure was given. A subsequent 10-min observation interval for measurement of FEV_1 and FVC was then followed, when indicated, by a further 1- to 2-min exposure. In subsequent tests, when there was no immediate reaction during this period and an unduly late reaction was not anticipated, a further 5-min exposure or more was given, providing a total exposure duration of 10 min or more. Ventilatory function tests were performed every 10 to 15 min for as long as 1 hour after the end of the test period and then hourly thereafter. After careful instruction, facilities were made available for some patients to perform the tests themselves during the evening or if awakened at night by symptoms.

Tests with Chemical Agents

The tests were made in a small cubicle that could be well ventilated at the end of the test, and preferably with a small lobby that could be ventilated to prevent escape of test materials into the atmosphere of the laboratory. This was desirable for protection of the staff and because the exquisitely high degree of sensitivity of some patients could result in confusing reactions.

Chemical dusts, vapors, fumes, and gases were not, as a rule, suitable for testing in solution as aerosols. In most cases, little is known about their capacity to elicit reactions; they may be irritant, toxic, insoluble, or highly allergenic. The effects of exposure, however, can be tested by simulating, under controlled conditions, the situation of the occupational or domestic exposure, thus making it possible to test each of a number of agents encountered in a complex exposure. The test result shows whether the particular agent is capable of provoking the subject's symptoms, when used in dosages so limited that it is unlikely to be acting as an irritant. In this respect, the provocation test is more definitive for diagnostic purposes than the demonstration of antibodies, which are evidence of sensitization and may only be suggestive evidence of a causal clinical relationship to the suspected agent. Antibodies to many of the chemical agents have not been found or, as yet, sought.

Tests with Chemical Dusts

Well-dried lactose powder, heated overnight at 105° C, is used as the vehicle for chemical dusts. When tipped from one receiver to another, the mixture gives rise to a cloud of dust, from which the patient inhales for controlled periods of time. The concentration of test agent is determined by the clinical history; our experience shows that the concentration should be very low for highly allergenic dusts, such as the complex salts of platinum encountered in the refining of platinum, and higher for other dusts, such as piperazine hydrochloride. Some dusts, such as wheat and rye flour and sawdusts from different woods, may not require dilution with lactose and can be used in the form in which they are encountered.

Ventilatory Function Tests

The patients were carefully instructed and supervised in the performance of ventilatory function tests. Bronchial reactions were mainly measured by FEV_1 and FVC. The FEV_1 and FVC were measured with a Vitalograph. The best of 3 readings was taken, and after a number of tests, most patients were able to perform the procedure adequately without supervision. Reactions were regarded as positive if the FEV_1 decreased by 15 per cent, and when there were large variations on control days, by a reading 15 per cent less than the value for the corresponding time of day. In tests for reactions in the peripheral lung tissues, as in extrinsic allergic alveolitis, measurements of CO gas transfer factor were useful; such tests were made during a number of the asthmatic reactions, and it was uncommon for there to be any changes.

These simple ventilatory function tests are almost universally available, and it would seem that they are adequate in most cases. More complex methods of testing pulmonary function and of performing the provocation test are likely to provide more information on the nature of the bronchial reactions, but may not necessarily contribute to the clinician's requirement for an unequivocal etiologic diagnostic test.

Patterns of Bronchial Reaction

The asthmatic reactions to provocation tests occur in 2 main patterns, immediate and nonimmediate (1–3, 5, 6, 9–12). Immediate reactions, of which there are at least 2 varieties, develop within minutes, are maximal at approximately 10 to 20 min, and resolve within 1.5 to 2 hours. There are also at least 3 patterns of nonimmediate reaction. The best known of these develops after several hours, is maximal at 5 to 8 hours, and usually resolves within 24 hours,

but may persist for days or weeks. More recently, other patterns of nonimmediate reaction have been observed; one develops after approximately 1 hour and resolves by 3 to 4 hours, and another, a much later asthmatic reaction, develops in the early hours of the morning, with a tendency to recur at approximately the same time on successive nights after a single test. The latter can be described as a recurrent, late reaction (13, 14; Davies, R. J.: Personal communication).

Reproducibility of Reactions

The degree of reaction is determined by the concentration of test material and the duration of exposure. When tests are repeated in the same way, the order of the reactions can be very close, indeed, as close as could be reasonably expected from a biologic test procedure. We have not observed either increased or decreased reactions in the tests made for such clinical purposes, although other workers using other methods have reported either decreased or increased reactions (3, 9). By testing on separate days with a stronger concentration or longer duration of exposure, we have been able to elicit reactions of sufficient magnitude to be unequivocal, without eliciting unnecessarily strong reactions, except on rare occasions. Consequently, there has seldom been a clinical need to reverse the reaction by bronchodilators or to use corticosteroids for prolonged reactions. This has made it possible to observe the evolution of the bronchial responses without modification. This was not always the case when other methods were used and when the order of reaction requiring reversal by treatment might have affected the patterns of bronchial reactivity, as will be discussed later.

Effects of Inhaled Bronchodilators,, Cromolyn Sodium, and Corticosteroids

In patients without undue bronchial lability on control days, given the reproducibility of the reactions, it was possible to examine the effects of inhaled bronchodilators, cromolyn sodium, and corticosteroids on reactions to bronchial challenge. The drug being evaluated was given 10 to 30 min before the allergen challenge, and in cases in which this had no effect, further tests were made with repeated 3 hourly administrations.

Cromolyn sodium was inhaled as a powder in a dose of 20 to 40 mg by means of a Spinhaler; the lactose vehicle was used as a placebo control. Corticosteroids were given by inhalation as a nebulized aerosol of 100 to 200 μg of beclomethasone dipropionate (Becotide®), and the vehicle propellant mixture was used as a placebo control. Isoproterenol and salbutamol were given as nebulized aerosols to assess their effect in reversing the asthmatic reactions.

Asthmatic Reactions to Common Allergens

Most reports on bronchial provocation tests deal with reactions to common allergens administered as aerosols of extract solutions. The reactions elicited will be dealt with in terms of immediate, nonimmediate (late), and dual reactions. Asthma may be classified as extrinsic or cryptogenic (intrinsic). Extrinsic asthma is commonly regarded as occurring in atopic subjects; however, better understanding of the patterns of asthmatic reaction that can be elicited has shown that this is not so and has created a need for terms to describe not only the patterns of reaction, but also their possible mechanisms in the different groups of subjects.

Immediate Asthmatic Reactions

Two possible mechanisms for Type I, immediate, allergic reactions were proposed (15), the first being mediated by the long-familiar reaginic antibody, now known as the immunoglobulin, IgE, and the second, mediated by short-term, sensitizing IgG antibody (STS-IgG). These will be discussed in more detail later. Problems of terminology arise from the fact that, whereas IgE antibody is a hallmark of atopic subjects, who are characterized by their capacity to become readily sensitized by ordinary exposure to common environmental allergens (16), this antibody is not confined to them, and its production may be induced in otherwise nonatopic subjects after intensive exposure to a particular allergen or by peculiarly potent allergens. Reactions mediated by IgE antibody can thus be described as reaginic.

One possible way of classifying extrinsic, immediate asthma is as follows: (*1*) extrinsic, reaginic (IgE), immediate asthma in (*a*) atopic subjects (the majority of those so affected), and (*b*) nonatopic subjects; (*2*) extrinsic, nonreaginic, STS-IgG, immediate asthma. There is now evidence that STS-IgG antibody may be present against common allergens, with or without the associated presence of IgE antibody (16–19). A role for STS-IgG antibody in the production of asthma is beginning to be understood (19), and it is now necessary to consider the possibility of reactions mediated by it, both without associated IgE antibody, mainly in nonatopic subjects, and in association with IgE antibody, mainly in atopic subjects.

Extrinsic, Reaginic (IgE), Immediate Asthma

The history, skin tests, and measurement of specific IgE antibody by the radioallergosorbent test (RAST) usually provide sufficient information about a possible causal relationship of relevant allergens to the patients' symptoms, although some workers contend that bronchial provocation tests are necessary for definitive etiologic diagnosis and as a guide to hyposensitization (7, 11). A better correlation has been found between bronchial reactions and the RAST than with skin (intracutaneous) tests (20–23); however, using the prick test with 4 common inhalant allergens, others have found a good correlation between prick test and bronchial reaction (21). No bronchial reactions were elicited in subjects with negative prick tests, in contrast to positive bronchial reactions in 9 per cent of subjects with a RAST test regarded as negative. Better correlation was found between the degree of bronchial and skin test reactivity than with the RAST (21). Extracts of common allergens are not, at present, adequately standardized, so that correlations among results of the various tests must take this into account. Nevertheless, significant associations have been found between the RAST and skin, nasal, and bronchial tests and the clinical history (21–24).

A typical example of an immediate asthmatic reaction to an inhalation test with an extract of *Dermatophagoides* species, to which the subject was allergic and against which specific IgE antibody was present by prick test and by RAST, is shown in figure 1. Also shown is the inhibitory effect of cromolyn sodium and the absence of effect of beclomethasone dipropionate given by inhalation before the test. The features of immediate reactions to common allergens will be contrasted later with those to a variety of chemical agents.

Extrinsic, Nonreaginic (STS-IgG), Immediate Asthma

In a group of 8 subjects who had an immediate cutaneous reaction to a prick test using an extract of *Dermatophagoides pteronyssinus*, and in whom STS-IgG, but not IgE, antibody was demonstrable, immediate asthmatic reactions were elicited by bronchial provocation tests (19). These subjects were also unresponsive to cromolyn sodium, in contrast to its blocking effect in those with specific IgE antibody and increased

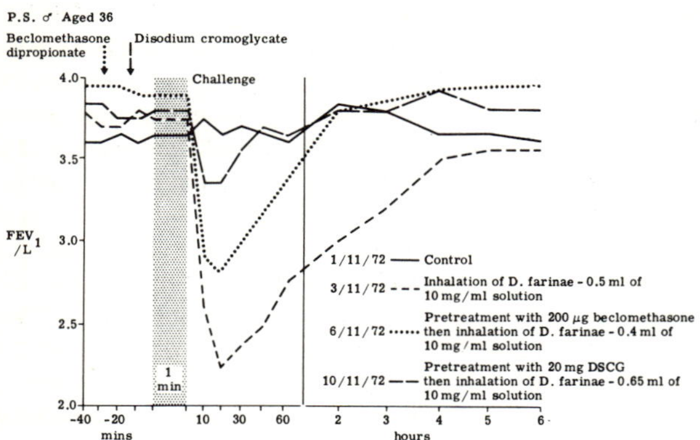

Fig. 1. Patient PS. There was no reaction to control, but an immediate asthmatic reaction to aerosol inhalation of an extract of *Dermatophagoides* sp in a sensitive subject. The reaction was blocked by pretest inhalation of cromolyn sodium, but not by 200 µg of beclomethasone dipropionate; (————) = control; (— — —) = *Dermatophagoides* sp extracts; (— — —) = pretest inhalation of cromolyn sodium; (· · · · ·) = pretest inhalation of beclomethasone dipropionate; FEV_1 = 1-sec forced expiratory volume; DSCG = disodium cromoglycate.

concentrations of IgE in the serum. The test procedure consisted of inhalation at one test session of the extract up to the full skin test strength for 20 min. This was a somewhat more intensive challenge than we have tended to use for such extracts. Such differences illustrate the importance, in analysis, of the method of testing. Differences in results may be related to the greater sensitizing capacity of the IgE than the IgG antibody and must be taken into account in any explanation of the apparent discordance between tests for IgE antibody and reactions to allergen exposure.

Isolated, Nonimmediate ("Late") Asthmatic Reactions

"Late" asthmatic reactions to provocation tests without evidence of preceding immediate reactions, as measured by the FEV_1, have been elicited by us mainly in nonatopic subjects. A typical example (figure 2) was seen in a nonatopic maltster who was sensitive to, had precipitins against, and gave Type III skin test reactions to extracts of *Aspergillus clavatus*, which contaminated the barley with which he worked. The reaction developed gradually and progressively, starting 2 to 3 hours after the test. Temporary reversibility of the reaction after isoproterenol inhalation was also evident. A number of similar reactions were elicited in nonatopic bird fanciers, who had also given typical Type III skin test reactions macroscopically and histologically (25, 26). In severe bronchial reactions, systemic reactions consisting of fever, malaise, and myalgia were present together with a leukocytosis and, in some cases, a moderate increase in the absolute blood eosinophil count.

The presence of precipitins and Type III skin test reactions that had a speed of appearance and a duration like those of the late asthmatic reaction suggested that the bronchial reaction might also be a Type III reaction. Both the Type III skin test and the late bronchial reaction could be effectively inhibited by corticosteroid drugs. In subjects with precipitins, the development of the late skin test reaction compatible with a Type III reaction was preceded by an immediate skin test reaction. When this occurred in atopic subjects with IgE antibody, as in allergic bronchopulmonary aspergillosis, the bronchial provocation test elicited immediate, followed by late, asthmatic reactions, as described in the previous section. In nonatopic subjects, however, the elicitation of an immediate skin test reaction tended to require a stronger dose and, as a rule, intracutaneous, rather than prick tests; IgE antibody was not readily demonstrable. It is postulated that other mast cell sensitizing antibodies, possibly STS-IgG antibody in one or more

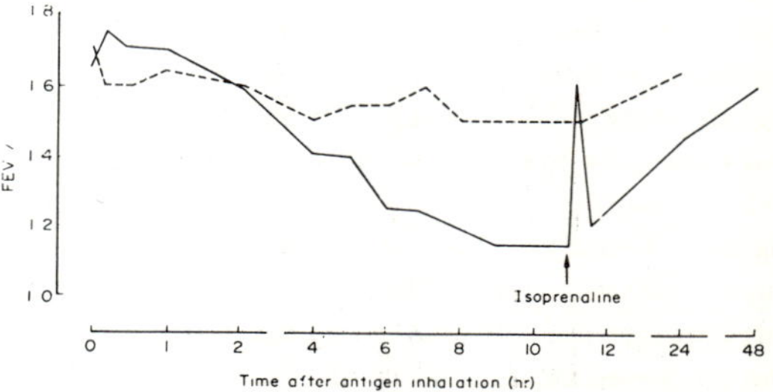

Fig. 2. There was no reaction to control inhalation of an aerosol of Coca's fluid, but a late asthmatic reaction to the test with an extract of *Aspergillus clavatus*, showing temporary reversibility by inhaled isoproterenol.

of the IgG subclasses, may be responsible. This antibody would be expected to mediate less release of tissue mediators from the reacting cells and, consequently, less evidence of an immediate bronchial reaction, at least with the challenge doses we used. That immediate reactions may, in fact, be occurring is indicated by the findings in subjects with asthma due to western red cedar, who showed evidence from the maximal expiratory flow at 50 per cent of vital capacity and 60 per cent of total lung volume of immediate changes in airway function not detected by measurements of FEV_1 or airway resistance (27, 28). If, indeed, the bronchial reaction is mediated by Type III allergy, such a reaction could, perhaps, serve as the immediate introductory component for the late reaction. Other possibilities must be considered and will be discussed later.

Dual, Immediate, and Nonimmediate Asthmatic Reactions to Extracts of Aspergillus fumigatus

Patients with allergic bronchopulmonary aspergillosis having both reagins and precipitins and giving typical Type III skin test reactions, as shown macroscopically and on histologic immunofluorescence examination (25), provide classic examples of dual asthmatic reactions, in which, as in the skin test, there is a typical immediate asthmatic reaction, followed by a late asthmatic reaction after an interval of some hours of apparent normality (29) (figure 3).

The findings in the immediate reactions in 21 subjects and the nonimmediate asthmatic reactions in 15 of them are presented in tables 1 and 2. In the immediate asthmatic reactions, highly significant differences were found in the following observations: the decreases in FEV_1 and FVC; the greater decrease in FEV_1 than FVC, also reflected in the decrease in FEV_1/FVC; the

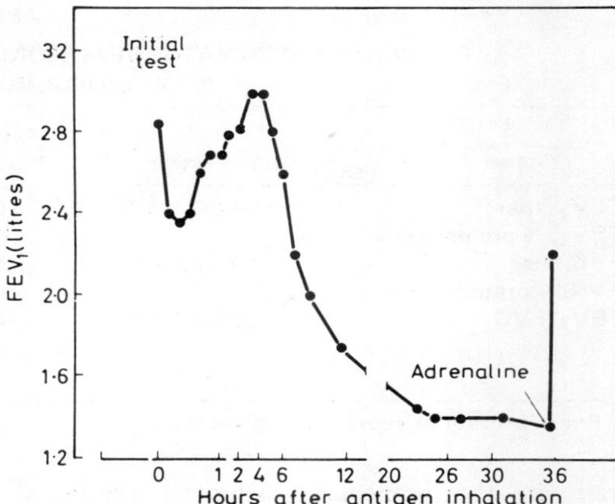

Fig. 3. Dual asthmatic reaction in a patient with allergic bronchopulmonary aspergillosis to inhalation of an aerosol of an extract of *Aspergillus fumigatus;* $FEV_1 = $ 1-sec forced expiratory volume.

reversibility of the reaction to more than 90 per cent of pretest values by inhalation of isoproterenol. The efficacy of the bronchodilator was further shown by FEV_1/FVC, for which there was no significant difference between values obtained before the test and those obtained after reversal of the reaction by isoproterenol.

In the nonimmediate asthmatic reactions, highly significant differences were found in the following measurements: the decreases in FEV_1, FVC, and FEV_1/FVC; the reversibility of the decreases in FEV_1 and FVC by isoproterenol inhalation, although this was only to 73.6 per cent of the pretest FEV_1 value. In the case of FEV_1/FVC, there were highly significant differences in the decrease after challenge and in the values obtained after inhalation of isoproterenol. It should be noted, however, that the ratio after inhalation of isoproterenol was highly significantly less than the pretest value; by con-

TABLE 1

IMMEDIATE ASTHMATIC REACTIONS IN 21 SUBJECTS WITH ALLERGIC BRONCHOPULMONARY ASPERGILLOSIS

Test	Pretest	After Bronchial Provocation Test	After Isoproterenol Inhalation	P Value (Paired t Tests)
FEV_1, liter	1.86 ± 0.6	1.2 ± 0.5		< 0.001
FEV_1, % pretest value		64.4 ± 10.7	91.4 ± 3.3	< 0.001
FVC, liter	3.20 ± 0.8	2.43 ± 1.0		< 0.001
FVC, % pretest value		78.3 ± 8.5	93.6 ± 20.9	< 0.02, > 0.01
FEV_1/FVC	59.47 ± 9.8	48.0 ± 8.9		< 0.001
		48.0 ± 8.9	57.9 ± 9.0	< 0.001
	59.47 ± 9.8		57.9 ± 9.0	No significant difference

Definition of abbreviations: FEV_1 = 1-sec forced expiratory volume; FVC = forced vital capacity.

TABLE 2
"LATE" ASTHMATIC REACTIONS IN 15 SUBJECTS WITH ALLERGIC BRONCHOPULMONARY ASPERGILLOSIS

Test	Pretest	After Bronchial Provocation Test	After Isoproterenol Inhalation	P Value (Paired t Test)
FEV_1, liter	1.86 ± 0.52	0.87 ± 0.50		< 0.001
FEV_1, % pretest value		47.7 ± 11.4	73.6 ± 10.9	< 0.001
FVC, liter	2.97 ± 1.33	1.99 ± 0.84		< 0.001
FVC, % pretest value		63.0 ± 13.7	86.4 ± 10.4	< 0.001
FEV_1/FVC	59.6 ± 9.6	42.3 ± 7.5		< 0.001
		42.3 ± 7.5	49.3 ± 9.8	$< 0.01, > 0.001$
	59.6 ± 9.6		49.3 ± 9.8	< 0.001

For definition of abbreviations, see table 1.

trast, in the immediate asthmatic reactions, FEV_1/FVC after isoproterenol was not significantly different from the pretest value. These findings show that the late reaction is less well reversed than the immediate reaction; furthermore, in some cases, the reversibility of the late reaction was only of short duration, compared to the permanent reversal of the immediate reaction. The greater reversibility of both FEV_1 and FVC in the immediate, as against the late, reactions was highly significant ($P < 0.001$). There was no significant difference between the 2 groups in initial FEV_1, FVC, or FEV_1/FVC, showing that they began from comparable baseline values.

Pretest inhalation of cromolyn sodium blocked the immediate and, in some instances, the late asthmatic reaction as well. In patients receiving systemic corticosteroid treatment, immediate, but not late, reactions were elicited.

Dual Asthmatic Reactions to Baker's Flour

Baker's asthma is a well-known entity in which there are immediate cutaneous and bronchial reactions to aqueous extracts. For present purposes, Baker's asthma provides an example of dual asthmatic reactions. In pursuance of occupational exposure type tests, we tested 2 bakers with the actual flours to which they were exposed at work and to which they gave dual asthmatic reactions (Hendrick, D. J., Davies, R. J., and Pepys, J.: Unpublished data). In one, who reacted to both wheat and rye flour, prick tests with aqueous extracts produced an immediate reaction, and intracutaneous tests produced dual reactions. In the second patient, who was tested only with wheat flour, a positive precipitin test was obtained, and an immediate reaction was elicited by prick test; an intracutaneous test was not done. The patterns of these dual asthmatic reactions are shown in figure 4. Both re-

actions were blocked by cromolyn sodium, whereas beclomethasone dipropionate had an inhibitory effect on the late reaction, and no effect on the immediate reaction. In tests with extracts of house dust (figure 31), there are reports of the same inhibitory effects of cromolyn sodium on dual reactions, and of systemic corticosteroids on the late reaction only (4, 12). It is suggested that blocking the immediate reaction

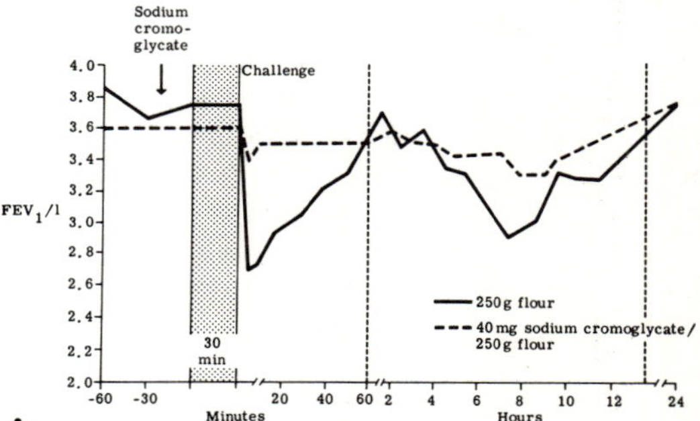

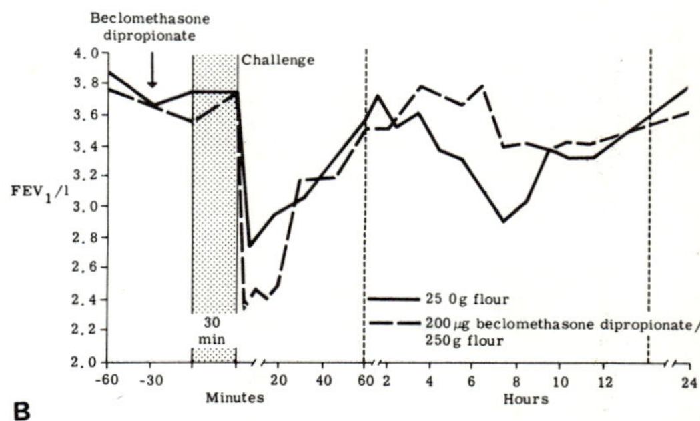

Fig. 4. A. Immediate and late asthmatic reactions to an "occupational" type exposure test with wheat flour. Both reactions were blocked by pre-test inhalation of 40 mg of cromolyn sodium; $FEV_1 = 1$-sec forced expiratory volume. B. Pretest inhalation of 200 μg of beclomethasone dipropionate blocked the late reaction and had no effect on the immediate reaction.

may interfere with a necessary introductory mechanism for the late reaction, by analogy with the dual mechanisms of the Type III allergic reaction. Blocking of "isolated" late reactions by pretest inhalation of cromolyn sodium has been reported (30), and it was postulated that an immediate reaction not measurable by changes in FEV_1 might have been present; if so, blocking this reaction could inhibit the development of the late asthmatic reaction, and as discussed in the previous section, evidence of immediate asthmatic reactions in such cases has been reported (27, 28).

Methods of Testing for Asthmatic Reactions to Chemical Dusts

Asthma Due to Complex Salts of Platinum

The complex salts of platinum, such as ammonium and sodium hexa- and tetrachlorplatinate, are mainly encountered in the refining of platinum and are among the most potent allergens known. Careful prick tests with solutions of these compounds show that positive reactions can be elicited in sensitive subjects with concentrations of 10^{-9} g per ml. Because the prick test introduces approximately 3×10^{-6} ml, the absolute skin test dose is less than 10^{-15} g, or approximately 100,000 molecules or fewer (31, 32). Despite this very high degree of sensitivity, careful occupational type provocation tests can be made safely and reproducibly.

In 16 workers who were investigated, 10 gave positive prick test reactions; 7 of 11 gave positive reactions to nasal tests, and 9 gave positive bronchial reactions (31). The bronchial tests were made with great care. Starting with 4 mg of platinum salt per kg of lactose, it was found that 40 mg of platinum salt per kg of lactose was an effective concentration. The different salts were tested to establish their allergenicity in individual subjects. Immediate, late, or dual reactions were produced in different subjects (figure 5). The absence of reaction to the lactose vehicle, the reproducibility of immediate reactions on repetition of the tests with the platinum salt, and the blocking of the reaction by pretest inhalation of cromolyn sodium are shown in figure 6. The immediate reaction to the platinum salt was similar to that elicited by common allergens in speed of appearance, duration, and inhibition by cromolyn sodium.

The differences among patients in their reactions to different platinum salts are shown in table 3, along with differences in the duration of exposure required to elicit reactions. Ammonium tetrachlorplatinate, $(NH_4)_2PtCl_4$, was the most potent of the salts and provoked reactions in all subjects. The least potent of the salts, Na_2PtCl_6, produced no reaction in 5 subjects after exposures as long as 30 min. In Patients 5 and 6, $(NH_4)_2PtCl_4$ provoked late asthmatic reactions, with neither subject reacting to the other 2 salts. The reproducibility of the reactions and the differences in the duration of challenge used for different subjects are shown in table 4. Also shown are the decreases in FEV_1 elicited in the initial test, and in the final test made after a lactose placebo and after block of the reaction by cromolyn sodium; all of these decreases were of an acceptably comparable order.

These findings show the usefulness of this form of test in distinguishing which, of a number of possible occupational agents, is more likely to be clinically relevant. This point was emphasized further in tests using dusts of antimicrobial agents.

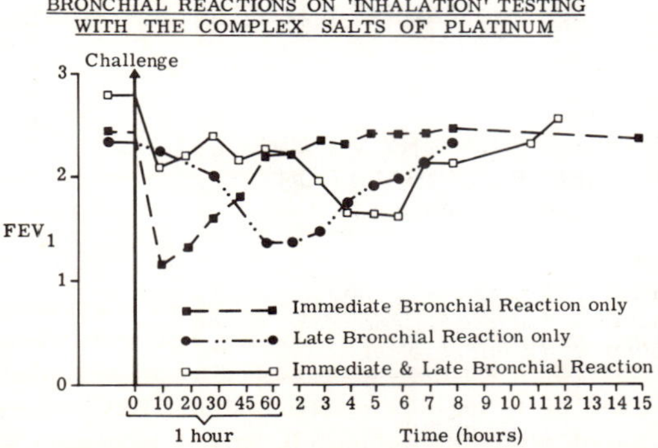

Fig. 5. Immediate, late, and dual patterns of reaction to occupational type tests with complex salts of platinum; $FEV_1 = $ 1-sec forced expiratory volume.

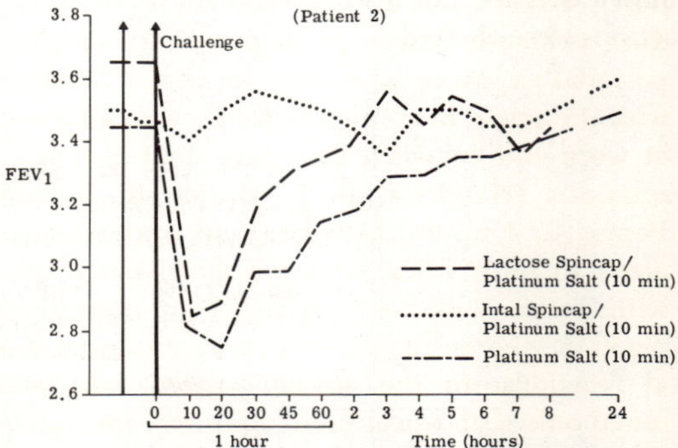

Fig. 6. Immediate asthmatic reactions to complex salts of platinum were blocked by pretest inhalation of cromolyn sodium (Intal®), but not by lactose placebo; $FEV_1 = $ 1-sec forced expiratory volume.

TABLE 3
COMPARISON OF ASTHMATIC REACTIONS TO COMPLEX PLATINUM SALTS

Patient	$(NH_4)_2PtCl_6$ Duration of Exposure *(min)*	Decrease in FEV_1 *(%)*	$(NH_4)_2PtCl_4$ Duration of Exposure *(min)*	Decrease in FEV_1 *(%)*	Na_2PtCl_6 Duration of Exposure *(min)*	Decrease in FEV_1 *(%)*
1	15	38	10	49	10	35
2	4	28	5	45	30	16
3	6	31	10	38	15	23
4	10	32	10	34	30	0
5	30	0	30	18*	30	0
6	30	0	30	15.5*	30	0
7	30	26	15	30	30	0
8	15	29	20	29	20	10
9	30	17	30	17	30	0

Definition of abbreviations: $(NH_4)_2PtCl_6$ = ammonium hexachlorplatinate; $(NH_4)_2PtCl_4$ = ammonium tetrachlorplatinate; Na_2PtCl_6 = disodium chlorplatinate; FEV_1 = 1-sec forced expiratory volume.

* Late asthmatic reactions.

Asthma Due to Manufacture of Antimicrobial Drugs

The analytic value of the occupational type test in identifying the cause of occupational asthma is well illustrated by the findings in workers engaged in the manufacture of antimicrobial drugs, who are exposed to a number of possible causes of asthma. Tests were initiated with concentrations of 10 mg of antimicrobial drug powder per 250 g of lactose. The concentration was increased 10-fold on successive days, or at intervals of days, to the effective concentration of 1 to 10 g per 250 g of lactose. We would now use such concentrations in future cases in which the patient's history does not suggest undue sensitivity. The duration of exposure required was 30 to 60 min. The large number of agents to be tested and our unfamiliarity with them meant that the period required for investigation of each in turn was lengthy, lasting several weeks in most cases. In 4 of 5 workers, late asthmatic reactions were elicited.

The production of late asthmatic reactions (14) to unpurified commercial ampicillin (figure 7), with only a small reaction to purified ampicillin and to unpurified, but not to purified, 6-amino-penicillanic acid preparations (figure 8) showed that this patient was sensitive to an impurity in these preparations. The late reaction was blocked by pretest inhalation of beclomethasone dipropionate (figure 9). Another worker had comparable and reproducible late asthmatic reactions to both purified and commercial ampicillins (figure 10). In this subject, a more slowly developing, reproducible, late reaction to 6-amino-penicillanic acid (figure 11) was similar in the time of maximal decrease and resolution between the reactions to those produced with commercial and purified preparations. These findings suggest that the side chain (phenylglycine) added to the 6-amino-penicillanic acid nucleus was an important allergenic determinant in this patient's reaction to the ampicillin. The patient was therefore sensitive to antigenic determinants

TABLE 4
PER CENT CHANGE IN 1-SEC FORCED EXPIRATORY VOLUME (FEV_1) AND DURATION OF CHALLENGE IN INHALATION TESTS WITH AMMONIUM HEXACHLORPLATINATE

Patient	Challenge Only (No Treatment) ΔFEV_1 *(% initial value)*	ΔFEV_1 after Pretreatment with Cromolyn Sodium *(% initial value)*	ΔFEV_1 after Pretreatment with Lactose Placebo *(% initial value)*	Duration of Challenge *(min)*
DL	38	7.5	41	15
CW	28	19	38	4
RB	31	7	28.5	6
FS	32	0	20.3	10
SH	17	0	36	13

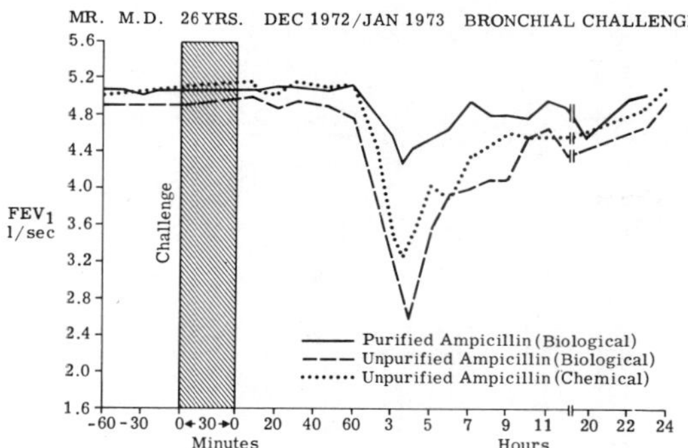

Fig. 7. Late asthmatic reactions to occupational type test with unpurified ampicillins, and small reaction to purified preparation; $FEV_1 = 1$-sec forced expiratory volume.

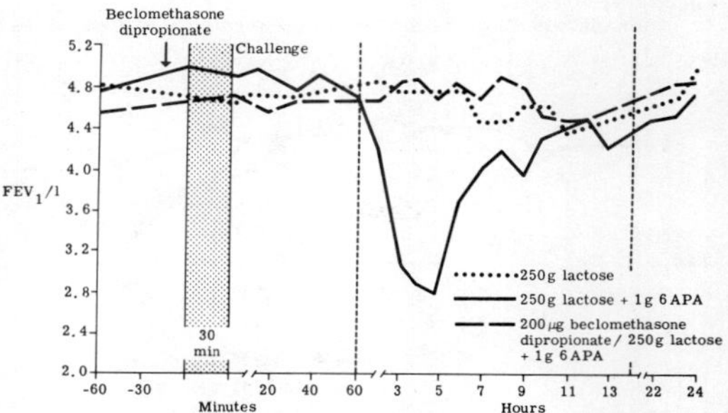

Fig. 9. No reaction to occupational type test with lactose vehicle, but late asthmatic reaction to test with 6-amino-penicillanic acid (6APA). The late reaction was inhibited by pretest inhalation of 200 µg of beclomethasone dipropionate; $FEV_1 = 1$-sec forced expiratory volume.

in the antimicrobial drug preparations themselves and not, as in the previous case, to impurities. In this patient, 3 hourly inhalation of beclomethasone dipropionate was required to block the reactions. After a single test, he also had a late reaction that appeared in the early hours of the morning the day after the test, and less strongly recurred again, at the same time the following night, with no reaction at other times of the day (figure 12). In other patients, this pattern has been observed to recur to a progressively decreasing degree for a number of nights (figures 26 and 27). It is necessary to recognize this phenomenon so as to allow time for the reaction to the particular test to have ceased completely before proceeding to further tests. Care is also needed in patients who come in for testing after recent occupational exposure, to which they may still be reacting in this way. This reaction may also be relevant to the

common clinical histories of nocturnal asthma and to episodes of persistent asthma in response to known or unrecognized exposure.

The differences among subjects in their reactions to the different agents and their reactions to oral ingestion of the relevant agent are listed in table 5. Oral ingestion (figure 13) of ampicillin and benzyl-penicillin elicited late asthmatic reactions comparable to those seen with the inhalation tests, as well as other allergic manifestations. It is probable that the patients swallowed some of the antimicrobial drug dusts during the inhalation tests, and it is possible that the asthmatic reaction either completely or in part might have been elicited in this way.

In a worker from a different factory, tests with all of the agents described to which he was exposed were negative, but a late asthmatic reac-

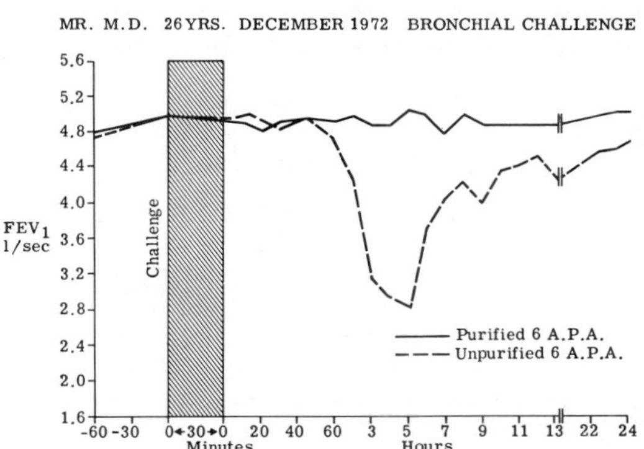

Fig. 8. Late asthmatic reaction to occupational type test with unpurified 6-amino-penicillanic acid (6 APA), and no reaction to purified preparation; $FEV_1 = 1$-sec forced expiratory volume.

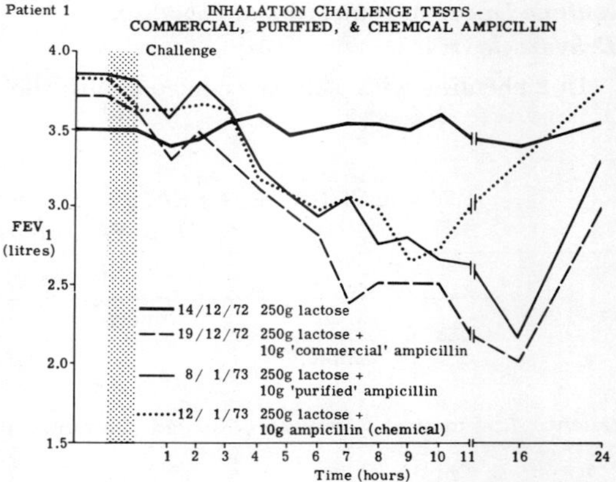

Fig. 10. No reaction to occupational type test with lactose, but late comparable asthmatic reactions to commercial and purified ampicillins. $FEV_1 = 1$-sec forced expiratory volume.

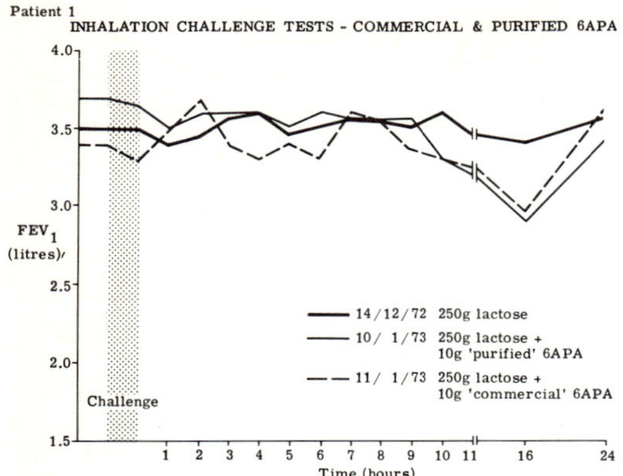

Fig. 11. Comparable late asthmatic reactions to commercial and purified 6-amino-penicillanic acid (6 APA). FEV_1 = 1-sec forced expiratory volume.

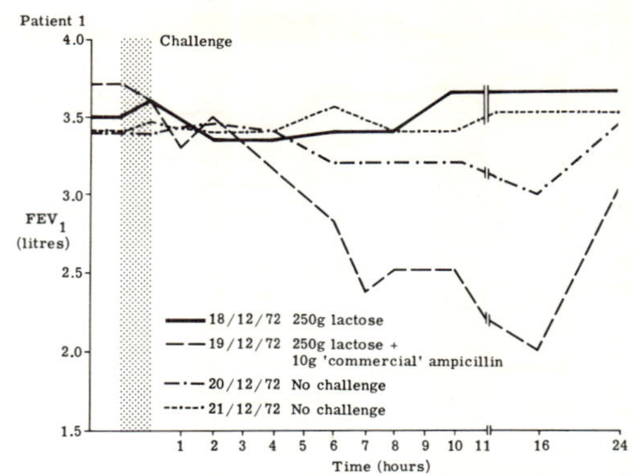

Fig. 12. Recurrent, nocturnal, late, asthmatic reaction at night, the day after the bronchial provocation test.

tion was elicited in tests with the macrolide antimicrobial agent, spiramycin (32a). The reproducibility of the late asthmatic reaction on repeat tests is shown in figure 14. The high degree of sensitivity that can be present is shown by this patient's asthmatic reaction, presumably to material contaminating the clothes of his wife, who continued to do clerical work in the factory. The patient's asthmatic reactions to the eating of eggs raised the possibility that spiramycin, used as an antimicrobial drug in laying hens and present in egg white at 3 ppm, might have been responsible.

In these cases, the relationship of the asthma to the occupation was evident from the history, but precise etiologic diagnosis would have been difficult, if not impossible, without the bronchial provocation tests.

Asthma Due to Manufacture of Piperazine Dihydrochloride

In 2 chemists with asthma associated with the manufacture of piperazine dihydrochloride, the approach to tests with a material of unknown potency is shown in the way an acceptable effective challenge concentration was established (33). Occupational type tests were made with a mixture of piperazine dihydrochloride powder, starting with 40 mg per kg of lactose, increasing to 400 mg, 4 g, 100 g, 250 g, and then to the effective concentration of 500 g per kg of lactose. The duration of exposure to the dust was 20 to 30 min. Future tests with this material can therefore be based on these findings, although in each case, a history indicating high or low degree of sensitivity must be taken into account. When degree of sensitivity is not known, it is better to begin with very low concentrations of the agent and arrive at an effective concentration by careful, patient testing.

The absence of reaction to the lactose control and the comparable order, on repetition of the test, of the speed of appearance of the late asthmatic reactions to piperazine dihydrochloride are shown in figure 15. Inhalation of cromo-

TABLE 5

INHALATION TEST REACTIONS TO AMPICILLIN, 6-AMINO-PENICILLANIC ACID (6APA), AND BENZYL PENICILLIN

	Late Asthmatic Reactions to Inhalation and Oral Challenge							Oral Challenge	
	Inhalation Challenge							Commercial	
	Ampicillin			6APA		Benzyl Penicillin			
Patient	Commerical	Chemical	Purified	Commercial	Purified	Commercial	Purified	Ampicillin	Benzyl Penicillin
1	+	+	+	±	±			0	
2	+	+	±	+	0	+		+	
3	+		+	0	0	+	+		+
4	0					0			

Definition of symbols: + = marked late asthmatic reactions; ± = weak late asthmatic reactions; 0 = no reaction.

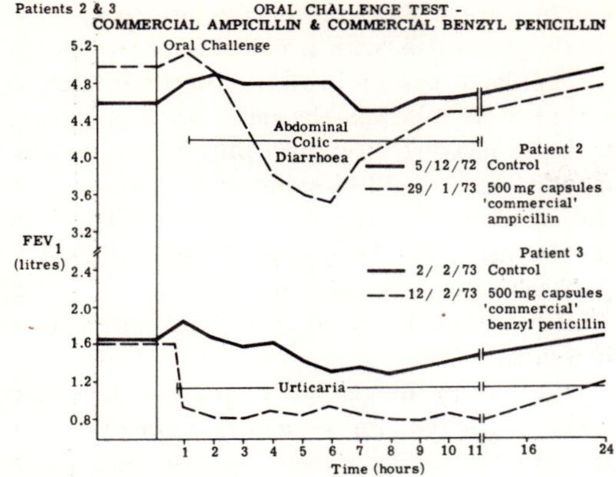

Fig. 13. Late asthmatic reactions to oral ingestion of ampicillin and benzyl-penicillin, comparable to those of the occupational type inhalation test. Note gastrointestinal and urticarial reactions as well.

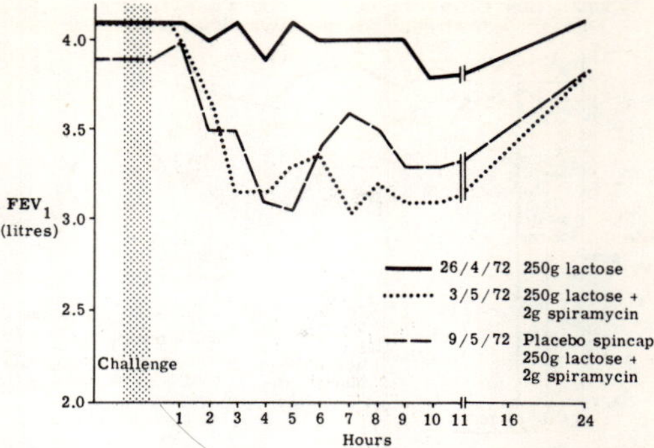

Fig. 14. No reaction to occupational type test with lactose, but late asthmatic reaction to spiramycin and comparable reaction to repeat test made after inhalation of lactose placebo. A Spinhaler was used as control for the test with cromolyn sodium, which had no effect on the reaction.

lyn sodium before and 3 hours after the test effectively inhibited the reaction, whereas when given only before the test, it did not. Poor reversibility of the late reaction by inhalation of isoproterenol is also shown.

Asthmatic Reactions to Wood Dusts

Bronchial provocation tests for the investigation of specific sensitivity to particular wood dusts have been made with the wood dusts themselves and with various extracts (27, 28, 34–36). These tests have elicited immediate, late, and dual reactions to such wood dusts as oak, mahogany, cedar, and iroko.

The late asthmatic reaction shown in figure 16 was elicited by 30-min occupational type exposure to the sawdust of iroko, but not to that of western red cedar, and responded poorly to bronchodilators. This reaction was not blocked by pretest inhalation of cromolyn sodium. In the

same patient, immediate asthmatic reactions were elicited by tests with a carbol saline and a toluene extract, showing how differences in the pattern of asthmatic reactions may result from the form in which the agent is tested.

The reactions of a patient in whom the roles of the wood dusts were reversed are shown in figure 17. In this case, a late asthmatic reaction was elicited by the western red cedar, but not by the iroko. In asthma produced by western red cedar (*Thuja plicata*), the active agent has been identified as plicatic acid, a small molecular component of the wood (27, 28). Here too, the occupational type test helped to identify the causal agent from among a mixture of possible causes.

Asthma Due to Gaseous Emanations of Toluene Diisocyanate

Toluene diisocyanate (TDI) is a classic example of a liquid that is not suitable for test-

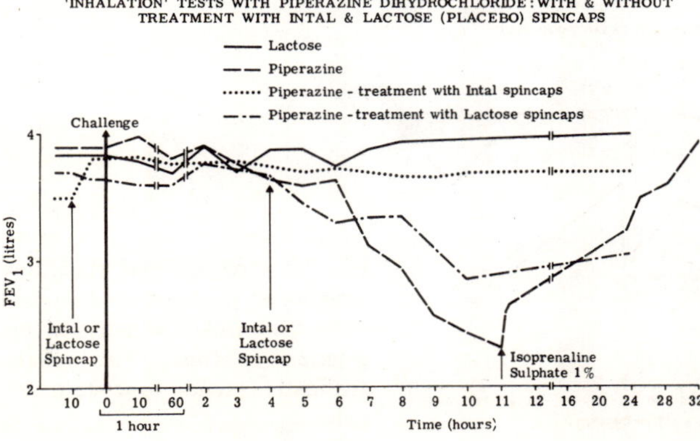

Fig. 15. No reaction to occupational type test with lactose, but late asthmatic reaction to piperazine dihydrochloride. The reaction was blocked by cromolyn sodium given before the test and 3 hours after the test, but not by lactose placebo. Note the poor reversibility of the late reaction by inhaled isoproterenol.

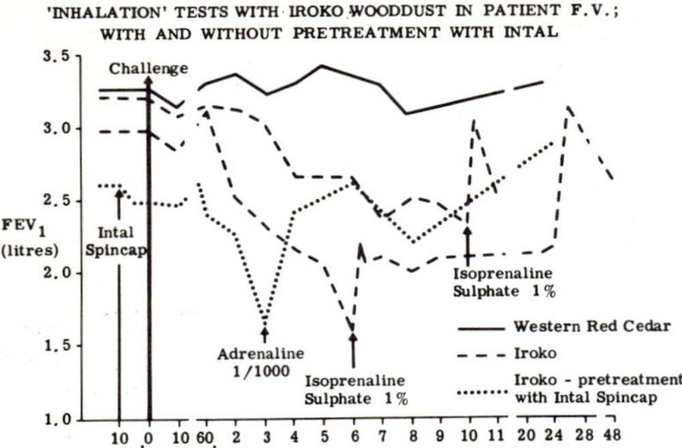

Fig. 16. Occupational type exposure to wood dusts of western red cedar and iroko. There was no reaction to the western red cedar, but there were late asthmatic reactions to 2 tests with the iroko dust and to a third test in which cromolyn sodium (Intal) given beforehand had no effect.

ing as an aerosol, because it is highly potent and cannot be satisfactorily diluted in an aqueous vehicle. This material is well known for its capacity to induce and provoke severe, persistent, and often refractory asthma in subjects heavily exposed at work, particularly to large spills. It may also sensitize subjects at much lower levels of exposure. The currently accepted factory atmospheric concentration is 0.02 ppm. It is important, however, to distinguish between levels that may sensitize and may be low, and those that can elicit reactions in already sensitized subjects; the latter concentrations are far lower, e.g., < 0.001 ppm in provocation tests. Because few exposed subjects are affected and develop increasingly high degrees of sensitivity to minimal exposure, it is probable that allergic mechanisms are responsible, rather than, or in addition to, irritant effects.

The occupational type exposure test to TDI is of great value (37). We have performed the test in 2 ways. First, use of a 2-part (pot) polyurethane varnish, with which the subject paints for regulated periods of time with the varnish as a control, is followed the next day by painting with the mixture of varnish plus TDI as recommended for use. The second method consists of the inhalation of fumes containing TDI from the burning, in the course of soldering, of a polyurethane film used for coating the wire. This has been described as an "old hazard in a new guise" (38).

Exposure to the gaseous emanations from the varnish elicited reproducible, immediate, or late reactions. The immediate reaction (figure 18) was blocked by pretest inhalation of cromolyn sodium. Late reactions were blocked by 3 hourly administration of either cromolyn sodium or beclomethasone dipropionate (figure 19).

Inhalation of the fumes from the soldering of polyurethane-coated wires used in the manufacture of transistors for television sets elicited late reactions that were also produced in the same subjects by the test with the mixture of varnish plus TDI. In some patients with suspected sensitivity to TDI, higher concentrations were sometimes needed to elicit reactions in patients with suggestive histories; therefore, whereas a positive reaction can be taken as evidence that the TDI could be a cause of the asthma, a negative test may yet have to be regarded with reserve.

A series of 5 workers exposed to very low concentrations of TDI in a printing factory dealing with plastics were found to be sensitive in our tests. The test thus confirmed what had been suspected from the fact that the material was being used for special inks, and made it possible to deal practically with a known, rather than an unproved, problem.

An extension of these findings was our obser-

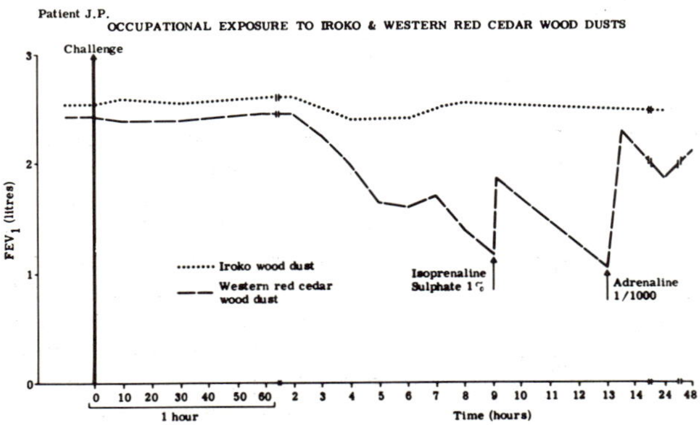

Fig. 17. Occupational type test with wood dusts of western red cedar and iroko. There was no reaction to iroko, but a late asthmatic reaction to western red cedar.

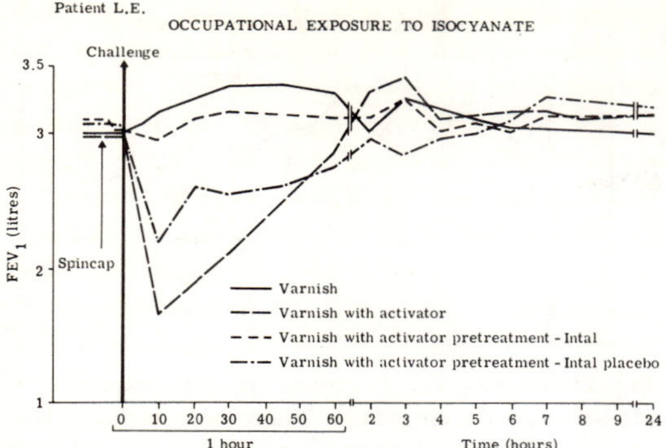

Fig. 18. Patient LE. Occupational type exposure to toluene di-isocyanate (TDI). There was no reaction to the control test with polyurethane varnish, but an immediate asthmatic reaction to the test with varnish plus TDI. Pretest inhalation of cromolyn sodium, but not lactose placebo, blocked the reaction.

vation that a group of 3 subjects were sensitized to TDI by exposure to exhaust fumes from a neighboring factory in which polyurethane foams were manufactured (Carroll, K. B., and Pepys, J.: Unpublished data). The fumes were aspirated into the air conditioning system of the factory in which the affected subjects were working (figure 20). The history of the presenting patient was of very severe asthma that was related to his place of work. His own factory appeared to be blameless, and further questioning revealed the presence of the neighboring factory. The occupational type test for TDI enabled us to make a definite etiologic diagnosis in 2 other workers,

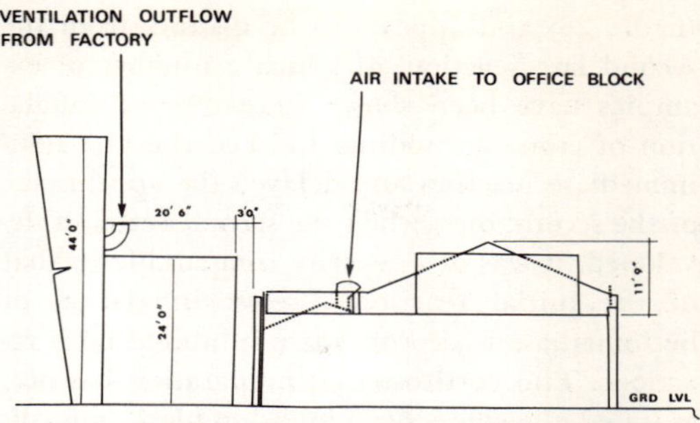

Fig. 20. Schematic illustration of a factory that emanated toluene di-isocyanate fumes and the air intake of the office block in which the subjects became sensitized. GRD LVL = ground level; ' = feet; " = inches.

whereas a fourth worker from the same factory with chronic bronchitis gave a negative reaction.

In the presenting case, there was no reaction to the polyurethane varnish itself (figure 21). The patient had 2 forms of nonimmediate asthmatic reaction to the test with the varnish plus TDI. One reaction started after 1 hour, was maximal at 2 to 3 hours, and showed marked reversal at 5 hours; it was followed by the progressive development of a second late reaction that was maximal at approximately 16 hours, when it began to resolve. The first nonimmediate reaction described here has also been observed in other cases in response to other allergens (30),

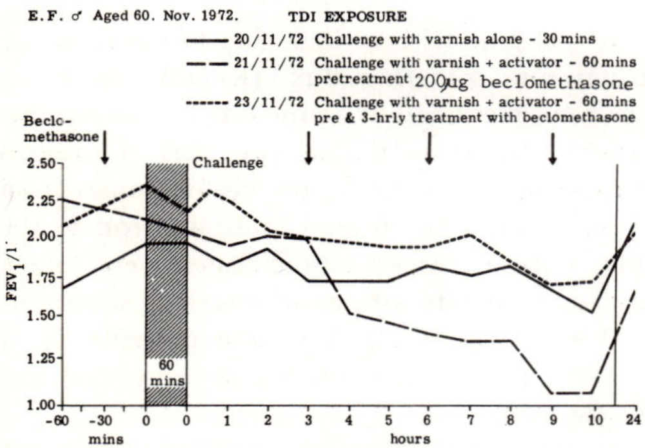

Fig. 19. Patient EF. Occupational type exposure to toluene di-isocyanate (TDI). There was no reaction to the test with polyurethane varnish. The late asthmatic reaction to the test with varnish plus TDI was not blocked by pretreatment with 200 µg of beclomethasone dipropionate, but was blocked by pretreatment and 3 hourly administration of the drug.

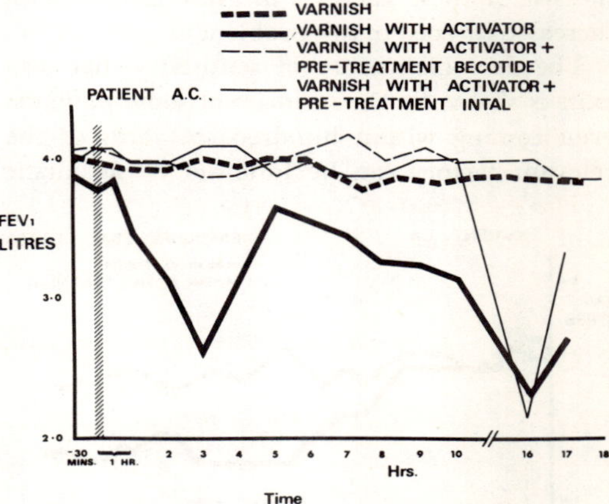

Fig. 21. Patient AC. Occupational type exposure to toluene di-isocyanate (TDI). There was no reaction to the test with polyurethane varnish, but 2 consecutive nonimmediate asthmatic reactions to the test with varnish plus TDI. Pretest administration of 40 mg of cromolyn sodium blocked the first nonimmediate reaction only. Pretest beclomethasone dipropionate (200 µg) blocked both reactions.

(figure 28) and appears to be distinct from the second late reaction, of which a number of examples have been shown here. Pretest inhalation of cromolyn sodium blocked the first nonimmediate reaction and delayed the appearance of the second one; when the second reaction developed, it was of a severity comparable to that of the initial reaction. Pretest inhalation of beclomethasone dipropionate inhibited both reactions. This corticosteroid preparation has not, as stated elsewhere, been found to block immediate asthmatic reactions in our tests, indicating that the first nonimmediate reaction, which only became evident after approximately 1.5 hours, was different in its mechanism from immediate reactions, which by that time are well on their way to resolution.

Another subject from this factory showed no reaction to the varnish itself, but a slowly developing, prolonged, late asthmatic reaction that became evident between 3 and 4 hours, was maximal at 6 hours, and was prolonged (figure 22).

All of these patients would have been regarded as having late-onset, so-called cryptogenic (intrinsic) asthma, were it not for identification of the causal agent. The possibility of environmental contamination with chemical dusts and fumes is often the subject of speculation in terms of asthma in industrial societies. Our findings with TDI show that this is a real possibility, but one that can be confirmed only with appropriate tests using known agents. It is probable that the list of these agents will grow rapidly with increased interest in this problem.

The very high order of sensitivity that may exist is shown by the histories of some patients; even coming within hundreds of yards of the relevant factory can be followed by asthmatic

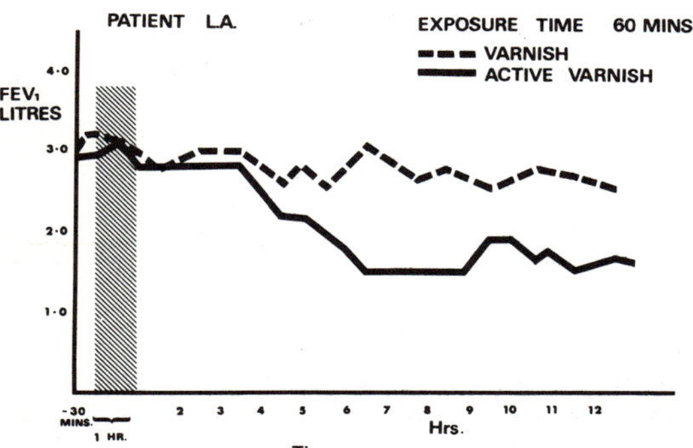

Fig. 22. Patient LA. Occupational type exposure to toluene di-isocyanate (TDI). There was no reaction to the test with polyurethane varnish, but a late asthmatic reaction to the test with varnish plus TDI.

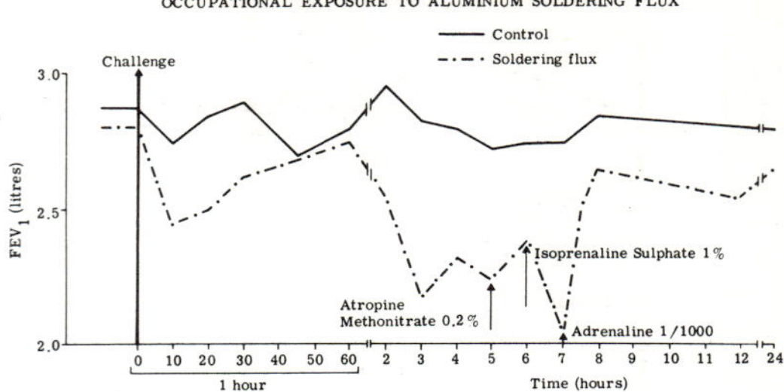

Fig. 23. Patient TB. Occupational type exposure to aluminum soldering flux. There was a dual asthmatic reaction to the test with fumes from soldering of aluminum flux containing amino-ethyl-ethanolamine. Note the poor reversibility by inhaled isoproterenol.

reactions that night or in the early hours of the next morning and by effective test concentrations of 0.001 ppm in the air. Reports of asthma after domestic use of TDI preparations have also been made (39). The home use of polyurethane materials is widespread, and although it is usually claimed that free TDI is absent from the finished materials, it should be appreciated that burning of such materials can liberate TDI into the air.

In further tests, we showed sensitivity in one subject to naphthalene di-isocyanate, but not to TDI (Newman-Taylor, A. J., and Pepys, J.: Unpublished data); again, this demonstrates the analytic value of this pragmatic form of testing in a situation in which a number of possible, often unproved, causes may be present.

Asthma Due to Fumes from Soldering Fluxes and from Natural and Synthetic Resins

In patients with asthma due to fumes of an aluminium soldering flux (Kynol), the cause has been identified as amino-ethyl-ethanolamine (40–42). In occupational type tests, 3 subjects were exposed to the barely visible fumes from application of the heated soldering iron to the flux; only 3 breaths of the fumes were taken, and dual or late asthmatic reactions were elicited (42) (figure 23). The poor reversibility of the late reaction by inhaled isoproterenol can also be seen.

In the course of tests for possible TDI sensitivity from the soldering of wires, we investigated a patient with asthma due to the fumes of a multicore solder. He gave a negative reaction in the TDI test, but as described later, the fumes of pine (colophony) resin in the multicore solder were the cause (Fawcett, I. W., and Pepys, J.: Unpublished data). In another patient who

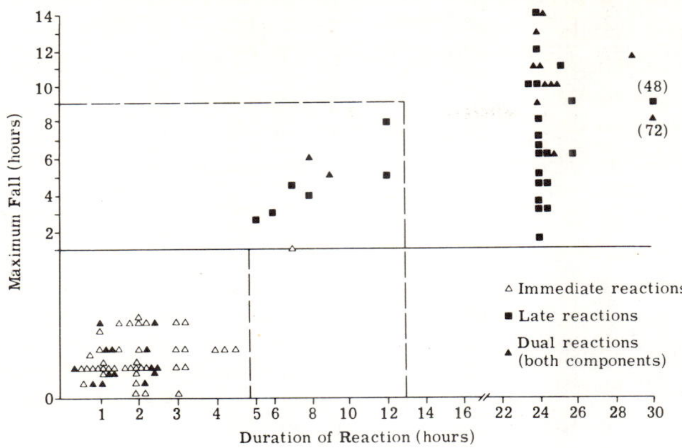

Fig. 24. Time to maximal decrease in 1-sec forced expiratory volume (FEV_1), and the duration of the reaction in immediate, late, and dual asthmatic reactions.

was already receiving compensation for presumed TDI sensitivity based on the history, tests with TDI were negative. The patient was, however, exquisitely sensitive to fumes from an epoxy resin to which he was exposed (Fawcett, I. W., and Pepys, J.: Unpublished data), thus showing the usefulness of the negative TDI test in leading to an accurate etiologic diagnosis. This was important, because the patient was severely asthmatic and was exposed to the unrecognized, relevant, causal material at work. These reactions to the epoxy resins are believed to be due to the different chemically reactive agents added to the epoxy resin, namely, phthalic anhydride, triethylenetetramine, and trimellitic acid. Many other such reactive materials are used with epoxy and other resins, and their potential roles as causes of asthma will no doubt require testing, probably by the occupational type exposure method described.

The possibility of an irritant effect of these agents must be kept in mind. Evidence against this being the chief cause includes the low incidence of affected subjects among workers exposed to much greater quantities of fumes for hours at a time, and the very limited exposure required to elicit asthmatic reactions in sensitized subjects, who may also show clinically their high degree of sensitivity. These arguments, however, do not exclude participation of an irritant effect in the over-all picture of industrial asthma.

Features of Immediate, Nonimmediate, and Combined Asthmatic Reactions

The features of immediate, nonimmediate, and combined asthmatic reactions elicited by common allergens, excluding *A. fumigatus* (discussed earlier), will be outlined and compared

with those elicited by the chemical agents previously described.

Immediate Asthmatic Reactions

Immediate asthmatic reactions start early (figure 24); the time to the maximal decrease in FEV_1 is 15 ± 13 min, and the duration of the reaction in most cases, 1 to 2 hours. Analysis of 39 immediate reactions showed a mean initial FEV_1 of 2.7 ± 1.1 liter with decreases in the control test with Coca's fluid of 0.1 ± 0.1 liter (6 ± 1 per cent) and decreases on allergen challenge of 1.0 ± 0.6 liter (37 ± 17 per cent) that were highly significant (P < 0.001) by the paired t test.

Among 31 subjects, comparable orders of decrease in FEV_1 were elicited in subjects with widely different ranges of initial FEV_1 (figure 25).

In 8 patients who showed variations in FEV_1

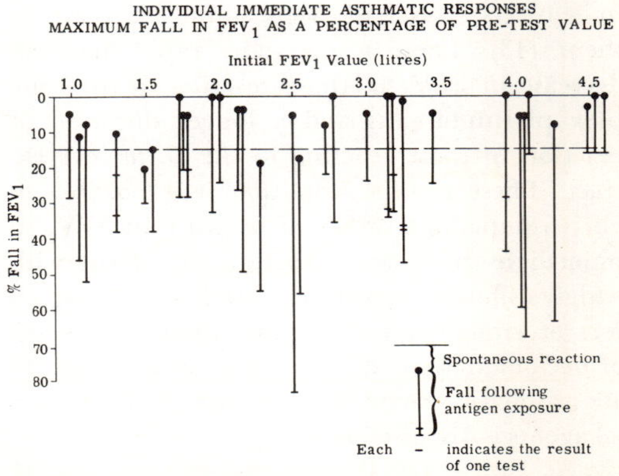

Fig. 25. Order of immediate asthmatic reactions in patients with range of different initial 1-sec forced expiratory volumes (FEV_1).

TABLE 6

COMPARISON OF CHANGES IN 1-SEC FORCED EXPIRATORY VOLUME (FEV$_1$) IN
IMMEDIATE ASTHMATIC REACTIONS TO *DERMATOPHAGOIDES FARINAE,*
COMPLEX PLATINUM SALTS, AND ALCOHOLIC BEVERAGES

	No. of Subjects	Mean Age (years)	Initial FEV$_1$ (liter)	Decrease in FEV$_1$		Time to Maximal Decrease (min)	Time to Recovery (hours)
				Actual	Percentage		
D. farinae	13	37	2.3	0.85	43	26	2.6
Complex platinum salts	14	37	3.1	0.95	33	12	1.8
Alcoholic beverages	5	31	2.6	0.9	37	25	1.5

greater than 10 per cent, it was possible to elicit unequivocal reactions. Thus, their mean initial FEV$_1$ was 1.7 ± 0.6 liter. The mean variation on the control day was 0.3 ± 0.1 liter (16 ± 4 per cent). The mean maximal decrease on challenge was 0.7 ± 0.5 liter (40 ± 13 per cent), a mean difference of 24 per cent. The differences between the control day decreases and maximal challenge decreases were significant in terms of actual measurement (P < 0.02) and in terms of per cent decrease (P < 0.001) by paired t tests.

Comparison of isolated immediate reactions and those occurring in association with nonimmediate reactions showed no significant differences in the initial FEV$_1$ values, the decreases in FEV$_1$, and the time required to reach the maximal decrease or the time to return to initial FEV$_1$ values.

Comparison of immediate reactions to common allergens and chemical agents. In table 6 are shown the over-all similarities of immediate asthmatic reactions to a common allergen, *Dermatophagoides farinae,* complex salts of platinum, and, as a matter of additional interest, the ingestion of different alcoholic beverages in subjects who had been found to react to them (43). There was a more rapid maximal decrease in FEV$_1$ in those reacting to the complex platinum salts and a longer duration of reaction in those reacting to the *D. farinae* extract. These results show that it is possible to elicit comparable orders of decrease in FEV$_1$ in immediate asthmatic reactions to tests with widely different agents. The similar blocking effect of cromolyn sodium and absence of effect of beclomethasone dipropionate on the immediate asthmatic reactions to the very different causal agents is discussed later.

Nonimmediate Asthmatic Reactions

There are at least 3 patterns of nonimmediate asthmatic reaction. They may present in isolation or in association with one another and with immediate reactions. We have found that the particular patterns of reaction, isolated or combined, are, as a rule, reproducible on repetition of the same challenge. They appear to be distinct from earlier reactions if present, because the FEV$_1$ returns to or near to the pretest value and remains there for a period of 1 or more hours before the next pattern of reaction develops.

There is clearly much to be learned about these reactions, and there is some difficulty in finding appropriate descriptive terms. It is preferable not to describe the nonimmediate reactions as "delayed," because this term is used for Type IV allergic reactions and carries unproved assumptions as to the mechanism of the nonimmediate reactions. The first nonimmediate reaction to be clearly recognized and described as a "late" reaction starts, in our experience, several hours after the challenge or after clinical exposure, is maximal at approximately 5 to 8 hours, and usually resolves within 24 hours, although it may occasionally take some days or even weeks for the FEV$_1$ to return spontaneously to pretest levels. An even later reaction that tends to develop in the early hours of the morning on the day after clinical exposure or challenge has been reported (13, 14, and Davies, R. J.: Personal communication). This reaction tends to be recurrent, occurring at approximately the same time on successive days without further challenge or exposure, and without evidence of asthmatic reaction at other times of the day, and could be termed a recurrent late reaction.

An example of this in response to a test with ampicillin powder in a sensitized subject has already been shown in figure 12. Another example of this quite remarkable asthmatic response to a single test shows (figure 26) that in a farmer who had an immediate asthmatic reaction of

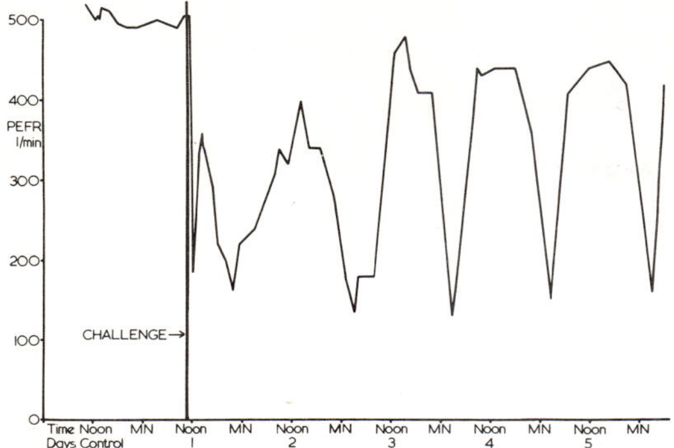

Fig. 26. Dual asthmatic reaction in a farmer to occupational type exposure to grain dust. The "late" reaction recurred without further testing during the early hours of the next 4 nights. PEF = Peak expiratory flow; MN = midnight.

short duration to a 30-min exposure to grain dust, a late reaction then developed (Davies, R. J.: Personal communication). Without any further exposure, there were recurrent, nocturnal, asthmatic reactions shortly after midnight for the next 4 nights. There were no asthmatic reactions during the daytime. In a third instance, this was seen to occur in a printer after actual exposure at work (Davies, R. J.: Personal communication). Within a few hours of starting work, the patient developed prolonged, severe, persistent, nonimmediate asthma. He came into hospital at the end of the day's work, when

the nocturnal reactions were recorded. The next day, without further exposure, the asthmatic reaction recurred at 10 P.M. and again at about 6 A.M., corresponding to two major times of decrease in the peak expiratory flow observed the previous day. The early morning decrease in his peak flow did not disappear until he had been away from work for 7 days.

These reactions must be taken into account in bronchial provocation tests, and we have found it necessary, on occasion, to delay further testing until they had resolved completely. As shown in figure 27, we also found that the delay was important in the investigation of workers who had recently been exposed at work and who needed to be observed for several days before control or challenge tests, to ensure that any reactions to the work exposure had completely resolved.

The other pattern of nonimmediate asthma, described earlier, starts approximately 1 hour after the test, is maximal at 2 to 3 hours, and resolves within another 1 to 2 hours. This reaction may be followed, after an interval of apparent normality, by the "late" reaction described previously. This associated pattern, seen in one of the TDI-sensitive subjects (figure 21), was also present, although it was not appreciated at the time, in a nonatopic bird fancier (figure 28). In the latter case, the reactions were inhibited by cromolyn sodium, so that the test

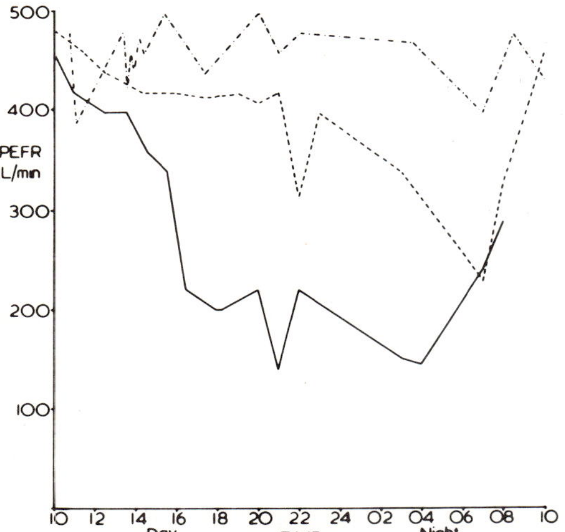

Fig. 27. Nonimmediate asthmatic reaction (continuous line) in a printer during his working day. Recurrent nocturnal reactions (hatched line) the following day without further exposure. Return to nonasthmatic state (interrupted line) after 7 days.

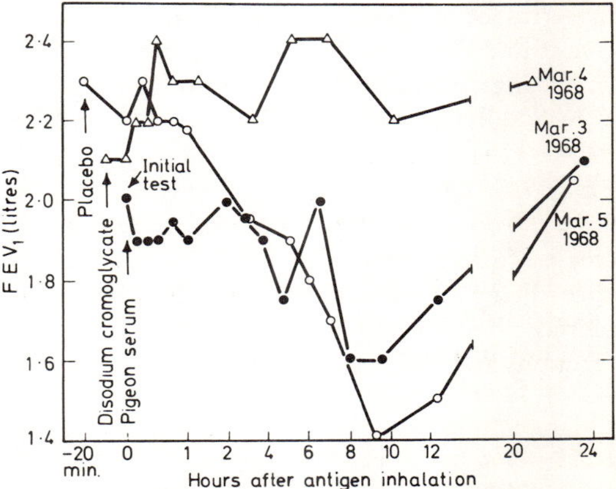

Fig. 28. Late asthmatic reactions to bronchial provocation test in a nonatopic pigeon fancier with precipitins. Note asthmatic reaction between 2 and 7 hours, followed by asthmatic reaction between 7 and 24 hours. Both reactions were blocked by pretest inhalation of cromolyn sodium. A more vigorous nonimmediate asthmatic reaction to a repeat test after lactose placebo started more than 1 hour after the test.

was repeated for control purposes after inhalation of a lactose placebo. On this occasion, a more vigorous asthmatic reaction developed that may have obscured the earlier nonimmediate reaction.

The features of nonimmediate asthmatic reactions are shown in figure 24. There were a small group of nonimmediate asthmatic reactions with maximal decreases at 2 to 5 hours, having started earlier, and resolving within 6 to 8 hours, and a larger group of reactions that were maximal after 4 to 5 hours and lasted for 24 hours. As discussed earlier, some patients may show both patterns of reaction, suggesting that they are distinct in their own right; but it is possible that different patterns of response may be elicited by a lower or greater challenge dose. Because our tests were designed to elicit positive reactions for etiologic diagnosis, we are unable to provide any information on this possibility.

In 34 late asthmatic reactions, the mean initial FEV_1 was 2.8 ± 0.9 liter, with a decrease on the control test day of 0.2 ± 0.1 liter (6 ± 6 per cent) in comparison with the highly significant challenge reaction mean decrease in FEV_1 of 1.1 ± 0.6 liter (36 ± 15 per cent) ($P < 0.001$ by paired t test). The time to maximal decrease was 7 ± 5 hours. This value includes data from some of the group described previously who started reacting earlier. In 26 subjects who had tests intended only to elicit positive reactions, so that the tests were not necessarily comparable in terms of dosage, comparable ranges of decrease in FEV_1 were elicited in patients with a wide range of initial FEV_1 values (figure 29).

In 7 subjects with decreases in FEV_1 greater than 10 per cent on the control day, the initial FEV_1 was 2.1 ± 0.5 liter; the control decrease, 0.8 ± 0.4 liter (46 ± 19 per cent), and the decrease after challenge, 1.1 ± 0.6 liter, the difference being highly significant ($P < 0.005$ by paired t test). Comparison of the isolated late reactions and those occurring in association with

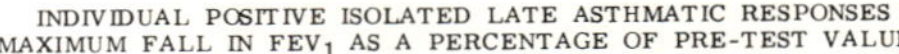
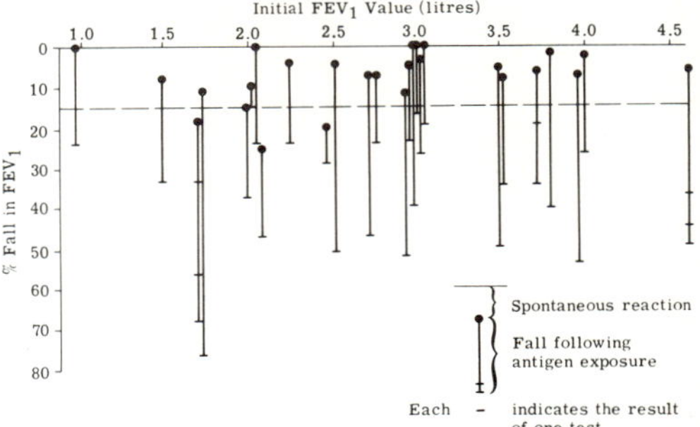

Fig. 29. Order of late asthmatic reactions in patients with range of different initial 1-sec forced expiratory volumes (FEV_1).

an immediate reaction showed that starting off with comparable initial FEV_1 measurements, there was no significant difference between the two groups in the order of decrease in FEV_1 or the time of maximal decrease.

Comparison of nonimmediate reactions to common allergens and chemical agents. The over-all similarity in the nonimmediate reactions to nebulized aerosols of common allergens and to occupational type tests with chemical dusts, vapors, and gases, except for a more rapid decrease to maximum with the chemical agents, is shown in table 7. The table also shows that it is possible, by the carefully graduated methods of testing used, to elicit nonimmediate reactions of comparable order to widely differing agents. The nonimmediate reactions to the chemical agents could be blocked by cromolyn sodium and corticosteroids, like those to aerosols of extracts of common allergens.

Combined (Dual) Immediate and Nonimmediate Asthmatic Reactions

The speed of appearance of the maximal decrease in FEV_1 of the immediate asthmatic reactions, their duration, and the time of maximal

TABLE 7

COMPARISON OF THE CHANGES IN 1-SEC FORCED EXPIRATORY VOLUME (FEV₁) IN LATE ASTHMATIC REACTIONS TO NEBULIZED COMMON ALLERGENS AND INDUSTRIAL AGENTS

	No. of Subjects	Mean Age *(years)*	Initial FEV₁ *(liter)*	Decrease in FEV₁ Actual	Decrease in FEV₁ Percentage	Time to Maximal Decrease *(hours)*	Time to Recovery *(hours)*
Nebulized extracts of common allergens	8	47	2.15	0.7	30	9	20
Industrial agents	23	40	3.55	1.25	38	6	23

decrease of the subsequent nonimmediate reaction are shown in figure 30. Most of the immediate reactions reached their maximum within 10 to 20 min, and all had resolved completely, or nearly so, by 2 hours. Most of the nonimmediate reactions that appeared after an interval of apparent normality were maximal between 4 and 12 hours. The orders of decrease in FEV_1 in the two reactions were similar, although, as shown earlier in the patients with allergic bronchopulmonary aspergillosis and in a number of examples of "late" asthmatic reactions to other agents, there was less effective and shorter-lasting reversibility of the late, compared to the immediate, reaction by the inhalation of isoproterenol. In 15 dual reactors, the decrease in the FEV_1 in the immediate reaction was highly significant ($P < 0.001$). In the recovery phase, after reversal by inhalation of isoproterenol, there was no significant difference from pretest values, whereas there were highly significantly lower values in the reversal of the "late" asthmatic reactions ($P < 0.001$ by paired t tests). There was no significant difference between isolated immediate or late reactions and the combined immediate and late asthmatic reactions, respectively, in the dual reactors.

Effect of Drugs on the Asthmatic Reactions to Provocation Tests

These effects will be discussed in terms of the need for drugs to reverse reactions and the effects of isoproterenol or salbutamol inhalation, cromolyn sodium, and corticosteroids on the different patterns of reaction.

Treatment given to relieve discomfort from

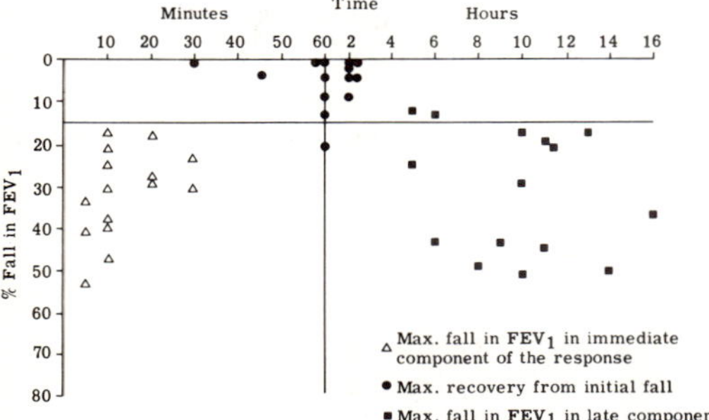

Fig. 30. Measurements of 1-sec forced expiratory volume (FEV_1) in dual asthmatic reactions. The speed of the maximal (Max.) decrease, the order of spontaneous reversibility in immediate reactions, and the time to the maximal decrease in late reactions are shown.

vigorous or prolonged reactions in a group of 91 positive bronchial tests consisted of the inhalation of isoproterenol or salbutamol in 5 of 42 isolated immediate reactions and 12 of 34 isolated late reactions; 3 patients from the latter group were given injections of epinephrine. Among 15 dual reactors, isoproterenol inhalation was given to one for reversal of the immediate and to 4, for the late reaction; 3 of the latter group were given injections of epinephrine. Reactions requiring reversal in this way were seldom of an unduly severe nature, and corticosteroids were not used; however, there are uncommon occasions when a sharper reaction than expected may be elicited, even with care, usually with the first test using an unfamiliar agent. It is necessary, therefore, to have the appropriate therapeutic agents available at all times during testing.

Inhaled Bronchodilators and Asthmatic Reactions

Immediate and nonimmediate reactions differ markedly in their response to inhalation of isoproterenol. As shown in allergic bronchopulmonary aspergillosis, immediate reactions of the order elicited by us are usually completely reversed, whereas late reactions of comparable intensity are usually reversed poorly, if at all, and then for only a short time. Immediate reactions in which IgE antibody is involved result from the liberation of tissue mediators by mast and basophil cells. It would seem that in the single period of allergen exposure of our tests, the effects of the mediators liberated can be blocked or reversed by the isoproterenol. In the nonimmediate reaction, however, the mechanisms by which there is support for a Type III allergic reaction are of an ongoing nature, as will be discussed later. In these circumstances, the bronchodilator is less likely to be effective.

The different effects of the isoproterenol in the two reactions may explain why, in the same subject, a bronchodilator works well at one time of the day and yet poorly at another. The fact that in our tests both reactions were elicited by a single challenge with extracts of even the most usual of allergens makes it highly probable that the same thing happens in clinical asthma, although the sequence is probably complicated by repeated exposures during the day.

Effects of Cromolyn Sodium on Bronchial Provocation Tests

The effect in 17 patients of pretest inhalation

TABLE 8

INHIBITION OF IMMEDIATE ASTHMATIC RESPONSE BY CROMOLYN SODIUM IN 17 PATIENTS

	Initial FEV_1	Maximal Decrease in FEV_1		
		Allergen Challenge	Cromolyn Sodium/ Allergen Challenge	Lactose Placebo/ Allergen Challenge
Actual value, liter	2.9 (1.4 − 4.75)	0.9 (0.4 − 1.6)	0.1 (0 − 0.6)	1.1 (0.4 − 1.7)
Percentage decrease		34.0 (12 − 65)	4.0 (0 − 15)	39.0 (21 − 61)

of 20 to 40 mg of cromolyn sodium on immediate asthmatic reactions to bronchial provocation tests is shown in table 8. In 17 subjects, the difference between the initial reaction and the reaction blocked by cromolyn sodium was significant ($P < 0.01$ by paired t test). In 13 subjects who were finally challenged again after inhalation of a lactose placebo, there was a significant difference ($P < 0.01$) from the inhibited reaction and no significant difference compared to the initial test reaction; the latter results illustrate the reproducibility of reactions on repetition of the tests.

The agents tested in this group of subjects ranged from common inhaled allergens, such as *Dermatophagoides* species extracts; flour; ingested agents, such as alcoholic beverages; chemical dusts, such as the complex platinum salts, piperazine dihydrochloride, wood dusts, and gaseous emanations from toluene diisocyanate (figures 1, 4A, 6, 15, and 18). The comparable inhibitory effect of cromolyn sodium on these reactions suggests that they are basically similar, and perhaps that they have the same or similar mechanisms, although this is not necessarily so. These possibilities will be discussed later.

Effect of Cromolyn Sodium on "Isolated" Late Asthmatic Reactions

Blocking of late asthmatic reactions by pretest inhalation of cromolyn sodium in a nonatopic pigeon fancier tested with pigeon serum is illustrated in figure 28. In 14 subsequent tests in other subjects who had late asthmatic reactions (table 9), these were blocked by pretest inhalation of 40 mg of cromolyn sodium in 5 cases, and in another 5 by pretest and 3 hourly administration. No further tests were made in the remaining 4, in whom the reaction was not blocked by pretest inhalation. The blocking effect of single or repeated treatment with cromolyn sodium or the absence of effect seemed related to the degree of the test reaction, as can be seen from the table. In practice, it has been

found (44) that more frequent inhalation of cromolyn sodium can be effective in children regarded as treaatment failures with the conventional regimen of 4 times per day.

Effects of Cromolyn Sodium on Combined (Dual) Immediate and Late Asthmatic Reactions

Tests in 5 patients showed that pretest inhalation of 40 mg of cromolyn sodium had a marked, significant inhibitory effect on the immediate and late reactions ($P < 0.05$). The immediate decrease in FEV_1 was reduced from 34 to 7 per cent, and the late reaction, from 30 to 10 per cent. In the final tests, lactose placebo was given before the challenge, and the late decrease in FEV_1 was 26 per cent compared with the late decrease in the initial test of 30 per cent. In addition to the effects of the cromolyn sodium, these findings show the reproducibility of the asthmatic reactions in repeat tests.

Blocking of both immediate and late reactions in a baker tested with flour is shown in figure 4A.

Effects of Inhaled Beclomethasone Dipropionate on Late Asthmatic Reactions

Inhibition of late reactions by systemic corticosteroids was reported soon after their introduction (9, 10); however, emphasis needs to be placed on the absence of effect of systemic (4) (figure 31) or inhaled corticosteroids (45) (figure 1) on the immediate reactions. In 4 of 6 subjects, pretest inhalation of 200 μg of beclomethasone dipropionate effectively inhibited the late asthmatic reaction ($P < 0.05$), reducing the decrease in FEV_1 from a mean of 30 to 3.5 per cent. In the remaining two, pretest followed by 3 hourly administration was required to inhibit the late asthmatic reaction, illustrating, in terms of this drug, a possible similarity to the point made with regard to frequency of use of cromolyn sodium, namely that when conventional 4 times per day administration fails, it may be

TABLE 9

EFFECT OF CROMOLYN SODIUM ON "LATE" ASTHMATIC REACTIONS

Block of Late Reaction by Cromolyn Sodium	No. of Subjects	Initial FEV_1 (liter)	Mean Maximal Decrease		Maximal Decrease after Cromolyn Sodium		Maximal Decrease after Lactose Placebo	
			(liter)	(%)	(liter)	(%)	(liter)	(%)
Pretest	5	2.5 (2.1 − 3.1)	0.5	20	0.1	3	0.6	25
Pretest and 3 hourly	5	4.0 (3.5 − 4.7)	0.95	25	0.1	4	0.7	18
Not blocked by pretest cromolyn sodium. No further tests	4	3.5 (2.15 − 4.1)	1.2 (0.65 − 2.2)	35	1.05 (0.4 − 2.3)	32		

worth trying more frequent administration. A number of examples are given of late asthmatic reactions, both to common allergens and to various chemical agents, in which inhaled corticosteroids blocked the reaction (figures 4B, 9, 19, 21, and 31), thus suggesting that there may be similar mechanisms in their production.

Immunopathologic Mechanisms of Asthmatic Reactions

In discussing the possible roles of allergic reactions in the production of asthmatic reactions to diagnostic tests with inhaled agents, it is not intended to imply that the causes of clinical asthma in such cases are purely and simply allergic, rather than multifactorial. There is evidence that the tendency to have asthma may be inherited (46); there are inherited factors related to the capacity to become sensitized, at present best understood for IgE antibody in atopy; and there are probably biochemical differences in the nature or amount of tissue mediators liberated and the responses to them (47).

Analysis of the possible participation of allergy in asthmatic reactions is based on 3 of the 4 main types of allergic reaction (48), i.e., Types I, III, and IV, and on agents that simulate them. It is hoped that it will become possible to classify asthmatic responses and other allergic disorders in terms of the immunopathologic mechanisms involved, thus giving greater precision. Until then, however, compromises in terminology are needed. Although some types of allergy are found predominantly in particular groups of subjects, these are not exclusive; furthermore, the different types of allergy may, and often do, coexist, and they may even be interdependent.

Type I, Immediate Allergy

There is now evidence in man, as in experimental animals, that immediate allergic reactions can be mediated, mainly by IgE antibody (49), and also to an extent yet to be determined by one or perhaps more of the subclasses of IgG antibody (18). The IgE antibody is heat-labile and is termed long-term homocytotropic antibody (LTS) because of its capacity to sensitize mast and basophil cells for prolonged periods of time from days to weeks, and because it is a feature of, although it is not confined to, atopic subjects, who produce it readily in response to limited exposures to allergens in ordinary life. It was to this antibody, although it was not recognized as such at the time, that the term "reagin" was first applied (50). It has been suggested (51) that it should be used solely for this purpose, rather than to include the STS-IgG antibody under the same heading. Whereas both are

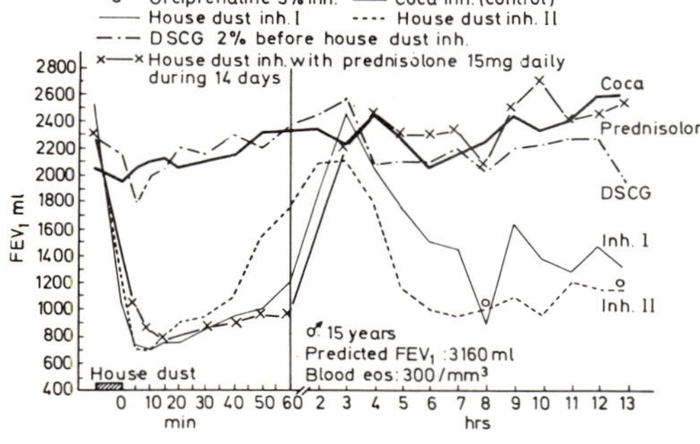

Fig. 31. Dual asthmatic reactions to house dust extract. Note lack of reaction to control test with Coca's fluid, comparable dual reactions to initial challenge and to final challenge, blocking of both reactions by pretest inhalation (inh.) of cromolyn sodium (DSCG), blocking only of late reaction by 15 mg of prednisolone given orally for 4 days, and poor reversibility of late reaction by inhaled metaproterenol. FEV_1 = 1-sec forced expiratory volume; blood eos = blood eosinophil count per mm³.

mast cell sensitizing antibodies, they have different properties and potential effects, as illustrated, in fact, by those who wish to group them together (19). The IgG antibody is heat-stable and is termed short-term homocytotropic antibody (STS) because it sensitizes these cells for short periods of a few hours. Much larger amounts of histamine are liberated in reactions mediated by IgE compared to those mediated by STS-IgG antibody (52).

The role of both of these mast cell sensitizing antibodies in asthmatic reactions is inferred from evidence of their presence in skin and serologic tests or in passive transfer tests, mainly to subhuman primates. The IgE-mediated reactions to inhalation tests may possibly be occurring with sensitized basophil cells lying on the surface of the bronchial mucosa, because there is some doubt as to whether, or how far, allergens penetrate into the mucosa to reach the tissue mast cells (53). It is also possible that some of the allergen given by inhalation is ingested and that the bronchial reaction results from blood-borne allergen reacting with sensitized tissue mast cells.

Subjects with evidence of Type I, IgE allergy, as shown by the presence of specific IgE antibodies in the serum, show a high correlation of these with immediate asthmatic reactions to bronchial tests. These reactions can be regarded as extrinsic, reaginic asthma. The demonstration of STS-IgG antibody in immediate skin test reactions in man (18) and the production of immediate asthmatic reactions to *Dermatophagoides* species in subjects with this antibody and without evidence of specific IgE antibody can be termed extrinsic, nonreaginic asthma (19) These findings have broadened the concept of Type I allergy as a mechanism for immediate asthma, so that acting on the assumption that this form of allergy is responsible for the bronchial reactions, one can refer to the immediate asthmatic reactions as either Type I, IgE- or Type I, STS-IgG-mediated, and it seems not unlikely that in some subjects, both may be present and possibly operating together. It has also been found that the Type I, STS-IgG reactors failed to respond to cromolyn sodium clinically and that it did not block the asthmatic reaction to challenge (19), in contrast to its blocking effect on Type I, IgE reactors.

The presence of both STS-IgG and IgE antibodies to common allergens in the same subject has been reported (16, 18, 19); in extensions of these studies, STS-IgG antibodies, in the absence of IgE antibodies, have been found against common allergens in subjects regarded as having cryptogenic (intrinsic) asthma, because of the late age of onset, absence of clinical history suggestive of extrinsic allergens, and, in these cases, negative skin test responses to a battery of common allergens (16). Approximately 20 per cent of patients with cryptogenic asthma so defined give histories suggestive of sensitivity to extrinsic allergens, but without the ready confirmation elicited in extrinsic asthma in atopic subjects. If these findings could be shown to be clinically relevant, it would mean the reclassification as extrinsic, nonreaginic asthma of the asthma of a number of patients at present termed cryptogenic. There is thus evidence of subjects with IgE antibody only to common allergens, others with STS-IgG only, and yet others with both types of antibody. A possible role for both types in providing an introductory immediate reaction in the development of Type III reactions will be discussed.

Reactions closely resembling Type I, immediate reactions can also be elicited by nonspecific agents capable of liberating histamine. There is little or no immunologic evidence for the various chemical agents like that for common allergens. The possibility that nonspecific irritation is responsible for the immediate reactions elicited must be taken into account, although not solely for the chemical agents, but also for extracts of common allergens. In the absence of supporting immunlogic evidence, the criteria for assuming an allergic, as against an irritant, mechanism are the traditional ones, namely that only a proportion, usually low, of exposed subjects are affected after repeated exposure and tend to show increasing and high degrees of sensitivity to amounts of the allergen less than the levels capable of causing irritation.

Type III, "Late" Allergic Reactions

The classic Type III reaction, the Arthus reaction, is mediated by soluble, toxic immune-complexes, formed in moderate excess of antigen over precipitating antibody, with fixation and enzymatic activation of the classic complement sequence, C1423. This reaction depends on the participation of neutrophil granulocytes in its early stages, although the characteristic infiltrating cell of the developed reaction is the mononuclear cell. In Arthus reactions in experimental animals, hemorrhage, fibrinoid necrosis, and perivascular, cellular infiltration are used as criteria. In man, however, it would be unacceptable to test in such a way as to elicit these changes. Such reactions were observed not infrequently in the past, when animal antisera were more widely used for treatment and when unequivocal Arthus reactions were elicited. Immunofluorescence studies of skin test reactions regarded as Type III to *A. fumigatus* and avian allergens have shown perivascular infiltration with small numbers of mononuclear cells, together with aggregates staining for IgG, IgM, IgA, and β_1C component of complement. These aggregates lay perivascularly, in or on mononuclear cells and in the vascular endothelium (25).

The classic features of the Type III skin test reaction consist of an extensive, ill-defined, soft, edematous reaction that becomes macroscopically evident after several hours and then becomes progressively larger, reaching its maximum at 5 to 8 hours, and resolving within approximately 24 hours. There may be some petechial hemorrhages in the center. There is usually little or no discomfort. The late asthmatic reaction starting after several hours, maximal at 5 to 8 hours, and resolving within 24 hours is compatible in speed of appearance, duration, and other features with this reaction. This asthmatic reaction could be described as extrinsic, "Type III" asthma, provided the assumptions made as to its mechanism were supported by further evidence.

An important element in the development of the Type III reaction is the participation, possibly an obligatory one, of a preceding immediate reaction (54) in experimental animals, suggesting that this plays a part in the vascular deposition of the immune complexes. In man it has been found that, with few exceptions, skin test reactions with these features are preceded by an immediate reaction (6).

In subjects with IgE antibody as well as precipitins, the IgE antibody could be responsible for the immediate reaction, and in bronchial tests, an immediate asthmatic reaction would be expected to precede the late reaction and is, indeed, found. In subjects without IgE antibody and precipitins, it seems possible, although this has not yet been established, that STS-IgG antibody might be responsible for the immediate reaction; this might require larger doses, as appears to be the case in eliciting skin test reactions (26). In such a case, the late asthmatic reaction might be expected to develop without obvious evidence, as measured by the FEV_1, of an immediate asthmatic reaction. More intensive challenge might elicit frank, immediate asthmatic reactions in such subjects, as was the case with the immediate asthmatic reactions attributed to STS-IgG antibody (19). The object of our tests, as stated earlier, was to establish, by gradual increase in doses on separate test days, only that amount capable of eliciting an unequivocally positive reaction.

Analysis of nonimmediate bronchial reactions in terms of associated Types I and III allergy is acceptable for common allergens, for which these mechanisms can be shown to be present, and, by assumption, are believed to be operative in the bronchial reactions. When such evidence is lacking, as for example with the chemical agents, it is the similarities that are striking. Thus, systemic corticosteroids effectively inhibit the Type III skin test reactions and the late asthmatic reactions, having, at the same time, little or no effect on the preceding Type I reactions, showing that these are two distinct reactions, whatever their mechanism. A possible explanation for the effectiveness of corticosteroids in Type III reactions that has been provided concerns their capacity to reinforce the phospholipid membrane of lysosomes and prevent the escape of their tissue-damaging enzyme content (55). Liberation of lysosomes from the neutrophil granulocytes is an early feature of Type III reactions, and it is likely that the corticosteroids exert some, perhaps much, of their protective effect at this point.

Other mechanisms for nonimmediate skin and bronchial reactions, like those described previously, are postulated (56–59) in patients who react in this way, but in whom precipitins are not demonstrable and examination of the late cutaneous reactions shows none of the features described earlier (25). These investigators suggest that a late "Type III-like" reaction to common allergens in the skin and the bronchi in these subjects may be part of an IgE-mediated reaction and may be dependent on dosage. They found, however, that the two reactions had distinctive features, like those discussed earlier, in that corticosteroids inhibited the late, but not the immediate, reaction (57). Inhalation tests (59) showed that in patients giving immediate asthmatic reactions only, tests with larger doses elicited both immediate and late reactions. Because in our tests we would have terminated the challenges on eliciting an immediate reaction, this phenomenon would not have been observed in at least some of our patients. There are, however, many questions yet to be resolved. The failure to demonstrate precipitins must be interpreted in the first instance as a negative test and not necessarily the absence of such antibodies. For example, immunoglobulins and complement have been found in skin biopsy specimens of reactions regarded as Type III to *A. fumigatus* in two subjects in whom precipitin tests were negative (25). We have also observed immediate and nonimmediate skin test reactions to purified protein fractions of *Candida albicans* in subjects in whom precipitins were not demonstrable, but who gave vigorous Type IV reactions 24 to 48 hours later. Among the lymphokines liberated from sensitized lymphocytes on antigen challenge is a skin reactive factor, which on introduction into the skin elicits a reaction with similar time sequence and appearance to the Type III reaction (60). Sensitized lymphocytes have been reported in subjects with Type I allergy, and it may be that the mechanism described could be re-

sponsible for reactions with macroscopic features of a Type III reaction, but lacking in supporting precipitin test evidence.

Activation of C3 complement by the "alternate" pathway by a variety of organic dusts and extracts of their organismal flora has been described (61, 62). The contribution of this observation to respiratory disease with features of a Type III reaction has yet to be established.

The participation of Type III reactions in allergic respiratory disease was first proposed in relation to farmer's lung and other forms of extrinsic allergic alveolitis. This has led some workers to question its possible role in nonimmediate bronchial reactions, because some of the features of the former were lacking. Although there is no explanation of why the reactions should present as asthma in one subject and al-

TABLE 10
OVER-ALL FEATURES OF BRONCHIAL PROVOCATION TESTS

Immediate Reactions	Late Reactions	
Acute, sharp, rapid decrease in 1-sec forced expiratory volume (FEV_1)	Slowly developing, progressively severe	
Clinically readily evident, subjectively and objectively	Often not obvious clinically except on exertion, until fully developed, when dyspnea and wheezing appear	
Tightness of chest, dyspnea, and wheezing		
Onset of reaction		
10–20 min	(A) Approximately 4–8 hours	(B) Approximately 1–2 hours
Maximal decrease in FEV_1		
10–20 min	(A) 8 hours	(B) 3 hours
Duration		
1–2 hours	(A) Approximately 24–96 hours	(B) 3 hours
Systemic reactions		
Usually none	Malaise, myalgia, fever often present	
White blood cell count		
LIttle or no change	Leukocytosis often present, especially with systemic reactions	
Eosinophilia		
Blood 0 to + or +	May be increased 0 to + or ++	
Reversibility by isoproterenol inhalation		
Readily and completely or almost completely reversible	Usually poorly or only temporarily reversible	
Reaction inhibitable by		
Inhalation of cromolyn sodium	Systemic of inhaled corticosteroids	
No inhibition by systemic or inhaled corticosteroids	Inhalation of cromolyn sodium	

veolitis in another, this does not exclude the possibility of Type III reaction in either of these or even in both together.

Type IV, Delayed Allergic Reactions

There is no evidence as yet for a role of Type IV lymphocyte-mediated allergy in asthma. The very late reactions described previously may perhaps reflect such a reaction, as may the prolonged persistence of nonimmediate reactions in some subjects. Lymphocyte sensitization to toluene diisocyanate conjugates has been reported (63).

Clinical Implications of Patterns of Asthmatic Reaction to Bronchial Provocation Tests

Features of the immediate and nonimmediate asthmatic reactions (64) are summarized in table 10, which emphasizes the differences in their modes of presentation with the acute, paroxysmal, clinically evident attacks of the immediate sort, in contrast to the slowly, progressively developing, and less obvious clinical presentation of the nonimmediate reaction. The mode of development of this reaction in response to a bronchial provocation test may not be recognized if frequent, hourly observations are not made, illustrating the difficulty of its clinical recognition in the ordinary way. When the causal exposure is known, however, it is possible to obtain histories of clinical asthma conforming to the patterns illustrated by the bronchial provocation tests made under controlled conditions. It is common for workers to complain at first of asthmatic symptoms coming on at the end of the day's work or at night, and some give a later history of acute attacks developing rapidly on exposure, suggesting that immunologic and, possibly, other as yet unrecognized mechanisms appropriate for such reactions had subsequently developed. It is also possible to elicit clinical histories of immediate reactions followed by a period of apparent normality and then the development of more persistent symptoms some hours later. Inhalation tests in 3 workers sensitized by heavy exposure to the enzymes of *Bacillus subtilis* (65) showed dual reactions in two cases and only a late reaction in the third. On repetition of the tests, however, the latter patient gave an immediate, as well as a nonimmediate, reaction accompanied after each test by an increase in the absolute eosinophil count.

In patients presenting with asthma without any clues as to possible causes, it is not possible to obtain histories of this sort, and other methods based on the findings in the provocation tests under controlled conditions may yet find a place. For example, poor reversibility by inhaled bronchodilators may suggest a nonimmediate asthmatic pattern of reaction. With corticosteroids, clinical control of the asthma would argue in favor of nonimmediate asthma, and when attacks continue to occur, the participation of immediate asthmatic reactions not affected by corticosteroids is possible. Analysis is complicated in clinical conditions by ignorance as to possible causal exposures and whether these may be occurring repeatedly at shorter or longer intervals during the period of observation.

When the controlled exposure elicits a vigorous late bronchial reaction, it is not uncommon for there to be pyrexia with malaise, myalgia, and leukocytosis. These are suggestive of infection, and once again, it would be difficult to evaluate in a clinical situation, except when the time of a known exposure can be established. It is probable that attempts to interpret the clinical history of the actual asthmatic episodes along these lines will add to our understanding of the individual patient, will act as a guide to lines of investigation, and will add to efficiency in the use of and interpretation of the effects of the various therapeutic agents.

Bronchial Provocation Tests for Extrinsic Allergic Alveolitis

In patients with farmer's lung, bird fancier's lung, and the other forms of extrinsic allergic alveolitis, precipitins are often present against the suspected agent, and Type III skin tests can be elicited when the test material is suitable (6). Inhalation tests made as described earlier for asthma may reproduce the features of the disease with systemic manifestations, such as fever, malaise, myalgia, cough, and dyspnea without wheezing, unless, uncommonly, asthma is present as well. Pulmonary function tests show a restrictive ventilatory defect with proportional decreases in the FEV_1 and FVC, so that the ratio may be unaltered, decrease in the CO gas transfer factor, and decreased lung compliance.

The speed of appearance and duration of the reaction are compatible with a Type III reaction, and the reactions to the challenge are blocked by corticosteroids, as is the case with nonimmediate asthmatic reactions in which Type III allergy may play a part.

There is controversy about the immunopathologic mechanisms in this disease, mainly because precipitins, which are, in the first place, evidence of exposure, may be present in exposed but unaffected subjects, and because epithelioid cell granulomas are a feature of the disease and are believed to indicate Type IV allergy. It seems more likely that the different types of allergic reaction may be participating either alone or together, and because the reaction is taking place in a particular part of the lung, the clinical features have much in common, whatever the causal agent and the mechanisms responsible. This is the same sort of problem that must be faced with bronchial reactions resulting in asthma. There are several possible mechanisms for the production of the characteristic granulomas. They may represent foreign body reactions to inhaled organic dusts, and some can be found in apparently healthy farmers; but they are more widespread and clearly related to an ongoing reaction in patients with allergic alveolitis. It has been reported (66) that insoluble immune complexes formed in antigen equivalence that do not fix complement stimulate the production of epithelioid cell granulomas on introduction into the tissues, whereas soluble complexes of the same antigens and precipitins formed in moderate excess fix complement and cause acute inflammatory reactions. The antigens from inhaled organic materials are readily diffusible, so that the tissues may be viewed as representing an agar-gel plate in which the visible precipitate is evidence of insoluble complexes of antigen and antibody, whereas on each side of the antigen and antibody wells, there are complexes soluble in antigen excess and in antibody excess, respectively.

A role for Type IV allergy is not excluded, and there are reports of lymphocyte transformation *in vitro* on challenge with, for example, avian antigens (67), although Type IV skin test reactions have not been observed (26), suggesting that the full picture of Type IV allergy is not present. Many of the organismal causes of allergic alveolitis represent particles that penetrate into the periphery of the lungs, where they may act in two ways. Their antigens may diffuse and react with precipitins, as discussed previously, and in their particulate form, they may react with sensitized lymphoid cells. It has been shown that bentonite particles coated with antigen elicit granulomas in sensitized animals (68). These reactions can be transferred passively by lymphoid cells from sensitized animals as for a Type IV reaction, but not by their antibody-containing serum. Such reactions with the resultant production of granulomas could be caused by spores of fungi, actinomycetes and other organisms causing allergic alveolitis.

Conclusions

Bronchial provocation tests in asthma and allergic alveolitis are a pragmatic means of etiologic diagnosis that, at the same time, reproduce some or all of the clinical manifestations. In this respect, the test reactions provide models of the clinical disorder and are useful in trying to interpret the variable history, in particular of clinical asthma, with which this review is mainly concerned. The findings discussed here, however, are based on single challenge procedures, and it is not known how the patterns of reaction might be modified by repeated or more continuous exposure once reactions have been initiated.

The identification of causal agents from the history, provocation tests, and other methods places the patient in the "extrinsic" group and, by definition, places those without such evidence in the cryptogenic (intrinsic) group. It is clear that some at least of the latter group will be reclassified when, for example, bronchial provocation tests elicit reactions to previously unsuspected agents or those for which test procedures were not previously available.

The term extrinsic asthma has been applied mainly in the past to asthma in atopic subjects with evidence of reagin, IgE antibody to the relevant allergens. Analyses of the asthmatic reactions to extrinsic agents promises, even with the many gaps in our knowledge, to broaden considerably the context of extrinsic asthma, and can be made taking into account, with many provisos (*1*) the immunologic classification of the subject as atopic or nonatopic (51); (*2*) the patterns of asthmatic reaction; (*3*) their possible immunopathologic mechanisms.

A comparison of asthmatic reactions in atopic and nonatopic subjects can be made as follows. (*1*) *Atopic subjects* are characterized by their capacity to become readily sensitized to common environmental allergens. (*a*) *"Immediate"* asthmatic reactions mediated by IgE antibody occur predominantly in this group, given that IgE antibody to a particular allergen may be produced in otherwise nonatopic subjects, and could be responsible for immediate asthmatic reactions. (*b*) *"Immediate plus nonimmediate"* asthmatic reactions, i.e., dual, or combined, reactions occur in subjects who have both IgE antibody and precipitating antibody.

(2) *Nonatopic subjects,* by definition, are not easily sensitized to common allergens. (*a*) *"Immediate"* asthmatic reactions are mediated by STS-IgG antibody in the absence of IgE antibody, given that there are subjects otherwise regarded as atopic in whom both classes of antibody to common allergens are present. (*b*) *"Nonimmediate"* asthmatic reactions are mediated, at least for some common allergens, by precipitating antibody. An association with antibodies other than IgE and, possibly, STS-IgG is postulated in view of the role of immediate reactions in the development of Type III reactions. (*c*) *"Immediate plus nonimmediate" asthmatic reactions,* i.e., dual, or combined, reactions occur to some common allergens in subjects with precipitins and possibly STS-IgG antibody, given that IgE antibody may also be produced in some of these subjects.

Combined or dual immediate and nonimmediate asthmatic reactions occur in (*a*) atopic subjects with Type I, IgE-mediated and Type III, precipitin-mediated allergy, given that in some subjects giving immediate asthmatic reactions, more intensive challenge may elicit dual reactions, without supporting evidence for a Type III reaction; (*b*) nonatopic subjects with, possibly, Type I STS-IgG and Type III, precipitin-mediated allergy. (*c*) A role for other mechanisms, immunologic or not, requires consideration.

Another analysis could be made along the following lines. (*1*) *Extrinsic reaginic, immediate, asthmatic reactions* are mediated by IgE antibody, and are a feature of atopic subjects. (*2*) *Extrinsic, nonreaginic, immediate asthmatic reactions* are mediated by STS-IgG antibody and are a feature of nonatopic subjects. (*3*) *Extrinsic combined reaginic/nonreaginic immediate asthmatic reactions,* as yet an unestablished pattern, must be considered because of the evidence for each of these independently, as in (*1*) and (*2*). (*4*) *Extrinsic, nonimmediate asthmatic reactions* are mediated by precipitins and possibly STS-IgG antibody or by other immunologic or nonimmmunologic factors. (*5*) *Extrinsic combined or dual asthmatic reactions* must take into account the various patterns of nonimmediate reaction, which may require yet other descriptive terms in the classification. This reaction could be mediated by Type I, IgE or STS-IgG antibodies, or both, plus precipitins, or by other immunlogic or nonimmunlogic factors.

This attempt to classify the asthmatic reactions can be clinically relevant, because, as has been shown, the patterns of asthmatic reaction determine how the subject is likely to respond to 3 of the main therapeutic agents for the treatment of asthma, namely, bronchodilator drugs, cromolyn sodium, and corticosteroids. The exercise of correlating these classifications, based on asthmatic reactions to tests under controlled conditions, with the obscure picture of clinical asthma is the challenge which faces us.

References

1. Colldahl, H.: A study of provocation tests in patients with bronchial asthma, Acta Allergol (Kbh), 1952, *5*, 133.
2. Gronemeyer, W., and Fuchs, E: Der inhalative antigen in pneumometric test als standard: Methode in der diagnose allergischer krankheiten, Int Arch Allergy, 1959, *14*, 217.
3. McAllen, M. K.: Bronchial sensitivity testing in asthma, Thorax 1961, *16*, 30.
4. Orie, N. G. M., Booij-Noord, H., Pelikan, Z., Snoek, W., van Lookeren Campagne, G., and De Vries, K.: Protective effect of disodium cromogly cate on nasal and bronchial reactions after allergen challenge, in *Disodium Cromoglycate in Allergic Airways Disease,* J. Pepys and A. W. Frankland, ed., Butterworths, London, 1970.
5. Pepys, J.: Hypersensitivity to inhaled organic antigens, Roy Coll Physcns, 1967, *2*, 42.
6. Pepys, J.: Hypersensitivity diseases of the lungs due to fungi and organic dusts, Monogr Allergy, no. 4, S. Karger, Basel, 1969.
7. Aas, K.: The Bronchial Provocation Test, Charles C Thomas, Springfield, Ill., 1975.
8. Spector, S. L., and Farr, R. J.: Comments on bronchial inhalation provocative tests, J Allergy Clin Immunol, 1971, *2*, 120.
9. Herxheimer, H.: The late bronchial reaction in induced asthma, Int Arch Allergy, 1952, *3*, 323.
10. Kim, C. J.: The bronchial provocation test: Its clinical evaluation and the course of induced asthma, J Allergy, 1965, *36*, 353.
11. Colldahl, H.: The importance of inhalation tests in the etiological diagnosis of allergic diseases of the bronchi and in the evaluation of the effects of specific hyposensitisation treatment, Acta Allergol (Kbh), 1967, *22* (Supplement 8).
12. Booij-Noord, H., De Vries, K., Sluiter, H. J., and Orie, N. G. M.: Late bronchial obstructive reaction to experimental inhalation of house dust extract, Clin Allergy, 1972, *2*, 43.
13. Mitchell, C. A., and Gandevia, B.: Respiratory symptoms and skin reactivity in workers exposed to proteolytic enzymes in the detergent industry, Am Rev Respir Dis, 1971, *104*, 1.
14. Davies, R. J., Hendrick, D. J., and Pepys, J.: Asthma due to inhaled chemical agents: Ampi-

cillin, benzyl penicillin, 6 amino-penicillanic acid and related substances, Clin Allergy, 1974, *4*, 227.

15. Parish, W. E., and Pepys, J.: The lung in allergic disease, in *Clinical Aspects of Immunology*, ed. 2, P. G. H. Gell and R. R. A. Coombs, ed., Blackwell Scientific Publications, Oxford, 1968, p. 959.

16. Pepys, J., Parish, W. E., Stenius, B., and Wide, L.: Long-term and short-term sensitising antibodies to common allergens in extrinsic and cryptogenic asthma (abstract), Clin Allergy, 1975, *5*, 237.

17. Parish, W. E.: Short-term anaphylactic IgG antibodies in human sera, Lancet, 1970, *2*, 591.

18. Parish, W. E.: A human heat-stable anaphylactic or anaphylactoid antibody which may participate in pulmonary disorders, in *Asthma*, K. F. Austen and L. M. Lichtenstein, ed., Academic Press Inc., New York, 1973, p. 72.

19. Bryant, D. H., Burns, M. W., and Lazarus, L.: New type of allergic asthma due to IgG "reaginic" antibody, Br Med J, 1973, *4*, 589.

20. Aas, K.: Bronchial provocation tests in asthma, Arch Dis Child, 1970, *45*, 221.

21. Bryant, D. H., Burns, M. W., and Lazarus, L.: The correlation between skin tests, bronchial provocation tests and the serum level of IgE specific for common allergens in patients with asthma, Clin Allergy, 1975, *5*, 145.

22. Berg, T., Bennich, H., and Johansson, S. G. O.: In vitro diagnosis of atopic allergy. I. A comparison between provocation tests and the radioallergosorbent test, Int Arch Allergy Appl Immunol, 1971, *40*, 770.

23. Ahlstedt, S., Eriksson, N., Lindgren, S., and Roth, A.: Specific IgE determination by RAST compared with skin and provocation tests in allergy diagnosis with birch pollen, timothy pollen and dog epithelium allergens, Clin Allergy, 1970, *4*, 131.

24. Stenius, B., Wide, L., Seymour, W. M., Holford-Strevens, V., and Pepys, J.: Clinical significance of specific IgE to common allergens, Clin Allergy, 1971, *1*, 37.

25. Pepys, J., Turner-Warwick. M., Dawson, P. L., and Hinson, K. F. W.: Arthus (Type III) skin test reactions in man: Clinical and immunopathological features, in *Allergology*, B. Rose, Sixth Congress of International Association of Allergology, Excerpta Medica Congress Series No. 162, 1968.

26. Hargreave, F. E., and Pepys, J.: Allergic respiratory reactions in bird fanciers provoked by allergen inhalation provocation tests, J Allergy Clin Immunol, 1972, *50*, 157.

27. Chan-Yeung, M., Barton, G. M., MacLean, L., and Grzybowski, S.: Occupational asthma and rhinitis due to western red cedar (*Thuja plicata*), Am Rev Respir Dis, 1973, *108*, 1094.

28. Chan-Yeung, M.: Maximal expiratory flow and airway resistance during induced bronchoconstriction in patients with asthma due to western red cedar (*Thuja plicata*), Am Rev Respir Dis, 1973, *108*, 1103.

29. McCarthy, D. S., and Pepys, J.: Allergic bronchopulmonary aspergillosis: Clinical immunology. 2. Skin, nasal and bronchial tests, Clin Allergy, 1971, *1*, 415.

30. Pepys, J., Hargreave, F. E., Chan, M., and McCarthy, D. S.: Inhibitory effects of disodium cromoglycate (Intal) on allergen inhalation tests, Lancet, 1968, *2*, 134.

31. Pepys, J., Pickering, C. A. C., and Hughes, E. G.: Asthma due to inhaled chemical agents: Complex salts of platinum, Clin Allergy, 1972, *2*, 391.

32. Cleare, M. J., Hughes, E. G., Jacoby, B., and Pepys, J.: Allergic response to platinum compounds, Clin Allergy, in press.

32a. Davies, R. J., and Pepys, J.: Asthma due to inhaled chemical agents: The macrolide antibiotic spiramycin, Clin Allergy, 1975, *5*, 99.

33. Pepys, J., Pickering, C. A. C., and Loudon, H. W. G.: Asthma due to inhaled chemical agents: Piperazine dihydrochloride, Clin Allergy, 1972, *2*, 189.

34. Sosman, A. J., Schlueter, D. P., Fink, J. N., and Barboriak, J. J.: Hypersensitivity to wood dust, N Engl J Med, 1969, *281*, 977.

35. Gandevia, B., and Milne, J.: Occupational asthma and rhinitis due to western red cedar (*Thuja plicata*) with special reference to bronchial reactivity, Br J Ind Med, 1970, *27*, 235.

36. Pickering, C. A. C., Batten, J. C., and Pepys, J.: Asthma due to inhaled wood dusts: Western red cedar and iroko, Clin Allergy, 1972, *2*, 213.

37. Pepys, J., Pickering, C. A. C., and Terry, D. J.: Asthma due to inhaled chemical agents: Tolylene di-isocyanate, Clin Allergy, 1972, *2*, 225.

38. Paisley, D. P. G.: Isocyanate hazard from wire insulation: An old hazard in a new guise, Br J Ind Med, 1969, *26*, 79.

39. Peters, J. M., and Murphy, R. L. H.: Hazards to health: Do-it-yourself polyurethane foam, Am Rev Respir Dis, 1971, *184*, 432.

40. McCann, J. K.: Health hazard from flux used in joining aluminum electricity cables, Lancet, 1964, *1*, 445.

41. Sterling, G. M.: Asthma due to aluminium soldering flux, Thorax, 1967, *22*, 533.

42. Pepys, J., and Pickering, C. A. C.: Asthma due to inhaled chemical fumes in amino ethyl ethanolamine in aluminium soldering flux, Clin Allergy, 1972, *2*, 197.

43. Breslin, A. B. X., Hendrick, D. J., and Pepys, J.: Effect of disodium cromoglycate on asthmatic reactions to alcoholic beverages, Clin Allergy, 1973, *3*, 71.

44. Konig, P., and Godfrey, S.: The effect of frequent administration of sodium cromoglycate to asthmatic children who previously respond-

ed poorly, Clin Allergy, 1973, *3*, 395.

45. Pepys, J., Davies, R. J., Breslin, A. B. X., Hendrick, D. J., and Hutchcroft, B. J.: The effects of inhaled beclomethasone dipropionate (Becotide) and sodium cromoglycate on asthmatic reactions to provocation tests, Clin Allergy, 1974, *4*, 13.

46. Schwartz, M.: Heredity in bronchial asthma: Clinical and genetic study of 191 asthma probands and 50 probands with baker's asthma, Acta Allergol (Kbh), 1952, *5*, (Supplement 2, p. 3).

47. Szentivanyi, A.: Effects of bacterial products and adrenergic blocking agents on allergic reactions, in *Immunological Diseases,* M. Samter, ed., Little, Brown, Boston, 1971, p. 356.

48. Gell, P. G. H., Coombs, R. R. A., and Lachmann, P. J.: Clinical Aspects of Immunology, ed. 3, Blackwell Scientific Publications, Oxford, 1975.

49. Ishizaka, K., Ishizaka, T., and Hornbrook, M. M.: Physico-chemical properties of reaginic antibody. IV. Presence of a unique immunoglobulin as a carrier of reaginic activity, J Immunol, 1966, *97*, 75.

50. Coca, A. E., and Grove, E.: Studies in hypersensitiveness. XIII. A study of the atopic reagins, J Immunol, 1925, *10*, 445.

51. Pepys, J.: Atopy, in *Clinical Aspects of Immunology,* ed. 3, P. G. H. Gell, R. R. A. Coombs, and P. J. Lachmann, ed., Blackwell Scientific Publications, Oxford, 1975, p. 877.

52. Grant, J. A., and Lichtenstein, L. M.: Reversed 'in vitro' anaphylaxis induced by anti-IgG: Specificity of the reaction and comparison with antigen-induced histamine release, J Immunol, 1972, *109*, 20.

53. Richardson, J. B., Hogg, J. C., Bouchard, T., and Hall, D. L.: Electron microscopic localisation of antigen in experimental bronchoconstriction in guinea pigs, Chest, 1973, *63* (Supplement, p. 445).

54. Cochrane, C. G.: Mechanisms involved in the deposition of immune-complexes in tissues, J Exp Med, 1971, *134* (Supplement, p. 75).

55. Weissman, G.: Effects of corticosteroids on the stability and fusion of biomembranes, in *Asthma,* K. F. Austen and L. M. Lichtenstein, ed., Academic Press Inc., New York, 1973, p. 221.

56. Dolovich, J., Hargreave, F. E., Chalmers, R., Shier, K. J., Gouldie, J., and Bienenstock, J.: Late cutaneous allergic responses in isolated

IgE-dependent reactions, J Allergy Clin Immunol, 1973, *52*, 38.

57. Umemoto, L., Poothullil, J., Dolovich, J., Hargreave, F. E., and Day, R. P.: Factors which influence the late cutaneous allergic response (LCAR), J Allergy Clin Immunol, 1975, *55*, 112.

58. Solley, G. O., Larson, J. B., Jordon, R. E., and Gleich, G. J.: Late cutaneous reactions due to IgE (abstract), J Allergy Clin Immunol, 1975, *55*, 112.

59. Killian, D., Hargreave, F. E., Dolovich, J., and Wolfe, R.: Factors which influence patterns of allergen-induced asthmatic responses (abstract), Clin Allergy, in press.

60. Turk, J. L.: Mechanisms in cell mediated immunity, Ann Sclavo, 1971, *13*, 748.

61. Edwards, J. H., Baker, J. T., and Davies, B. J.: Precipitin test negative farmer's lung-activation of the alternative pathway of complement by mouldy hay dusts, Clin Allergy, 1974, *4*, 379.

62. Marx, J. J., and Flaherty, D. K.: Alternate pathway activation of complement by antigens associated with hypersensitivity pneumonitis (abstract), J Allergy Clin Immunol, 1975, *55*, 70.

63. Konzen, R. B., Craft, B. F., and Scheel, L. D.: Human response to low concentrations of p.p. diphenylmethane di-isocyanate (MDI), Am Ind Hyg Assoc J, 1966, *27*, 121.

64. Pepys, J.: Non-immediate type of hypersensitivity in bronchial asthma, in *Allergology,* Proc. 8th Int. Congr. Allergology, Tokyo, 1973, Y. Yamamura, ed., Excerpta Medica International Congress Series no. 323, 1974, p. 84.

65. Pepys, J., Hargreave, F. E., Longbottom, J. L., and Faux, J.: Allergic reactions of the lungs to enzymes of *Bacillus subtilis,* Lancet, 1969, *1*, 1181.

66. Spector, W. G., and Heesom, W: The production of granulomata by antigen-antibody complexes, J Pathol Bact, 1969, *98*, 31.

67. Hansen, P., and Penny, R.: Immune mechanisms and diagnosis of pigeon breeder's disease, Med J Aust, 1974, *1*, 984.

68. Boros, D. L., and Warren, K. F.: Bentonite granuloma characterisation of a model system for infection and foreign body granulomatous infiltration using soluble mycobacterial, histoplasma and schistosoma antigens, Immunology, 1973, *24*, 511.

 ————————————————————

General Anesthesia and the Lung[1,2]

KAI REHDER, ALAN D. SESSLER, and H. MICHAEL MARSH

Contents

Interest in lung function during general anesthesia arises because the incidence of pulmonary problems in clinical practice is high and because the lung is the site of uptake and elimination of volatile and gaseous anesthetics. Concern for pulmonary problems has existed from the time of "ether pneumonias" to the present, when atelectasis and arterial hypoxemia remain among the major causes of postoperative morbidity (1, 2). Death rates with anesthesia have been estimated to be as frequent as 1 in 1,560 cases (3), and hypoxia has been said to be an attributable cause in one half of all deaths associated with anesthesia (4).

Most investigators agree that general anesthesia interferes with pulmonary gas exchange. Impairment of oxygenation and CO_2 elimination during anesthesia has been thoroughly reviewed (4–6). Impaired pulmonary gas exchange may result from increased venous admixture, or changes in cardiac output, O_2-carrying characteristics of hemoglobin, and dead space. The contributions of these factors to the impairment of pulmonary gas exchange will be discussed, and some of the possible mechanisms will be reviewed, with major emphasis placed on alterations in pulmonary mechanics and the effects of these alterations on intrapulmonary gas distribu-

---

[1] From the Mayo Clinic and Mayo Foundation, Rochester, Minn. 55901.

[2] This investigation was supported in part by Research Grants HL-12090 and RR-585 from the National Institutes of Health, U. S. Public Health Service, and by a grant from the Parker B. Francis Foundation, Kansas City, Mo.

tion as induced by anesthesia with or without muscle paralysis.

Pulmonary Gas Exchange

Factors that affect arterial oxygenation and CO_2 elimination during general anesthesia include (*1*) the inspired concentrations of O_2 and CO_2; (*2*) the volume of alveolar ventilation; (*3*) the alveolar gas concentrations as influenced by pulmonary inert gas exchange, with second-gas and concentration effects during uptake (7–9), and dilution effect during elimination of volatile or gaseous anesthetics (10); (*4*) the magnitude of venous admixture; (*5*) the content of gases of mixed venous blood.

During anesthesia, concentrations of inspired O_2 and CO_2 are influenced by the breathing circuit of the anesthesia machine, including increased dead space, normal function of the CO_2 absorber, the competency of the respiratory valves, and the fresh gas inflows. These factors are controlled by the anesthesiologist and can be excluded as causes of impaired gas exchange if attention is paid to the proper regulation and function of the equipment.

A small transient increase in alveolar Po_2 and arterial Po_2 may result from concentration and second-gas effects during general anesthesia. Similarly, an increase in arterial Po_2 may occur if mixed venous O_2 content ($C\bar{v}_{O_2}$) is increased, although the magnitude of the right-to-left shunt and the alveolar Po_2 remain unchanged. The resulting increase in arterial Po_2 is usually of little clinical consequence, and the factors that tend to decrease arterial Po_2 are far more important.

Impaired Oxygenation

Arterial Po_2 can be reduced by supplying a hypoxic inspiratory gas mixture, by permitting alveolar hypoventilation from an obstructed airway, or by allowing pharmacologic or metabolic depression of respiratory drive. Appropriate inspiratory O_2 concentrations, endotrachael intubation, and mechanical ventilation usually can prevent reduction in arterial Po_2 by these mechanisms. Arterial Po_2 also can be reduced by an increased venous admixture, which commonly occurs during general anesthesia. The effect of the increased venous admixture cannot be corrected, and its mechanisms remain unclear.

Venous admixture. Venous admixture, or physiologic shunt, results from anatomic shunts and from "shunt-like" effects, i.e., perfusion of poorly ventilated or nonventilated alveoli and

perfusion of alveoli in which diffusion is impaired.

Anatomic Shunting

Anatomic shunting through right-to-left vascular connections occurs in the heart and lungs. Blood from anterior cardiac and thebesian veins, together with blood from giant pleural capillaries and bronchial veins flowing into pulmonary veins, constitutes a shunt of approximately 2 per cent of the total cardiac output in normal, conscious man.

Anatomic pathways less frequently considered for shunting through the lungs have been described by von Hayek (11, 12). Small anastomoses exist between the bronchial and pulmonary arteries. These anastomotic vessels (rami pulmobronchiales) have walls of thick longitudinal musculature that apparently can totally occlude their lumina. Thus, they have been called "Sperrarterien," i.e., blocking arteries. Three types of vessels originate from these rami pulmobronchiales, or "Sperrarterien": (*1*) rami alveolares to alveoli and thence to pulmonary veins; ·(*2*) rami bronchiales to bronchial walls and thence to bronchial and pulmonary veins; (*3*) vasa vasorum to the walls of the pulmonary artery, but not communicating with its lumen. Von Hayek suggested that the lumina of these arteries can be occluded to block flow from the bronchial arteries, thus remaining open only to flow from the pulmonary artery, thereby constituting a right-to-left shunt. On the basis of anatomic measurements, he estimated that as much as 10 per cent of the cardiac output could take this path, whereas as much as 10 per cent more could be shunted through giant pleural capillaries. Blood flow through these vessels seems to be small in normal, conscious man; but at present, nothing is known concerning their function during anesthesia. If the patency of these vessels were affected by general anesthetics, major intrapulmonary shunts could open.

"Shunt-like" Effects

Mismatching of ventilation to perfusion may contribute to venous admixture during general anesthesia, thus producing "shunt-like" effects.

Ventilation-perfusion relationships. Twelve years after Lilienthal and co-workers (13) presented an analysis of the alveolar-to-arterial Po_2 difference ($[A\text{-}a]Po_2$) into a diffusion or membrane component and a venous admixture component, and 9 years after Riley and Cournand (14) and Rahn (15) independently introduced their analyses of ventilation-perfusion relationships ($\dot{V}/\dot{Q}$), Campbell and co-workers (16) in 1958 suggested that $\dot{V}/\dot{Q}$ mismatching was a probable cause for the increased venous admixture and widened (A-a)Po_2 during general anesthesia and mechanical ventilation. They studied 6 healthy, supine subjects during awake, spontaneous ventilation and again during general anesthesia with mechanical ventilation and determined (A-a)Po_2 during room air breathing, physiologic dead space, and total respiratory system compliance. They concluded that there was little increase in (A-a)Po_2 in the group as a whole while breathing room air, but that with the considerable individual differences seen, various abnormal patterns of $\dot{V}/\dot{Q}$ occurred in some subjects during mechanical ventilation, resulting in abnormal $\dot{V}/\dot{Q}$ during general anesthesia and mechanical ventilation. Despite much work in this area since Campbell and co-workers' original paper, controversy continues regarding the contribution of $\dot{V}/\dot{Q}$ mismatching to impaired oxygenation during general anesthesia.

Finley and co-workers (17), on the basis of indirect evidence obtained in dogs during pentobarbital anesthesia, suggested that spontaneous collapse of lung areas caused the major part of the observed (A-a)Po_2 during spontaneous breathing. Similar conclusions for anesthetized man were drawn by Bendixen and associates (18), who found a progressive decrease in Pa_{O_2} during ventilation with small tidal volumes. Nunn (19) and Nunn and co-workers (20) confirmed the increase in (A-a)Po_2 during anesthesia, but stressed that the increase was not progressive and not always reversible with large breaths. They attributed the increased (A-a)Po_2 that occurred during general anesthesia with spontaneous breathing or with mechanical ventilation to increased $\dot{V}/\dot{Q}$ mismatching. Bergman (21) found evidence for increased shunting, but not for significant $\dot{V}/\dot{Q}$ mismatching during general anesthesia in supine man on the basis of the (A-a)Po_2 measured while patients breathed 25 and 100 per cent O_2. During that study, however, measurable inert gas exchange, causing an increased alveolar Po_2 by the second-gas effect, occurred in the subjects' lungs, precluding detection of small degrees of $\dot{V}/\dot{Q}$ mismatching.

That $\dot{V}/\dot{Q}$ mismatching may occur and contribute to the (A-a)Po_2 while breathing 100 per cent O_2 was re-emphasized by studies based on analysis of pulmonary N_2 clearance curves obtained simultaneously with data that indicated the rate of increase of arterial Po_2. With this method, a larger spread of $\dot{V}/\dot{Q}$ throughout the lung than occurs in awake man was found in anesthetized, paralyzed, and mechanically ventilated man in the lateral decubitus position (22). Increased $\dot{V}/\dot{Q}$ mismatching during anesthesia, however, could not be demonstrated by this technique in subjects in the supine position.

Interest in the mechanism for increased shunting and increased $\dot{V}/\dot{Q}$ mismatching has been rekindled by the concept of airway closure. Airway closure is believed to affect pulmonary gas exchange either by creating poorly ventilated regions, when it occurs within the tidal breathing range, or by leading to cessation of ventilation if opening volume exceeds end-inspiratory lung volume (23–25). If the distribution of pulmonary blood flow is not adjusted to this altered gas distribution, areas with low or zero $\dot{V}/\dot{Q}$ would develop, leading to impaired oxygenation. Evidence for the occurrence of airway closure in anesthetized man is incomplete.

Using intravenous injections of xenon-133 in 8 anesthetized, spontaneously ventilating, nonobese, supine human subjects, Couture and associates (26) found a decreased ventilation in dependent lung regions that they attributed to airway closure. The decreased ventilation correlated with changes in physiologic shunt. Weenig and associates (27) found no significant increase in (A-a)Po_2 while breathing 100 per cent O_2 after induction of anesthesia if preoperative, supine closing capacity (CC), i.e., the absolute lung volume at which the onset of phase IV occurs, was smaller than end-inspiratory lung volume during anesthesia: CC < functional residual capacity (FRC) + tidal volume (VT). In another group of patients, they found that (A-a)Po_2 while breathing 100 per cent O_2 increased significantly if VT was reduced so that end-inspiratory lung volume was less than preoperative CC, i.e., CC > FRC + VT. Don and co-workers (28) found small volumes of trapped gas during anesthesia when FRC was larger than preoperative CC, but found significantly larger volumes when FRC was less than CC. They suggested that the increased trapping was due to airway closure and that absorption with collapse may occur in alveoli that contain trapped gas. Hence, pulmonary shunting through open capillaries past such regions may occur.

In normal, awake, spontaneously breathing man, CC does not change with continuous positive airway pressure (CPAP), but FRC increases. Because reductions in FRC in supine, anesthetized man have been repeatedly demonstrated

(29–39), attempts have been made using CPAP to increase the difference between FRC and CC during general anesthesia, on the assumption that CC does not increase, or increases less than FRC. For instance, Wyche and co-workers (36), studying the effect of mechanical ventilation with positive end-expiratory pressure (PEEP) on arterial P_{O_2} in anesthetized subjects, demonstrated an average increase in arterial P_{O_2} of 1.6 mm Hg per cm H_2O of end-expiratory pressure in anesthetized, paralyzed patients who had arterial P_{O_2} values less than 100 mm Hg at a fraction of inspired O_2 ($F_{I_{O_2}}$) of 0.3; patients with arterial P_{O_2} values greater than 100 mm Hg showed a variable response. The results of that study support the much earlier work of Frumin and co-workers (40) in 1959. Colgan and co-workers (41) found no change in (A-a)P_{O_2} in anesthetized dogs that breathed 100 per cent O_2 spontaneously at CPAP or were mechanically ventilated with O_2 at PEEP. However, they found a significant decrease in right-to-left shunting ($\dot{Q}_s/\dot{Q}_t$) with PEEP in the same dogs. Reductions in cardiac output with alterations in $C\bar{v}_{O_2}$ may have masked the effects of PEEP on the (A-a)P_{O_2} while breathing 100 per cent O_2 in that study.

Although "airway closure" may seem an attractive explanation for impaired oxygenation during general anesthesia, valid experimental proof for its contribution to hypoxemia is lacking. First, it is still undecided whether closure of airways (42), dynamic compression of airways (43), or other mechanisms produce the onset of phase IV. A recent study (44) produced some evidence that was consistent with both theories and some that was inconsistent with both. Second, in the studies previously cited (27, 28), CC during general anesthesia was assumed to remain unchanged from that in the awake state. This may be invalid. The elastic recoil of the lung, the major determinant of CC, i.e., the volume at the onset of phase IV, is increased during general anesthesia (31), and therefore the possibility of reductions in CC must be considered.

One must conclude that further studies are required before the relationship of FRC and CC and their influence on Pa_{O_2} during general anesthesia can be clearly understood or predicted. These studies must include the demonstration of phase IV and comparative measurements of CC in awake and anesthetized man. Certainly, CPAP and PEEP should not be considered as routine adjuvants for general anesthesia and should not be used without gauging the response

of the Pa_{O_2} and the circulatory system to its application.

The techniques used for obtaining continuous distributions of ventilation and perfusion relative to volume throughout the lung pioneered by Gómez (45), Lenfant and Okubo (46), and Okubo and Lenfant (47) and the foreign gas elimination technique of Wagner and associates (48, 49) may provide more information concerning the distribution of $\dot{V}/\dot{Q}$ throughout the lung during anesthesia. These methods also may be helpful in distinguishing shunts from lung regions that have very low $\dot{V}/\dot{Q}$. Such methods, however, do not permit regional localization of the shunt or of regions with low $\dot{V}/\dot{Q}$. This information may be obtained by the use of radioactive isotopes such as [133]Xe.

Diffusion. Piiper and associates (50), on the basis of experiments in anesthetized dogs at various $F_{I_{O_2}}$, concluded that unequal distribution of diffusion to perfusion was the main factor increasing (A-a)P_{O_2} while breathing room air. Dollery and co-workers (51) showed a gradient of diffusion per unit lung volume between apex and base using $C^{15}O$ in normal, sitting man. Staub (52), noting the large disparity between reported diffusing capacities for CO ($D_{L_{CO}}$) and O_2 ($D_{L_{O_2}}$), concluded that the diffusion component of (A-a)P_{O_2} could not be reliably differentiated from the total (A-a)P_{O_2}, but that on theoretic grounds, $D_{L_{O_2}}$ was probably higher than previously believed. He also emphasized that regional variations in capillary transit times are more important than membrane variations because of a higher diffusion resistance of the blood than of the alveolar membrane.

Fukuma and co-workers (53) investigated the effects of 6 different anesthetic regimens on $D_{L_{O_2}}$ in dogs. They concluded that there was no noticeable difference in $D_{L_{O_2}}$ among the various regimens. The effect of general anesthesia on diffusing capacity has received scant attention in man. Bergman (54) compared $D_{L_{CO}}$ measured in the awake state and again during halothane anesthesia in man. He reported no significant change from awake values for the same subjects, using the method of Filley and associates (55) to calculate mean alveolar P_{CO}. Estimations of uneven distribution of pulmonary blood flow to diffusing capacity during general anesthesia, using the method of Hyde and co-workers (56), have not, to our knowledge, been reported.

Evidence is accumulating that CO and O_2 transfer may be partially carrier-mediated in the human lung (57). If such facilitated diffusion occurs, an effect of anesthetics on CO and O_2 transfer might be anticipated in view of a possible competition between CO or O_2 and the anesthetic for cytochrome P-450 (58, 59).

Other influences on arterial Po_2. Factors that affect $C\bar{v}_{O_2}$ may alter arterial Po_2. These include cardiac output and the O_2-carrying characteristics of hemoglobin.

Cardiac Output

A reduced cardiac output ($\dot{Q}$) may be accompanied by a decreased $C\bar{v}_{O_2}$ if total O_2 consumption ($\dot{V}o_2$) is not concurrently decreased or if arterial O_2 content (Ca_{O_2}) is not increased. This is illustrated by expressing the Fick equation with $C\bar{v}_{O_2}$ as the dependent variable:

$$C\bar{v}_{O_2} = Ca_{O_2} - \frac{\dot{V}o_2}{\dot{Q}}.$$

If the percentage of shunt flow ($\dot{Q}_s/\dot{Q}_t$) remains unaltered, Ca_{O_2} must decrease during O_2 breathing in the presence of a decreased $C\bar{v}_{O_2}$ if alveolar Po_2 and thus end-capillary O_2 content (Cc'_{O_2}) remain unchanged, because, from a rearrangement of the shunt equation,

$$Ca_{O_2} = Cc'_{O_2}\left[1 - \frac{\dot{Q}_s}{\dot{Q}_t}\right] + C\bar{v}_{O_2}\frac{\dot{Q}_s}{\dot{Q}_t}.$$

Thus, if the O_2 dissociation curve is not shifted to the right, $(A-a)Po_2$ will increase.

It has been proposed that reductions in cardiac output without major changes in either shunt fraction or $\dot{V}/\dot{Q}$ matching are responsible for increases in $(A-a)Po_2$ during anesthesia (60). This view was influenced by a study (61) suggesting that, during anesthesia, cardiac output may consistently decrease to very low levels, a condition that has not been confirmed (62).

Changes in O_2-Carrying Characteristics of Hemoglobin

A shift or change in the slope of the oxyhemoglobin dissociation curve affects the relationship between Po_2 and O_2 content. A left shift of the curve results in a decreased Po_2 for a given O_2 content. Thus, a fixed shunt fraction would increase $(A-a)Po_2$ and could reduce arterial Po_2.

Several investigators have examined the possibility that anesthetics cause a left shift of the O_2-dissociation curve and thus lead to an increased $(A-a)Po_2$. A retrospective review of data from anesthetized man suggested that a right shift of the dissociation curve occurred with N_2O, cyclopropane, halothane, or enflurane anesthesia

(63), and a right shift also was observed with human blood exposed *in vitro* to 3 per cent halothane (64). Careful *in vitro* studies failed to demonstrate any such shift of the curve for human blood exposed to halothane (65), cyclopropane (65), methoxyflurane (66), diethyl ether (67), or N_2O (67). One would conclude that most of the evidence shows that *in vitro*, there is no shift of the dissociation curve seen in the presence of anesthetics. *In vivo*, the situation remains unclear, because the effects of the anesthetics on hemoglobin may be compounded by complex biochemical and physiologic alterations.

Impaired CO_2 Elimination

Severinghaus and co-workers (68) first demonstrated the impaired elimination of CO_2 during anesthesia, reporting an increase of 2 to 3 mm Hg in arterial to end-tidal Pco_2 differences ($[a-A]Pco_2$) in 5 patients mechanically ventilated during anesthesia with diethyl ether.

Analysis of the mechanisms underlying this change in $(a-A)Pco_2$ awaited quantification of the components of the physiologic dead space (V_D). Campbell and associates (16) demonstrated a significant increase in V_D in 6 anesthetized and mechanically ventilated patients. They could not distinguish increases in anatomic dead space ($V_{D_{anat}}$) from increases in alveolar dead space ($V_{D_{alv}}$) ($V_D = V_{D_{anat}} + V_{D_{alv}}$) because they did not measure anatomic dead space. This distinction was later made by Nunn and Hill (69), who found that the value of anatomic dead space was close to predicted values in both spontaneously breathing and mechanically ventilated anesthetized subjects. They concluded, therefore, that the alveolar dead space was increased, and they estimated that it ranged from 15 to 231 ml.

The anatomic dead space also may be affected during anesthesia, being reduced by one-half with intubation or tracheostomy, increased by atropine (70), and altered by the position of the neck and lower jaw. With an extended neck and protruded jaw, the anatomic dead space will be twice that seen with a flexed neck and depressed chin (71). This is of clinical importance, because extension and protrusion are commonly used to maintain a patent airway during general anesthesia in nonintubated subjects.

Askrog and associates (72) found a consistent increase in $(a-A)Pco_2$ and in the ratio of physiologic dead space to tidal volume (V_D/V_T) in 18 patients anesthetized with halothane, cyclopropane, or N_2O. The increase in V_D/V_T was progressive with time and apparently unrelated to the agent used. Thornton (73) confirmed this progressive increase in physiologic dead space with time. It was not found by Kain and co-workers (74), who did, however, observe an increase in V_D/V_T with increasing concentrations of halothane.

Askrog (75) later examined the relationship between (a-A)P_{CO_2} and induced changes in pulmonary artery pressure in patients anesthetized with 1 per cent halothane and found an increase in (a-A)P_{CO_2} of 4 to 6 mm Hg 1 hour after induction of anesthesia. There was a linear negative correlation between pulmonary artery pressure and (a-A)P_{CO_2} regardless of how pulmonary artery pressure was changed. Askrog suggested that the major factor responsible for the increased (a-A)P_{CO_2} during anesthesia was an altered distribution of pulmonary blood flow related to moderate pulmonary hypotension, presumably resulting in underperfusion of nondependent lung regions. His observations were substantiated and extended by studies that showed similar increases in (a-A)P_{CO_2} with the administration of ganglion-blocking agents (72, 76) and with hemorrhagic shock (77–79). It should be recalled that an increase in calculated alveolar dead space also may result from either an increase in anatomic shunt or an altered ventilation-perfusion relationship, or from both.

Conclusion

Oxygenation and elimination of CO_2 are impaired during general anesthesia. This may be attributed to an increased right-to-left shunt, increased alveolar dead space, and probably an altered ventilation-perfusion relationship. Other factors, such as changes in cardiac output, O_2-carrying characteristics of hemoglobin, diffusion-perfusion relationships, and an altered relationship between FRC and CC may contribute to an increased (A-a)P_{O_2} during anesthesia.

Intrapulmonary Gas Distribution

Mismatching of ventilation to perfusion occurs if the distribution of either ventilation or perfusion is altered without appropriate adjustment in the other. The distribution of pulmonary blood flow will not be discussed, because the bulk of evidence suggests that regional distribution of pulmonary blood flow remains primarily gravity dependent during general anesthesia, although some effects of anesthetics on pulmonary blood vessels have been demonstrated. Consideration will be given to the intrapulmonary distribution of inspired gas during general anesthesia with and without mechanical ventilation.

Uniform distribution of intrapulmonary gas has been defined by Fowler (80) as occurring when "during inspiration each alveolus would receive at the same time gas of the same chemical composition and of the same volume (in relation to its previous pre-inspiratory volume) and that this gas would mix almost instantaneously with the functional residual gas in the alveolus." The gas volume inspired by an individual lung unit is directly proportional to the forces for expansion of that unit and the admittance to that unit. Admittance is the inverse of impedance, impedance being the total opposition to gas flow into the lungs and consisting of elastic, flow-resistive, and inertial forces of the respiratory system. Nonuniform intrapulmonary gas distribution per unit lung volume may occur when either the applied forces or the mechanical properties of the respiratory system are unequally distributed throughout the lung relative to one another.

Nonuniform distribution of ventilation per unit lung volume has been demonstrated in the lungs of normal man (80–82), such that dependent lung regions receive a larger ventilation per unit volume than do nondependent regions. The mechanism for the nonuniform distribution has been ascribed to a gravity-dependent, linear, vertical gradient in pleural pressure that leads to regional differences in preinspiratory lung volumes (81, 82), which in turn cause differences in regional compliances. A vertical pleural pressure gradient was demonstrated in dogs by Krueger and co-workers (83) and calculated from intrapulmonary gas distribution studies with ^{133}Xe by Milic-Emili and co-workers (81). Glazier and co-workers (84) freeze-fixed the lungs of dogs *in situ* and showed differences in alveolar size between dependent and nondependent lung regions, an observation that is consistent with a vertical pleural pressure gradient.

On the basis of regional differences in compliance and on the assumption of uniform pleural pressure changes during inspiration for each lung unit, as well as identical pressure-volume (P-V) characteristics for each lung unit, a nonuniform distribution of ventilation per unit lung volume can be predicted. As has been pointed out by Anthonisen and co-workers (85), however, given the above assumptions plus a single exponential P-V characteristic of the lung, synchronous emptying of the lungs should occur. Apparently, this does not happen. As indicated by the commonly observed upslope of phase III, asynchronous emptying seems to occur. Therefore, one must have some reservations concerning the validity of the assumed model, i.e., whether the pleural pressure gradient is the only determinant for intrapulmonary gas distribution, although, in general, intrapulmonary gas distribution follows the pattern predicted by the model.

Intrapulmonary Gas Distribution in Anesthetized Man

Only in recent years has intrapulmonary gas distribution during anesthesia been closely examined.

Spontaneous ventilation during anesthesia. Wulff and Aulin's (86) work with ^{133}Xe suggested that intrapulmonary gas distribution during anesthesia with spontaneous ventilation did not differ significantly from that found in supine, awake man. Froese and Bryan (87), in anesthetized man, observed a cephalad displacement of the end-expiratory position of the diaphragm and during spontaneous inspiration, a greater movement of its dependent region similar to that occurring in awake man. The observation suggests that a larger ventilation of dependent lung regions occurs during spontaneous ventilation in anesthetized man, as it does in awake man. As Froese and Bryan recognized, however, this may not always occur during anesthesia, particularly in the presence of the reduced FRC seen with general anesthesia.

Our group studied the distribution of inspired gas between left and right lungs by bronchospirometry in anesthetized man during spontaneous ventilation in the lateral decubitus positions (88). We argued that FRC is known to decrease (table 1) during general anesthesia in recumbent positions. Therefore, the possibility exists that an altered intrapulmonary distribution of ventilation per unit lung volume may occur. We found an intrapulmonary gas distribution similar to that in the awake man who initiates inspiration voluntarily from a low lung volume (82), namely a preferential distribution of ventilation to the nondependent lung. Comparing the ratios of FRC to total lung capacity (TLC) of individual lungs with those seen in awake subjects (96), we found them significantly lower in the anesthetized subjects. We hypothesized that the nondependent lung therefore may be functioning on the steeper part of its P-V curve, whereas the dependent lung may be down on the flatter part of the curve, thus resulting in the different gas distribution.

Mechanical ventilation during anesthesia. Doerfel (97) measured the distribution of the tidal volume between the lungs by bronchospirometry in anesthetized, paralyzed, mechanically ventilated man. With the subject in the lateral decubitus position, he found that the dependent lung received a smaller share of the tidal volume than did the nondependent lung; this finding is contrary to observations made in the awake state. He attributed this to a reduced mobility of the dependent hemidiaphragm during anesthesia. Potgieter (98) examined the mechanisms for the frequent development of postoperative atelectases (99) in the dependent lung of patients undergoing upper urinary tract surgery in the lateral decubitus position. He observed that the dependent lung was not adequately ventilated during mechanical ventilation. This lack of ventilation was considered to be caused by a downward shift of the mediastinum, particularly toward the lung base, and an elevated dependent hemidiaphragm. A preferential ventilation of the nondependent lung was also observed by bronchospirometry in anesthetized, paralyzed, mechanically ventilated dogs in the lateral decubitus position (100, 101).

Bergman (30) studied the intrapulmonary gas distribution by measuring the rate of N_2 elimination during N_2 clearance in 9 supine patients, first awake during spontaneous ventilation, then during anesthesia with spontaneous ventilation, and finally during mechanical ventilation. Because he found no significant differences among the rates of N_2 elimination for these 3 states, and no differences among the calculated indices for distribution and efficiency of over-all pulmonary ventilation after the method of Fowler and associates (102), he concluded that the distribution of ventilation was unaltered by anesthesia with and without muscle paralysis and mechanical ventilation. This view was accepted by other investigators at that time.

Close examination of Bergman's data (30) reveals a considerable variability of several determinants of the rate of pulmonary N_2 clearance, and recalculation of the pulmonary N_2-clearance delay revealed variable results. The variability of the determinants of pulmonary N_2 clearance was probably sufficient to obscure differences that might have existed between the awake and the anesthetized state. Indeed, the 3 subjects whose tidal volumes when anesthetized and paralyzed were within 10 per cent of corresponding volumes while awake showed evidence of faster clearance

TABLE 1

FUNCTIONAL RESIDUAL CAPACITY (FRC) DURING ANESTHESIA

Reference	Male/ Female	Age, years Weight, kg Height, cm	Anesthetic Agent	Muscle Relaxant	Body Position	Method of Measurement	FRC (liter) Mean ± SE	Control, FRC (liter) Mean ± SE
89 (1955)	6	... ...	...	Succinylcholine	...	Measurement of resting expiratory level (REL)	Increase of 0.26 in REL	...
90 (1957)	10	15–59 50–84 155–177	Pentothal	Yes	...	Measurement of REL	Decrease of 0.18 ± 0.04 in REL*	...
91 (1957)	1	... ...	Pentothal	Spontaneous respiration	Supine	Measurement of REL	Decrease of 0.20 in REL	...
91 (1957)	4	... ...	Pentothal	Succinylcholine	Supine	Measurement of REL	No change in REL	...
30 (1963)	5/0	23–74 66–92 ...	Pentothal	Spontaneous respiration	Supine	N_2 washout (Darling method)	1.81 ± 0.34	2.71 ± 0.62 (n = 6)
30 (1963)	5/0	23–74 66–92 ...	Pentothal	Succinylcholine	Supine	N_2 washout (Darling method)	1.68 ± 0.30	2.71 ± 0.62 (n = 6)
92 (1967)	2	... ...	Yes	Yes	...	Continuous pneumograph recording of abdominothoracic circumference change	Less than 0.15 reduction	...
93 (1968)	8	... ...	Halothane	Spontaneous respiration	Supine	Helium dilution	2.33 ± 0.26	2.26 ± 0.19
33 (1968)	2/6	16–59 47–83 ...	Pentothal	Succinylcholine	Supine	Helium dilution	1.84 ± 0.15	2.08 ± 0.18
34 (1970)	4/2	19–56 47–106 152–180	Pentothal, halothane in 100% O_2	Spontaneous respiration	Supine	Helium dilution	1.39 ± 0.12†	2.27 ± 0.28
34 (1970)	0/5	18–65 45–73 152–172	Pentothal, halothane in 30% O_2	Spontaneous respiration	Supine	Helium dilution	1.31 ± 0.12	1.80 ± 0.10
29 (1971)	12/4	23–33 54–97 164–188	Pentothal, meperidine	Succinylcholine	Supine	N_2 washout (Darling method)	2.28 ± 0.18 (n = 10)	2.65 ± 0.22 (n = 11)
			Pentothal, meperidine	Succinylcholine	Lateral	N_2 washout (Darling method)	2.46 ± 0.15 (n = 12)	2.71 ± 0.13 (n = 13)
94 (1972)	9	... ...	Pentothal, meperidine	Succinylcholine	Sitting	N_2 washout (Darling method)	3.29 ± 0.24	3.26 ± 0.26
95 (1973)	16	21–74	Pentothal, halothane	Spontaneous respiration	...	Helium dilution	2.18 ± 0.21 (after 20–40 min of anesthesia) 2.01 ± 0.17 (after 50–70 min of anesthesia)	2.50 ± 0.13 2.50 ± 0.13
31 (1973)	5/0	24–29 60–92 166–189	Pentothal, meperidine	Spontaneous respiration	Supine	Body plethysmography	2.38 ± 0.15	3.08 ± 0.22
			Pentothal, meperidine	Succinylcholine	Supine	Body plethysmography	2.31 ± 0.25	3.08 ± 0.22
38 (1974)	26/0	19–68 53–93 165–194	Pentothal, halothane, 35% O_2	...	Supine	Helium dilution	1.89 ± 0.12	2.28 ± 0.15
39 (1974)	13	22–64 54.5–82.0 154–175	Pentothal, halothane, 35% O_2, pancuronium	...	Supine	Helium dilution	1.72 ± 0.21	2.02 ± 0.25
32 (1974)	5/0	23–28 71–80 176–189	Isoflurane	Succinylcholine	Supine	N_2 washout (Darling method)	2.45 ± 0.16	2.65 ± 0.14
32 (1974)	4/0	23–28 71–79 178–189	Isoflurane	Succinylcholine	Supine	N_2 washout (Darling method)	2.70 ± 0.10	2.75 ± 0.11
27 (1974)	33	... ...	Pentothal, halothane	Succinylcholine, d-tubocurarine	Supine	Helium dilution	2.57 ± 0.17 (tidal volume = 5 ml/kg) 2.54 ± 0.16 (tidal volume = 10 ml/kg)	2.60 ± 0.14

*REL was decreasing in 6 subjects and increasing in 3 subjects. In one subject, the airway was obstructed.
†No change in REL with pentothal or succinylcholine.

and more uniform intrapulmonary gas distribution. For this reason, and in the light of further evidence (103), studies were undertaken to re-evaluate the pulmonary N_2 clearance of awake and anesthetized volunteers (29). These studies concluded that an altered, probably more uniform intrapulmonary gas distribution within the tidal volume range existed during anesthesia, paralysis, and mechanical ventilation than was present during awake, spontaneous ventilation. This conclusion was supported both by significant differences in calculated indices for distribution and efficiency and by decreases in the slopes of phase III for the initial tidal breaths during N_2 washout in the anesthetized, mechanically ventilated state.

To define these changes more clearly, bronchospirometric studies were performed that measured simultaneously pulmonary N_2 clearances from individual lungs of anesthetized, paralyzed, mechanically ventilated volunteers (104) for comparison with similar data previously obtained by Lillington and co-workers (105) in awake, spontaneously ventilating subjects. The conclusions reached were that, during anesthesia and mechanical ventilation (1) uniformity of gas distribution was increased within each lung in the supine position, and (2) a greater uniformity for N_2 clearance between dependent and nondependent lungs was seen for the subjects in the lateral decubitus position. These conclusions suggest that anesthesia and mechanical ventilation induce a more uniform distribution of ventilation per unit lung volume within the tidal breathing range (figure 1).

Brendstrup (103) used regional clearance rates after the intravenous injection of ^{133}Xe to compare the distribution of ventilation in supine, anesthetized, paralyzed, mechanically ventilated subjects with that in awake, spontaneously breathing man. He found a larger ventilation per unit lung volume in dependent than in nondependent regions of the lungs in awake man, whereas ventilation per unit lung volume was nearly equal between dependent and nondependent regions with anesthesia and mechanical ventilation. Using ^{133}Xe, Couture and co-workers (26) later confirmed this, and Wulff and Aulin

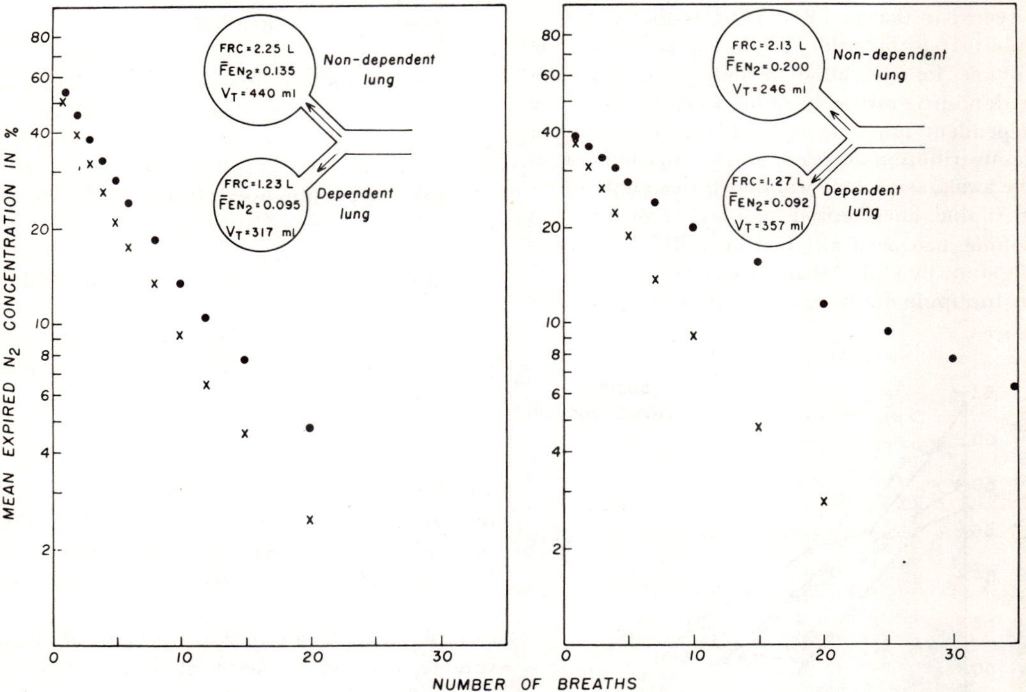

Fig. 1. Nitrogen (N_2) clearance curves for dependent (x) and nondependent (●) lungs calculated from mean data. *Left.* Subject anesthetized, paralyzed, and mechanically ventilated. *Right.* Subject awake and breathing spontaneously. Both patients in lateral decubitus position. Data plotted from Lillington and co-workers (105). The figures for mean expired N_2 concentration ($\bar{F}_{EN_2}$) refer to the tenth breath during N_2 clearance. Note the faster pulmonary N_2 clearance of the dependent lung and the more similar clearances of the two lungs in figure 1 *left.* Both diagrams show the similarity of functional residual capacity (FRC), tidal volume (V_T), and $\bar{F}_{EN_2}$ of the dependent lungs. In the nondependent lung, values for FRC were similar in the two conditions; however, there was a marked difference in V_T and in $\bar{F}_{EN_2}$ of the tenth breath. During anesthesia, paralysis, and mechanical ventilation (*left*), values for $\bar{F}_{EN_2}$ in the two lungs were similar, whereas in awake, spontaneously breathing subjects (*right*), there was a large difference between the values for $\bar{F}_{EN_2}$, representing a more uniform gas distribution in the two lungs during anesthesia, paralysis, and mechanical ventilation. (From Rehder, K., Hatch, D. J., Sessler, A. D., and Fowler, W. S.: The function of each lung of anesthetized and paralyzed man during mechanical ventilation, Anesthesiology, 1972, *37*, 16. By permission of J. B. Lippincott Company.)

(86) also found a reduction in the relative ventilation of the dependent lung during general anesthesia and mechanical ventilation in man in the lateral decubitus position. Hulands and co-workers (106), making their measurements at 1 liter more than FRC, found a greater uniformity in ventilation per unit lung volume in only one of 4 supine subjects. The failure to demonstrate an altered gas distribution in that study may have been fortuitous. In the lateral decubitus position during anesthesia, paralysis, and mechanical ventilation, the proportion of total ventilation to the nondependent lung decreases with increasing airway pressure, i.e., with increasing lung volume (figure 2) (107); the proportion of total FRC in the nondependent lung also decreases. The relative decrease in VT, however, is larger than that in FRC. Thus, in the lateral decubitus position, the ventilation per unit lung volume for the nondependent lung decreases with positive airway pressure, whereas that of the dependent lung increases. Thus, uniformity of gas distribution decreases and approaches that in the awake state. One wonders if this might occur in supine, anesthetized man and if such a lung volume had been attained in 3 of 4 subjects in the study by Hulands and associates (106), wherein intrapulmonary gas distribution was similar

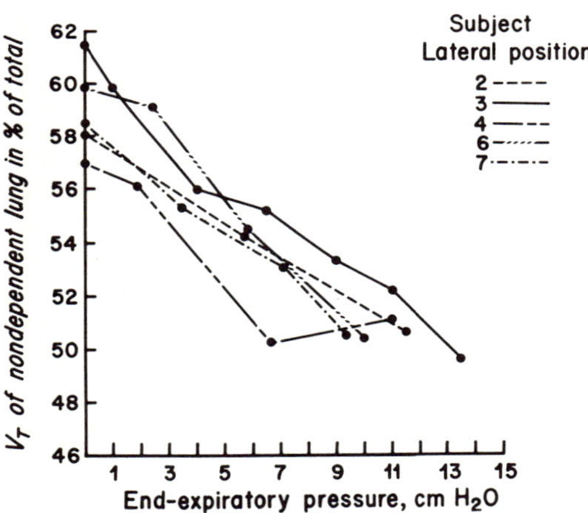

Fig. 2. Tidal volume (VT) of nondependent lung in per cent of total in the lateral decubitus position, plotted as a function of end-expiratory pressure. The relative ventilation of nondependent lung decreased consistently with increasing end-expiratory pressure. (From Rehder, K., Wenthe, F. M., and Sessler, A. D.: Function of each lung during mechanical ventilation with ZEEP and with PEEP in man anesthetized with thiopental-meperidine, Anesthesiology, 1973, *39*, 597. By permission of J. B. Lippincott Company.)

during anesthesia and muscle paralysis and spontaneous ventilation.

Conclusion

One can conclude that general anesthesia results in an altered intrapulmonary gas distribution in both spontaneously breathing and mechanically ventilated subjects in the supine and lateral decubitus positions. Although this altered gas distribution may be partly due to alterations in regional ratios of FRC/TLC that accompany the decrease in over-all FRC seen with general anesthesia or muscle paralysis (or both), changes in the mechanics of the respiratory system seem to have a major role.

Mechanisms Underlying Altered Intrapulmonary Gas Distribution

Considered here will be the alterations in the forces for expansion and in the compliance of the respiratory system that may be induced by general anesthesia, muscle paralysis, and mechanical ventilation. Flow-resistive and inertial forces will not be discussed. It should be recalled, however, that airway resistance is inversely related to lung volume, and presumably this is also true of regional resistances. Commentary will be confined to anesthesia-induced changes in FRC (that is, preinspiratory lung volume), pleural pressure gradient, and compliance of the respiratory system.

Functional Residual Capacity

The FRC is reduced during anesthesia in man in the recumbent positions (table 1). The reduction in FRC occurs with or without muscle relaxation and does not seem to be progressive with time; its mechanisms remain unclear. Possibilities include an increase in central blood volume, a change in chest-wall mechanical properties, gas trapping, and increased elastic recoil of the lung, as may occur with atelectasis.

Central blood volume is usually decreased during general anesthesia (108) and therefore cannot directly cause a reduction in FRC, because an increase and not a decrease in FRC would result.

Changes in the mechanical properties of the chest wall have been suggested as a possible mechanism for the reduction in FRC. Westbrook and co-workers (31) found, by a plethysmographic method, a significant reduction in FRC shortly after induction of anesthesia. They suggested that changes in chest-wall properties, i.e., a right shift of the P-V curve, might occur on induction of anesthesia (figure 3), which may lead secondarily to a reduction of FRC. Studies in man, comparing pulmonary mechanics in the awake state to that during isoflurane anesthesia, demonstrated a shift to the right of the chest-wall P-V curve (32). In interpreting these two studies, it must be noted that a shift in the P-V curve of the chest wall may, in part, reflect an incomplete respiratory muscle relaxation of the untrained awake subjects, rather than a change due to anesthesia; however, this was not considered to be a major factor.

Evidence for a change in the mechanical properties of the chest wall has been added by Froese and Bryan's (87) study of the position and movement of the diaphragm during general anesthesia and muscle paralysis. They observed a cephalad shift in the end-expiratory position of the diaphragm (particularly in the dependent regions), a different motion during ventilation, and an altered tension. Although the study supports a change in the P-V characteristics of the chest wall during anesthesia, it does not necessarily explain the mechanism of the observed right shift of the

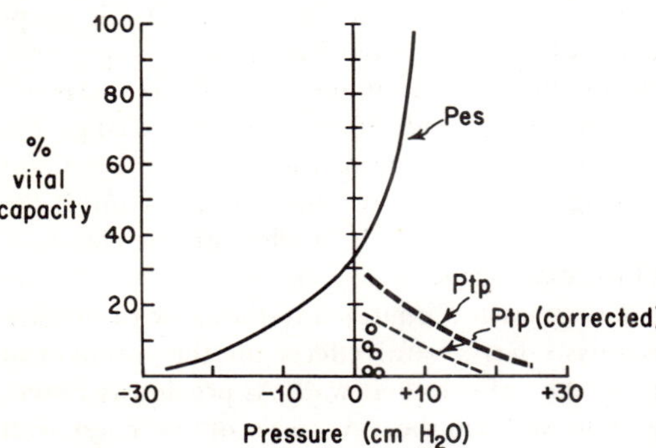

Fig. 3. Normal pressure-volume (P-V) curve of chest wall in relaxed supine subjects. Heavy dashed line represents static lung recoil pressures (Ptp) that would be required to balance the chest wall if functional residual capacity (FRC) decreased with no change in the chest wall pressure-volume characteristic. Circles indicate static Ptp measured in 5 anesthetized subjects at FRC. Light dashed line represents the Ptp curve corrected for "artifacts" in supine subjects. Even with this correction, the measured values were lower than the predicted values, suggesting a rightward shift in the chest wall P-V curve. (From Westbrook, P. R., Stubbs, S. E., Sessler, A. D., Rehder, K., and Hyatt, R. E.: Effects of anesthesia and muscle paralysis on respiratory mechanics in normal man, J Appl Physiol, 1973, *34*, 81. By permission of the American Physiological Society.)

P-V curve. The effect of anesthesia and muscle paralysis on the mechanical properties of the other components of the chest wall (rib cage and abdominal wall) and their interaction with the diaphragm have been incompletely studied. That the reduction in FRC may be due to altered mechanics of the diaphragm is supported by another observation. The FRC is apparently not reduced in sitting, anesthetized man (94), when both hemidiaphragms work under the same gravitational forces and uniform transdiaphragmatic pressure. Therefore, under these conditions, a change in the end-expiratory position of the diaphragm by the mechanisms suggested by Froese and Bryan (87) is unlikely. Interestingly, the compliance of the lung was not reduced in that study (94). The finding that FRC is not reduced in seated, anesthetized man was not confirmed by Shah and co-workers (109); however, their measurements were made by body plethysmography during the first 2 minutes of N_2O anesthesia. The changes observed, therefore, may largely reflect uptake of N_2O by the blood during airway obstruction that was required for the measurement, rather than a real change in FRC.

Gas trapping was proposed as a cause for the decrease in FRC by Don and co-workers (28). The demonstration of a significant positive correlation between the ratio of preoperative closing capacity to FRC and the decrease in FRC seen with anesthesia in a group of volunteers given isoflurane anesthesia (32) seems to support gas trapping as a contributing factor. Trapping of gas, however, does not explain entirely the reduction in FRC, because the sum of FRC plus volume of trapped gas was substantially less during anesthesia than in the awake state (28), indicating a reduction in lung volume. Furthermore, the studies by Westbrook and co-workers (31) did not demonstrate significant differences in FRC measured by body plethysmography and by the N_2-clearance method.

Another cause for the reduction in FRC may be the development of miliary atelectasis during anesthesia. Atelectasis and its relationship to the decreased lung compliance observed during anesthesia will be discussed later.

Thus, one must conclude that, whereas changes in the chest-wall properties seem at present to be the dominant cause for the decrease in FRC, gas trapping may be a contributory factor.

Pleural Pressure Gradient

A vertical pleural pressure gradient has been repeatedly demonstrated (110–113). Apparently this gradient, as measured from the differences between mouth and esophageal pressures, is not uniform down the lung (113–115).

The vertical pleural pressure gradient is largely the result of the forces necessary for the lungs to adapt to the configuration of the chest wall (116, 117). It is also caused by the gravitational forces associated with the support of the weight of the lungs and with the interaction of the weight of the abdominal contents with the chest wall.

The gravity-related pleural pressure gradient has a role in the distribution of intrapulmonary gas, but certain evidence suggests that other mechanisms also may be important. For instance, there is a wide variation among the ratios of volume to ventilation in all anatomic divisions of the lungs of normal subjects (that is, lobes, segments, and subsegments) (118) that cannot be adequately explained by the vertical pleural pressure gradient. In addition, closing capacity is similar in the erect and recumbent positions (25). In these positions, a different closing capacity would be anticipated from the different vertical heights of the lung.

Agostoni and co-workers (119) and Agostoni and Miserocchi (120) observed a decrease and even a disappearance of the vertical pleural pressure gradient in anesthetized, paralyzed animals exposed to increasing airway pressure. They suggested that this change might alter the distribution of gas during mechanical ventilation. To examine this possibility, CPAP of 11 and 20 cm H_2O was applied in conscious, seated, nonparalyzed human subjects. No significant alteration of the vertical pleural pressure gradient (measured as the difference between airway opening and esophageal pressures) was found (113), suggesting that the distortion of the thoracic configuration by CPAP in conscious man probably was not sufficient to abolish the vertical pleural pressure gradient. This conclusion is supported by additional indirect evidence. Neither the slope of phase III (the alveolar plateau) (121, 122) nor the onset of phase IV (121) is changed by the application of CPAP in conscious man, suggesting an unaltered distribution of intrapulmonary gas.

Compliance of the Respiratory System

Nims and co-workers (89) rendered patients apneic by hyperventilation or muscle paralysis to relax their respiratory muscles completely for measurement of the P-V characteristics of the total respiratory system. Because neuromuscular blockade without general anesthesia can be extremely unpleasant, subjects were given a general anesthetic before receiving muscle relaxants. Compliance of the respiratory system was less in anesthetized, paralyzed patients than had been reported by Rahn and co-workers (123) for conscious, voluntarily relaxed subjects. Some of Nims and co-workers' (89) subjects had a reduced compliance of the respiratory system after induction of anesthesia and muscle paralysis. They concluded that the values obtained during anesthesia and muscle paralysis may be closer to the actual P-V characteristics for the respiratory system. Subsequently, their observations were confirmed by numerous investigators (16, 31, 32, 91, 124–132), but not by all (table 2) (92, 133, 134).

To assess the individual contributions of the lung and chest wall, the P-V behavior of the respiratory system was partitioned into its components. Most investigators found a low or reduced lung compliance during general anesthesia and muscle paralysis (31, 32, 90, 135, 136), but some detected no change (92, 133) in supine subjects (table 3). In evaluating these studies, one must note that estimates of esophageal pressure from a balloon may not accurately reflect the pleural pressure or the over-all elastic properties of the lung, particularly in the supine position; however, accurate comparative measurements can be made if one does not change the position and volume of the esophageal balloon during the comparative measurements and if the anesthetics have no direct effect on the elastance of the esophagus.

Chest wall. General anesthesia with muscle paralysis has several effects on the mechanical properties of the chest wall. As previously noted, a right shift of the P-V curve of the chest wall during anesthesia and muscle paralysis was suggested by Westbrook and co-workers (31) and demonstrated in a study using isoflurane anesthesia (32). The cephalad shift of the diaphragm on induction of anesthesia with or without muscle paralysis also was mentioned (87). In addition, the pattern of diaphragmatic motion is reversed during mechanical ventilation (figure 4). In contrast to spontaneous breathing, mechanical ventilation causes a greater displacement in the nondependent region of the diaphragm as compared with the dependent region. In the paralyzed subjects, diaphragmatic motion is accomplished presumably by a relatively uniform pressure applied to the thoracic side of the diaphragm, which is opposed by a nonuniform

TABLE 2

COMPLIANCE OF RESPIRATORY SYSTEM

Reference	Male/ Female	Age, years Weight, kg Height, cm	Anesthetic Agent	Muscle Relaxant	Body Position	Method of Measurement	Compliance of Respiratory System $(liter/cm\ H_2O)$ Mean $\pm$ SE	Compliance of Total Respiratory System Control $(liter/cm\ H_2O)$ Mean $\pm$ SE
89 (1955)	4/20	20–66 44–108 148–185	Pentothal, cyclopropane, diethyl ether, N_2O	Succinylcholine, decamethonium, hyperventilation	Supine	Expiratory P-V measurements	0.065 $\pm$ 0.004 (Pao† = 20 cm H_2O)	0.111 (n = 12) (Pao = 20 cm H_2O)
129 (1956)	11		Diethyl ether, pentothal, cyclopropane	Succinylcholine, decamethonium, hyperventilation	Supine	Average slope of expiratory and inspiratory P-V curve	0.047 $\pm$ 0.003 (average slope of P-V curve)	0.170 $\pm$ 0.020
133 (1957)	10	21–48	Pentothal	Succinylcholine	...	Pressure on spirometer bell for 2–5 sec	0.090 $\pm$ 0.010 (mean of compliance at Pao = 5 and 10 cm H_2O)	...
90 (1957)	28/13	18–67 39–95 155–185	Pentothal	Gallamine	Supine	Inspiratory P-V curve in 200-ml increments to 2–3 liter more than FRC	0.098 $\pm$ 0.002 (between FRC and 2.0 liter more than FRC) 0.087 $\pm$ 0.002 (between FRC and 1.0 liter more than FRC)	...
90 (1957)	19/10	38 (avg)	Pentothal	Gallamine	Supine	Inspiratory P-V curve in 200-ml increments to 2–3 liter more than FRC	0.101 for men; 0.088 for women (between FRC and 2 liter more than FRC)	...
91 (1957)	12	$\geqslant$ 13	Pentothal	Succinylcholine, gallamine, d-tubocurarine	Supine	Prolonged positive pressure	0.078 (Pao = 20 cm H_2O)	...
91 (1957)	9/6	18–63	Pentothal	Succinylcholine, gallamine, d-tubocurarine	Supine	Cyclic positive pressure	0.057 $\pm$ 0.003 (Pao = 20 cm H_2O) 0.065 $\pm$ 0.003 (slope of P-V curve)	0.117 (n = 5)
130 (1958)	83	20–71	Pentothal, N_2O	Succinylcholine or hyperventilation	Supine	Inspiratory P-V measurement at predetermined airway pressures	0.070 (range: 0.026–0.125) (Pao = 15 cm H_2O)	...
16 (1958)	4/2	23–42 57–80 152–178	Pentothal	d-Tubocurarine	Supine	Dynamic compliance	0.056 $\pm$ 0.004 (tidal volume range)	...
126 (1959)	15/39	16–70 41–126 ...	Pentothal, cyclopropane, meperidine, diethyl ether, N_2O	Succinylcholine, d-tubocurarine	Supine	Inflation of lungs with 1.0 liter for 5 sec	0.056 (range 0.025–0.093) (between FRC and 1.0 liter more than FRC)	...
124 (1963)	36	15–84 41–81 150–180	Diethyl ether, N_2O, cyclopropane, halothane, no anesthesia	Curare, succinylcholine	Supine; lateral decubitus or Trendelenburg	After inflation of lungs with 500 ml	0.039 $\pm$ 0.002 (between FRC and 500 ml more than FRC)*	...
125 (1965)	6/14	29–60 52–86 152–185	Pentothal, N_2O	Succinylcholine	Supine	After constant flow inflation for 0.7–1.0 sec	0.076 $\pm$ 0.003 (between FRC and 1 liter more than FRC)	...
92 (1967)	39/0	29–68 ... 160–183	Pentothal	Succinylcholine	Supine	Inspiratory P-V curve in 500-ml increments to 3.0 liter more than FRC	0.111 (range 0.075–0.166) (between FRC and 1.5 liter more than FRC)	...
128 (1968)	10/4	32–74 42–96 154–183	Pentothal, N_2O	d-Tubocurarine	...	Dynamic compliance	0.043 $\pm$ 0.002 (tidal volume range)	...
127 (1970)	0/5	... ...	Pentothal, N_2O	Succinylcholine	Supine	Expiratory P-V curve from 1.0 liter more than FRC in 200-ml decrements	0.062 (between FRC and 1.0 liter more than FRC)	...
127 (1970)	0/5	... ...	Pentothal, N_2O	Succinylcholine	Lithotomy	Expiratory P-V curve from 1.0 liter more than FRC in 200-ml decrements	0.058 (between FRC and 1.0 liter more than FRC)	...
31 (1973)	5/0	24–29 60–92 166–189	Pentothal, meperidine	Succinylcholine	Supine	Expiratory P-V curve from Pao = 35 – 40 cm H_2O	0.099 $\pm$ 0.011 (between 44-54% awake TLC)	0.121 $\pm$ 0.009
32 (1974)	5/0	23–28 71–80 176–189	Isoflurane Isoflurane	Succinylcholine	Supine	Expiratory P-V curve from Pao = 30 cm H_2O	0.087 $\pm$ 0.005 0.086 $\pm$ 0.006 (n = 4) (between FRC and FRC + 10% awake TLC)	0.113 $\pm$ 0.010 (n = 4) 0.113 $\pm$ 0.010

*No difference in compliance of respiratory system between patients who were breathing spontaneously and those whose lungs were ventilated mechanically.
†Pao = pressure at airway openings.

pressure on the abdominal side of the diaphragm. The latter is not uniform because of the hydrostatic pressure gradient generated by the abdominal contents. The result is that the nondependent leaf of the diaphragm has the greater excursion during anesthesia, paralysis, and mechanical ventilation.

The results of Froese and Bryan's (87) study confirmed and extended previous studies on gas distribution between individual lungs in anesthetized, paralyzed, and mechanically ventilated subjects in the lateral decubitus position (104).

TABLE 3

LUNG COMPLIANCE

Reference	Male/Female	Age, years Weight, kg Height, cm	Anesthetic Agent	Muscle Relaxant	Body Position	Method of Measurement	Lung Compliance (liter/cm H₂O) Mean ± SE	Lung compliance (Control) (liter/cm H₂O) Mean ± SE
90 (1957)	21/12	18–67 39–90 155–185	Pentothal	Gallamine	Supine	Inspiratory P-V curve in 200-ml increments to 2–3 liter more than FRC	0.153 ± 0.008 (between FRC and 2.0 liter more than FRC)	...
133 (1957)	10	21–48	Pentothal	Succinylcholine	...	Inflate lung by pressure on spirometer bell for 2–5 sec	0.171 ± 0.016 (mean of compliance at Pao = 5 and 10 cm H₂O)	0.149 ± 0.009
91 (1957)	9/6	18–63	Pentothal	Succinylcholine, gallamine, d-tubocurarine	Supine	Cyclic positive pressure	0.084 ± 0.006 (Pao = 10 cm H₂O)	...
91 (1957)	4	... ...	Pentothal	Succinylcholine, gallamine, d-tubocurarine	Supine	Cyclic positive pressure	0.109 (range: 0.095–0.144)	0.154 (range: 0.120–0.200)
136 (1965)	15/22	19–59 53–104 148–183	Pentothal, halothane, N₂O	None	Supine	Dynamic lung compliance; average of 25 consecutive spontaneous breaths	0.08 ± 0.01 (VT range)	0.12 ± 0.01
135 (1965)	13	... ...	Pentothal, light halothane, N₂O	None	Supine	Dynamic lung compliance; average of 25 consecutive spontaneous breaths	0.088 (range: 0.05–0.16; VT range)	0.107 (range: 0.04–0.33)
136 (1965)	20	... ...	Pentothal, halothane, N₂O	None	Supine	Dynamic lung compliance; average of 25 consecutive breaths	0.083 (during spontaneous breathing, VT range) 0.063 (during mechanical ventilation, VT range)	...
135 (1965)	5/8	22–58 50–84 155–180	Pentothal, halothane, methoxyflurane	None	Supine	Dynamic lung compliance; average of 25 consecutive spontaneous breaths	0.10 ± 0.02 (VT range)	0.12 ± 0.02
92 (1967)	20/0	29–62 ... 160–185	Pentothal	Succinylcholine	Supine	Inspiratory P-V curve in 500-ml increments to 3 liter more than FRC	0.203 ± 0.019 (between FRC and 1.5 liter more than FRC)	0.196 ± 0.014
93 (1968)	8	... ...	Halothane	None	Supine	Dynamic lung compliance	0.091 ± 0.012 (VT range)	0.109 ± 0.010
127 (1970)	0/5	... ...	Pentothal, N₂O	Succinylcholine	Supine	Expiratory P-V curve from 1.0 liter more than FRC in 200-ml decrements	0.136 (between FRC and 1.0 liter more than FRC)	...
127 (1970)	0/5	... ...	Pentothal, N₂O	Succinylcholine	Lithotomy	Expiratory P-V curve from 1.0 liter more than FRC in 200-ml decrements	0.158 (between FRC and 1.0 liter more than FRC)	...
94 (1972)	9	... ...	Pentothal, meperidine	Succinylcholine	Sitting	Dynamic lung compliance; average of 7–29 consecutive breaths	0.153 ± 0.034 (VT range)	0.182 ± 0.025
31 (1973)	5/0	24–29 60–92 166–189	Pentothal, meperidine	Succinylcholine	Supine	Expiratory P-V curve from Pao = 35–40 cm H₂O	0.140 ± 0.016 (between 44 and 54% awake TLC)	0.204 ± 0.007
31 (1973)	5/0	24–29 60–92 166–189	Pentothal, meperidine	None	Supine	Expiratory P-V curve from Pao = 35–40 cm H₂O	0.143 ± 0.014 (between 44 and 54% awake TLC)	0.204 ± 0.007
32 (1974)	5/0	23–28 71–80 176–189	Isoflurane	Succinylcholine	Supine	Expiratory P-V curve from Pao = 30 cm H₂O	0.167 ± 0.013 (between FRC and FRC + 10% awake TLC)	0.215 ± 0.011
32 (1974)	4/0	23–28 71–79 178–189	Isoflurane	Succinylcholine	Supine	Expiratory P-V curve from Pao = 30 cm H₂O	0.181 ± 0.003 (between FRC and FRC + 10% awake TLC)	0.215 ± 0.011

In that study (104), driving pressure during inspiration was kept equal for both lungs, and the distribution of gas between the two lungs, therefore, was indirectly proportional to the relative impedances of the two hemithoraces. Because compliance (C) for each individual hemithorax was measured and inertia was assumed to be negligible (137, 138), pulmonary resistances (R) for each hemithorax could be calculated from the time constants (T = RC). These resistances were estimated for each hemithorax from the expiratory flows during passive exhalation, which were plotted as a function of cumulative expired volume. The calculated resistances of the left and the right hemithorax differed considerably. Yet, the calculated end-inspiratory-alveolar pressures in the two lungs were similar because of the relatively long duration of inspiration. It follows that the measured differences between the respiratory compliances in the two hemithoraces were primarily responsible for the relative distribution of the tidal volume between the two lungs. This method of analysis was limited by its inability to partition the compliance into lung and chest-wall components of individual hemithoraces.

Recently, Grimby and co-workers (139) studied the compliance of the chest wall and its components during mechanical ventilation in anesthetized, nonparalyzed subjects. They found that the chest wall was slightly more compliant than the lungs and that the compliance of the rib cage was greater than the compliance of the diaphragm-abdomen. The chest wall became more compliant with ventilation at larger tidal volumes and was less compliant at lower pressures, resembling the P-V curves obtained at low lung volumes in awake, supine subjects during voluntary relaxation. Grimby and co-workers suggested that this similarity may reflect the reduced FRC during general anesthesia. They also compared the relative contribution of abdominal and rib-cage displacements during spontaneous ventilation in conscious subjects and in anesthetized and mechanically ventilated subjects. Whereas in the conscious and spontaneously breathing subjects the rib-cage displacement accounted for only 40 per cent of tidal volume, such displacement increased to 72 per cent during mechanical ventilation and was not altered significantly by increasing the tidal volume from 0.39 to 1.1 liter. These investigators pointed out that the relationship of rib-cage and abdomen-diaphragm expansions during mechanical ventilation is similar to the one calculated for uniform expansion of the lung on the basis of the area of diaphragm in contact with the lung, namely, approximately 28 per cent of the external pleural surface of the lung (140).

From these studies, one can conclude that the static and dynamic mechanics of the chest wall are different during anesthesia, muscle paralysis, and mechanical ventilation than during awake spontaneous breathing.

Lung. Because of the curvilinear relationship between pressure and volume and a failure to relate lung compliance to absolute lung volume in a number of the earlier studies, confusion existed concerning the effect of anesthesia on lung compliance. There is now reliable evidence

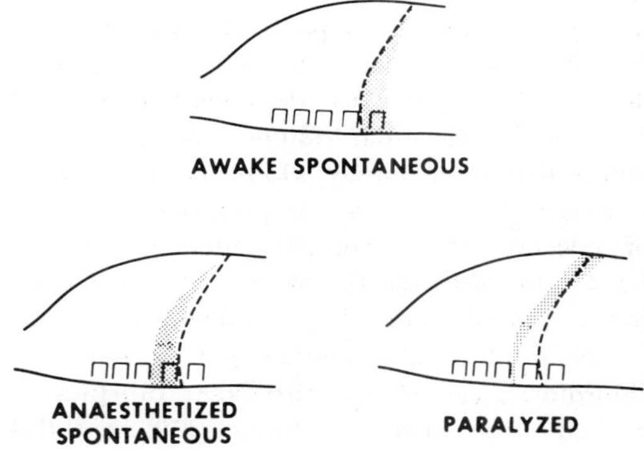

Fig. 4. Position and displacement of diaphragm during tidal breathing in supine subject. Dashed line represents control functional residual capacity position of the diaphragm. Stippled area represents diaphragmatic excursion during tidal breathing. (From Froese, A. B., and Bryan, A. C.: Effects of anesthesia and paralysis on diaphragmatic mechanics in man, Anesthesiology, 1974, *41,* 242. By permission of J. B. Lippincott Company.)

that anesthesia alters lung compliance (table 3). These changes may be caused by numerous mechanisms, including a direct effect of anesthetics on the lung, airway closure, development of atelectasis, changes in surfactant with altered air-space configuration, an altered intrapulmonary gas distribution, and accumulation of interstitial fluid.

Anesthetic Effects

Anesthetics, muscle relaxants, premedicants, and other drugs administered during anesthesia may have a direct pharmacologic effect on lung compliance, possibly by the constriction of alveolar ducts or respiratory bronchioles (141, 142). Although a direct effect cannot be ruled out, the failure to demonstrate significant differences in compliance with various agents and levels in the depth of anesthesia (126) and the unchanged lung compliance in sitting, anesthetized man (94) argue against it. In dogs, however, *d*-tubocurarine has been shown to have an effect on lung compliance, presumably by releasing histamine (143). More work on this mechanism is needed.

Airway Closure

Airway closure may reduce lung compliance by decreasing the number of distensible units accessible to ventilation. As has been pointed out, evidence exists for increased airway closure, leading to gas trapping during anesthesia; however, simultaneous measurements of lung volume by body plethysmography and gas dilution (31) failed to confirm increased gas trapping. Questions regarding the contribution of increased airway closure to reductions in lung compliance remained unanswered.

Atelectasis

Reduced lung compliance during anesthesia has been frequently attributed to atelectasis, despite lack of radiographic evidence.

Bernstein (144), studying anesthetized, paralyzed rabbits, found that the P-V characteristics of the total respiratory system differed substantially between the first and subsequent inflations of the lung. When the inflations were performed in rapid succession, there was an increase in compliance in the subsequent inflations that was attributed to recruitment of distensible respiratory units after the first inflation (144). Mead and Collier (145) observed a progressive reduction in lung compliance both in spontaneously breathing and mechanically ventilated dogs; this could be almost completely reversed with one hyperinflation. Progressive reductions in compliance were not seen when periodic hyperinflations were given, and if they were discontinued, lung compliance decreased progressively again. The reduced compliance in these animals was attributed in part to atelectasis, which was demonstrated in dependent lung regions at postmortem examination.

Bendixen and co-workers (18) followed this with studies in man in which they related the decrease in arterial Po_2 in surgical patients to the ventilatory pattern and the decreased compliance of the total respiratory system. Finding a progressive decrease in arterial Po_2 reversible by hyperinflation and preventable by use of large tidal volumes, Bendixen and co-workers (18) and Egbert and associates (124) suggested that collapse of air spaces in the lung was the cause for most of the decrease in lung compliance. Subsequent studies in dogs (146–150) also suggested the development of atelectasis during anesthesia.

Favorable conditions exist for the development of atelectasis during anesthesia. In the alveoli, the relatively soluble anesthetic gases or vapors and high concentrations of inspired O_2 displace the less soluble N_2. If gas trapping occurs or if regions are poorly ventilated and continue to be perfused, absorption with collapse may result. The importance of alveolar N_2 was documented by Déry and co-workers (151), who observed a reduction in FRC during general anesthesia only if 100 per cent O_2 was being inspired, but not when gas mixtures containing N_2 were administered. This is consistent with the work of Finley and co-workers (17) in anesthetized dogs, which showed that the rate of increase in $(A-a)Po_2$ on changing from positive pressure breathing to spontaneous breathing was inversely proportional to the increase in inspired N_2 concentration.

Surfactant

If the reduction in lung compliance with anesthesia is due solely to fewer participating distensible units, then one might expect a proportional reduction in lung volume or an increase in transpulmonary pressure or both. Mead and Collier (145), Collier and Mead (146), Velasquez and Farhi (147), Farhi and Velasquez (148), and Laver and associates (149) have all noted a disproportionately larger reduction in lung compliance than in lung volume in anesthetized dogs. This finding suggests that another mechanism, such as a change in surface tension in lung units, may have contributed to a reduced lung compliance. Williams and co-workers (152), observing a progressive reduction in lung compliance in anesthetized, paralyzed rabbits and newborn lambs ventilated with constant tidal volumes, also ascribed this to a change in surface tension.

As lung volume decreases at low transpulmonary pressure, the alveolar surface area decreases and the surface tension in small air spaces may become lower than the "equilibrium" value for the surfactant film. If one assumes that the "equilibrium" surface tension for the film is similar *in vivo* and *in vitro*, and if the surface area remains unchanged, then surfactant molecules will leave the surface. *In vivo*, however, the surface area of the air space may decrease, resulting in a change of the air space configuration (153), which could proceed to total collapse of the air space.

Young and co-workers (154) could not detect alterations in air space configurations in excised rat lungs kept at a low transpulmonary pressure of 3 cm H_2O. They suggested that the most likely mechanism for the decreased compliance that developed at low transpulmonary pressures was a decrease in compliance of the surface-lining film of the lung.

High transpulmonary pressures also may result in abnormal surface tension in the lung. Overinflation of the lungs of anesthetized dogs for 1 hour may deplete or alter the surfactant material, and 2 hours of overinflation may result in diffuse atelectasis that may be undetectable immediately, but develops 24 hours later (155). No changes in forces at the lung surface were detected in anesthetized dogs ventilated for 8 hours with large tidal volumes (50 ml per kg) and killed immediately (156); however, early killing of the dogs may have precluded detection of atelectasis. Depressed surfactant action also has been found after ventilating excised canine (157) or rat (158) lungs with large tidal volumes.

The lipid-soluble anesthetics, halothane and chloroform, can change surfactant function in excised, unperfused dog lungs (159), but this effect seems small when compared with the effects of overinflation and decreased pulmonary blood flow (160). Reduction in pulmonary blood flow during anesthesia, with impairment of surfactant function, may result from a reduced cardiac output due to a myocardial depressant effect of anesthetics, reduced venous return secondary to hypovolemia, increased mean intrathoracic pressure, or some combination of these.

Intrapulmonary Gas Distribution

Howell and Peckett (91) first suggested that values for lung compliance in anesthetized, paralyzed, mechanically ventilated man may not be comparable to values for conscious and probably unconscious spontaneously breathing subjects because of a different intrapulmonary gas distribution. This possibility was later considered by others (29, 125, 149, 161).

Regional differences in diaphragmatic movement (87) during paralysis and mechanical ventilation may result in different regional lung volume histories. The limited excursion of the diaphragm against the dependent lung under these conditions may reduce regional and over-all lung compliance. Studies in anesthetized man suggested that, during mechanical ventilation, lung compliance may be lower than during spontaneous breathing (136). In anesthetized dogs, this difference could not be shown (145), but in excised canine lungs that were alternately subjected to uniform and nonuniform transpulmonary pressure, a consistent difference in the P-V characteristics has been demonstrated (162, 163).

Interstitial Fluid

Marshall and Wyche (164) studied pulmonary extravascular water volume during halothane anesthesia in dogs. During 3 hours of halothane anesthesia, they found no significant change in pulmonary extravascular water volume, as estimated by double indicator-dilution techniques. To our knowledge, there is little other information available, and no comparative measurements of pulmonary extravascular water volumes between conscious and anesthetized states and their relationship to lung compliance have been published.

Conclusion

General anesthesia results in an alteration in the mechanical properties of both the lung and the chest wall, leading to reductions in FRC in the recumbent, but probably not in the sitting, position. Anesthesia also results in an imbalance between the forces that expand the lung and the forces that oppose expansion, leading to an altered intrapulmonary gas distribution, both with spontaneous and with mechanical ventilation. Changes in the lung mechanical properties seem to be secondary to those in the chest wall.

General Conclusions

In this review, an attempt has been made to select, evaluate, and interpret the pertinent literature relative to general anesthesia and the lung. Concepts of intrapulmonary gas exchange and respiratory system mechanics were synthesized, emphasizing the importance of changes in intrapulmonary gas distribution that are induced by general anesthesia and exploring the possible underlying mechanisms of these changes. The area of control mechanisms and the effects of anesthesia on respiratory regulation were not discussed, nor was the distribution of pulmonary blood flow examined. The following general conclusions can be reached: *(1)* impaired gas exchange occurs during general anesthesia, with both impaired oxygenation and CO_2 elimination; *(2)* increased venous admixture and increased alveolar dead space impair gas exchange; *(3)* the distribution of ventilation is changed during general anesthesia, and this change is related to a decrease in FRC in the recumbent positions and to altered chest-wall mechanics. Numerous questions regarding the effect of anesthesia on the lung remain unanswered. The close relationship between advances in pulmonary physiology and the pulmonary effects of anesthetic actions is increasingly apparent, as is the importance of this knowledge in applying mechanical ventilation and end-expiratory pressure to patients with pulmonary disease.

References

1. Stein, M., and Cassara, E. L.: Preoperative pulmonary evaluation and therapy for surgery patients, JAMA, 1970, *211*, 787.
2. Wightman, J. A. K.: A prospective survey of the incidence of postoperative pulmonary complications, Br J Surg, 1968, *55*, 85.
3. Beecher, H. K., and Todd, D. P.: A study of the deaths associated with anesthesia and surgery, based on a study of 599,548 anesthesias in ten institutions 1948-1952, inclusive, Ann Surg, 1954, *140*, 2.
4. Bendixen, H. H., and Laver, M. B.: Hypoxia in anesthesia: A review, Clin Pharmacol Ther, 1965, *6*, 510.
5. Nunn, J. F.: Elimination of carbon dioxide by the lung, Anesthesiology, 1960, *21*, 620.
6. Marshall, B. E., and Wyche, M. Q., Jr.: Hypoxemia during and after anesthesia, Anesthesiology, 1972, *37*, 178.
7. Markello, R., Maceda, L., and Goplerud, D.: Diffusion hyperoxia, a "concentrating" effect, Anesth Analg (Cleve), 1974, *53*, 233.
8. Heller, M. L., Watson, T. R., Jr., and Imredy, D. S.: Effect of nitrous oxide uptake on arterial oxygenation, Anesthesiology, 1967, *28*, 904.
9. Eger, E. I., II: Effect of inspired anesthetic concentration on the rate of rise of alveolar concentration, Anesthesiology, 1963, *24*, 153.

10. Fink, B. R.: Diffusion anoxia, Anesthesiology, 1955, *16*, 511.

11. Von Hayek, H.: Über einen Kurzschlusskreislauf (arteriovenöse Anastomosen) in der menschlichen Lunge, Z Anat Entwicklungsgesch, 1940, *110*, 412.

12. Von Hayek, H.: Kurz- und Nebenschlüsse des menschlichen Lungenkreislaufes in der Pleura, Z Anat Entwicklungsgesch, 1942, *112*, 221.

13. Lilienthal, J. L., Jr., Riley, R. L., Proemmel, D. D., and Franke, R. E.: An experimental analysis in man of the oxygen pressure gradient from alveolar air to arterial blood during rest and exercise at sea level and at altitude, Am J Physiol, 1946, *147*, 199.

14. Riley, R. L., and Cournand, A.: 'Ideal' alveolar air and the analysis of ventilation-perfusion relationships in the lungs, J Appl Physiol, 1949, *1*, 825.

15. Rahn, H.: A concept of mean alveolar air and the ventilation-bloodflow relationships during pulmonary gas exchange, Am J Physiol, 1949, *158*, 21.

16. Campbell, E. J. M., Nunn, J. F., and Peckett, B. W.: A comparison of artificial ventilation and spontaneous respiration with particular reference to ventilation-bloodflow relationships, Br J Anaesth, 1958, *30*, 166.

17. Finley, T. N., Lenfant, C., Haab, P., Piiper, J., and Rahn, H.: Venous admixture in the pulmonary circulation of anesthetized dogs, J Appl Physiol, 1960, *15*, 418.

18. Bendixen, H. H., Hedley-Whyte, J., and Laver, M. B.: Impaired oxygenation in surgical patients during general anesthesia with controlled ventilation: A concept of atelectasis, N Engl J Med, 1963, *269*, 991.

19. Nunn, J. F.: Factors influencing the arterial oxygen tension during halothane anaesthesia with spontaneous respiration, Br J Anaesth, 1964, *36*, 327.

20. Nunn, J. F., Bergman, N. A., and Coleman, A. J.: Factors influencing the arterial oxygen tension during anaesthesia with artificial ventilation, Br J Anaesth, 1965, *37*, 898.

21. Bergman, N. A.: Components of the alveolar-arterial oxygen tension difference in anesthetized man. Anesthesiology, 1967, *28*, 517.

22. Marsh, H. M., Rehder, K., Sessler, A. D., and Fowler, W. S.: Effects of mechanical ventilation, muscle paralysis, and posture on ventilation-perfusion relationships in anesthetized man, Anesthesiology, 1973, *38*, 59.

23. Holland, J., Milic-Emili, J., Macklem, P. T., and Bates, D. V.: Regional distribution of pulmonary ventilation and perfusion in elderly subjects, J Clin Invest, 1968, *47*, 81.

24. Craig, D. B., Wahba, W. M., Don, H. F., Couture, J. G., and Becklake, M. R.: "Closing volume" and its relationship to gas exchange in seated and supine positions, J Appl Physiol, 1971, *31*, 717.

25. Leblanc, P., Ruff, F., and Milic-Emili, J.: Effects of age and body position on "airway closure" in man, J Appl Physiol, 1970, *28*, 448.

26. Couture, J., Picken, J., Trop, D., Ruff, F., Lousada, N., Houseley, E., and Bates, D. V.: Airway closure in normal, obese, and anesthetized supine subjects (abstract), Fed Proc, 1970, *29*, 269.

27. Weenig, C. S., Pietak, S., Hickey, R. F., and Fairley, H. B.: Relationship of preoperative closing volume to functional residual capacity and alveolar-arterial oxygen difference during anesthesia with controlled ventilation, Anesthesiology, 1974, *41*, 3.

28. Don, H. F., Wahba, W. M., and Craig, D. B.: Airway closure, gas trapping, and the functional residual capacity during anesthesia, Anesthesiology, 1972, *36*, 533.

29. Rehder, K., Hatch, D. J., Sessler, A. D., Marsh, H. M., and Fowler, W. S.: Effects of general anesthesia, muscle paralysis, and mechanical ventilation on pulmonary nitrogen clearance, Anesthesiology, 1971, *35*, 591.

30. Bergman, N. A.: Distribution of inspired gas during anesthesia and artificial ventilation, J Appl Physiol, 1963, *18*, 1085.

31. Westbrook, P. R., Stubbs, S. E., Sessler, A. D., Rehder, K., and Hyatt, R. E.: Effects of anesthesia and muscle paralysis on respiratory mechanics in normal man, J Appl Physiol, 1973, *34*, 81.

32. Rehder, K., Mallow, J. E., Fibuch, E. E., Krabill, D. R., and Sessler, A. D.: Effects of isoflurane anesthesia and muscle paralysis on respiratory mechanics in normal man, Anesthesiology, 1974, *41*, 477.

33. Laws, A. K.: Effects of induction of anaesthesia and muscle paralysis on functional residual capacity of the lungs, Can Anaesth Soc J, 1968, *15*, 325.

34. Don, H. F., Wahba, M., Cuadrado, L., and Kelkar, K.: The effects of anesthesia and 100 per cent oxygen on the functional residual capacity of the lungs, Anesthesiology, 1970, *32*, 521.

35. Pietak, S., Weenig, C. S., Hickey, R. F., and Fairley, H. B.: Anesthetic effects on ventilation in patients with chronic obstructive pulmonary disease, Anesthesiology, 1975, *42*, 160.

36. Wyche, M. Q., Jr., Teichner, R. L., Kallos, T., Marshall, B. E., and Smith, T. C.: Effects of continuous positive-pressure breathing on functional residual capacity and arterial oxygenation during intra-abdominal operations: Studies in man during nitrous oxide and *d*-tubocurarine anesthesia, Anesthesiology, 1973, *38*, 68.

37. Kallos, T., and Smith, T. C.: Measurement of the pulmonary diffusing capacity in anesthe-

tized man (abstract), American Society of Anesthesiologists Annual Meeting, Abstracts of Scientific Papers, 1969, pp. 73-74.

38. Hewlett, A. M., Hulands, G. H., Nunn, J. F., and Heath, J. R.: Functional residual capacity during anaesthesia. II. Spontaneous respiration, Br J Anaesth, 1974, 46, 486.

39. Hewlett, A. M., Hulands, G. H., Nunn, J. F., and Milledge, J. S.: Functional residual capacity during anaesthesia. III. Artificial ventilation, Br J Anaesth, 1974, 46, 495.

40. Frumin, M. J., Bergman, N. A., Holaday, D. A., Rackow, H., and Salanitre, E.: Alveolar-arterial O_2 differences during artificial respiration in man, J Appl Physiol, 1959, 14, 694.

41. Colgan, F. J., Barrow, R. E., and Fanning, G. L.: Constant positive-pressure breathing and cardiorespiratory function, Anesthesiology, 1971, 34, 145.

42. Burger, E. J., Jr., and Macklem, P.: Airway closure: Demonstration by breathing 100% O_2 at low lung volumes and by N_2 washout, J Appl Physiol, 1968, 25, 139.

43. Hyatt, R. E., Okeson, G. C., and Rodarte, J. R.: Influence of expiratory flow limitation on the pattern of lung emptying in normal man, J Appl Physiol, 1973, 35, 411.

44. Rehder, K., Frazier, A. R., Sessler, A. D., Rodarte, J. R., and Hyatt, R. E.: Closing volume for individual lungs (abstract), Fed Proc, 1975, 34, 403.

45. Gómez, D. M.: A mathematical treatment of the distribution of tidal volume throughout the lung, Proc Natl Acad Sci USA, 1963, 49, 312.

46. Lenfant, C., and Okubo, T.: Distribution function of pulmonary blood flow and ventilation-perfusion ratio in man, J Appl Physiol, 1968, 24, 668.

47. Okubo, T., and Lenfant, C.: Distribution function of lung volume and ventilation determined by lung N_2 washout, J Appl Physiol, 1968, 24, 658.

48. Wagner, P. D., Saltzman, H. A., and West, J. B.: Measurement of continuous distributions of ventilation-perfusion ratios: Theory, J Appl Physiol, 1974, 36, 588.

49. Wagner, P. D., Naumann, P. F., and Laravuso, R. B.: Simultaneous measurement of eight foreign gases in blood by gas chromatography, J Appl Physiol, 1974, 36, 600.

50. Piiper, J., Haab, P., and Rahn, H.: Unequal distribution of pulmonary diffusing capacity in the anesthetized dog, J Appl Physiol, 1961, 16, 499.

51. Dollery, C. T., Dyson, N. A., and Sinclair, J. D.: Regional variations in uptake of radioactive CO in the normal lung, J Appl Physiol, 1960, 15, 411.

52. Staub, N. C.: Alveolar-arterial oxygen tension gradient due to diffusion, J Appl Physiol, 1963, 18, 673.

53. Fukuma, S., Wildeboer-Venema, F. N., Horie, S., Yokota, H., Honda, Y., Schuurmans Stekhoven, J. H., and Kreuzer, F.: Pulmonary diffusing capacity in the dog as influenced by anesthesia and ventilatory regime, Respir Physiol, 1970, 8, 311.

54. Bergman, N. A.: Pulmonary diffusing capacity and gas exchange during halothane anesthesia, Anesthesiology, 1970, 32, 317.

55. Filley, G. F., MacIntosh, D. J., and Wright, G. W.: Carbon monoxide uptake and pulmonary diffusing capacity in normal subjects at rest and during exercise, J Clin Invest, 1954, 33, 530.

56. Hyde, R. W., Marin, M. G., Rynes, R. I., Karreman, G., and Forster, R. E.: Measurement of uneven distribution of pulmonary blood flow to CO diffusing capacity, J Appl Physiol, 1971, 31, 605.

57. Summer, W., and Gurtner, G. H.: Evidence for partially carrier mediated CO transfer in the human lung (abstract), Physiologist, 1973, 16, 466.

58. Gurtner, G. H., and Burns, B.: The role of cytochrome P-450 of placenta in facilitated oxygen diffusion, Drug Metab Dispos, 1973, 1, 368.

59. Burns, B., and Gurtner, G. H.: A specific carrier for oxygen and carbon monoxide in the lung and placenta, Drug Metab Dispos, 1973, 1, 374.

60. Kelman, G. R., Nunn, J. F., Prys-Roberts, C., and Greenbaum, R.: The influence of cardiac output on arterial oxygenation: A theoretical study, Br J Anaesth, 1967, 39, 450.

61. Prys-Roberts, C., and Kelman, G. R.: Haemodynamic influences of graded hypercapnia in anaesthetized man (abstract), Br J Anaesth, 1966, 38, 661.

62. Theye, R. A., Milde, J. H., and Michenfelder, J. D.: Effect of hypocapnia on cardiac output during anesthesia, Anesthesiology, 1966, 27, 778.

63. Smith, T. C., Colton, E. T., III, and Behar, M. G.: Does anesthesia alter hemoglobin dissociation?, Anesthesiology, 1970, 32, 5.

64. Gillies, I. D. S., Bird, B. D., Norman, J., Gordon-Smith, E. C., and Whitwam, J. G.: The effect of anaesthesia on the oxyhaemoglobin dissociation curve (abstract), Br J Anaesth, 1970, 42, 561.

65. Millar, R. A., Beard, D. J., and Hulands, G. H.: Oxyhaemoglobin dissociation curves in vitro with and without the anaesthetics halothane and cyclopropane, Br J Anaesth, 1971, 43, 1003.

66. Cohen, P. J., and Behar, M. G.: The *in vitro* effect of anesthesia on the oxyhemoglobin dissociation curve (abstract), Fed Proc, 1970, 29, 329.

67. Prime, F. J.: Oxygen dissociation curves of whole blood in the presence of anaesthetic gases,

Br J Anaesth, 1951, *23*, 171.

68. Severinghaus, J. W., Stupfel, M. A., and Bradley, A. F.: Alveolar dead space and arterial to end-tidal carbon dioxide differences during hypothermia in dog and man, J Appl Physiol, 1957, *10*, 349.

69. Nunn, J. F., and Hill, D. W.: Respiratory dead space and arterial to end-tidal CO_2 tension difference in anesthetized man, J Appl Physiol, 1960, *15*, 383.

70. Severinghaus, J. W., and Stupfel, M.: Respiratory dead space increase following atropine in man, and atropine, vagal or ganglionic blockade and hypothermia in dogs, J Appl Physiol, 1955, *8*, 81.

71. Nunn, J. F., Campbell, E. J. M., and Peckett, B. W.: Anatomical subdivisions of the volume of respiratory dead space and effect of position of the jaw, J Appl Physiol, 1959, *14*, 174.

72. Askrog, V. F., Pender, J. W., Smith, T. C., and Eckenhoff, J. E.: Changes in respiratory dead space during halothane, cyclopropane, and nitrous oxide anesthesia, Anesthesiology, 1964, *25*, 342.

73. Thornton, J. A.: Physiological dead space: Changes during general anaesthesia, Anaesthesia, 1960, *15*, 381.

74. Kain, M. L., Panday, J., and Nunn, J. F.: The effect of intubation on the deadspace during halothane anaesthesia, Br J Anaesth, 1969, *41*, 94.

75. Askrog, V.: Changes in (a-A)CO_2 difference and pulmonary artery pressure in anesthetized man, J Appl Physiol, 1966, *21*, 1299.

76. Eckenhoff, J. E., Enderby, G. E. H., Larson, A., Edridge, A., and Judevine, D. E.: Pulmonary gas exchange during deliberate hypotension, Br J Anaesth, 1963, *35*, 750.

77. Gerst, P. H., Rattenborg, C., and Holaday, D. A.: The effects of hemorrhage on pulmonary circulation and respiratory gas exchange, J Clin Invest, 1959, *38*, 524.

78. Freeman, J., and Nunn, J. F.: Ventilation-perfusion relationships after haemorrhage, Clin Sci, 1963, *24*, 135.

79. Rehder, K., Teichert, P., Hessler, O., and Carveth, S. W.: Pulmonary gas exchange after hemorrhage during intermittent positive pressure breathing, Anesth Analg (Cleve), 1965, *44*, 618.

80. Fowler, W. S.: Intrapulmonary distribution of inspired gas, Physiol Rev, 1952, *32*, 1.

81. Milic-Emili, J., Henderson, J. A. M., Dolovich, M. B., Trop, D., and Kaneko, K.: Regional distribution of inspired gas in the lung, J Appl Physiol, 1966, *21*, 749.

82. Kaneko, K., Milic-Emili, J., Dolovich, M. B., Dawson, A., and Bates, D. V.: Regional distribution of ventilation and perfusion as a function of body position, J Appl Physiol, 1966, *21*, 767.

83. Krueger, J. J., Bain, T., and Patterson, J. L., Jr.: Elevation gradient of intrathoracic pressure, J Appl Physiol, 1961, *16*, 465.

84. Glazier, J. B., Hughes, J. M. B., Maloney, J. E., and West, J. B.: Vertical gradient of alveolar size in lungs of dogs frozen intact, J Appl Physiol, 1967, *23*, 694.

85. Anthonisen, N. R., Robertson, P. C., and Ross, W. R. D.: Gravity-dependent sequential emptying of lung regions, J Appl Physiol, 1970, *28*, 589.

86. Wulff, K. E., and Aulin, I.: The regional lung function in the lateral decubitus position during anesthesia and operation, Acta Anaesthesiol Scand, 1972, *16*, 195.

87. Froese, A. B., and Bryan, A. C.: Effects of anesthesia and paralysis on diaphragmatic mechanics in man, Anesthesiology, 1974, *41*, 242.

88. Rehder, K., and Sessler, A. D.: Function of each lung in spontaneously breathing man anesthetized with thiopental-meperidine, Anesthesiology, 1973, *38*, 320.

89. Nims, R. G., Conner, E. H., and Comroe, J. H., Jr.: The compliance of the human thorax in anesthetized patients, J Clin Invest, 1955, *34*, 744.

90. Butler, J., and Smith, B. H.: Pressure-volume relationships of the chest in the completely relaxed anaesthetised patient, Clin Sci, 1957, *16*, 125.

91. Howell, J. B. L., and Peckett, B. W.: Studies of the elastic properties of the thorax of supine anaesthetized paralysed human subjects, J Physiol, 1957, *136*, 1.

92. Van Lith, P., Johnson, F. N., and Sharp, J. T.: Respiratory elastances in relaxed and paralyzed states in normal and abnormal men, J Appl Physiol, 1967, *23*, 475.

93. Colgan, F. J., and Whang, T. B.: Anesthesia and atelectasis, Anesthesiology, 1968, *29*, 917.

94. Rehder, K., Sittipong, R., and Sessler, A. D.: The effects of thiopental-meperidine anesthesia with succinylcholine paralysis on functional residual capacity and dynamic lung compliance in normal sitting man, Anesthesiology, 1972, *37*, 395.

95. Hickey, R. F., Visick, W. D., Fairley, H. B., and Fourcade, H. E.: Effects of halothane anesthesia on functional residual capacity and alveolar-arterial oxygen tension difference, Anesthesiology, 1973, *38*, 20.

96. Svanberg, L.: Influence of posture on the lung volumes, ventilation and circulation in normals: A spirometric-bronchospirometric investigation, Scand J Clin Lab Invest, 1957, *9* (Supplement 25, p. 1).

97. Doerfel, G.: Bronchospirometrische Messungen während chirurgischer Eingriffe am offenen Thorax, Thoraxchirurgie, 1959, *7*, 393.

98. Potgieter, S. V.: Atelectasis: Its evolution during

upper urinary tract surgery, Br J Anaesth, 1959, *31*, 472.

99. Faulconer, A., Jr., Gaines, T. R., and Grove, J. S.: Atelectasis during operations on the upper urinary tract, Anesthesiology, 1946, *7*, 635.

100. Rehder, K., Theye, R. A., and Fowler, W. S.: Function of each lung of dogs during intermittent positive-pressure breathing, Am J Physiol, 1964, *206*, 1031.

101. Seed, R. F., and Sykes, M. K.: Differential lung ventilation, Br J Anaesth, 1972, *44*, 758.

102. Fowler, W. S., Cornish, E. R., Jr., and Kety, S. S.: Lung function studies. VIII. Analysis of alveolar ventilation by pulmonary N_2 clearance curves, J Clin Invest, 1952, *31*, 40.

103. Brendstrup, A.: The effect of artificial respiration on the regional distribution of ventilation examined with xenon-133, Acta Anaesthesiol Scand [Suppl], 1966, *23*, 180.

104. Rehder, K., Hatch, D. J., Sessler, A. D., and Fowler, W. S.: The function of each lung of anesthetized and paralyzed man during mechanical ventilation, Anesthesiology, 1972, *37*, 16.

105. Lillington, G. A., Fowler, W. S., Miller, R. D., and Helmholz, H. F., Jr.: Nitrogen clearance rates of right and left lungs in different positions, J Clin Invest, 1959, *38*, 2026.

106. Hulands, G. H., Greene, R., Iliff, L. D., and Nunn, J. F.: Influence of anaesthesia on the regional distribution of perfusion and ventilation in the lung, Clin Sci, 1970, *38*, 451.

107. Rehder, K., Wenthe, F. M., and Sessler, A. D.: Function of each lung during mechanical ventilation with **ZEEP** and with **PEEP** in man anesthetized with thiopental-meperidine, Anesthesiology, 1973, *39*, 597.

108. Johnson, S. R.: The effect of some anaesthetic agents on the circulation in man, with special reference to the significance of pulmonary blood volume for the circulatory regulation, Acta Chir Scand [Suppl], 1951, *158*, 1.

109. Shah, J., Jones, J. G., Galvin, J., and Tomlin, P. J.: Pulmonary gas exchange during induction of anaesthesia with nitrous oxide in seated subjects, Br J Anaesth, 1971, *43*, 1013.

110. Daly, W. J., and Bondurant, S.: Direct measurement of respiratory pleural pressure changes in normal man, J Appl Physiol, 1963, *18*, 513.

111. Banchero, N., Schwartz, P. E., and Wood, E. H.: Intraesophageal pressure gradient in man, J Appl Physiol, 1967, *22*, 1066.

112. Hoppin, F. G., Jr., Green, I. D., and Mead, J.: Distribution of pleural surface pressure in dogs, J Appl Physiol, 1969, *27*, 863.

113. Rehder, K., Abboud, N., Rodarte, J. R., and Hyatt, R. E.: Positive airway pressure and vertical transpulmonary pressure gradient in man, J Appl Physiol, 1975, *38*, 896.

114. Sheehan, W. C., and Hyatt, R. E.: Effect of oxygen breathing on regional lung perfusion in patients with chronic obstructive pulmonary disease (abstract), J Lab Clin Med, 1970, *76*, 1029.

115. Milic-Emili, J., Mead, J., and Turner, J. M.: Topography of esophageal pressure as a function of posture in man, J Appl Physiol, 1964, *19*, 212.

116. Grassino, A., and Anthonisen, N. R.: Effects of distortion of the human rib cage on the distribution of regional lung volumes and ventilation (abstract), Fed Proc, 1974, *33*, 323.

117. Minh, V. D., Kurihara, N., Friedman, P. J., and Moser, K. M.: Reversal of the pleural pressure gradient during electrophrenic stimulation, J Appl Physiol, 1974, *37*, 496.

118. Suda, Y., Martin, C. J., and Young, A. C.: Regional dispersion of volume-to-ventilation ratios in the lung of man, J Appl Physiol, 1970, *29*, 480.

119. Agostoni, E., D'Angelo, E., and Bonanni, M. V.: Topography of pleural surface pressure above resting volume in relaxed animals, J Appl Physiol, 1970, *29*, 297.

120. Agostoni, E., and Miserocchi, G.: Vertical gradient of transpulmonary pressure with active and artificial lung expansion, J Appl Physiol, 1970, *29*, 705.

121. Abboud, N., Rehder, K., Rodarte, J. R., and Hyatt, R. E.: Lung volumes and closing capacity with continuous positive airway pressure, Anesthesiology, 1975, *42*, 138.

122. Martin, R. R., Wilson, J. E., Ross, W. R. D., and Anthonisen, N. R.: The effect of added external resistance on regional pulmonary filling and emptying sequences, Can J Physiol Pharmacol, 1971, *49*, 406.

123. Rahn, H., Otis, A. B., Chadwick, L. E., and Fenn, W. O.: The pressure-volume diagram of the thorax and lung, Am J Physiol, 1946, *146*, 161.

124. Egbert, L. D., Laver, M. B., and Bendixen, H. H.: Intermittent deep breaths and compliance during anesthesia in man, Anesthesiology, 1963, *24*, 57.

125. Don, H. F., and Robson, J. G.: The mechanics of the respiratory system during anesthesia: The effects of atropine and carbon dioxide, Anesthesiology, 1965, *26*, 168.

126. Safar, P., and Aguto-Escarraga, L.: Compliance in apneic anesthetized adults, Anesthesiology, 1959, *20*, 283.

127. Marx, G. F., Murthy, P. K., and Orkin, L. R.: Static compliance before and after vaginal delivery, Br J Anaesth, 1970, *42*, 1100.

128. Norlander, O., Herzog, P., Nordén, I., Hossli, G., Schaer, H., and Gattiker, R.: Compliance and airway resistance during anaesthesia with controlled ventilation, Acta Anaesthesiol Scand, 1968, *12*, 135.

129. Brownlee, W. E., and Allbritten, F. F., Jr.: The

significance of the lung-thorax compliance in ventilation during thoracic surgery, J Thorac Surg, 1956, *32*, 454.

130. Bromage, P. R.: Total respiratory compliance in anaesthetized subjects and modifications produced by noxious stimuli, Clin Sci, 1958, *17*, 217.

131. Douglas, F. G. V., Cocco, J., Brindle, F., Gilbert, R. G. B., and Becklake, M. R.: Pulmonary mechanics and gas exchange during neurosurgical anaesthesia, Can Anaesth Soc J, 1969, *16*, 7.

132. Wu, N., Miller, W. F., and Luhn, N. R.: Studies of breathing in anesthesia, Anesthesiology, 1956, *17*, 696.

133. Foster, C. A., Heaf, P. J. D., and Semple, S. J. G.: Compliance of the lung in anesthetized paralyzed subjects, J Appl Physiol, 1957, *11*, 383.

134. Waltemath, C. L., and Bergman, N. A.: Total respiratory compliance during general anesthesia (abstract), American Society of Anesthesiologists Annual Meeting, Abstracts of Scientific Papers, 1971, pp. 37-38.

135. Gold, M. I., and Helrich, M.: Mechanics of breathing during anesthesia. 2. The influence of airway adequacy, Anesthesiology, 1965, *26*, 751.

136. Gold, M. I., and Helrich, M.: Pulmonary compliance during anesthesia, Anesthesiology, 1965, *26*, 281.

137. Mead, J.: Measurement of inertia of the lungs at increased ambient pressure, J Appl Physiol, 1956, *9*, 208.

138. DuBois, A. B., Brody, A. W., Lewis, D. H., and Burgess, B. F., Jr.: Oscillation mechanics of lungs and chest in man, J Appl Physiol, 1956, *8*, 587.

139. Grimby, G., Hedenstierna, G., and Löfström, B.: Chest wall mechanics during artificial ventilation, J Appl Physiol, 1975, *38*, 576.

140. Keith, A.: The mechanism of respiration in man, in *Further Advances in Physiology*, L. Hill, ed., Edward Arnold, London, 1909, p. 182.

141. Nadel, J. A., Colebatch, H. J. H., and Olsen, C. R.: Location and mechanism of airway constriction after barium sulfate microembolism, J Appl Physiol, 1964, *19*, 387.

142. Clarke, S. W., Graf, P. D., and Nadel, J. A.: In vivo visualization of small-airway constriction after pulmonary microembolism in cats and dogs, J Appl Physiol, 1970, *29*, 646.

143. Safar, P., and Bachman, L.: Compliance of the lungs and thorax in dogs under the influence of muscle relaxants, Anesthesiology, 1956, *17*, 334.

144. Bernstein, L.: The elastic pressure-volume curves of the lungs and thorax of the living rabbit, J Physiol (Lond), 1957, *138*, 473.

145. Mead, J., and Collier, C.: Relation of volume history of lungs to respiratory mechanics in anesthetized dogs, J Appl Physiol, 1959, *14*, 669.

146. Collier, C. R., and Mead, J.: Pulmonary exchange as related to altered pulmonary mechanics in anesthetized dogs, J Appl Physiol, 1964, *19*, 659.

147. Velasquez, T., and Farhi, L. E.: Effect of negative-pressure breathing on lung mechanics and venous admixture, J Appl Physiol, 1964, *19*, 665.

148. Farhi, L. E., and Velasquez, T.: Changes in compliance associated with changes in shunt flow in the lung (abstract), Fed Proc, 1960, *19*, 96.

149. Laver, M. B., Morgan, J., Bendixen, H. H., and Radford, E. P., Jr.: Lung volume, compliance, and arterial oxygen tensions during controlled ventilation, J Appl Physiol, 1964, *19*, 725.

150. Hedley-Whyte, J., Laver, M. B., and Bendixen, H. H.: Effect of changes in tidal ventilation on physiologic shunting, Am J Physiol, 1964, *206*, 891.

151. Déry, R., Pelletier, J., Jacques, A., Clavet, M., and Houde, J.: Alveolar collapse induced by denitrogenation, Can Anaesth Soc J, 1965, *12*, 531.

152. Williams, J. V., Tierney, D. F., and Parker, H. R.: Surface forces in the lung, atelectasis, and transpulmonary pressure, J Appl Physiol, 1966, *21*, 819.

153. Tierney, D. F., and Clements, J. A.: Surface forces, compliance and airspace configuration of the lung (abstract), Physiologist, 1964, *7*, 271.

154. Young, S. L., Tierney, D. F., and Clements, J. A.: Mechanism of compliance change in excised rat lungs at low transpulmonary pressure, J Appl Physiol, 1970, *29*, 780.

155. Greenfield, L. J., Ebert, P. A., and Benson, D. W.: Effect of positive pressure ventilation on surface tension properties of lung extracts, Anesthesiology, 1964, *25*, 312.

156. Woo, S. W., and Hedley-Whyte, J.: Macrophage accumulation and pulmonary edema due to thoracotomy and lung overinflation, J Appl Physiol, 1972, *33*, 14.

157. Faridy, E. E., Permutt, S., and Riley, R. L.: Effect of ventilation on surface forces in excised dogs' lungs, J Appl Physiol, 1966, *21*, 1453.

158. McClenahan, J. B., and Urtnowski, A.: Effect of ventilation on surfactant, and its turnover rate, J Appl Physiol, 1967, *23*, 215.

159. Woo, S. W., Berlin, D., and Hedley-Whyte, J.: Surfactant function and anesthetic agents, J Appl Physiol, 1969, *26*, 571.

160. Woo, S. W., Berlin, D., Büch, U., and Hedley-Whyte, J.: Altered perfusion, ventilation, anesthesia and lung-surface forces in dogs, Anesthesiology, 1970, *33*, 411.

161. Opie, L. H., Spalding, J. M. K., and Stott, F. D.: Mechanical properties of the chest during intermittent positive-pressure respiration, Lancet,

1959, *1*, 545.

162. Glaister, D. H., Schroter, R. C., Sudlow, M. F.,
and Milic-Emili, J.: Bulk elastic properties of
excised lungs and the effect of a transpulmonary
pressure gradient, Respir Physiol, 1973, *17*, 347.

163. Glaister, D. H., Schroter, R. C., Sudlow, M. F.,
and Milic-Emili, J.: Transpulmonary pressure
gradient and ventilation distribution in excised
lungs, Respir Physiol, 1973, *17*, 365.

164. Marshall, B. E. ,and Wyche, M. Q.: Pulmonary
extravascular water volume during halothane-
oxygen anesthesia in dogs, Anesthesiology, 1970,
32, 530.